BASIC AND CLINICAL SCIENCE COURSE

Master Index

2006–2007

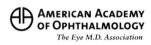
AMERICAN ACADEMY
OF OPHTHALMOLOGY
The Eye M.D. Association

LEO

LIFELONG
EDUCATION FOR THE
OPHTHALMOLOGIST®

American Academy of Ophthalmology Staff

Richard A. Zorab, *Vice President, Ophthalmic Knowledge*
Hal Straus, *Director, Publications Department*
Carol L. Dondrea, *Publications Manager*
Christine Arturo, *Acquisitions Manager*
Ruth Modric, *Production Manager*
Stephanie Tanaka, *Medical Editor*
Katie Loftus, *Administrative Coordinator*

Index by Katherine Pitcoff, Fort Bragg, California

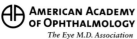

**AMERICAN ACADEMY
OF OPHTHALMOLOGY**
The Eye M.D. Association

655 Beach Street
Box 7424
San Francisco, CA 94120-7424

Basic and Clinical Science Course
2006–2007

Thomas J. Liesegang, MD, Jacksonville, Florida, *Senior Secretary for Clinical Education*

Gregory L. Skuta, MD, Oklahoma City, Oklahoma, *Secretary for Ophthalmic Knowledge*

Louis B. Cantor, MD, Indianapolis, Indiana, *BCSC Course Chair*

Section 1   *Update on General Medicine*
    Chair: Eric P. Purdy, MD, Fort Wayne, Indiana

Section 2   *Fundamentals and Principles of Ophthalmology*
    Chair: Gerhard Cibis, MD, Kansas City, Missouri

Section 3   *Clinical Optics*
    Chair: Kevin M. Miller, MD, Los Angeles, California

Section 4   *Ophthalmic Pathology and Intraocular Tumors*
    Chair: Debra J. Shetlar, MD, San Francisco, California

Section 5   *Neuro-Ophthalmology*
    Chair: Lanning B. Kline, MD, Birmingham, Alabama

Section 6   *Pediatric Ophthalmology and Strabismus*
    Chair: John W. Simon, MD, Albany, New York

Section 7   *Orbit, Eyelids, and Lacrimal System*
    Chair: John Bryan Holds, MD, St. Louis, Missouri

Section 8   *External Disease and Cornea*
    Chair: John E. Sutphin, Jr, MD, Iowa City, Iowa

Section 9   *Intraocular Inflammation and Uveitis*
    Chair: Ramana S. Moorthy, MD, Indianapolis, Indiana

Section 10   *Glaucoma*
    Chair: Steven T. Simmons, MD, Slingerlands, New York

Section 11   *Lens and Cataract*
    Chair: Steven I. Rosenfeld, MD, Delray Beach, Florida

Section 12   *Retina and Vitreous*
    Chair: Carl D. Regillo, MD, Philadelphia, Pennsylvania

Section 13   *Refractive Surgery*
    Chair: Jayne S. Weiss, MD, Detroit, Michigan

Master Index

(*i* = image; *t* = table. Numbers in **boldface** indicate Section numbers.)

A

A-beta-42, in Alzheimer disease, **1**:286
A constant, in power prediction formulas, **3**:219–220, 220*t*, **11**:149
A-pattern deviations, **6**:87, 119–125, 121*i*
  definition of, **6**:119, 122
  esotropia, **6**:87, 121*i*, 122
    treatment of, **6**:124–125
  exotropia, **6**:121*i*, 122
    treatment of, **6**:125
  surgical treatment of, **6**:122–124, 123*i*, 124–125, 182
A-scan ultrasonography/echography, **3**:310–312, 310*i*, 311*i*
  in choroidal/ciliary body melanoma, **4**:226, 228*i*
  in choroidal hemangioma, **4**:243*i*, 245
  in IOL selection, **3**:217
  in metastatic eye disease, **4**:273
a-wave, of electroretinogram, **5**:101, **12**:28*i*, 29, 205. *See also* Electroretinogram
AA. *See* Arachidonic acid
AAION. *See* Arteritic anterior ischemic optic neuropathy
Abacavir, **1**:41
  for postexposure HIV prophylaxis, **1**:46–47*t*
Abbe number (V number), **3**:50
ABC classification, for retinoblastoma, **6**:396, 397*t*
ABC transporters. *See* ATP binding cassette (ABC) transporters
ABCA4 gene
  in cone–rod dystrophy, **12**:215
  in Stargardt disease, **12**:216
Abciximab, **1**:111, 115, 123
Abducens nerve. *See* Cranial nerve VI
Abducens nerve palsy. *See* Sixth nerve (abducens) palsy
Abduction, **6**:34
  extraocular muscles in
    inferior oblique, **6**:16, 30*t*, 31
    lateral rectus, **6**:13–14, 30*t*
    superior oblique, **6**:15, 30*t*, 31, 34*i*
  in Möbius syndrome, **6**:154, 154*i*
  nystagmus and (dissociated nystagmus), **6**:168
Aberrations. *See also specific type and* Wavefront aberrations
  chromatic, **3**:40, 102–103, 104*i*
    duochrome test and, **3**:140
    prisms producing, **3**:89
  higher-order, **3**:93, 101–102, 103*i*, 238–241, **13**:15–17, 17*i*, 18*i*, 19*i*
  optical, **3**:93–104
  prism, **3**:89
  regular astigmatism, **3**:93–98, 94*i*
  of retinoscopic reflex, **3**:133
  spherical, **3**:93, 101–102, 103*i*, 231–234, 232*i*, 233*i*, 234*i*
Aberrometry. *See* Wavefront aberrometry
Abetalipoproteinemia
  Leber congenital amaurosis and, **6**:335

microsomal triglyceride transfer protein defects causing, **2**:351
retinal degeneration and, **12**:241–242
vitamin supplements in management of, **2**:281
Ablepharon, **8**:285
Abnormal polarity, definition of, **8**:247*t*
Abrasions, corneal, **4**:19–20, **8**:406–407
  cataract surgery in diabetic patients and, **11**:205
  in children, **6**:445
Abrevia. *See* Nedocromil
Abscesses, orbital, **7**:42–44, 45*i*
Absence epilepsy, **1**:282
Absidia infection, **8**:130–131
Absorptiometry, dual-photon x-ray, **1**:243
Absorption, light, **3**:14
  in lasers, **3**:19, 21*i*
  spectra of for visual pigments, **12**:313, 314*i*
Absorptive lenses, **3**:165–167. *See also* Sunglasses
Abstinence (withdrawal) syndrome, **1**:267. *See also specific drug*
  hypertension and, **1**:97–98
ABT-773. *See* Cethromycin
Abuse
  child, ocular trauma and, **6**:442–445, 443*i*, 444*i*, **12**:301–302, 302*i*
  elder, **1**:236–237
AC. *See* Accommodative convergence
AC/A esotropia. *See* High accommodative convergence/ accommodative esotropia
AC/A ratio. *See* Accommodative convergence/ accommodation ratio
ACA. *See* Anterior cerebral artery
ACAID. *See* Anterior chamber–associated immune deviation
Acanthamoeba, **8**:131, 131*i*, 187
  cytologic identification of, **8**:70*i*
  keratitis/ocular infection caused by, **4**:66, 67*i*, **8**:119*t*, 131, 187–189, 188*i*
    contact lens wear and, **3**:207, **4**:66, 67*i*, **8**:187
    herpes simplex keratitis differentiated from, **8**:188–189
    isolation techniques for diagnosis of, **8**:136
    treatment of, **2**:444–445, **8**:188–189
  polyphaga, **8**:131
  stains and culture media for identification of, **8**:137*t*
Acantholysis, definition of, **4**:169
Acanthosis, definition of, **4**:168, **8**:247*t*
Acarbose, **1**:212*t*, 213
Acceptor splice site, **2**:181
Accessory lacrimal glands, **2**:29*t*, 34, 289–290, 289*i*
  aqueous component/tears secreted by, **8**:56
  of Krause, **2**:24*i*, 29*t*, 34, 290, **4**:168*t*, **7**:140*i*, 145, 253
  of Wolfring, **2**:24*i*, 29*t*, 34, 290, **4**:168*t*, **7**:140*i*, 145, 253
Accessory molecules, in immune processing, **9**:22
Accolate. *See* Zafirlukast
Accommodating intraocular lenses, **3**:229, **13**:165, 178–180, 179*i*

Accommodation, 2:73–74, 3:119, 119*i*, 179–180,
   11:21–23, 22*t*, 13:167–171
   aging affecting, 11:21–22, 23. *See also* Presbyopia
   amplitude of, 3:119, 150, 11:22
      aging affecting, 3:147, 148*t*
      binocular, 3:119, 150, 151, 152
      measuring, 3:150–151
      monocular, 3:119
      premature loss of (accommodative insufficiency),
         3:147
   catenary (hydraulic support) theory of, 13:171
   changes with, 5:314, 11:22, 22*t*
   clinical problems of, 3:147–150, 148*t*
   contact lens correction affecting, 3:149–150, 179–180
   definition of, 3:119
   evaluation of before cataract surgery, 11:81
   Helmholtz (capsular) theory of, 13:167–168, 168*i*
   muscarinic drugs affecting, 2:394, 398
   near point of, measuring, 3:150
   in near reflex, 2:111
   paralysis, for refraction in infants and children,
      3:146
   pupils and, 5:313–314
   range of, 3:119
      measuring, 3:151
   relaxing. *See also* Cycloplegia/cycloplegics
      in children, 3:146
      for gradient method of accommodative
         convergence/accommodation ratio
         measurement, 3:149
   Schachar theory of, 11:23, 13:168–171, 169*i*, 170*i*
      scleral expansion for presbyopia correction and,
         13:177
   spasm of (ciliary muscle spasm), 5:314
      accommodative excess caused by, 3:148
   spectacle lens correction affecting, 3:149–150,
      179–180
   stimulating, for gradient method of accommodative
      convergence/accommodation ratio measurement,
      3:149
   terminology for, 3:119
Accommodative amplitude. *See* Accommodation,
   amplitude of
Accommodative convergence, 6:38
   in refractive accommodative esotropia, 6:101
Accommodative convergence/accommodation ratio,
   3:148–149, 6:38, 87
   in high accommodative convergence/accommodative
      esotropia, 6:102
   in intermittent exotropia, 6:111
   measurement of, 6:87–88
Accommodative effort, 3:119
Accommodative esotropia, 6:98*t*, 101–104
   high accommodative convergence/accommodative
      (nonrefractive), 6:98*t*, 102–104
   muscarinic agents for management of, 2:398
   partially accommodative, 6:98*t*, 104
   refractive, 6:98*t*, 101–102
   refractive surgery in patient with, 13:195–196
Accommodative excess, 3:148
Accommodative insufficiency, 3:147
Accommodative range, and dioptric power of bifocal
   segment, occupation and, 3:163

Accommodative response, 3:119. *See also*
   Accommodation
   loss of, aging and, 3:147
Accommodative rule, 3:151
Accupril. *See* Quinapril
Accuracy, of screening/diagnostic test, 1:354
Accuretic. *See* Quinapril
Accutane. *See* Isotretinoin
ACE. *See* Angiotensin-converting enzyme
ACE inhibitors. *See* Angiotensin-converting enzyme
   (ACE) inhibitors
Acebutolol, 1:88*t*
Acenorm. *See* Captopril
Aceon. *See* Perindopril
Acephalgic migraine (migraine equivalent), 5:294–295.
   See also Migraine headache
Acetazolamide, 2:411*t*, 412, 413
   for cystoid macular edema in uveitis, 9:239
   for glaucoma, 10:162*t*, 168
      in children, 6:283
   for idiopathic intracranial hypertension, 5:119
Acetohexamide, 1:212*t*
Acetylcholine
   clinical use of, 2:395, 396*i*
   drugs affecting receptors for, 2:394–403, 395*i*, 396*i*.
      See also Cholinergic agents
   in iris–ciliary body, 2:308, 308*t*
   sphincter activity affected by, 2:309, 310
   synthesis/release/degradation of, 2:395, 397*i*
   in tear secretion, 2:290, 292, 292*i*
Acetylcholine receptor antibody tests, for myasthenia
   gravis, 5:328, 7:213
Acetylcholinesterase. *See* Cholinesterase/
   acetylcholinesterase
Acetylcholinesterase inhibitors. *See* Cholinesterase/
   acetylcholinesterase inhibitors
Acetylcysteine, for filamentary keratopathy, 2:393,
   8:75–76
Acetylsalicylic acid. *See* Aspirin
Ach. *See* Acetylcholine
Achromatic automated perimetry, in glaucoma, 10:57
Achromatopsia, 12:196–198
   cerebral, 5:194
   in children, 6:335–336, 455
   electroretinogram in, 12:30*i*, 196
   gene defects causing, 2:350
   with myopia, racial and ethnic concentration of,
      2:260
Achromycin. *See* Tetracyclines
Acid, ocular injuries caused by, 8:391
   in children, 6:445
Acid-fast staining, 8:65*t*, 123
Acidic fibroblast growth factor, in aqueous humor,
   2:320
ACL syndrome, congenital corneal keloids in, 8:299
ACLS. *See* Advanced cardiac life support
Acne rosacea. *See* Rosacea
Acoustic neurofibromas (NF2), 5:337, 6:408–409. *See
   also* Neurofibromatosis, bilateral acoustic (type 2)
Acoustic neuroma, of cerebellopontine angle, 5:284,
   285*i*
ACPIOL (anterior chamber phakic intraocular lenses).
   See Phakic intraocular lenses, anterior chamber
Acquired (adaptive) immunity, 9:9–10. *See also*
   Adaptive immune response

Acquired immunodeficiency syndrome. *See* HIV infection/AIDS
Acral-lentiginous melanoma, **4:**185
Acridine orange staining, **8:**65*t*
Acrocentric chromosome, **2:**182
Acrocephalopolysyndactyly, **8:**351*t*
Acrocephalosyndactyly (Apert syndrome), **6:**425–426, 427*i*, **7:**38, **8:**351*t*
   V-pattern deviations associated with, **6:**119–121, 429, 430*i*
Acrocephaly, **6:**421
Acrochordons (skin tags), **7:**163, 164*i*
Acrodermatitis chronica atrophicans, in Lyme disease, **1:**19
Acromegaly, **1:**228
Acropachy, in Graves ophthalmopathy, **7:**53
Acrospiroma, eccrine (clear cell hidradenoma), **7:**167
Acrylic, for foldable intraocular lenses, **3:**213
ACS. *See* Acute coronary syndrome; Anterior ciliary sclerotomy
ACTH (adrenocorticotropic hormone)
   pituitary adenoma producing, **1:**228–229
   in tear secretion, **2:**293
Actin, in immunohistochemistry, **4:**37
Actin filaments, **2:**327
Actinic injury. *See* Photochemical injury
Actinic (Labrador) keratopathy (spheroidal degeneration), **4:**68, 69*i*, **8:**368–369
Actinic (solar) keratosis, **4:**176–177, 177*i*, **7:**172–173, 172*i*
Actinomyces, **8:**128
   canaliculitis caused by, **7:**276
Actinomycin-D (dactinomycin), **1:**257, 259*t*
Action potential
   in ganglion cells, **12:**11
   in photoreceptors, **12:**10
Activase. *See* Alteplase; Tissue plasminogen activator
Activated (stimulated) macrophages, **9:**50, 51*i*, 52–53
Activated protein C, **1:**164, 165
   deficiency of, **1:**170
Activated protein C resistance, **1:**170
Activation
   lymphocyte, **9:**22–24, 23*i*, 25
   macrophage, **9:**14–15, 48–54, 51*i*
   polymorphonuclear leukocyte, **9:**49–50, 49*i*
Activators, **2:**392
Active force generation, **6:**89
Active immunization, **1:**303
Active medium, laser, **3:**17, 19, 21, 22*i*
Active transport
   across retinal pigment epithelium, **2:**361–362
   aqueous humor composition affected by, **2:**316
   in aqueous humor dynamics, **2:**304–305
   in lens, **2:**328–329, **11:**19–20
   in pump-leak theory, **11:**20–21, 21*i*
Activities of daily living (ADL), assessment of, **1:**233, 234
Activities of Daily Vision Scale (ADVS), cataract surgery outcome evaluated with, **11:**160
Actos. *See* Pioglitazone
Acuity. *See* Brightness acuity; Visual acuity
Acuity meter, potential. *See* Potential acuity meter
Acular. *See* Ketorolac tromethamine

Acute coronary syndrome, **1:**113–115. *See also* Myocardial infarction
   hypercholesterolemia and, **1:**143
   management of, **1:**111, 122–125
Acute hemorrhagic conjunctivitis, **8:**163
Acute idiopathic blind-spot syndrome, **5:**107, **12:**176
Acute lymphoblastic leukemia, orbital involvement in, **7:**94–95
Acute macular neuroretinopathy, **9:**182
Acute phase reactants, in innate immune response, **9:**47
Acute posterior multifocal placoid pigment epitheliopathy (APMPPE), **9:**177*t*, 178, 179*i*, **12:**173–175, 174*t*, 175*i*
Acute retinal necrosis, **4:**123, 124*i*, **9:**154–156, 155*i*, 156*i*, **12:**185–186, 185*i*
Acute retinal pigment epitheliitis (ARPE/Krill disease), **9:**177*t*, 178, 179*i*
Acute zonal occult outer retinopathy (AZOOR), **5:**107, **9:**180, **12:**179–180, 180*i*
Acyclovir, **1:**65*t*, 76–77, **2:**440*t*, 441–442, 441*i*
   for acute retinal necrosis, **9:**155, **12:**186
   for herpes simplex virus infections, **1:**28, 76, **8:**142*t*
      epithelial keratitis, **8:**145
      in infants and children, **6:**220, 226
      stromal keratitis, **8:**148–150, 149*t*
   for herpes zoster infections, **1:**28, 76–77, **8:**155
Acylureidopenicillins, **1:**67
AD. *See* Alzheimer disease
Adalat. *See* Nifedipine
Adalimumab, **1:**199
Adaptation, dark, sunglasses affecting, **3:**165
Adaptive immune response, **9:**9–10
   effector reactivities of, **9:**25, 54–74, 55*t*. *See also specific type*
      antibody-mediated, **9:**54–63, 55*t*
      combined antibody and cellular, **9:**55*t*, 70–74
      lymphocyte-mediated, **9:**55*t*, 63–70
   immunization and, **9:**17–31. *See also* Immune response arc
   immunoregulation of, **9:**87–89
   innate immunity and
      differences from, **9:**10–11
      similarities to, **9:**10–11
   mediator systems affecting, **9:**74–86, 75*t*
   triggers of, **9:**9–11
   in viral conjunctivitis, **9:**35
Adaptometer, Goldmann-Weekers, for dark adaptation testing, **12:**41–42, 42*i*
ADCC. *See* Antibody-dependent cellular cytotoxicity
"Additivity error," **3:**142
Adduction, **6:**34
   elevation deficiency in (double elevator palsy), **6:**137–138, 138*i*, **7:**214
   extraocular muscles in
      inferior rectus, **6:**14, 28, 30, 30*t*, 33*i*
      lateral rectus, **6:**31*i*
      medial rectus, **6:**13, 30*t*, 31*i*
      superior oblique, **6:**31
      superior rectus, **6:**14, 28, 30, 30*t*, 32*i*
   in Möbius syndrome, **6:**154, 154*i*
   overdepression in, **6:**129
   overelevation in, **6:**128
   underelevation in, **6:**135
Adefovir, **1:**41, 77

Adenine arabinoside. *See* Vidarabine
Adenocarcinoma
  of retinal pigment epithelium, 4:147, 241–242
  sebaceous, 7:180–182, 180*i*, 181*i*
    medial canthal/lacrimal sac involvement and,
      7:284
Adenoid cystic carcinoma (cylindroma)
  of eyelid, 7:168
  of lacrimal glands, 4:192–194, 194*i*, 7:90–91
Adenoma
  of ciliary epithelium, 4:241–242
  Fuchs (pseudoadenomatous hyperplasia), 4:147,
    241–242
  pituitary, 1:228–229
    chiasmal syndromes caused by, 5:161–162, 162*i*
    MR imaging of, 1:229, 5:73*i*
  pleomorphic (benign mixed tumor)
    of eyelid, 7:167
    of lacrimal gland, 4:192–193, 193*i*, 7:89
  of retinal pigment epithelium, 4:147
  sebaceous (sebaceum), 7:167
    in tuberous sclerosis, 5:338, 339*i*, 6:410, 410*i*
Adenomatous polyposis, familial (Gardner syndrome),
  retinal manifestations of, 2:173, 4:122–123, 230,
  6:390, 12:236–237, 237*i*
Adenosine
  in atrial flutter diagnosis, 1:138
  for atrial tachycardia, 1:136–137
Adenoviruses, 8:120–121, 157
  immune response to, 9:35
  ocular infection caused by, 8:120–121, 157–159, 158*i*,
    159*i*, 160*i*
    in children, 6:225–226
    epidemic keratoconjunctivitis, 6:225–226, 8:158,
      158*i*, 159, 159*i*, 160*i*
    follicular conjunctivitis, 8:157, 158
    herpes simplex infection differentiated from,
      8:140, 158–159
    pharyngoconjunctival fever caused by, 6:226,
      8:157–158
Adenylyl/adenylate cyclase
  alpha-adrenoceptor binding and, 2:408
  in signal transduction in iris–ciliary body, 2:311,
    312*i*
  in tear secretion, 2:293, 293*i*
Adherence, as microbial virulence factor, 8:116
Adherence syndrome, after strabismus surgery, 6:188
Adhesins, 8:116, 123, 179
Adhesion, in neutrophil recruitment and activation,
  9:48, 49*i*
Adie's pupil (tonic pupil), 5:266–267, 267*i*, 268*i*
  pharmacologic testing for, 2:395–396
Adipose tissue, in orbit, 6:19*i*, 23
Adipose tumors, of orbit, 4:201
Adjustable refractive surgery (ARS), 13:156, 157*t*. *See
  also* Bioptics
Adjustable suture techniques, 6:175–176
Adnexa. *See* Ocular adnexa
Adolescents. *See also* Children
  hypertension in, 1:81, 91
  low vision in, 3:267
Adrenergic agents, 2:404–411, 404*i*. *See also specific
  agent*
  centrally acting, for hypertension, 1:89*t*, 93–94

  for glaucoma, 10:160–161*t*, 169–171, 170*i*
    in children, 6:283
  for heart failure, 1:130
  inhibitors. *See* Alpha-blockers; Beta-blockers
  as miotics, 2:314*t*, 408
  modes of action of, 2:314*t*
  as mydriatics, 2:309–310
Adrenergic neurons, 2:308
Adrenergic receptors, 2:308, 404–405, 404*i*
  adrenergic drug action and, 2:404–405, 404*i*,
    408–409
  in iris–ciliary body, 2:308, 308*t*
    signal transduction and, 2:311–312, 312*i*, 313*i*,
      314*t*
  in tear secretion, 2:292, 292*i*, 293, 293*i*
Adrenochrome deposition, corneal pigmentation
  caused by, 8:376–378, 377*i*, 377*t*
Adrenocorticotropic hormone (ACTH)
  pituitary adenoma producing, 1:228–229
  in tear secretion, 2:293
Adrenoleukodystrophy, neonatal, 12:233*t*, 234, 236,
  242, 242*i*
Adriamycin. *See* Doxorubicin
ADRP. *See* Retinitis, pigmentosa, autosomal dominant
Adult gangliosidosis (GM₁ gangliosidosis type III),
  6:437*t*
Adult-onset diabetes. *See* Diabetes mellitus, type 2
Adult-onset foveomacular vitelliform dystrophy,
  12:219–220, 219*i*
  age-related macular degeneration differentiated
    from, 12:67, 68*i*
Adult-onset myopia, 3:120–121
Adult-onset vitelliform lesions, 12:219–220, 219*i*, 220*i*,
  221*i*
Adult Treatment Panel (ATP) reports, 1:144, 144*t*
Advance directives, surgery in elderly patients and,
  1:238
Advanced cardiac life support (ACLS), 1:317
Advanced Glaucoma Intervention Study (AGIS), 10:90*t*
Advanced glycosylation end products, diabetes
  complications and, 1:217
Advancement flaps, 8:438
  for canthal repair, 7:192
  for eyelid repair, 7:190*i*, 192
Advancing (extraocular muscle insertion), 6:174
Advil. *See* Ibuprofen
ADVS. *See* Activities of Daily Vision Scale
Aerial image
  in fundus photography, 3:276*i*, 278, 279*i*
  in indirect ophthalmoscopy, 3:272, 273*i*, 277*i*, 279*i*
    binocular observation and, 3:275, 276*i*, 279*i*
AeroBid. *See* Flunisolide
Aerolate. *See* Theophylline
Affective disorders (mood disorders), 1:265–266
  drugs for treatment of, 1:277
Afferent fibers
  somatic, 2:117
  visceral, 2:117
Afferent lymphatic channels, 9:8, 19
Afferent phase of immune response arc, 9:17, 18*i*,
  19–22, 20*i*, 21*i*
  response to poison ivy and, 9:29, 30
  response to tuberculosis and, 9:30–31
Afferent pupillary defects
  relative. *See* Relative afferent pupillary defect

in traumatic optic neuropathy, 7:107
Afferent pupillary pathway, 2:110
Afferent visual pathways, 5:23–31, 269
  cortex, 5:28–29, 30*i*, 31, 31*i*
  in functional visual disorder evaluation, 5:305–311
  optic chiasm, 5:27
  optic nerve, 5:25–27
  optic tract, 5:27–28, 28*i*
  retina, 5:23–25, 25*i*
Affinity constant (K_m), "sugar" cataract development
  and, 11:14–16
aFGF. *See* Acidic fibroblast growth factor
AFL. *See* Anterior focal length
Afocal systems, 3:81–84, 82*i*, 83*i*
Afterimage test, retinal correspondence evaluated with,
  6:63–64, 64*i*
Afterload, 1:129
  reduction of for heart failure, 1:130
"Against" motion, in retinoscopy, 3:127–128, 127*i*, 129,
  130*i*
Against-the-rule astigmatism, 3:117–118
Age/aging, 1:233–249
  accommodative response/presbyopia and, 2:73–74,
    3:119, 147, 148*t*, 11:22, 23, 13:167
  angioid streaks and, 12:83
  angle closure and, 10:123
  angle-closure glaucoma and, 10:11
  cataracts related to, 11:45–49. *See also* Age-related
    cataracts
  of conjunctiva, 8:361
  of cornea, 8:362
    donor corneas and, 8:450
    stromal corneal degenerations and, 8:369–370
  Descemet's membrane affected by, 2:301
  elder abuse and, 1:236–237
  electroretinogram affected by, 12:31
  extrinsic, 7:236
  facial changes caused by
    cosmetic surgery and, 7:235–248. *See also specific*
      procedure
    pathogenesis of, 7:236
    physical examination of, 7:236
  falls and, 1:247, 248*t*
  hypertension and, 1:96
  intrinsic, 7:236
  lens changes associated with, 11:5, 45–49, 46*i*. *See*
    also Age-related cataracts
    presbyopia and, 3:147
  lens proteins affected by, 11:13
  Lisch nodule prevalence and, 6:264
  macular changes associated with, 5:104, 12:55, 56*i*.
    See also Age-related macular degeneration
  medication use and, 1:235–236
  mitochondrial DNA diseases and, 2:217–218
  myopia onset and, 3:120–121
  open-angle glaucoma and, 10:7–8, 10, 86, 91*t*
  osteoporosis and, 1:240–247, 242*t*, 243*t*, 245*t*
  outpatient visits and, 1:236
  parental, chromosomal aberrations in Down
    syndrome and, 2:250
  pharmacologic principles affected by, 2:381
  physiologic/pathologic eye changes and, 1:235
  posterior vitreous detachment and, 12:256, 279
  psychology/psychopathology of, 1:238–240, 265
    normal changes and, 1:238–239

refractive status affected by, 3:119–120, 6:199–200,
  201*i*
refractive surgery and, 13:42
  outcome of radial keratotomy and, 13:61
  overcorrection in PRK and, 13:100
of sclera, 8:363, 378, 379*i*
surgical considerations and, 1:237–238
syneresis and, 4:108, 108*i*
systemic disease incidence and, 1:247–249
transient visual loss and, 5:171
vitreous changes associated with, 2:89
Age-related cataracts, 11:45–49. *See also specific type of*
  cataract
  cortical, 11:46–48, 48*i*, 49*i*, 50*i*, 51*i*, 52*i*
  epidemiology of, 11:71–74, 72*t*
  nuclear, 11:45–46, 47*i*
  posterior subcapsular (cupuliform), 4:99, 99*i*,
    11:48–49, 53*i*
Age-Related Eye Disease Study (AREDS), 2:369, 373,
  11:72, 73, 12:60–61
Age-related macular degeneration/maculopathy (senile
  macular degeneration), 4:137–139, 137*i*, 138*i*, 139*i*,
  5:104, 12:54–79
  central serous chorioretinopathy differentiated from,
    12:53, 59, 68–69, 69*i*
  choroidal neovascularization in, 12:20*i*, 63, 64–67,
    65*i*. *See also* Choroidal neovascularization
  clinical studies in, 12:77*t*
  drusen associated with, 4:137–139, 137*i*, 138*i*,
    12:55–57, 56*i*
  dry (nonexudative), 4:139
  fluorescein angiogram patterns of, 12:58–59
  hyperfluorescent lesions in, 12:58–59
  hypofluorescent lesions in, 12:59
  management of, 12:59–62, 70–78, 71–72*t*, 73*i*, 74*i*,
    77*t*
  melanoma differentiated from, 4:229–230
  neovascular, 12:63–78
    choroidal neovascularization and, 12:20*i*, 63,
      64–67, 65*i*
    differential diagnosis of, 12:67–70, 67*t*, 68*i*, 69*i*
    management of, 12:70–78, 71–72*t*, 73*i*, 74*i*, 77*t*
    signs and symptoms of, 12:63
  nonneovascular, 12:55–62
    differential diagnosis of, 12:59
    management of, 12:59–62
  photocoagulation for, 12:70–73, 71–72*t*, 73*i*, 74*i*
    prophylactic, 12:61–62
  photodynamic therapy for, 12:71–72*t*, 73–76,
    320–322
  retinal pigment epithelium abnormalities associated
    with, 2:363, 12:57–58
  statin drugs and, 1:143, 150–151, 349
  wet (exudative), 4:139
Agenerase. *See* Amprenavir
Agenesis, 2:125, 6:205
Agglutinization, antibody, 9:58, 58*i*
Aggrastat. *See* Tirofiban
Aggrecan, 8:14
Aging. *See* Age/aging
Agnosia
  in Alzheimer disease, 1:288
  object, 5:192
  parietal lobe lesions and, 5:166
Agonist, receptor, 2:392

Agonist muscles, **6:**34
Agranulocytosis, clozapine causing, **1:**271
Agraphia, alexia without, **5:**192, 193*i*, 194
AHC. *See* Acute hemorrhagic conjunctivitis
Ahmed implant, for childhood glaucoma, **6:**281
AICA. *See* Anterior inferior cerebellar artery
Aicardi syndrome, **2:**269, **6:**337, 338*i*
AIDS. *See* HIV infection/AIDS
AIDS-dementia complex (HIV encephalopathy), **1:**37,
    5:361. *See also* HIV infection/AIDS
AIDS-related virus (ARV), **1:**36–37. *See also* HIV
    infection/AIDS; Human immunodeficiency virus
AION (anterior ischemic optic neuropathy). *See*
    Anterior optic neuropathy, ischemic
Air, refractive index of, **3:**40*t*
Air cells, ethmoidal, **5:**9, 9*i*
Air–cornea interface, reflection at, **3:**13
Air–glass interface, reflection at, **3:**13, 13*i*
Air-puff tonometers, **10:**28–29
Air–tear film interface, optical power of eye and, **13:**5
Air-ventilated scleral lenses, **3:**201
Airway management, in CPR, **1:**314
Airy disk, **3:**11–12, 12*i*
AJCC (American Joint Committee on Cancer),
    definitions/staging of ocular tumors by, **4:**285–293*t*
AK. *See* Arcuate keratotomy; Astigmatic keratotomy
AK Beta. *See* Levobunolol
AK-Chlor. *See* Chloramphenicol
AK-Dex. *See* Dexamethasone
AK-Dilate. *See* Phenylephrine
AK-Mycin. *See* Erythromycin
AK-Pentolate. *See* Cyclopentolate
AK-Pred. *See* Prednisolone
AK-Sulf. *See* Sulfacetamide
AK-T-Caine. *See* Tetracaine
AK-Tain. *See* Proparacaine
AK-Tracin. *See* Bacitracin
Akarpine. *See* Pilocarpine
AKC. *See* Atopic keratoconjunctivitis
Akinetopsia, **5:**192
    in Alzheimer disease, **1:**288
Akkommodative ICU, **13:**178, 179–180
AKPro. *See* Dipivefrin
Alagille syndrome
    posterior embryotoxon in, **6:**252
    retinal degeneration and, **12:**232*t*
Alamast. *See* Pemirolast
Albaconazole, **1:**76
Albinism, **2:**176–178, 177*i*, 262*t*, **4:**119–120, **6:**345–348,
    346–347*t*, **12:**239–240, 240*i*
    brown, **6:**346*t*
    in Chédiak-Higashi syndrome, **6:**347*t*, 348
    Cross syndrome (oculocerebral hypopigmentation),
        6:346*t*
    with deafness, **6:**347*t*
    enzyme defect in, **2:**262*t*, 263
    in Hermansky-Pudlak syndrome, **6:**346*t*, 348
    in infants/children, **6:**345–348, 346–347*t*
    iris transillumination in, **6:**270, 345
    minimal pigment, **6:**347*t*
    ocular, **2:**176, **6:**347*t*
        autosomal recessive, **6:**347*t*
        ocular findings in carriers of, **2:**176, 270*t*, 271*i*
        X-linked (Nettleship-Falls), **6:**345, 347*t*
            ocular findings in carriers of, **2:**270*t*, 271*i*, 272

    oculocutaneous, **2:**176, 177*i*, 362, **6:**345, 347*t*
        racial and ethnic concentration of, **2:**260
    with pigment, **6:**346*t*
    retinal manifestations of, **6:**345
    temperature-sensitive, **6:**347*t*
    tyrosinase-negative/positive, **2:**176, 243, **6:**345, 346*t*,
        12:240
    X-linked, **6:**345, 347*t*
Albinoidism, **4:**119
Albright hereditary osteodystrophy, **8:**351*t*
Albright syndrome, **7:**81
Albumin
    in aqueous humor, **2:**304, 319
    in vitreous, **2:**337
Albuterol, **1:**157, 157*t*
    with ipratropium, **1:**157*t*
Alcain. *See* Proparacaine
Alcian blue stain, **4:**35, 36*t*
Alcohol (ethanol)
    hypertension affected by, **1:**85, 87*t*
    use/abuse of, **1:**268*t*, 269–270
        maternal, malformations associated with, **1:**270,
            2:160–161, 161*i*, 162*i*, **6:**433–434, 434*i*
    optic neuropathy caused by, **5:**152
Alcohol abstinence syndrome, **1:**269–270
Aldactazide. *See* Spironolactone
Aldactone. *See* Spironolactone
Aldehyde dehydrogenase, in cornea, **2:**299
Aldochlor. *See* Methyldopa
Aldomet. *See* Methyldopa
Aldoril. *See* Methyldopa
Aldose reductase
    in cataract formation, **2:**331–332, 354, **11:**14–16, 60
    in lens glucose/carbohydrate metabolism, **2:**331*i*,
        11:14, 15*i*
Aldose reductase inhibitors
    cataract prevention/management and, **11:**77
    for diabetes mellitus, **1:**217, 218
Aldosterone-receptor blockers, for hypertension, **1:**88*t*
Alendronate, for osteoporosis, **1:**245*t*
Aleve. *See* Naproxen
Alexander's law, **5:**244, 246, 248, **6:**160
Alexia, without agraphia, **5:**192, 193*i*, 194
Alfenta. *See* Alfentanil
Alfentanil, perioperative, **1:**332*t*, 335
Alignment
    ocular
        in infant with decreased vision, **6:**452
        tests of. *See also specific type*
            in children, **6:**80–86
            confounding factors and, **6:**86
            Vernier acuity and, **3:**111
        unsatisfactory, after strabismus surgery, **6:**184
    for retinoscopy, **3:**126
Alizarin red stain, **4:**36*t*
ALK. *See* Automated lamellar keratoplasty/automated
    lamellar therapeutic keratoplasty
Alkalis (alkaline solutions), ocular injuries caused by,
    8:389–391, 390*i*
    cataract and, **11:**57
    in children, **6:**445
    vitamin C and, **8:**94, 392
Alkapton, corneal pigmentation caused by, **8:**377*t*
Alkaptonuria, **2:**261–263, 262*t*, **8:**309*t*, 345
Alkeran. *See* Melphalan

Alkylating agents, 9:96
  for cancer chemotherapy, 1:258*t*
  for uveitis, 9:119*t*
    in children, 6:321–322
All-*trans*-retinaldehyde, 2:359, 360*i*
Allele-specific marking (genetic imprinting), 2:188, 210
Allele-specific oligonucleotides, 2:182
  in mutation screening, 2:231, 233*i*
Alleles, 2:182, 242–244, 8:307
  human leukocyte antigen, 9:91–93. *See also* Human
    leukocyte (HLA) antigens
Allelic association. *See* Linkage disequilibrium
Allelic heterogeneity, 2:182, 241, 347
Allen pictures, for visual acuity testing in children,
  6:78*t*, 79
Allergens, 9:74
Allergic aspergillosis, 5:365
  sinusitis and, 7:46–47
Allergic conjunctivitis, 8:207–209, 9:74
  in children, 6:234
  drugs for, 2:423–425, 424*t*
Allergic granulomatosis and angiitis (Churg-Strauss
  syndrome), 1:189*t*, 193
Allergic reactions. *See also specific type and*
  Hypersensitivity reactions
  anaphylaxis as, 1:319–320, 8:198–200, 199, 199*t*
  atopic keratoconjunctivitis, 6:235, 9:74
  in children, 6:233–236, 236*t*
  conjunctivitis, 6:234, 8:207–209, 9:74
  contact lens wear and, 8:107, 107*i*
  to cycloplegics, 6:95
  to drugs, 1:319–320
  drugs for, 1:319, 6:235–236, 236*t*. *See also*
    Antihistamines
    mediators as target of, 8:200, 200*t*
    ocular effects of, 1:325*t*
  in eyelid
    atopic dermatitis, 8:207
    contact dermatoblepharitis, 8:205–207, 206*i*
  immunization and, 1:303, 305
  to insulin, 1:211
  keratoconjunctivitis
    atopic, 8:211–213, 212*i*, 213*i*
    vernal, 8:209–211, 209*i*, 210*i*
  to latex, in ocular surgery candidate, 1:330
  to local anesthetics, 1:330–331
  to penicillin, 1:67–68
  to suture materials, in strabismus surgery, 6:186,
    187*i*
  to topical medications, 8:205, 206*i*
  vernal keratoconjunctivitis, 6:234–235, 235*i*, 9:13
Allergic shiners, 6:234
Allografts
  corneal, 8:453. *See also* Keratoplasty, penetrating
    rejection of, 8:448, 449, 466–470, 468*i*, 469*i*, 9:39,
      40*i*, 41. *See also* Rejection (graft)
  limbal, 8:423*t*, 433
    for chemical burns, 8:392
    indications for, 8:423*t*
Alloplastic intracorneal implants
  corneal biomechanics affected by, 13:23–24, 25*i*
  corneal inlays
    for keratophakia, 13:72–73, 73*i*
    for presbyopia, 13:175–176

corneal onlays, for epikeratoplasty (epikeratophakia),
  13:77
Allylamines, 1:64*t*, 76
ALMS1 mutation, cone–rod dystrophy and, 12:215
Alocril. *See* Nedocromil
Alomide. *See* Lodoxamide
Alpha-adrenergic agents, 2:405–408, 406*i*, 407*t*
  agonists, 2:407*t*
    direct-acting, 2:405
    for glaucoma, 10:161*t*, 170–171
    indirect-acting, 2:405–408, 406*i*, 407*t*
    in suppression of aqueous formation, 10:19
  antagonists, 2:309, 408. *See also* Alpha-blockers
Alpha-adrenergic receptors, 2:404, 404*i*
  blocking, 2:309, 408
  in iris–ciliary body, 2:308, 308*t*
  signal transduction and, 2:311–312, 312*i*, 313*i*, 314*t*
  in tear secretion, 2:292, 292*i*
Alpha$_1$-antitrypsin, in aqueous humor, 2:319
Alpha-blockers, 2:309, 408
  for heart failure, 1:130
  for hypertension, 1:89*t*, 93
    with beta-blockers, 1:89*t*, 93
Alpha chemokines, 9:81*t*
Alpha-chymotrypsin, for ICCE, 11:105
Alpha (α)-crystallins, 2:326, 326*t*, 11:11–12, 11*i*
Alpha-galactosidase A gene, in Fabry disease, 12:244
Alpha-glucosidase inhibitors, 1:212*t*, 213
Alpha (α) helix, 2:206
Alpha (α)-hemolytic bacteria, endocarditis prophylaxis
  and, 1:7, 8–11*t*
Alpha (α)-interferon, 1:261, 9:82*t*
  for Behçet syndrome, 1:193
  in cancer therapy, 1:260*t*, 261
  for capillary hemangioma, 7:66
  for hepatitis C, 1:31
  for orbital hemangiomas in children, 6:378
Alpha (α)-ketoglutarate reductase, deficiency of in
  hyperlysinemia, 6:308
Alpha$_2$ (α_2)-macroglobulin
  in aqueous humor, 2:319
  in innate immune response, 9:47
Alpha-melanocyte-stimulating hormone (α-MSH),
  8:198*t*
  in tear secretion, 2:293
Alpha (α)-thalassemia, 1:161
Alpha-tocopherol. *See* Vitamin E
Alphagan. *See* Brimonidine
Alport disease/syndrome, 6:349
  lenticonus in, 11:30
  pleiotropism in, 2:259
  renal disease and, 12:236
Alprazolam, ocular effects of, 1:324*t*
Alrex. *See* Loteprednol
Alström syndrome
  cone–rod dystrophy and, 12:215
  renal disease and, 12:236
Altace. *See* Ramipril
Alteplase, for ST-segment elevation acute coronary
  syndrome, 1:124
Alternate cover test (prism and cover test), 6:82, 83*i*
  simultaneous, 6:82
Alternating bifocal contact lenses, 3:182–183, 198–199,
  198*i*
  concentric (annular), 3:198–199, 198*i*

segmented, 3:198–199, 198*i*
Alternating cross-over test, for ocular misalignment, 5:214
Alternating fixation, 6:11
Alternating gaze deviation, periodic, in comatose patients, 5:256
Alternating heterotropia, 6:81
Alternating nystagmus, periodic, 6:165
Alternating skew deviation, 5:223
Alternating suppression, 6:55
Alternative splicing, 2:203, 209
ALTK. *See* Automated lamellar keratoplasty/automated lamellar therapeutic keratoplasty
Alu repeat sequence, 2:182, 203
Aluminum, foreign body of, 12:298
Alveolar nerve, posterior, 5:52, 53*i*
Alveolar rhabdomyosarcoma, 4:198, 199*i*, 6:373, 7:80
Alzheimer disease, 1:240, 284, 285–289
    recent developments in, 1:263
Amacrine cells, 2:352, 5:24, 12:11
    differentiation of, 2:142
Amantadine, 1:65*t*, 77
    for Parkinson disease, 1:280
Amaryl. *See* Glimepiride
Amaurosis
    acquired, 6:456–459, 457*t*
    fugax, 5:175. *See also* Monocular transient visual loss
        carotid artery disease and, 1:107, 5:172
        in central retinal artery occlusion, 12:149
        embolic cause of, 5:176
        Horner syndrome and, 5:265
        hypoperfusion causing, 5:183
        vasculitis causing, 5:183
    Leber congenital (congenital retinitis pigmentosa), 6:334–335, 335*i*, 452, 454–455, 12:211–212, 233–234
        guanylate cyclase mutations causing, 2:349
        RPE65 gene defects causing, 2:350, 6:335
Amber codon, 2:182
Ambien. *See* Zolpidem
Ambient light toxicity, 12:309. *See also* Light toxicity
    retinopathy of prematurity and, 12:132
AmBisome. *See* Amphotericin B
Amblyopia, 5:111, 6:67–75
    abnormal visual experiences and, 6:49–52, 50*i*, 51*i*, 67–68
    ametropic, 6:70
    anisometropic, 3:118, 147, 6:69–70
        refractive surgery and, 13:195
        visual development affected by, 6:50
    aphakia correction in prevention of, 11:199–200
    in bilateral congenital cataracts, 11:195
    cataract surgery planning and, 11:195
    in classic congenital (essential infantile) esotropia, 6:98
    classification of, 6:68–70
    compliance with therapy and, 6:74
    in congenital ptosis, 7:211
    contrast sensitivity affected in, 3:115
    in craniofacial syndromes, 6:429
    deprivation, 6:70
        eye trauma and, 6:441–442
        visual development affected by, 6:49–52, 50*i*, 51*i*, 67–68

    diagnosis of, 6:70–71, 77–95. *See also* Ocular motility, assessment of
    history/presenting complaint in, 6:77–78
    meridional, 6:70
    in monofixation syndrome, 6:57
    occlusion, 6:70
        eye trauma and, 6:441–442
    penetrating keratoplasty and, 8:470
    recurrence of, 6:75
    refractive error and, 6:69–70, 72
    refractive surgery in patient with, 13:193–195
    in retinopathy of prematurity, 6:331
    screening for, 6:67
    strabismic, 6:68–69, 69*i*
        visual development and, 6:51–52, 51*i*
    treatment of, 6:71–75
        complications of, 6:73–75
        pediatric cataract surgery and, 6:71–72, 302
    unresponsiveness to therapy and, 6:74–75
Amblyopia ex anopsia. *See* Deprivation amblyopia
Amblyoscope testing, 6:64–65, 64*t*, 84, 86
Ambulatory blood pressure monitoring, 1:92, 292
AMD. *See* Age-related macular degeneration
AMD-3100, 1:42
Amdoxovir (DADP), 1:41
Amebic keratitis. *See* Acanthamoeba, keratitis/ocular infection caused by
American Joint Committee on Cancer (AJCC), definitions/staging of ocular tumors by, 4:285–293*t*
Ametropia, 3:116. *See also* Refractive errors
    of aphakic eye, 3:116, 118–119, 177–178
    correction of
        in children, 3:145–146
        contact lens, image size and, 3:173, 176*i*
        spectacle, 3:143–145, 144*i*, 145*i*
            cylindrical lenses for, 3:145–146
            far point concept and, 3:143–145, 144*i*
            spherical lenses for, 3:143–145, 144*i*
            vertex distance and, 3:143–145, 144*i*
Ametropic amblyopia, 6:70
Amicar. *See* Aminocaproic acid
Amikacin, 1:62*t*, 70, 2:428*t*, 435
    for endophthalmitis, 9:217, 217*t*
Amikin. *See* Amikacin
Amiloride, 1:88*t*, 90*t*
Amino acids
    disorders of
        corneal changes and, 8:343–345
        retinal degeneration and, 12:244–245
    symbols for, 2:200*t*
    in tear film, 2:290
Aminocaproic acid/ε-aminocaproic acid, 2:453
    for hyphema, 6:448, 8:402
Aminocyclitols. *See* Aminoglycosides
Aminoglycosides, 1:61–62*t*, 70–71, 2:434–435. *See also* specific agent
    for Acanthamoeba keratitis, 8:189
    for endophthalmitis, 9:217
    macular infarction and, 11:178
    ototoxicity of, mitochondrial DNA mutations and, 2:220
p-Aminohippuric acid, in aqueous humor dynamics, 2:305
Aminopenicillins, 1:67
Aminophylline, for medical emergencies, 1:316*t*

Amiodarone
    cornea verticillata caused by, 8:375
    for heart failure, 1:131
    keratopathy caused by, 4:70
    lens changes caused by, 11:54
    ocular effects of, 1:141, 325t
    optic neuropathy caused by, 5:152
Amlodipine
    for angina, 1:120
    for heart failure, 1:130
    for hypertension, 1:89t, 90t
AMN. See Acute macular neuroretinopathy
Amniocentesis, 2:278
Amniotic fluid embolism, Purtscher-like retinopathy
    and, 12:95
Amniotic membrane transplantation, 8:423t, 425, 439
    for chemical burns, 8:392–393, 439
    indications for, 8:423t
Amniotocele, lacrimal sac (congenital dacryocele),
    6:240–241, 240i
AMO. See Array multifocal lens
Amorphous corneal dystrophy, posterior, 8:297
Amoxicillin, 1:56t, 67, 2:429
    with clavulanic acid, 1:56t, 69
    for endocarditis prophylaxis, 1:10t, 11t
Amoxil. See Amoxicillin
Amphetamines, abuse of, 1:268t, 270
Amphotec. See Amphotericin B
Amphotericin B, 1:25, 64t, 76, 2:437, 438t
    for aspergillosis, 5:365
    for coccidioidomycosis, 9:226–227
    for endophthalmitis, 9:217t, 219
        Aspergillus, 9:225–226, 12:189
    for fungal keratitis, 8:186, 187
Ampicillin, 1:56t, 67, 2:428t, 429
    for endocarditis prophylaxis, 1:10t, 11t
        Haemophilus influenzae resistance and, 1:12
    intravenous administration of, 2:389, 428t
    with sulbactam, 1:56t, 69–70
Amplifying cells, transient, in corneal epithelium, 2:45
Amplitude
    of accommodation, 3:119, 150, 11:22
        aging affecting, 3:147, 148t
        binocular, 3:119, 150, 151, 152
        measuring, 3:150–151
        monocular, 3:119
        premature loss of (accommodative insufficiency),
            3:147
    fusional, 6:43, 43t
    of light wave, 3:3, 4i
Amprenavir, 1:42
    for postexposure HIV prophylaxis, 1:46–47t
Ampullectomy, 7:274
Amsler grid testing
    in low vision evaluation, 5:90
    in vision rehabilitation, 3:252–253
Amyloid AA, 8:348, 349
Amyloid AL, 8:348
Amyloid beta peptide immunization, for Alzheimer
    disease, 1:288
Amyloid degeneration, 8:372. See also Amyloidosis/
    amyloid deposits
    polymorphic, 8:370
Amyloid plaques, in Alzheimer disease, 1:285, 286
Amyloid precursor protein (APP), 1:286

Amyloid SAA, 8:348
Amyloidosis/amyloid deposits, 1:166, 8:345–349, 347t,
    348i, 372
    conjunctival, 4:50, 51i, 8:348, 348i
    corneal, 8:345–349, 347t, 372
        in Avellino dystrophy, 4:72–73
        in gelatinous droplike dystrophy, 8:321, 321i, 347t,
            348–349
        in lattice dystrophy, 4:71–72, 75i, 8:318, 349
    in eyelid, 4:171–174, 173t, 174i
    orbital, 4:191, 192i
    primary familial (gelatinous droplike dystrophy),
        8:310t, 321, 321i, 347t, 348–349
    primary localized, 8:347t, 348–349, 348i
    primary systemic, 8:347t, 349
    secondary localized, 8:347t, 349, 372
    secondary systemic, 8:347t, 349
    vitreous involvement in, 4:110–111, 110i, 12:286–287
ANA. See Antinuclear (antineutrophil) antibodies
Ana-Kit, 1:320
Anabolism, glucose, 1:202
Anaerobes, as normal ocular flora, 8:115t
Anaerobic glycolysis
    in corneal glucose metabolism, 2:297
    in lens glucose/carbohydrate metabolism, 2:330,
        11:14, 15i
Anakinra, 1:199
Analgesics. See also specific agent
    ocular effects of, 1:324t
    rebound headache and, 5:296
Anaphase lag, mosaicism caused by, 2:252
Anaphylactic hypersensitivity (type I) reaction,
    8:198–200, 199, 199t, 9:27, 54t, 72–73, 73i. See also
        Allergic reactions; Anaphylaxis
    fluorescein angiography and, 12:21
    topical medication and, 8:205, 206i
Anaphylactoid reactions, 1:319
    from fluorescein angiography, 12:21
Anaphylatoxins, 9:60, 75
    retinal vasculitis in systemic lupus erythematosus
        and, 9:61
Anaphylaxis, 1:319–320, 8:198–200, 199, 199t, 9:73,
    73i. See also Anaphylactic hypersensitivity (type I)
        reaction
    penicillin allergy causing, 1:68
    slow-reacting substance of, 8:200t
Anaplasia, definition of, 8:246, 247t
Anaplasma phagocytophilum, 1:19
Anaplastic carcinoma, of thyroid gland, 1:227
Anaprox. See Naproxen
Anatomic reattachment surgery, for retinal
    detachment, 12:273
ANCA. See Antinuclear (antineutrophil) antibodies
Ancef. See Cefazolin
ANCHOR Study, 12:77t
Ancobon. See Flucytosine
Ancotil. See Flucytosine
Ancrod, for stroke, 1:104–105
Ancylostoma caninum (dog hookworm), diffuse
    unilateral subacute neuroretinitis caused by, 12:190
Anderson-Kestenbaum procedure, 5:255, 6:168–170,
    170i
Androgens, in tear secretion, 2:293–294, 8:79
Anecortave acetate (RETAANE), 2:455, 12:76, 77t

Anemia, 1:160–163
    aplastic, chloramphenicol causing, 1:74, 2:434
    of chronic disease, 1:161
        iron deficiency differentiated from, 1:159
    diabetic retinopathy and, 12:105
    in elderly, 1:247
    hemolytic, 1:162–163
        autoimmune, 1:163
    iron deficiency, 1:159, 161
    pernicious, 1:162
    sickle cell. See Sickle cell disease
    sideroblastic, 1:162
Anergy, 9:88
Anesthesia, corneal
    congenital, 8:299
    herpes simplex epithelial keratitis and, 8:114
    neurotrophic keratopathy caused by, 8:102, 151
Anesthesia (anesthetics)
    for blepharoplasty, 7:231
    for cataract surgery, 11:93–97, 95i, 96i
        in diabetic patient, 11:205
        general, 11:94
            in arthritis patients, 11:203
        local, 11:94, 95i, 96i
        topical, 11:94–96
            minimizing bleeding risk and, 11:202
    for corneal transplantation in children, 8:470
    in elderly patients, 1:238
    examination under. See Examination, under
        anesthesia
    for eyelid surgery, 7:150–151
    general
        for cataract surgery, 11:94, 203
        for extraocular muscle surgery, 6:183
        for eyelid surgery, 7:150
    local (topical/regional), 2:445–449, 445t, 446t
        abuse of, 8:105–106, 106i
        in adjustable suture technique, 6:176
        adverse reactions to, 1:321–323, 330–331,
            335–336, 8:101
            allergic, 1:330–331
            toxic overdose, 1:321–323, 331, 336
        for anterior segment surgery, 2:448
        for blepharoplasty, 7:231
        for cataract surgery, 11:94, 95i, 96i
        for examination in ocular trauma, 6:441
        for extraocular muscle surgery, 6:176, 183
        for eyelid surgery, 7:150
        for foreign-body removal in children, 6:5
        keratoconjunctivitis caused by, 8:393–395
        maximum safe dose of, 1:322t
    malignant hyperthermia caused by, 1:329–330,
        336–337, 337t, 6:191–192, 193t
    for phakic IOL insertion, 13:147
    for photocoagulation, 12:317
    retrobulbar
        adverse reactions to, 1:322, 323, 335–336
        for extraocular muscle surgery, 6:183
        needle perforation and, 12:296
        strabismus after, 6:157
    tear production affected by, 8:81t
Aneuploidy, 2:182. See also specific disorder
    of autosomes, 2:249–251
    of sex chromosomes, 2:249
Aneurysmal bone cyst, orbital involvement and, 6:380

Aneurysms
    basilar artery, 5:355
    berry (saccular), 1:105–106, 5:350
    cerebral, 5:350–354, 350i
        clinical presentation of, 5:351, 352i
        laboratory investigation of, 5:351–352, 353i
        prognosis of, 5:352–353
        ruptured, 5:351, 352i
            intracranial hemorrhage caused by, 1:105, 106
        treatment of, 5:353–354
    contrast angiogram of, 5:68i
    cranial nerve III, 2:109
    internal carotid, 5:350–351
        chiasmal syndromes caused by, 5:162
        third nerve palsy and, 5:228–229, 229i
    intracavernous carotid, 5:351
    Leber miliary, 4:121–122
    retinal arterial
        in HIV infection/AIDS, 9:248
        macroaneurysms, 12:158–160, 160i
            age-related macular degeneration differentiated
                from, 12:67, 68i
        microaneurysms
            ischemia causing, 4:131, 132i
            in nonproliferative diabetic retinopathy, 12:103,
                104i
Angelman syndrome, imprinting abnormalities
    causing, 2:210
Angiitis
    in Churg-Strauss syndrome, 1:193
    cutaneous leukocytoclastic, 1:189t
Angina pectoris, 1:113. See also Ischemic heart disease
    ECG changes in, 1:113, 116
    stable, 1:113
        management of, 1:120–122
        risk stratification for, 1:121t
    unstable, 1:114
    variant (Prinzmetal), 1:113
Angioedema, 8:217t
Angiofibromas, facial, in tuberous sclerosis, 6:410, 410i
Angiogenesis, vitreous as inhibitor of, 2:338–339
Angiogenesis inhibitors, in cancer therapy, 1:251, 257
Angiographic cystoid macular edema, 12:154
Angiography
    in carotid stenosis, 5:179
    in cerebrovascular ischemia, 1:104
    computerized tomographic, 5:67–68
        definition of, 5:78
        limitations of, 5:77t
    conventional/catheter/contrast, 5:66, 68i
    coronary, 1:115, 119–120, 123–124
    fluorescein. See Fluorescein angiography
    indocyanine green. See Indocyanine green
        angiography
    magnetic resonance, 5:66–67
        in cerebral ischemia/stroke, 1:103–104
        definition of, 5:80
        limitations of, 5:77t
    in orbital evaluation, 7:34
        for arteriovenous fistulas, 7:70
        magnetic resonance, 7:34
    retinal, 12:18–23, 20i, 22i. See also Fluorescein
        angiography; Indocyanine green angiography
    in subarachnoid hemorrhage, 1:106

Angioid streaks, **12:**83–84, 83*i*
in pseudoxanthoma elasticum, **12:**83, 83*i*, 237
in sickle cell hemoglobinopathies, **12:**83, 123
Angiokeratoma corporis diffusum universale (Fabry
disease), **2:**262*t*, **6:**436*t*, 438, **8:**340–341, 341*i*
cataract and, **6:**288*t*
ocular findings in carriers of, **2:**270*t*
plasma infusions in management of, **2:**281
retinal degeneration and, **12:**244, 246*i*
Angiomas (angiomatosis). *See also* Hemangiomas
(hemangiomatosis)
cerebellar, **5:**340
encephalofacial/cerebrofacial/encephalotrigeminal.
See Sturge-Weber disease/syndrome
racemose (Wyburn-Mason syndrome), **4:**248, 249*i*,
5:336*t*, 342–343, 343*i*, **6:**402*t*, 419–420, 420*i*,
12:163
retinal. *See* von Hippel disease/syndrome
Angiomatous tumors, **4:**243–249, 249*i*. *See also specific
type*
Angioplasty, percutaneous transluminal coronary
(PTCA/balloon angioplasty)
for angina, **1:**121
for ST-segment elevation acute coronary syndrome,
1:125
troponin levels in determining need for, **1:**117
Angiopoietin 1, nevus flammeus and, **8:**270
Angiotensin-converting enzyme (ACE), in sarcoidosis,
7:36
Angiotensin-converting enzyme (ACE) inhibitors
for heart failure, **1:**130
for hypertension, **1:**88*t*, 90*t*, 92
for non-ST-segment elevation acute coronary
syndrome, **1:**123
ocular effects of, **1:**142
in perioperative setting, **1:**333
Angiotensin II receptor blockers
for heart failure, **1:**130
for hypertension, **1:**88*t*, 90*t*, 93
Angle, **3:**32–33, 33*i*
anterior chamber. *See* Anterior chamber angle
Brewster, **3:**13, 13*i*
critical, **3:**47–48, 48*i*
of deviation, prisms producing, **3:**84–85, 84*i*
prism diopter and, **3:**84–85, 85*i*
of incidence, **3:**13–14, 13*i*, 43–44, 43*i*, 45*i*, 46
critical angle and, **3:**42–44, 43*i*, 48*i*
kappa (positive and negative), **3:**235, **6:**86, 87*i*
in retinopathy of prematurity, **6:**86, 331, 331*i*
of reflection, **3:**43*i*, 44
of refraction, **3:**43*i*, 44*i*
of transmission, **3:**44, 45*i*, 46
Angle closure. *See also* Angle-closure glaucoma
chronic, **10:**126–127
creeping, **10:**126
definition of, **10:**120
intermittent, **10:**125–126
iris-induced, **10:**122
mechanisms of, **10:**120, 121*t*
primary, **10:**122–128
with pupillary block, lens-induced, **10:**128–132, 129*i*,
131*i*, 131*t*
without pupillary block, **10:**121–122, 121*t*
subacute, **10:**125–126

Angle-closure glaucoma, **10:**119–146. *See also*
Glaucoma
categories of, **10:**120
central retinal vein occlusion and, **12:**143
childhood (congenital/infantile/juvenile)
with iris bombé, **6:**280
topiramate causing, **6:**279
management of, **10:**207–209, 208*i*, 209*i*
goniotomy in, **10:**207–209, 208*i*, 209*i*
trabeculotomy in, **10:**207–209, 208*i*, 209*i*
ciliary block (malignant/aqueous misdirection),
10:140–141, 140*i*
cataract surgery and, **11:**166, 182
classification of, **10:**5, 6*t*, 8*i*
mechanisms of outflow obstruction in, **10:**9*t*
cornea plana and, **8:**291
definition of, **10:**120
described, **10:**119–120
genetics of, **10:**15
history of, **10:**119
iris-induced, **10:**122
lens-induced, **10:**122
management of
in children, **10:**207–209, 208*i*, 209*i*
medical, **10:**175–176
surgical, **10:**197–200, 198*i*
cataract extraction in, **10:**200
chamber deepening in, **10:**200
goniosynechialysis in, **10:**200
incisional, **10:**200
laser gonioplasty in, **10:**199–200
laser iridectomy, **10:**197–199, 198*i*
microcornea and, **8:**289
microspherophakia and, **11:**33
nanophthalmos and, **8:**287
pain caused by, **5:**298
pars planitis and, **9:**151
pathogenesis of, **10:**120–122, 121*i*, 121*t*
pathophysiology of, **10:**120–122, 121*i*, 121*t*
persistent hyperplastic primary vitreous and, **12:**282
phakic, **10:**132
prevalence of, **10:**119
primary, **10:**122–128
acute, **10:**124–125
characteristics of, **10:**6*t*
age and, **10:**11, 123
chronic, **10:**6*t*, 126–127
definition of, **10:**122
epidemiology of, **10:**10–12
family history and, **10:**123–124
gender and, **10:**11, 123
hereditary factors in, **10:**12
intermittent, **10:**125–126
ocular biometrics and, **10:**123
race and, **10:**11, 122–123
refraction and, **10:**12, 124
with relative pupillary block, characteristics of,
10:6*t*
risk factors for, **10:**122–124
subacute, **10:**6*t*, 125–126
pseudophakic, **10:**132
pupillary block in, **10:**120–121, 121*i*
retinopathy of prematurity and, **12:**131
secondary
central retinal vein occlusion and, **10:**144

drug-induced, **10**:145–146
epithelial downgrowth and, **10**:141–143
fibrous downgrowth and, **10**:141–143
flat anterior chamber and, **10**:145
inflammation and, **10**:138–140, 139*i*
nanophthalmos and, **10**:145
nonrhegmatogenous retinal detachment and,
  10:141
persistent hyperplastic primary vitreous and,
  10:145
with pupillary block, **10**:128–132, 129*i*, 131*i*, 131*t*
  characteristics of, **10**:6*t*
  ectopia lentis, **10**:130, 131*i*, 131*t*
  lens-induced, **10**:128–132, 129–131*i*, 131*t*
  microspherophakia and, **10**:130, 131*i*
without pupillary block, **10**:132–146
  characteristics of, **10**:6*t*
  retinal surgery and, **10**:143–144
  retinal vascular disease and, **10**:143–144
  retinopathy of prematurity and, **10**:145
  trauma and, **10**:143
  tumors and, **10**:138
  uveal effusions and, **10**:141
types of, **10**:119–120
Angle kappa (positive and negative) , **3**:235, **6**:86, 87*i*
  in retinopathy of prematurity, **6**:86, 331, 331*i*
Angle recession, posttraumatic, **4**:25, 25*i*
  glaucoma and, **4**:82–84, 83*i*, **10**:113–114, 113*i*
Angular artery, **5**:13, **7**:255
  eyelids supplied by, **2**:29, 32*i*, **7**:147
  orbit supplied by, **2**:39*i*
Angular magnification, **3**:30, 34. *See also* Transverse
  magnification
Angular vein, **5**:20, 22*i*, **7**:255
  eyelids drained by, **7**:147
Anhedonia, **1**:265
Anhidrosis, **5**:262
Anhidrotic ectodermal dysplasia, **8**:89
Anidulafungin, **1**:76
Animal bites, eyelid injuries caused by, **7**:187
Animal cap, **2**:125, 130
Aniridia, **2**:125, 170, **4**:151, **5**:259, **6**:261–262, 262*i*,
  277–278, **8**:309*t*, **10**:153–154, **11**:33, 34*i*
  cataract and, **6**:293*i*
  mutation rate of, **2**:256
  nystagmus and, **6**:162, 262
  pediatric glaucoma and, **6**:277–278
  short arm 11 deletion syndrome/*PAX6* gene
    mutations and, **2**:170, 254–255
  Wilms tumor and, **6**:262, 277–278
Aniseikonia, **3**:118
  anisometropia correction causing, **3**:118
    contact lens optics and, **3**:177–178
  contact lenses for management of, **3**:177–179
  intraocular lenses and, **3**:216
  meridional (meridional magnification). *See also*
    Distortion
    astigmatic spectacle lenses causing, **3**:145
      avoidance of with contact lenses, **3**:178–179
    distortion caused by, **3**:145
      avoidance of with contact lenses, **3**:181–182
  monocular aphakia and, **3**:178
Anisocoria, **2**:125, 169–170, **5**:260–269
  Adie's tonic pupil and, **5**:266–267, 267*i*, 268*i*
  equal in dim and bright light, **5**:260

evaluation of, flowchart in, **5**:261*i*
greater in bright light, **5**:265–269
greater in dim light, **5**:260, 262–265, 263*i*
in Horner syndrome, **5**:262–265, 263*i*, 264*i*
iris damage in, **5**:265–266
pharmacologic, **5**:262, 266
physiologic (simple/essential), **5**:260, 261*i*, 262
post-cocaine, **5**:262
in posterior synechiae, **5**:262
third nerve palsy in, **5**:267, 269
Anisohyperopia, amblyopia in conjunction with, **3**:147
Anisometropia, **3**:118
  aniseikonia caused by correction of, **3**:118
  anisophoria caused by correction of, **3**:118, 156–157,
    158–160, 158*i*. *See also* Anisophoria, induced
  image size and, with contact lenses, **3**:177–178
  in infants and children, **3**:118, 147
    amblyopia caused by (anisometropic amblyopia),
      3:118, 147, **6**:69–70
    refractive surgery and, **13**:195
    visual development affected by, **6**:50
  prismatic effect of bifocal lenses in, **3**:155, 158*i*
  triple procedure and, **11**:209
Anisomyopia, amblyopia in conjunction with, **3**:147
Anisophoria, induced (anisometropia correction),
  3:118, 156–157, 158–160, 158*i*
  calculating, **3**:160, 160*i*
  compensating for, **3**:158–162, 160*i*, 161*i*
Anisoylated plasminogen streptokinase activator
  complex (APSAC), for ST-segment elevation acute
  coronary syndrome, **1**:124
Ankyloblepharon, **6**:210, 210*i*, **7**:154–156, 155*i*, **8**:285
  filiforme adnatum, **6**:210, 210*i*
Ankylosing spondylitis, **1**:175–176, **9**:127*i*, 129–130,
  130*i*
  cataract surgery in patients with, **11**:203, 203*i*
  HLA in, **9**:94–95, 125–130
  juvenile, **1**:178
Anlage (primordium), **2**:125, 127
Annular keratopathy, traumatic, **8**:396
Annular zones, in multifocal intraocular lenses,
  3:226–227, 227*i*
Annulus of Zinn, **2**:10–12, 16, 17*i*, 18*t*, 101, **5**:26, 41,
  7:14, 14*i*, 15
Anomalies, congenital. *See specific type and* Congenital
  anomalies
Anomaloscope, red-green color defects tested with,
  12:43
Anomalous retinal correspondence, **6**:41, 53, 54*i*, 55–57
  harmonious, **6**:60, 64, 65*i*
  testing for, **6**:56–57, 58–65
  unharmonious, **6**:60, 65, 65*i*
Anomalous trichromats, **12**:195, 196*t*, 197*i*
Anophthalmic ectropion, **7**:126–127
Anophthalmic ptosis, **7**:127
Anophthalmic socket, **7**:119–129. *See also specific aspect*
  complications and treatment of, **7**:124–127, 124*i*,
    125*i*, 126*i*
  contracted, **7**:125–126, 126*i*
  enucleation and, **7**:119–122
  evisceration and, **7**:119, 123–124
  exenteration and, **7**:119, 127–129, 128*i*
Anophthalmos (anophthalmia), **2**:125, 162, 164*i*, **7**:37
Ansa subclavia, **5**:57
Ansaid. *See* Flurbiprofen

Anspor. *See* Cephradine
Antagonist, receptor, **2**:392
Antagonist muscles, **6**:35
    contralateral, **6**:37
Antazoline/naphazoline, **2**:423, 424*t*
Anterior banded zone, of Descemet's membrane, **2**:47, 48*i*
Anterior basement membrane dystrophy, **4**:70–71, 72*i*
Anterior border layer, of iris, **2**:62, 63*i*
Anterior capsular fibrosis and phimosis, **11**:187
    Nd:YAG laser capsulotomy for, **11**:187, 187–191, 189*i*
Anterior capsulotomy. *See* Capsulotomy, anterior
Anterior cerebral artery, **5**:16
Anterior chamber, **2**:43, 43*i*, 52–54, 53*i*, 55*i*. *See also* Anterior segment
    congenital anomalies of, **2**:168–169, 168*i*, 169*i*, 170*i*, **4**:78–79, 78*i*, 79*i*
    degenerations of, **4**:79–84
    depth of, **2**:52
        in IOL selection, **3**:218
            phakic IOLs and, **13**:146–147
    development of, **2**:153–154, 153*i*
    disorders of, **4**:77–85. *See also specific type*
        neoplastic, **4**:84, 85*i*
    evaluation of
        before cataract surgery, **11**:82
        in glaucoma, **10**:34–36, 34*i*, 35*i*, 35*t*
    flat or shallow
        cataract surgery and, **11**:163–166
            intraoperative complications, **11**:163–165
            postoperative complications, **11**:165–166
            preoperative considerations, **11**:82
        penetrating keratoplasty and, **8**:460
        refractive surgery and, **13**:44
        secondary angle-closure glaucoma and, **10**:145
    gonioscopy of, **2**:59–61
    immune response in, **9**:34*t*, 36–39
    Onchocerca volvulus microfilariae in, **9**:196
    in persistent hyperplastic primary vitreous, **12**:281, 282
    phacoemulsification in, **11**:128
    topography of, **2**:43, 43*i*, **4**:77–78, 77*i*, 78*i*
    in uveitis, **9**:102–105, 103*t*, 104*i*. *See also* Anterior uveitis
Anterior chamber angle, **2**:52, 52*i*, 53*i*, 55*i*, 56*i*, **10**:127
    development of, **2**:153–154, 153*i*
        abnormalities of, cataract surgery and, **11**:212
    gonioscopy of, **2**:59–61
    narrow, **10**:127
    neovascularization of, in diabetic patients, **12**:111
    occludable, **10**:127
    traumatic recession of, **4**:25, 25*i*
        glaucoma and, **4**:81–84, 82*i*, 83*i*
    in uveitis, **9**:103*t*
Anterior chamber–associated immune deviation (ACAID), **9**:37–39
    corneal graft tolerance and, **8**:448
    lens crystallins tolerance and, **9**:90
    therapeutic potential of immune privilege and, **9**:39
Anterior chamber cleavage syndrome. *See* Anterior segment, dysgenesis of
Anterior chamber intraocular lenses. *See* Intraocular lenses
Anterior chiasmal syndrome, **5**:158, 159*i*

Anterior choroidal artery, **5**:16
Anterior ciliary arteries, **2**:36, 38–40, 39*i*, 40*i*, 67, **5**:15, **6**:16
    anterior segment ischemia after strabismus surgery and, **6**:189, 189*i*
Anterior ciliary sclerotomy, for presbyopia, **13**:176
Anterior clinoid process, **5**:13, 15, 26
Anterior communicating artery, **5**:16
Anterior corneal dystrophies, **8**:311–315. *See also specific type*
Anterior elastic tendons, **2**:67
Anterior ethmoidal air cells, **5**:9, 9*i*
Anterior ethmoidal artery, **5**:13, 15
Anterior ethmoidal foramen, **5**:10
Anterior focal length (AFL), **3**:79
Anterior focal plane, **3**:69–71
Anterior focal point, **3**:69–71
Anterior inferior cerebellar artery, **2**:117, **5**:18, 19*i*
Anterior lacrimal crest, **2**:5, 7*i*
Anterior lamella, **2**:27*i*
Anterior lenticonus, **4**:97, **11**:30
Anterior lentiglobus, **11**:31
Anterior megalophthalmos, **6**:250
Anterior microphthalmos, **8**:289
Anterior optic neuropathy
    ischemic, **5**:120–124, 121*t*, 347
        arteritic, **5**:120–122, 121*i*, 121*t*
        nonarteritic, **5**:121*t*, 122–124, 123*i*, 124*t*
    with optic disc edema, **5**:111–113, 115–129
    without optic disc edema, **5**:129–141
Anterior orbitotomy, **7**:109–114
    inferior approach for, **7**:110–111, 112*i*, 113*i*
    medial approach for, **7**:111–114
    superior approach for, **7**:109–110
Anterior pigmented layer, of iris, **2**:64, 65*i*
Anterior polar cataract (APC), **6**:288, 288*i*
    hereditary factors in, **6**:287*t*
Anterior (peripheral) retina, **12**:8
Anterior segment, **5**:23. *See also specific structure and* Anterior chamber
    development of, **6**:249, **8**:6
    disorders of
        developmental anomalies, **8**:288–298
        in infants and children, **6**:249–260, 453
        Th1 delayed hypersensitivity and, **9**:68*t*
        toxic keratoconjunctivitis from medications and, **8**:393–395
        traumatic, **8**:387–420. *See also* Anterior segment, trauma to
    dysgenesis of, **6**:251–253, 251*i*, 253*i*. *See also specific type and* Neurocristopathy
        glaucoma and, **6**:271, 278
        Peters anomaly and, **11**:32
    examination of, **5**:258–259. *See also* Biomicroscopy, slit-lamp
        in congenital/infantile glaucoma, **6**:275, 276*i*
        echography in, **8**:37
        fluorescein angiography in, **8**:37
        in pediatric cataract, **6**:295
        in penetrating trauma, **6**:446, 446*i*
        photography in, **8**:35–38, 36*i*, 38*i*
        before refractive surgery, **13**:44
    function of, **8**:5
    immune response in, **9**:34*t*, 36–39
    ischemia of, after strabismus surgery, **6**:189, 189*i*

leukemic infiltration of, **6**:344
metastatic disease of, **4**:268–269
posterior segment complications of surgery on,
  vitrectomy for, **12**:328–340
topical anesthetics for surgery of, **2**:448
trauma to, **8**:387–420
  animal and plant substances causing, **8**:395–396
  chemical injuries, **8**:389–393
  concussive, **8**:396–403
  nonperforating mechanical, **8**:403–407
  perforating, **8**:407–418. *See also* Perforating
    injuries
  surgical, **8**:418–420
  temperature and radiation causing, **8**:387–389
  in uveitis, **9**:102–105, 102*t*, 104*i*, 105*i*. *See also*
    Anterior uveitis
  wound healing/repair in, **8**:383–386, 424. *See also*
    Wound healing/repair
Anterior stromal micropuncture, for recurrent corneal
  erosions, **8**:99–100, 100*i*
Anterior sutures, **11**:9
Anterior synechiae
  in glaucoma, **10**:5, 7
    gonioscopy in identification of, **10**:39
  in sarcoidosis, **9**:198
Anterior uvea. *See* Uvea
Anterior uveitis, **9**:106–107, 127–146. *See also specific*
  cause and Iridocyclitis; Iritis; Uveitis
  acute, **9**:127–141
  causes of, **9**:112*t*
  in children, **6**:311, 312–316, 312*t*, 313*t*, 314*i*, 316*t*
    differential diagnosis of, **6**:312*t*
    in juvenile idiopathic (chronic/rheumatoid)
      arthritis, **6**:311, 312–315, 313*t*, 314*i*
    laboratory tests for, **6**:321*t*
    masquerade syndromes and, **6**:320*t*
    sarcoidosis and, **6**:315
    treatment of, **6**:319–322
    tubulointerstitial nephritis and, **6**:315–316
  chronic, **9**:141–146
  circulating immune complexes and, **9**:59
  differential diagnosis of, **9**:110*t*
  granulomatous, iris nodules in, **4**:219*t*
  herpetic disease and, **9**:138–140
  HLA association and, **1**:175, 176, **9**:93, 94*t*, 128–132
  in inflammatory bowel disease, **9**:131–132
  juvenile idiopathic (chronic/rheumatoid) arthritis
    and, **9**:141–144, 142*i*, 144*t*
  in onchocerciasis, **9**:185–197
  signs of, **9**:102–105, 103*t*, 104*i*, 105*i*
  in spondyloarthropathies, **1**:175, 178
  Th1 delayed hypersensitivity and, **9**:68*t*
Anterior vascular capsule (pupillary membrane), **11**:29,
  29*i*
  persistent, **6**:267–268, 268*i*
Anterior vestibular artery, **5**:18
Anterior vitreous detachment, contusion injury
  causing, **12**:254
Anteriorization (extraocular muscle), and recession,
  6:175*t*
Anthracyclines, in cancer chemotherapy, **1**:257
Antiangiogenic agents
  for age-related macular degeneration, **12**:76, 77*t*
  for retinal capillary hemangioma, **4**:247

Antianxiety drugs, **1**:273–277, 274*t*
  ocular effects of, **1**:324*t*
  preoperative, **1**:335
Antiarrhythmic drugs, tear production affected by,
  8:81*t*
Antibacterial agents, **1**:54–72, 55–63*t*. *See also specific*
  agent and Antibiotics
Antibiotic-associated colitis, *Clostridium difficile*
  causing, **1**:8
Antibiotics, **1**:53–78, 55–65*t*, **2**:427–437, 428*t*, 431*t*. *See*
  also specific type and agent
  for *Acanthamoeba* keratitis, **2**:444–445, **8**:189
  for bacterial keratitis, **8**:181–183, 182*t*
  beta- (β) lactam, **1**:54–66, 67–70
  in cancer chemotherapy, **1**:257, 259*t*
  for cat-scratch disease, **5**:368
  in combination preparations with anti-inflammatory
    agents, **2**:432*t*
  for endophthalmitis, **9**:215, 217–219, 218*t*, 219,
    12:328, 329, 331
  for gonococcal conjunctivitis, **8**:171–172
  intraocular injection of, **2**:386–387
  intravenous administration of, **2**:389
  intravitreal administration of, for postoperative
    endophthalmitis, **12**:328, 329, 331
  after LASIK, **13**:115
  for Lyme disease, **5**:364
  new/new classes of, **1**:63–65*t*, 74–75, **2**:457
  ocular effects of, **1**:324*t*
  ototoxicity of, mitochondrial DNA mutations and,
    2:220
  for perforating injury, **8**:410, 416
  after PRK/LASEK, **13**:96, 97
  prophylactic
    before cataract surgery, **11**:98
      macular infarction and, **11**:178
    for endocarditis, **1**:10*t*
      ocular surgery and, **1**:334
    for endophthalmitis, **12**:300
    for PRK/LASEK, **13**:92
    for tuberculosis reactivation, **1**:24
  for recurrent corneal erosions, **8**:99
  resistance to, **1**:3, 66. *See also specific agent and*
    specific organism
    new drug classes and, **1**:74–75
  for scleritis, **8**:192
  for septic shock, **1**:319
Antibodies, **9**:7, 25. *See also* Immunoglobulins
  definition of, **9**:7
  immune complex formation and, **9**:58–59, 58*i*
  local production of, **9**:63
  monoclonal, **9**:56
  polyclonal, **9**:56
  stimulatory, **9**:62
  structural and functional properties of, **9**:54–55, 56*i*,
    57*t*
Antibody-dependent cellular cytotoxicity, **8**:200,
  9:70–72
Antibody isotypes. *See* Isotypes
Antibody-mediated immune effector responses,
  9:54–63, 55*t*
  B-cell tissue infiltration and local antibody
    production and, **9**:63

immune complexes in
  circulating, **9**:58–59, 58*i*
    anterior uveitis and, **9**:59
    tissue-bound, **9**:59–62, 60*i*
  immunoglobulin structure and function and,
    9:54–55, 56*i*, 57*t*
  terminology associated with, **9**:56
Anticardiolipin antibodies, in antiphospholipid
  antibody syndrome, **1**:182, 183
Anti-CCP antibodies. *See* Anti-citrulline–containing
  peptide antibodies
Anticholinergic agents
  dry eye caused by, **8**:80, 81*t*
  for ocular deviation, **5**:212
  for Parkinson disease, **1**:279–280
  for pulmonary diseases, **1**:157–158, 157*t*
Anticholinesterase agents. *See* Cholinesterase/
  acetylcholinesterase inhibitors
Anticipation (genetic), **2**:182, 257
Anti-citrulline–containing peptide antibodies, in
  rheumatoid arthritis, **1**:174
Anticoagulant therapy, **1**:171–172. *See also specific agent*
  for antiphospholipid antibody syndrome, **1**:184
  for carotid artery disease, **5**:182
  cataract surgery and, **11**:98, 168–169, 201–202
  for central retinal vein occlusion, **12**:144
  for cerebral ischemia/stroke, **1**:104
  for non-ST-segment elevation acute coronary
    syndrome, **1**:123
  in perioperative setting, **1**:331–332
  after PTCA with stenting, **1**:121
  tailoring dosages and, **1**:165
Anticodon (triplet recognition site), **2**:211
Anticodon loop, **2**:211
Anticonvulsant drugs, **1**:282–283, 283*t*
  as mood stabilizers, **1**:277
  ophthalmic side effects of, **1**:263, 284, 324*t*
  in perioperative setting, **1**:334
Anticytokine therapy, **1**:199–200
Antidepressants, **1**:274–276, 275*t*
  apraclonidine/brimonidine interactions and, **2**:408
  ocular effects of, **1**:324*t*
    tear production and, **8**:81*t*
Antidiabetic agents. *See* Insulin therapy; Oral
  hypoglycemic agents
Anti-double-stranded DNA (dsDNA) antibodies, in
  systemic lupus erythematosus, **1**:181, 181*t*
Anti-elevation syndrome, **6**:129
Antiemetic agents, for migraine, **5**:296
Antiepileptic drugs, **1**:282–283, 283*t*
  as mood stabilizers, **1**:277
  ophthalmic side effects of, **1**:263, 284, 324*t*
  in perioperative setting, **1**:334
Antifibrinolytic agents, **2**:453
  for hyphema, **6**:448, **8**:402
Antifibrotic agents, **2**:425–427
  toxic keratoconjunctivitis caused by, **8**:394
  in trabeculectomy, **10**:188, 190–192
    in children, **6**:281
Antifungal agents, **1**:64–65*t*, 75–76, **2**:437–439, 438*t*.
  See also specific type
Antigen–antibody complexes. *See* Immune
  (antigen–antibody) complexes
Antigen-presenting cells, **9**:7, 19–22, 20*i*, 21*i*
  locations of, **9**:34*t*

in processing, **9**:23*i*
Antigen receptors
  in adaptive immune response, **9**:11
  B- and T-cell, **9**:87
  in innate immune response, **9**:12
Antigenic surface variation, as microbial virulence
  factor, **1**:4
Antigens, **9**:7, 19
  adaptive immunity triggered by, **9**:9, 10
  histocompatibility, **8**:447
  processing of, **9**:22–24, 23*i*
  self, tolerance to, **9**:87–89
  transplantation, **8**:447, **9**:93–94
  tumor, **8**:249
Antiglaucoma agents, **10**:159–174, 160–164*t*, 170*i*. *See
  also* Glaucoma, management of
  adrenergic agonists, **10**:160–161*t*, 169–171, 170*i*
    alpha-adrenergic agonists, **2**:407–408, **10**:161*t*,
      170–171
    beta-adrenergic agonists, **2**:408–409, 410*t*
  beta-blockers, **2**:409–411, 410*t*, **10**:159, 160*t*,
    165–166
  calcium channel blockers, **2**:310
  carbonic anhydrase inhibitors, **2**:305, 411–413, 411*t*,
    10:162–163*t*, 168–169
  combined preparations, **2**:414–415, **10**:164*t*, 173
  hypotensive lipids, **10**:163–164*t*, 171–172
  latanoprost, **2**:413–414, 414*t*
  osmotic agents, **2**:415–416, 415*t*, **10**:164*t*, 173–174
  parasympathomimetics, **10**:161–162*t*, 166–168
  prostaglandin analogs, **2**:413–414, 414*t*
  receptors in mode of action of, **2**:312–313, 314*t*
Antihistamines, **1**:319, **2**:424*t*, 425. *See also specific
  agent*
  for ocular allergies, **6**:235, 236, 236*t*
    conjunctivitis, **8**:208
    vernal keratoconjunctivitis, **8**:211
  ocular effects of, **1**:325*t*
  tear production affected by, **8**:81*t*
Anti-HIV antibody tests, **1**:39
Antihypertensive drugs, **1**:86, 87–94, 88–89*t*, 90*t*, 91*i*,
  91*t*. *See also specific agent*
  for children and adolescents, **1**:97
  combination, **1**:90*t*
  high-risk conditions affecting selection of, **1**:86, 91*t*
  for hyphema, **8**:401–402
  new developments and, **1**:81
  in older patients, **1**:96
  parenteral, **1**:94
  in perioperative setting, **1**:333
  during pregnancy, **1**:96–97
  tear production affected by, **8**:81*t*
  withdrawal from, rebound hypertension and,
    1:97–98
Anti-idiotypic antibodies, **9**:56
Anti-infective agents, **1**:53–78, 55–65*t*, **2**:427–437, 428*t*,
  431*t*. *See also specific type and* Antibiotics
Anti-inflammatory agents, **2**:416–427. *See also specific
  agent and* Corticosteroids; Nonsteroidal anti-
  inflammatory drugs
  arachidonic acid release affected by, **2**:418
  in combination preparations with antibiotics, **2**:432*t*
  for keratoconjunctivitis sicca, **2**:295–296, 295*i*
  ocular effects of, **1**:324*t*
  for pulmonary diseases, **1**:157*t*, 158

Anti-La (SSB) autoantibodies
  in aqueous tear deficiency, 8:73–74
  in Sjögren syndrome, 1:186, 187t, 8:73–74, 79t
Antimetabolites, 2:425–427, 9:96
  in cancer chemotherapy, 1:258t
  for rheumatic disorders, 1:200
  for uveitis, 9:119t
    in children, 6:321
Antimicrobial prophylaxis
  before cataract surgery, 11:98
    macular infarction and, 11:178
  for endocarditis, 1:7, 8–11t
    ocular surgery and, 1:334
  for endophthalmitis, 12:300
  for PRK/LASEK, 13:92
Antimicrobial susceptibility testing, 1:66–67
Antimicrobial therapy, 1:53–78, 55–65t. See also specific
    agent
Antimuscarinic agents, 2:400–402, 401t, 402i
Antineoplastic drugs. See Chemotherapy
Antinuclear (antineutrophil) antibodies
  in aqueous tear deficiency, 8:73
  in juvenile idiopathic (chronic/rheumatoid) arthritis,
    1:178, 6:314, 9:141, 144t
  in scleroderma, 1:185
  in Sjögren syndrome, 8:73, 78
  in systemic lupus erythematosus, 1:180–182, 181t
  testing for, 8:202t
  in Wegener granulomatosis, 1:192, 7:36, 60–61
Antioncogenes. See Tumor-suppressor genes
Antioxidants
  age-related macular degeneration and, 12:60–61
  in lens, 2:368–369, 369i, 11:17
  in retina and retinal pigment epithelium, 2:369i,
    371–373, 373i, 374i
  retinitis pigmentosa and, 12:213
  retinopathy of prematurity and, 12:132
  supplemental, 2:373–375, 374t, 454
Antiparkinson agents, tear production affected by,
    8:81t
Antiphospholipid antibody syndrome (phospholipid
    antibody syndrome), 1:171, 182–184
Antiplatelet therapy. See also Aspirin
  for carotid disease, 1:107, 5:182
  for central retinal vein occlusion, 12:144
  for cerebral ischemia/stroke, 1:104
  in perioperative setting, 1:331
  after PTCA with stenting, 1:121
Antipsychotic drugs, 1:271–273, 272t
  atypical, 1:263, 271–272, 272t
  idiosyncratic reaction to, 5:212
  ocular side effects of, 1:272–273
Antipyrimidines
  in cancer chemotherapy, 1:258t
  for rheumatic disorders, 1:199
Antirecoverin antibodies, cancer-associated retinopathy
    and, 9:61
Antireflection films, interference and, 3:8–9, 9i
Antiretroviral therapy, 1:40–45, 2:244, 9:246–248, 247t
  drug resistance and, 1:41, 43, 44
  HAART, 1:43–44, 9:246
    CMV retinitis and, 1:3, 48, 9:253, 12:193
    immune reconstitution syndromes and, 1:51
  prophylactic, 1:45, 46–47t
  recent developments in, 1:3, 42, 44

Anti-Ro (SSA) autoantibodies
  in aqueous tear deficiency, 8:73–74
  in Sjögren syndrome, 1:186, 187t, 8:73–74, 79t
Antisense DNA, 2:182, 202
Antisense oligonucleotides
  in gene therapy, 2:238, 238i
  for glaucoma, 10:177
Antisense primer, for PCR, 2:230
Anti-Smith (anti-Sm) antibodies, in systemic lupus
    erythematosus, 1:181, 181t
Antispasmodics, tear production affected by, 8:81t
Antithrombin III, 1:164, 165
  deficiency of, 1:170
Antithrombin therapy, for non-ST-segment elevation
    acute coronary syndrome, 1:123
Antithyroid antibodies, testing for, 1:223
Antitoxoplasma antibodies, 9:167
α_1-Antitrypsin, in aqueous humor, 2:319
Antitumor antibiotics, 1:257, 259t
Antiulcer agents, tear production affected by, 8:81t
Anti-VEGF agents
  for age-related macular degeneration, 12:76, 77t
  for diabetes mellitus, 1:217
Antiviral agents, 1:65t, 76–77, 2:439–444, 440t, 441i
  for acute retinal necrosis, 9:155
  for Bell's palsy, 5:284
  for herpetic eye disease, 2:440–444, 8:141, 142t
    herpes simplex epithelial keratitis, 8:145–146
    herpes zoster ophthalmicus, 8:155
    stromal keratitis, 8:148–150, 149t
  for HIV infection/AIDS, 1:40–45, 2:244, 9:246–248,
    247t. See also Antiretroviral therapy
  intravitreal administration of, 2:387
  before laser skin resurfacing, 7:238
  systemic, 2:441–444, 441i
  topical, 2:439, 440t
  for uveitis, 9:140
Anton syndrome, 5:195
Antoni A pattern/Antoni B pattern, in schwannomas,
    7:79
Anwar's big bubble, 8:475
Anxiety, 1:266–267
  drugs for management of (antianxiety drugs/
    anxiolytics), 1:273–277, 274t
    ocular effects of, 1:324t
  preoperative, 1:335
Anxiolytics. See Anxiety, drugs for management of
Aortic arch, 5:17, 178i
Aortic arch (Takayasu) arteritis, 1:189t, 191
Aortic coarctation, hypertension in, 1:83, 84t
Aortic dissection, cerebral ischemia/stroke and, 1:102
Aortitis syndrome (Takayasu arteritis), 1:189t, 191
APC. See Activated protein C; Anterior polar cataract;
    Antigen-presenting cells
Apert syndrome (acrocephalosyndactyly), 6:425–426,
    427i, 7:38, 8:351t
  V-pattern deviations associated with, 6:119–121, 429,
    430i
Apex, cornea, 3:175
Aphakia, 3:116
  ametropia and, 3:116, 118–119, 177–178
  aniseikonia and, 3:118, 178
  congenital, 6:304, 11:30
  contact lenses for correction of, 3:178–179
    in children, 6:300, 11:199

epikeratoplasty (epikeratophakia) for, 13:76
intraocular lenses for correction of, 3:216. *See also*
    Intraocular lenses
    in adults, 11:139–156
    in children, 6:301, 11:156–157, 199–200
    monocular/unilateral, 3:118–119
        aniseikonia and, 3:178
        cataract surgery outcome and, 6:303
    posterior vitreous detachment and, 12:257
    prophylactic treatment of retinal breaks and, 12:267
    spectacle lenses for correction of, 3:118–119,
        164–165. *See also* Aphakic spectacles
        in children, 6:300–301, 11:199
Aphakic glaucoma, 6:279–280, 280*i*, 10:132
    cataract surgery and, 6:279–280, 302–303
Aphakic spectacles, 3:118–119, 164–165
    for children, 6:300–301, 11:199
    refracting technique for, 3:164–165
    Ultra Thin lens for, 3:168
Apical alignment, 3:180, 181*i*, 192–193, 193*i*
Apical bearing, 3:180, 181*i*, 193
Apical clearance, 3:180, 181*i*, 192–193
Apical zone (optic cap), 3:174, 205, 8:38
Apidra. *See* Glulisine insulin
Aplasia, 2:125. *See also specific structure affected*
Aplastic anemia, chloramphenicol causing, 1:74, 2:434
APMPPE. *See* Acute posterior multifocal placoid
    pigment epitheliopathy
Apocrine glands of eyelid, 7:166
    tumors arising in, 7:167–168, 169*i*
Apolipoprotein D, in aqueous humor, 2:319
Apolipoprotein E ε3 and ε4 genes, in Alzheimer
    disease, 1:287
Apolipoprotein E mutation, in hyperlipoproteinemia,
    8:338, 339*t*
Aponeurosis, levator. *See* Levator aponeurosis
Aponeurotic ptosis, 7:215, 216*i*, 217*t*
Apoplexy, pituitary, 1:229–230
Apoptosis, 2:125, 181, 182, 6:206, 8:247*t*, 248
    by cytotoxic T lymphocytes, 9:68, 69*i*
    in DNA repair, 2:213
    Fas ligand in, 9:38, 68, 69*i*
Apostilb, 3:15, 16*t*
APP. *See* Amyloid precursor protein
APP gene, in Alzheimer disease, 1:286–287
Appendage neoplasms, 4:180–182, 181*i*
Applanation tonometer/tonometry, 3:289–292, 290*i*,
    292*i*, 10:25–28, 26*i*, 27*i*, 28*t*. *See also* Goldmann
        applanation tonometry
    in congenital/infantile glaucoma, 6:274
    corneal thickness affecting, 8:34
    fluorescein for, 8:20
    sources of error in, 10:28*t*
Appositional growth, in development of lamellae, 2:151
Approximations, for analysis of optical system,
    3:55–56. *See also specific type and* First-order optics
Apraclonidine, 2:407, 407*t*, 408
    for glaucoma, 10:161*t*, 170–171
        in children, 6:283
    in Horner syndrome diagnosis, 5:263
Apraxia
    definition of, 5:207
    of eyelid opening, 5:278–279
    ocular motor, 5:207–208
        acquired, 5:194, 207–208

congenital, 5:207, 6:156
    parietal lobe lesions and, 5:166
Apresazide. *See* Hydralazine
Apresoline. *See* Hydralazine
APS. *See* Antiphospholipid antibody syndrome
APSAC. *See* Anisoylated plasminogen streptokinase
    activator complex
Aptamers, in cancer chemotherapy, 1:257
Aqueous cellular reaction, in uveitis, 9:102
Aqueous-cornea interface, reflection at, 3:13
Aqueous flare, in uveitis, 9:102, 104*i*, 105*i*
Aqueous humor, 2:52–54, 315–322
    biochemistry and metabolism of, 2:304–305,
        315–322
    carbohydrates in, 2:316*t*, 318
    carbon dioxide in, 2:322
    composition of, 2:315–317, 316*t*, 10:18–19
    dynamics of, 2:304–305
    formation of, 10:17–20, 19*i*
        process in, 10:18
        rate of, 10:20
        suppression of, 10:19–20
    glutathione in, 2:318
    growth modulatory factors in, 2:320–321
    immune response and, 9:36
    inorganic ions in, 2:316*t*, 317
    intraocular pressure and, 10:17–23
    organic anions in, 2:316*t*, 317–318
    outflow of, 10:20–22, 21*i*
        measurement of, tonography in, 10:22
        trabecular, 10:19*i*, 20–22
        uveoscleral, 10:22
    oxygen in, 2:322
    proteins in, 2:304, 305, 316–317, 318–320
    refractive index of, 3:40*t*
    separation of from blood. *See* Blood–aqueous barrier
    specimen collection from, 9:215–216
    urea in, 2:318
Aqueous misdirection (malignant/ciliary block
    glaucoma; posterior aqueous diversion syndrome),
    10:140–141, 140*i*
    cataract surgery and, 11:166, 182
Aqueous penicillin, 1:55*t*
Aqueous phase (component), tear film, 2:44, 288*i*,
    289–291, 289*i*, 8:56
    deficiency of. *See* Aqueous tear deficiency
    secretion of, 8:57
    tests of, 8:62–63, 62*i*, 62*t*
Aqueous tear deficiency, 2:294, 8:56, 57, 71–80, 72*t*. *See
    also* Dry eye syndrome
    clinical presentation of, 8:71–72, 73*i*
    laboratory evaluation of, 8:73–74, 74*t*
    medications causing, 8:76, 80, 81*t*
    non–Sjögren syndrome, 8:72*t*, 80
    refractive surgery and, 13:44, 45*i*
    Sjögren syndrome, 8:72*t*, 78–80, 79*t*
    in staphylococcal blepharitis, 8:164
    systemic diseases associated with, 8:74*t*
    tear composition assays in, 8:63
    tear production tests in, 8:62–63, 62*i*, 62*t*
    tests of, 8:62–63, 62*i*, 62*t*
    treatment of
        medical management, 8:74–76, 75*t*
        surgical management, 8:75*t*, 76–77, 76*i*, 77*i*
Aqueous veins, 2:59, 60*i*

Ara-A. *See* Vidarabine
Ara-C. *See* Cytarabine
Arachidonic acid (arachidonate)
    in eicosanoid synthesis, 2:305, 306*i*, 9:77, 78*i*
    nonsteroidal anti-inflammatory drug derivation and,
        2:420–421
    release of, 2:305, 306*i*
        anti-inflammatory drugs affecting, 2:418
    in retinal pigment epithelium, 2:358
    in vitreous, 2:337
Arachnodactyly, in Marfan syndrome, 6:306
Arachnoid cysts, nystagmus caused by, 6:159*t*
Arachnoid mater, optic nerve, 2:101*i*, 102, 4:203, 204*i*,
        5:26
Arachnoid villi, 5:20
Arachnoidal gliomatosis, 6:406
Aralen. *See* Chloroquine
Arava. *See* Leflunomide
ARBs. *See* Angiotensin II receptor blockers
ARC. *See* Anomalous retinal correspondence;
        Lymphadenopathy syndrome
Arc of contact, 6:28
ARC-T trial, 13:68
Arc welding, occupational light injury and, 12:309
Arcade retinal artery, inferior/superior, 5:15
Arcade retinal vein, 5:20, 21–22*i*
Archeocerebellum, 5:39
Arcuate fibers, 5:111, 114*i*
Arcuate keratotomy, 13:21*t*, 66, 68–69
    after penetrating keratoplasty, 13:66, 67*i*, 68, 187
Arcuate (Bjerrum) scotoma, 10:60, 62*i*
Arcus (corneal)
    in dyslipoproteinemia/hyperlipoproteinemia, 1:151,
        293, 8:338, 339*t*, 369
    juvenilis, 2:127, 8:302, 338, 339*t*, 369
    in Schnyder crystalline dystrophy, 8:322, 322*i*
    senilis, 8:369
Arcus marginalis, 7:12
Arden ratio, 12:36–37, 38*i*
    in Best disease, 12:37–38, 219
Area centralis, 2:86, 87*i*, 12:9*t*. *See also* Macula
AREDS (Age-Related Eye Disease Study), 2:369, 373,
        11:72, 73, 12:60–61
Areolar choroidal dystrophy, central, 12:226, 227*i*
Arginine, restriction of, in gyrate atrophy, 12:225
Argon-fluoride excimer laser, 3:22–23. *See also* Lasers
    for photoablation, 13:29, 87, 88–89*i*. *See also*
        Photoablation
Argon laser, 3:22–23. *See also* Lasers
Argon laser therapy. *See also* Photocoagulation
    for branch retinal vein obstruction, 12:139–140,
        139*i*, 140*i*
    for choroidal hemangioma, 4:164
    for coronary revascularization, 1:122
    for diabetic retinopathy/macular edema, 4:136, 136*i*,
        12:114, 115*i*, 116*t*
    ocular damage (laser burns) caused by, 8:420
    for punctal occlusion, 7:274
    for trichiasis, 7:208
Argyll-Robertson–like pupil, 5:270
Argyll-Robertson pupil, 5:270
    in syphilis, 9:190
Argyriasis, corneal pigmentation in, 8:376, 377*t*
Aricept. *See* Donepezil
Arion sling, 5:286

Aristocort. *See* Triamcinolone
Arlt's line, 8:175, 175*i*
Armaly-Drance screening perimetry, 10:78, 79*i*
ARN. *See* Acute retinal necrosis
Arnold-Chiari malformation, downbeat nystagmus
        caused by, 5:248–249, 248*i*
ARPE. *See* Acute retinal pigment epitheliitis
Array multifocal lens, 13:163–164, 163*i*, 173
Arrestin, 2:343, 344*t*
    mutations in, 2:227, 349
Arrhythmias, 1:132–141. *See also specific type*
    heart failure and, 1:131–132
    sudden cardiac death and, 1:115
ARRP. *See* Retinitis, pigmentosa, autosomal recessive
ARS. *See* Adjustable refractive surgery
Artane. *See* Trihexyphenidyl
Arterial circles, 2:40, 64, 5:15
    development of, 2:155
Arterial dissections, 5:354–355, 354*i*. *See also specific
        type or artery affected*
Arterial occlusive disease
    carotid. *See* Carotid occlusive disease
    retinal. *See* Occlusive retinal disease, arterial
Arterial plexus, ciliary body, 2:67
Arteries. *See also specific type or structure supplied and*
        Vascular system
    anatomy of, 5:11–20
Arteriography. *See* Angiography
Arteriohepatic dysplasia (Alagille syndrome), retinal
        degeneration and, 12:232*t*
Arteriovenous anastomoses, retinal, in Takayasu
        arteritis, 1:191
Arteriovenous fistulas
    glaucoma associated with, 10:32
    orbital, 7:70, 71*i*
Arteriovenous malformations, 5:355, 356*i*, 357
    congenital retinal, 4:248, 249*i*, 12:164
    diagnosis of, 5:357
    intracranial hemorrhage caused by, 1:105, 106
    migraine with, 5:295, 295*i*
    orbital, 6:379, 7:69–70
    transient visual loss and, 5:185
    treatment of, 5:357
    in Wyburn-Mason syndrome, 5:342–343
Arteritic anterior ischemic optic neuropathy,
        5:120–122, 121*i*, 121*t*
Arteritis
    cerebral ischemia/stroke and, 1:102
    giant cell (temporal), 1:188–190, 189*t*, 7:59–60
        anterior ischemic optic neuropathy and,
            5:120–122
        central retinal artery occlusion and, 12:149–150
        choroidal perfusion abnormalities and, 12:166,
            169*i*
        facial pain associated with, 5:299
        headache with, 5:292
        optic nerve affected in, 4:205
    Takayasu (aortic arch arteritis/aortitis syndrome/
        pulseless disease), 1:189*t*, 191
Arthritis
    in Behçet syndrome, 1:193
    cataract surgery in patients with, 11:203
    enteropathic, 1:177
    juvenile. *See* Juvenile idiopathic (chronic/
        rheumatoid) arthritis

Lyme, 1:19
mutilans, 1:178
psoriatic, 1:178, 9:132, 133*i*
   in children, uveitis and, 6:313*t*, 314
reactive (Reiter syndrome), 1:176–177, 8:227–228,
   9:130–131, 131*i*, 132*i*
   HLA association in, 9:94*t*, 130
rheumatoid, 1:173–174
   cataract surgery in patients with, 11:206–207
   juvenile. *See* Juvenile idiopathic (chronic/
     rheumatoid) arthritis
   peripheral ulcerative keratitis and, 8:203, 229, 232*i*
   in systemic lupus erythematosus, 1:179, 181*t*
Arthro-ophthalmopathy, hereditary progressive. *See*
   Stickler syndrome
Arthropods, ocular infection caused by, 8:133–134,
   133*i*
Arthrotec. *See* Diclofenac, with misoprostol
Arthus reaction, 8:201, 9:60, 60*i*
   acute, 9:60, 60*i*
   chronic, 9:63
   retinal vasculitis in systemic lupus erythematosus
     and, 9:61
Artifacts, in visual field testing, 10:70–71, 72*i*, 73*i*
Artificial tears, 2:449–450, 5:286. *See also* Lubricants
   for dry eye, 8:74, 75, 75*t*
   for hay fever and perennial allergic conjunctivitis,
     8:208
   for Stevens-Johnson syndrome, 6:237, 8:218
   for Thygeson superficial punctate keratitis, 8:225
ARV. *See* AIDS-related virus
AS. *See* Ankylosing spondylitis
Ascending optic atrophy, 4:206
Ascending t●act of Deiters, 5:34
Ascertainment, 2:182
Ascorbate. *See* Ascorbic acid
Ascorbic acid (vitamin C)
   for age-related macular degeneration, 12:60–61
   in aqueous humor, 2:316*t*, 317–318
   for chemical burns, 8:94, 392
   deficiency of (scurvy), 1:166, 8:94
   in lens, 2:369, 11:17
   oral supplements and, 2:373, 374*t*, 454
   in retina and retinal pigment epithelium, 2:372
   in tear film, 2:290
Ash-leaf spot (hypopigmented macule), in tuberous
   sclerosis, 5:339, 6:409–410, 410*i*
Asian eyelid, epicanthus tarsalis and, 7:156
ASO. *See* Allele-specific oligonucleotides
Asparaginase, 1:260*t*
Aspart insulin, 1:209, 209*t*
Aspergilloma (fungus ball), 5:365, 366*i*
Aspergillus (aspergillosis), 5:365, 366*i*, 7:46–47
   endogenous endophthalmitis caused by, 9:225–226,
     225*i*, 12:188–189, 189*i*
   flavus, 9:225–226, 225*i*
   fumigatus, 9:225–226, 225*i*
   keratitis caused by, 8:186
   ocular infection caused by, 8:130
   orbital infection caused by, 4:189, 189*i*
Aspiration
   in ECCE, 11:109
   in phacoemulsification, 11:118–121, 119*i*, 120*i*, 137
     definition of, 11:115
     instrument settings for, 11:135*t*, 136–137

Aspiration (respiratory), during surgery, prevention of,
   1:331
Aspiration biopsy. *See* Fine-needle aspiration biopsy
Aspiration flow rate, in phacoemulsification, 11:115
   vacuum rise time and, 11:121, 122*i*
Aspirin, 1:197*t*, 2:421–422, 421*t*
   for carotid artery disease, 1:107
   cataract surgery in patient taking, 11:202
   for central retinal vein occlusion, 12:144
   for cerebral ischemia/stroke, 1:101, 104
   discontinuing before surgery, 1:331–332
   for non-ST-segment elevation acute coronary
     syndrome, 1:122
   ocular effects of, 1:324*t*
   platelet function affected by, 1:167–168, 331–332
   prostaglandin synthesis affected by, 2:306
Assassination (cell), by cytotoxic T lymphocytes, 9:68,
   69*i*
Association (genetic), 2:221–222, 6:205
Assortative mating, 2:183
Asteroid bodies, 4:110, 110*i*
   in sarcoidosis, 4:155, 9:198
Asteroid hyalosis, 4:110, 110*i*, 12:285–286, 286*i*
Asthenopia
   corrective treatment of intermittent exotropia and,
     6:112
   strabismus surgery and, 6:173
Asthma, 1:153–154
   drug treatment for, 1:158
     ocular effects of, 1:325*t*
Astigmatic dial refraction, 3:134–136, 135*i*
Astigmatic keratotomy, 13:21*t*, 66–69, 67*i*, 69*t*
   for astigmatism/refractive errors after penetrating
     keratoplasty, 8:465*t*, 466
   cataract surgery and, 11:102–103
   wound healing/repair and, 13:28
Astigmatic lenses. *See* Cylinders; Spherocylindrical
   lenses
Astigmatic photorefractive keratectomy, 13:98–99. *See
   also* Photorefractive keratectomy
Astigmatism, 3:116–118, 8:309*t*
   against-the-rule, 3:117–118
   amblyopia and, 6:69–70
   in cataract patient, toric intraocular lenses for,
     13:161–163
   after clear lens extraction/refractive lens exchange,
     13:158–159
   corneal topography in detection/management of,
     8:46, 48, 13:9, 10–11, 12
   correction of
     cataract surgery wound construction and,
       11:102–103
     clear corneal incisions and, 11:100–101
     with contact lenses, 3:181–182
       distortion reduction and, 3:181–182
       flexible lenses for, 3:181–182
     with cylindrical spectacle lenses, 3:145. *See also*
       Cylinders; Spherocylindrical lenses
       distortion and, 3:145. *See also* Distortion
   hyperopic
     conductive keratoplasty for, 13:140
     LASIK for, 13:118
     PRK for, 13:99

irregular, **3:**101–102, 118, 236–242. *See also*
Wavefront aberrations
corneal topography in detection/management of,
8:46, 48, **13:**9, 10–11
keratorefractive surgery and, **3:**102, **13:**10–11, 47,
48*i*
retinoscopy of, **3:**133, **8:**49
wavefront analysis and, **3:**237–240, 237*i*, 238*i*,
239*i*, 240*i*, 241*i*, 318–320, 319*i*, 321*i*, 322*i*,
8:49, **13:**13–17. *See also* Wavefront analysis
lenticular, contact lenses and, **3:**182
mixed
LASIK for, **13:**118
PRK for, **13:**99
myopic
LASIK for, **13:**117–118
wavefront-guided laser ablation for, **13:**133–135
oblique, **3:**118
after penetrating keratoplasty
arcuate keratotomy for, **13:**66, 67*i*, 68, 187
control of, **8:**464–466, 465*t*, 467*i*
corneal topography in management of, **13:**12
refractive surgery for, **13:**187–189
after radial keratotomy, **13:**63, 64*i*
refractive, contact lenses and, **3:**182
regular, **3:**93–98, 94*i*, 117–118
retinoscopy of, **3:**129–133, 131*i*, 132*i*, 133*i*
wavefront aberration produced by, **13:**15, 16*i*
retinoscopy in detection of, **8:**49
secondary, wavefront aberration produced by, **13:**17,
18*i*
surgical correction of
arcuate keratotomy for, **13:**66, 68–69
conductive keratoplasty for, **13:**139, 140
hyperopia and, **13:**118
incisional corneal surgery for, **13:**66–69, 67*i*, 69*t*
LASIK for
hyperopia and, **13:**118
mixed astigmatism and, **13:**118
myopia and, **13:**117–118
light-adjustable IOLs for, **13:**165–166
limbal relaxing incisions for, **13:**66, 67*i*, 68–69, 69*t*
after penetrating keratoplasty, **8:**465*t*
PRK/LASEK for, **13:**98–99
hyperopia and, **13:**99
mixed astigmatism and, **13:**99
toric intraocular lenses for, **13:**161–163
transverse keratotomy for, **13:**66–67, 67*i*
suture-induced, cataract surgery and, **11:**184
toric lenses and, **3:**195, 197, 197*t*
visual acuity testing and, **8:**15
wavefront analysis and, **3:**237–240, 237*i*, 238*i*, 239*i*,
240*i*, 241*i*, 318–320, 319*i*, 321*i*, 322*i*, **8:**49,
13:13–17. *See also* Wavefront analysis
with-the-rule, **3:**117–118
after strabismus surgery, **6:**184
Astrocytes, **4:**203
optic nerve, **2:**98
retinal, **2:**83, 84, 353, **5:**24
Astrocytoma (astrocytic hamartoma)
malignant, **5:**151
nystagmus caused by, **6:**159*t*
optic. *See* Optic nerve (optic pathway) glioma
of orbit, **6:**381

pilocytic, **5:**148–151, 149*i*, 150*t*
juvenile, of optic nerve, **4:**208, 209*i*
retinal, optic disc drusen differentiated from,
5:132–134, 133*i*
retinoblastoma differentiated from, **4:**255–258, 258*i*,
6:394
in tuberous sclerosis, **5:**339, **6:**410, 411*i*
Astronomical telescope
in operating microscope, **3:**296, 297*i*
in slit-lamp biomicroscope, **3:**280, 281*i*
AT. *See* Ataxia-telangiectasia
AT III. *See* Antithrombin III
Atacand. *See* Candesartan
Ataxia
Friedreich's, retinal degeneration and, **12:**232*t*, 235
intermittent, **2:**262*t*
with neuropathy and retinitis pigmentosa, **12:**245
mitochondrial DNA mutations and, **2:**218, 219*i*,
220
optic, **5:**194
Ataxia-telangiectasia (Louis-Bar syndrome), **5:**336*t*,
340, 342, 342*i*, **8:**91–92, 270
ATM mutation in, **2:**213, **6:**417–418
in children, **6:**402*t*, 416–418, 417*i*
Atazanavir, **1:**42
ATD. *See* Aqueous tear deficiency
Atenolol, **1:**88*t*, 90*t*
Atevirdine, **1:**41
Atheroma, transient visual loss and, **5:**176–177, 178*i*
Atheroma-cutting blades, for coronary
revascularization, **1:**122
Atherosclerosis
central retinal artery occlusion and, **12:**148, 149
coronary artery (coronary heart disease), **1:**111. *See
also* Ischemic heart disease
in diabetes, **1:**218
hypercholesterolemia and, **1:**143, 143–144
risk factors for, **1:**112–113
screening for, **1:**293–294
ocular ischemic syndrome and, **12:**150, 151
ATM gene mutation, **2:**213, **6:**417–418
Atopic dermatitis, **8:**207
cataracts associated with, **11:**66
keratoconjunctivitis and, **8:**211–213, 212*i*, 213*i*
Atopic hypersensitivity (immediate/type I) reaction,
8:198–200, 199, 199*t*, **9:**27, 54*t*, 72–73, 73*i*. *See also*
Allergic reactions
fluorescein angiography and, **12:**21
topical medication and, **8:**205, 206*i*
Atopic keratoconjunctivitis, **6:**235, **8:**211–213, 212*i*,
213*i*, **9:**74
Atorvastatin, for hypercholesterolemia, **1:**149*t*, 150*t*
heart disease prevention and, **1:**148
Atovaquone
for *Pneumocystis carinii* (*Pneumocystis jiroveci*)
pneumonia, **1:**45
for toxoplasmosis, **6:**217, **9:**168
ATP binding cassette (ABC) transporters
in rods, **2:**344, 344*t*
mutations in, **2:**349
in Stargardt disease, **6:**338, **12:**216
ATP production
in lens, **2:**330
in rod outer segments, **2:**344
ATP reports. *See* Adult Treatment Panel (ATP) reports

ATPase-6 gene, in neuropathy with ataxia and retinitis
  pigmentosa, 2:219*i*, 220
Atrial complexes, premature (PACs), 1:135
Atrial fibrillation, 1:138
  heart failure and, 1:131, 132
  stroke and, 1:102
Atrial flutter, 1:137–138
Atrial tachycardia, paroxysmal, 1:136–137
Atrioventricular block, 1:134
Atrioventricular (AV) junction, 1:133
Atrioventricular junctional rhythm, 1:133
Atrophia bulbi
  with disorganization (phthisis bulbi), 4:29, 29*i*
  with shrinkage, 4:28
  without shrinkage, 4:28, 29*i*
Atrophic retinal holes, 12:253
  treatment of, 12:265, 266, 266*t*, 267*t*
Atrophy
  definition of, 8:247*t*
  gyrate, 2:262*t*, 12:225–226, 226*i*
    ornithine amino transferase defects causing, 2:351,
      12:225
    retinal pigment epithelium in, 2:363
  optic. *See* Optic atrophy
Atropine, 2:310, 400, 401, 401*t*, 402*i*, 3:142
  accommodation affected by, 11:22
  for amblyopia, 6:73
  for cholinergic stimulation in toxic overdose, 1:323
  for cycloplegia/cycloplegic refraction, 3:142*t*, 6:94,
    94*t*
  in Down syndrome patients, pharmacogenetics and,
    2:279
  for medical emergencies, 1:316*t*
  side effects of, 3:142, 6:95
  systemic absorption of, 2:383, 401–402, 402*i*
  for uveitis, 9:114
Atropine-Care. *See* Atropine
Atropisol. *See* Atropine
Atrovent. *See* Ipratropium
Attachment, as microbial virulence factor, 1:4
Atypia, cellular
  definition of, 8:247*t*
  in primary acquired melanosis, 4:57–58, 57*i*, 58*i*
Atypical antipsychotic agents, 1:263, 271–272, 272*t*
Atypical mycobacteria, 1:23, 8:127, 185
  in HIV infection/AIDS, 1:23, 49–50
Atypical necrotizing retinitis, diagnosis of, 9:63
Auditory aids, for low vision patient, 3:261
Auditory artery, internal, 5:18
Auditory meatus, internal, 2:118
Auditory nerve. *See* Cranial nerve VIII
Augmentin. *See* Amoxicillin, with clavulanic acid
Aura
  without headache (acephalgic migraine/migraine
    equivlent), 5:294–295
  with headache (classic migraine), 5:185, 293–294,
    293*i*
  headache without (common migraine), 5:294
  seizures and, 1:281
Auricular chondritis, in relapsing polychondritis, 1:187
Auscultation, in orbital disorders, 7:27
Autism, MMR vaccine and, 1:306
Autoantibodies. *See also specific type*
  in aqueous tear deficiency, 8:73–74
  in diabetes mellitus, 1:203

  in juvenile idiopathic (chronic/rheumatoid) arthritis,
    6:314, 9:141, 144*t*
  in Sjögren syndrome, 1:186, 187*t*, 8:73–74, 79*t*
  in systemic lupus erythematosus, 1:180–182, 181*t*
    retinal vasculitis and, 9:61, 173–175
  in Wegener granulomatosis, 1:192, 7:36, 60–61
    scleritis/retinal vasculitis and, 9:62, 175
Autocrine action, of cytokines, 9:80
Autofluorescence, 12:21. *See also* Hyperfluorescence
  in drusen, 5:131
Autografts
  conjunctival, 8:423*t*, 429–433. *See also* Conjunctiva,
    transplantation of
  indications for, 8:423*t*
    for wound closure after pterygium excision,
      8:430*i*, 431–432
  corneal, 8:453, 471–472. *See also* Keratoplasty,
    penetrating
  limbal, 8:109, 423*t*, 425, 433, 434–435*i*
    for chemical burns, 8:392, 393
    indications for, 8:423*t*
Autoimmune diseases. *See also specific type*
  Graves hyperthyroidism as, 1:224
  molecular mimicry and, 9:91
  Mooren ulcer in, 8:232–234, 233*i*, 234*i*
  peripheral keratitis in, 8:229–232, 230*t*, 232*i*
  scleritis in, 8:234–241
  systemic lupus erythematosus as, 1:179
  thyroiditis. *See* Thyroid ophthalmopathy
  tolerance and, 9:87–89
  uveitis, 9:91
Autoimmune hemolytic anemia, 1:163
Automated DNA sequencing, 2:231, 232*i*
Automated lamellar keratoplasty/automated lamellar
  therapeutic keratoplasty, 8:472, 13:107
Automated perimetry
  achromatic, 10:57
  in functional visual disorder evaluation, 5:310, 311*i*
  short-wavelength (SWAP), 10:58, 70, 71*i*
  standard (SAP), 10:57
  static, 5:92–93, 93*i*, 94*i*, 95*i*, 96, 10:59, 65–68, 66*i*,
    68*i*
    artifacts seen on, 10:70–71, 72*i*, 73*i*
    in glaucoma, 10:57
    learning effect and, 10:74, 75*i*
    screening tests, 10:67
    testing strategy in, categories of, 10:65–67
Automated refraction, 3:312–314, 313*i*, 314*i*, 315*i*
Automatic lensmeters, 3:307–308, 308*i*
Automatisms, 1:281
Autonomic pathways
  cholinergic drug action and, 2:394, 395*i*
  ocular, 5:56–60
    parasympathetic, 5:57, 59–60, 59*i*, 60*i*
    sympathetic, 5:56–57, 58*i*
Auto-oxidation, 2:366, 367*i*
  in lens, 2:368
Autoregulation, vascular, disturbances of, in glaucoma,
  10:51
Autosomal dominant inheritance, 2:265–266, 267*t*
  of retinitis pigmentosa. *See* Retinitis, pigmentosa,
    autosomal dominant
Autosomal dominant optic atrophy, 5:136–137, 137*i*,
  6:364

Autosomal recessive inheritance, 2:261–265, 265t
    of retinitis pigmentosa. See Retinitis, pigmentosa,
        autosomal recessive
Autosomes, 2:183, 242
    aneuploidy of, 2:249–251. See also specific disorder
AV block. See Atrioventricular block
AV junction. See Atrioventricular junction
Avalide. See Irbesartan
Avandamet. See Rosiglitazone, with metformin
Avandia. See Rosiglitazone
Avapro. See Irbesartan
Avellino dystrophy, 4:72–73, 8:310t, 317
Avelox. See Moxifloxacin
Average versus individual effect, 1:361–362
Avilamycin, 1:63t, 75
AVMs. See Arteriovenous malformations
Awareness of vision, problems with, 5:195–196
Axenfeld anomaly/syndrome, 2:168, 169, 169i, 4:79,
    79i, 6:278. See also Axenfeld-Rieger syndrome
Axenfeld loop, 2:50, 51i, 8:14
Axenfeld-Rieger syndrome, 2:169, 169i, 4:78–79,
    6:252–253, 252i, 253i, 278, 8:292, 293i, 10:152, 153t
    differential diagnosis of, 10:153t
    glaucoma associated with, 4:78–79, 6:253, 271, 278,
        10:32, 152, 153t
    posterior embryotoxon in, 6:251i, 252, 253
    pseudopolycoria in, 6:269, 269i
Axes
    cylinder
        locating, 3:130–132, 130i, 131i, 132i
        refinement of, 3:136–139
    of Fick, 6:27–28, 27i
    optical, 3:29–30, 29i, 11:5, 7i
    visual, 6:29–30, 41
Axial ametropia, 3:116
Axial curvature, 8:43
    power and, 13:6–7, 7i
Axial displacement of globe, in orbital disorders, 7:23
Axial distance, 8:42, 13:6
Axial length, in infants and children, 6:199, 200i
    congenital glaucoma and, 6:276
Axial (longitudinal) magnification, 3:30, 34
Azactam. See Aztreonam
Azalides, 1:60t, 71. See also specific agent
Azar intraocular lenses, 11:141i, 143, 144
Azathioprine, 1:200
    for Behçet syndrome, 1:194
    for cicatricial pemphigoid, 8:223
    for uveitis, 9:119, 119t
        in children, 6:321
AZD2563, 1:75
Azelastine, 2:423, 424t, 425
Azidodeoxythymidine. See Zidovudine
Azidothymidine. See Zidovudine
Azithromycin, 1:60t, 71, 2:436
    for chlamydial conjunctivitis, 8:177
    for endocarditis prophylaxis, 1:10t
    for trachoma, 8:177
Azlocillin, 1:67, 2:429
Azmacort. See Triamcinolone
AZOOR. See Acute zonal occult outer retinopathy
Azopt. See Brinzolamide
AZT (azidothymidine). See Zidovudine
AZTEC. See Zidovudine
Aztreonam, 1:59t, 70

Azulfidine. See Sulfasalazine

B

B&B stain (Brown and Brenn stain), 4:36t
B&H stain (Brown and Hopps stain), 4:36t
B-cell antigen receptors, 9:87
B-cell lymphomas
    conjunctival, 8:274–275, 274i
    in HIV infection/AIDS, 1:50
    intraocular, 4:277–279
    marginal zone, 7:85, 86t
    orbital, 4:194–196, 195i
B cells (B lymphocytes), 4:15, 9:15
    activation of, 9:19–22, 21i, 24
    cytologic identification of, 8:67
    in external eye, 8:196t
    in HIV infection/AIDS, 1:37
    infiltration of into tissues, in antibody-mediated
        immune response, 9:63
    maturation of, in bone marrow, 9:15
    monoclonal proliferation of, 8:349–350
    tumor immunology and, 8:249
B-scan ultrasonography/echography, 3:310–312, 311i
    anterior segment (ultrasound biomicroscopy), 2:54,
        55i, 8:37, 38i
    before cataract surgery, 11:84
    in choroidal/ciliary body melanoma, 4:226–227, 228i
    in choroidal hemangioma, 4:243i, 245
    in differentiating drusen from papilledema, 5:131,
        132i
    in metastatic eye disease, 4:273
b-wave, of electroretinogram, 5:101, 12:28i, 29, 205. See
    also Electroretinogram
    vascular disease and, 12:34i, 35, 35i
Babesiosis, 1:19
BAC (bacterial artificial chromosome), 2:183
Bacampicillin, 2:429
Bacille Calmette-Guérin (BCG) vaccination, 1:302
    PPD test affected by, 1:24, 9:195
Bacillus, 8:126
    cereus, 8:126
        endogenous bacterial endophthalmitis caused by,
            12:183
    as normal ocular flora, 8:115t
    ocular infection caused by, 8:126
        after perforating injury, 8:410
    traumatic endophthalmitis caused by, 9:208t, 212,
        12:300
Bacitracin, 2:428t, 431t, 437
    in combination preparations, 2:431t, 432t
Background, wavelength of, perimetry affected by,
    10:65
Baclofen, for nystagmus, 5:255
Bacteria, 8:122–123. See also specific organism or type of
    infection
    conjunctivitis caused by, 4:46–47, 48i, 8:169–174,
        170i, 172i
        in children, 6:224–225, 8:169–172, 170t, 172i
        classification of, 8:170t
        in neonates, 6:222–223, 222i, 8:172–174
    corneal infections caused by, 4:65–67
    cytologic identification of, 8:70, 70i

endophthalmitis caused by
  endogenous, 9:213, 12:183–184, 183*i*
  vitreous affected in, 4:107
eyelid infections caused by, 4:169–171
innate immunity triggered by molecules derived
  from, 9:43–47, 44*t*
keratitis caused by, 4:65–66, 8:51*t*, 179–185, 180*i*,
  181*i*, 181*t*, 182*t*
  intrauterine infection and, 8:298–299
ocular infection caused by, 8:119*t*, 122–128, 163–192
  of cornea and sclera, 8:179–192, 191*i*
  of eyelid margin and conjunctiva, 8:163–179
  invasion and, 8:116–117
  isolation techniques for diagnosis of, 8:136
  specimen collection for diagnosis of, 8:135*t*
orbital infections caused by, 4:188–189
  cellulitis, 7:42–43
  necrotizing fasciitis, 7:44–45
panuveitis caused by, 9:187–195
scleritis caused by, 8:191–192, 191*i*
treatment of infection caused by. See Antibiotics
Bacterial artificial chromosome (BAC), 2:183
Bacterial cell wall, 8:123
  innate immune response and, 9:44
Bactericidal drugs, 1:54
Bacteriology, 8:119*t*, 122–128. See also Bacteria
Bacteriophage, 2:183
Bacteriostatic drugs, 1:54
Bactrim. See Trimethoprim-sulfamethoxazole
Badal principle, 3:80–81, 305
Baerveldt implant, for childhood glaucoma, 6:281
Bagolini striated glasses, in suppression/anomalous
  retinal correspondence evaluation, 6:60–61, 62*i*
Baily-Lovie visual acuity chart, 3:112
BAL (British antilewisite), for Wilson disease, 2:281
BAL9141, 1:68
"Balance lens," in severe low vision, 3:256
Balint syndrome, 5:195, 208
  in Alzheimer disease, 1:288
Balloon angioplasty. See Percutaneous transluminal
  coronary angioplasty
Balloon catheters, in dacryocystorhinostomy, 7:283
Balloon dacryoplasty (balloon catheter dilation), for
  congenital tearing/nasolacrimal duct obstruction,
  6:246, 7:264–265
Baltimore Eye Survey, 10:86, 91*t*, 11:72
Bamboo spine, in ankylosing spondylitis, 1:176
Band cells, cytologic identification of, 8:66
Band keratopathy, 4:67–68, 68*i*
  calcific (calcium hydroxyapatite deposition), 8:356,
    373–374, 374*i*
  in sarcoidosis, 8:88
  in juvenile idiopathic (chronic/rheumatoid) arthritis,
    6:314, 314*i*, 9:142, 142*i*, 143
  surgery for, 6:322
Bandage contact lenses, 3:202, 8:441
  for chemical burns, 8:392
  contraindications to in exposure keratopathy, 8:95
  for corneal abrasion, 8:407
  with cyanoacrylate adhesives, 8:442
  for dry eye, 8:75*t*
  after LASIK, for epithelial erosions, 13:122
  for perforating injury, 8:410
  for peripheral ulcerative keratitis, 8:231

after PRK/LASEK, 13:96, 97, 206
  overcorrection and, 13:100
  sterile infiltrates associated with, 13:104, 104*i*
for recurrent corneal erosions, 8:99
for Thygeson superficial punctate keratitis, 8:225
Barbados Eye Study (BES), 11:73
Barbiturates, 1:274*t*. See also Sedative-hypnotics/
  sedation
  abuse of, 1:268*t*, 269
Bardet-Biedl syndrome, 12:232*t*, 234, 235*i*
  pleiotropism in, 2:259
  renal disease and, 12:236
Bare sclera, wound closure after pterygium excision
  and, 8:429, 430*i*
Bariatric surgery, for obesity in type 2 diabetes,
  1:208–209
Barium enema, in cancer screening, 1:298
Baroreceptors, phenylephrine affecting, 2:405
Barr body, 2:183, 242, 271
Barraquer erysiphake, 11:91, 93*i*
Barraquer intraocular lens, 11:140*i*, 143
Barrett esophagus, 1:297
Barrier devices, for basic life support, 1:314, 315
Barron corneal vacuum trephine system, 8:456
Bartonella henselae (*Rochalimea* spp)
  cat-scratch disease caused by, 5:368, 6:229,
    12:184–185, 185*i*
  ocular infection caused by, 8:127, 178
Basal cell carcinoma
  of eyelid, 4:179–180, 179*i*, 7:174–179, 175*i*
    intraocular extension of, 4:275
  medial canthal/lacrimal sac involvement and, 7:284
Basal cell nevus syndrome (Gorlin syndrome), 7:174
  eyelid manifestations of, 4:176*t*
Basal ganglia, in Parkinson disease, 1:278
Basal lamina (basal cell layer)
  ciliary body, 2:66–67, 68*i*
  corneal, 2:45, 46*i*, 47, 48*i*. See also Descemet's
    membrane/layer
  drusen of (cuticular drusen), 4:138, 12:221
    age-related macular degeneration differentiated
      from, 12:59
    vitelliform exudative macular detachment and,
      12:220, 220*i*
  lens. See Lens capsule
Basal laminar deposits, 12:55, 56*i*
Basal linear deposits, 12:55, 56*i*
Basal skull fracture, arteriovenous fistula caused by,
  7:70
Base curve, contact lens, 3:174, 174*i*, 177, 192–193
  apical alignment, 3:180, 181*i*, 192–193, 193*i*
  apical bearing, 3:180, 181*i*, 193
  apical clearance, 3:180, 181*i*, 192–193
  changing, 3:175, 176*i*
  power determined by, 3:194
Base-out prism test, in functional visual disorder
  evaluation, 5:307
Base pair, 2:183, 199, 200–201
  mutations of, 2:214
    conserved, 2:214
Baseline probability of outcome, 1:361
Basement membrane dystrophies, corneal epithelial,
  8:310*t*, 311–313, 312*i*
  cataract surgery in patients with, 11:208, 209*i*
Basic (acquired) esotropia, 6:98*t*, 104–105

Basic fibroblast growth factor, 2:456
  in aqueous humor, 2:320
Basic life support, 1:313–317
  medications used in, 1:316t
  for ventricular fibrillation, 1:140
Basic secretion test/basic secretors, 2:291, 8:62, 62i
Basilar artery, 5:11, 18, 19i, 178i
  aneurysm of, 5:355
  caudal, 5:18
  dissection of, 5:354
  median perforators of, 5:18
Basilar-type (complicated) migraine, 5:293–294. See also Migraine headache
Basilar vein of Rosenthal, 5:22
Basophil hypersensitivity, cutaneous, 9:66
Basophils, 9:13–14
  cytologic identification of, 8:65t, 66
    in immune-mediated keratoconjunctivitis, 8:203t
  in inflammation, 4:13, 14i
Bassen-Kornzweig syndrome
  Leber congenital amaurosis and, 6:335
  ornithine amino transferase defects causing, 2:351
Batson's venous plexus, 2:117
Batten disease, 12:233t, 234, 236, 241, 241i
Battle's sign, 5:285
BAX gene, in DNA repair, 2:213
Bayes' theorem, 1:358
Baylisascaris procyonis (raccoon ascarid), diffuse unilateral subacute neuroretinitis caused by, 9:172, 12:190
BB isoenzyme, in myocardial infarction, 1:117
BCG (Bacille Calmette-Guérin) vaccination, 1:302
  PPD test affected by, 1:24, 9:195
BDUMP. See Bilateral diffuse uveal melanocytic proliferation
Beaded filament, 2:327
Bear tracks (grouped pigmentation of retina), 2:173, 4:230, 232i, 6:390, 12:264
Beaver Dam Eye Study, 1:360, 11:72, 72t
BEB. See Benign essential blepharospasm
Beclomethasone, for pulmonary diseases, 1:157t
Beclovent. See Beclomethasone
Bee stings, ocular injury caused by, 8:395
Behavioral/psychiatric disorders, 1:264–277. See also specific type
  aging and, 1:239–240
  anxiety disorders, 1:266–267
  cataract surgery in patients with, 11:200–201
  mental disorders due to general medical condition, 1:264
  mood (affective) disorders, 1:265–266
  noncompliance and, 1:277
  ophthalmic considerations and, 1:277
  pharmacologic treatment of, 1:271–277, 272t, 274t, 275t
    ocular side effects and, 1:277
    recent developments and, 1:263
  schizophrenia, 1:264–265
  somatoform disorders, 1:266
  substance abuse disorders, 1:267–271, 268t
Behçet syndrome, 1:193–194, 9:132–135, 134i, 12:181
  HLA association in, 1:193, 9:94t, 134, 12:181
  hypopyon in, 9:107, 132, 133, 134i
Behr optic atrophy, 6:364
Bell's palsy, 5:280, 283–284

Benadryl. See Diphenhydramine
Benazepril, 1:88t, 90t
Bence Jones protein, corneal deposition of, 8:349–350
Benedikt syndrome, 5:227
Benicar. See Olmesartan
Benign episodic pupillary mydriasis, 5:270–271
Benign essential blepharospasm, 7:226
Benign hereditary intraepithelial dyskeratosis, 8:255t, 309t
Benign lymphoid folliculosis, 8:26, 28i
Benign melanosis, 4:56t, 8:264, 264i, 267t
Benign mixed tumor (pleomorphic adenoma)
  of eyelid, 7:167
  of lacrimal gland, 4:192–193, 193i, 7:89
Benign monoclonal gammopathy, corneal deposits in, 8:350
Benign paroxysmal positional vertigo, 5:247
Benign reactive lymphoid hyperplasia. See Lymphoid hyperplasia
Benign retinal vasculitis, 5:128, 128i
Benoxinate, 2:446t, 448
Benzalkonium
  absorption affected by, 2:385
  toxic reactions to, 2:381, 8:101, 393
Benzathine penicillin, 1:55t
Benzodiazepines, 1:273–274, 274t
  abuse of, 1:269, 273
  for seizures, 1:283t
Benztropine, for Parkinson disease, 1:279
Benzylamines, 1:65t, 76
Bergmeister papillae, 2:91, 175, 4:107, 6:361, 12:280. See also Hyaloid artery/system, persistence/remnants of
Berlin disease/edema (commotio retinae), 4:28, 12:291, 292i
Berlin nodules, in uveitis, 9:105, 105i
Bernasconi-Cassinari artery, 5:13
Bernheimer-Seitelberger disease (GM$_2$ gangliosidosis type III), 6:351, 437t
Berry (saccular) aneurysm, 1:105–106, 5:350
Best disease (vitelliform macular dystrophy/vitelliruptive macular degeneration), 6:339–340, 339i, 12:218–219, 218i
  bestrophin defect causing, 2:350, 6:340, 12:218
  electrooculogram in, 6:340, 12:37–38, 219
  retinal pigment epithelium in, 2:363
Bestrophin, mutations in, 2:350, 6:340, 12:218
Beta-adrenergic agents, 2:408–411, 410t
  agonists, 2:408–409, 410t
    for pulmonary diseases, 1:157, 157t
  antagonists, 2:404i, 409–411, 410t. See also Beta-blockers
  for glaucoma, 2:305
Beta-adrenergic receptors, 2:404–405, 404i
  in iris–ciliary body, 2:308t
    signal transduction and, 2:311, 314t
  in tear secretion, 2:293, 293i
Beta-blockers, 2:404i, 409–411, 410t
  adverse reactions to topical use of, 8:101
  for angina, 1:120–121
  cholesterol levels affected by, 1:150
  for glaucoma, 10:159, 160t, 165–166
    in children, 6:282–283
    side effects of, 10:160t, 165
  for heart failure, 1:131

for hypertension, 1:88*t*, 90*t*, 92
  with alpha-blockers, 1:89*t*, 93
for hyperthyroidism, 1:225
for non-ST-segment elevation acute coronary
    syndrome, 1:122
ocular effects of, 1:141–142, 325*t*
in perioperative setting, 1:329, 333
in suppression of aqueous formation, 10:19
Beta (β) carotene
  for age-related macular degeneration, 12:60–61
  antioxidant effect of, 2:369
    oral supplements and, 2:374, 374*t*, 454
Beta (β) cells, pancreatic, in diabetes mellitus, 1:202
  genetic defects and, 1:204*t*
Beta chemokines, 9:81*t*
Beta (β)-crystallins, 2:326–327, 326*t*, 11:11, 11*i*, 12
Beta (β)-hemolytic group A streptococci (*Streptococcus
    pyogenes*), 1:6, 8:124
  orbital cellulitis caused by, 6:231
  orbital necrotizing fasciitis caused by, 7:44–45
  preseptal cellulitis caused by, 6:230
Beta (β)-interferon, 1:261
Beta (β)-lactam antibiotics, 1:54–66, 67–70. *See also
    specific agent*
Beta (β)-lactam ring, 1:54, 67
Beta (β)-lactamase inhibitors, 1:69–70. *See also specific
    antibiotic combination*
Beta (β) lactamases, 2:427
Beta (β)-thalassemia, 1:161
  bone marrow transplantation for, 1:159, 161
Betadine. *See* Povidone-iodine
Betagamma (β,γ) crystallins, 2:326–327, 326*t*, 11:11,
    11*i*, 12
Betagan. *See* Levobunolol
Betaine, for homocystinuria, 6:438
Betamethasone
  for capillary hemangioma, 7:66
  for uveitis, 9:115*t*
Betaxolol, 1:88*t*, 2:410, 410*t*
  for glaucoma, 10:160*t*, 165
  in children, 6:282–283
Bethanechol, 2:396*i*
Betimol. *See* Timolol
Betoptic. *See* Betaxolol
Bextra. *See* Valdecoxib
bFGF. *See* Basic fibroblast growth factor
BFU-E. *See* Burst-forming unit–erythroid
Biapenem, 1:69
Bias (statistical)
  measurement, 1:343
  recall, 1:349
  selection, 1:341
    in case-control studies, 1:349
    in case series, 1:346
Biaxin. *See* Clarithromycin
Biber-Haab-Dimmer dystrophy, 8:319
Bicarbonate
  in aqueous humor, 2:316*t*, 317
  in ciliary epithelium, 2:411
  for malignant hyperthermia, 1:337*t*, 6:193*t*
  for medical emergencies, 1:316*t*
  for shock, 1:318
  in tear film, 2:290

Bicentric grinding (slab-off), for induced anisophoria,
    3:160–161, 161*i*
  reverse, 3:161
Bichrome (red-green/duochrome) test, 3:140
  before refractive surgery, 13:43
    PRK/LASEK, 13:91
Bicillin. *See* Benzathine penicillin
Bick procedure, 7:198
BiCNU. *See* Carmustine
Biconvex indirect lenses, for retinal examination, 12:17
Bielschowsky head-tilt test, 6:92
  in superior oblique muscle palsy, 6:132, 133*i*
Bietti crystalline corneoretinal dystrophy/retinopathy,
    8:342–343, 12:232*t*
Bietti nodular dystrophy, 8:368–369. *See also
    Spheroidal degeneration*
Bifixation, in monofixation syndrome, 6:57, 61–62
Bifocal add. *See also* Bifocal lenses
  determining power of, 3:150–154
    with lensmeter, 3:306–307, 306*i*
  selecting, 3:151–152
Bifocal lenses. *See also* Bifocal add
  contact, 3:198–199
    alternating, 3:182–183, 198–199, 198*i*
    simultaneous vision, 3:182–183, 198–199, 199*i*
  for high accommodative convergence/
      accommodative esotropia, 6:102, 103–104
  intraocular, 3:226, 11:146–147
  for overcorrection of intermittent exotropia, 6:113
  spectacle
    decentration and, 3:163–164, 170
    design of, 3:154*i*, 155–162, 156*i*, 163
    fused, 3:152, 153*i*
    image displacement and, 3:155–157, 159*i*
    image jump and, 3:157–158, 159*i*
    induced anisophoria and, 3:158–162, 160*i*, 161*i*
    for magnification in low vision, 3:255–256
    occupation and, 3:163–164
    one-piece, 3:152, 153*i*
    prismatic effects of, 3:155
    reading position and, 3:156, 157*i*, 158*i*
    types of, 3:152, 153*i*, 154*i*
Bifonazole, 1:76
BIGH3 (keratoepithelin) gene, 8:305, 307, 317
  in amyloidosis, 8:347*t*
  in granular dystrophy, 8:316, 317
  in lattice dystrophy, 8:318
Biglycan, 8:14
Biguanides, 1:212*t*, 213
  for *Acanthamoeba* keratitis, 2:444, 8:189
Bilateral acoustic neurofibromatosis. *See
    Neurofibromatosis, bilateral acoustic (type 2)*
Bilateral complete blindness, evaluation of, as
    functional disorder, 5:305–306, 306*i*
Bilateral diffuse uveal melanocytic proliferation, 9:233,
    12:165–166, 165*i*
Bilateral ptosis, 5:226. *See also* Ptosis
Bilateral visual loss, unilateral visual loss compared
    with, 5:83
Bile acid sequestrants, for hypercholesterolemia, 1:149*t*
Bimatoprost, 2:414, 414*t*, 10:162*t*, 171–172
  for childhood glaucoma, 6:283
Binary fission, in bacterial replication, 8:123
Binkhorst intraocular lens, 11:140*i*, 143

Binocular amplitude of accommodation, 3:119, 150, 152
Binocular balance, in subjective refraction, 3:140–141
Binocular eye movements, 6:36–38. *See also specific type*
  conjugate (versions), 6:36–38, 37*i*
  disconjugate (vergences), 6:38
    in infants, 6:451
Binocular indirect ophthalmoscope (BIO), in retinal examination, 12:17. *See also* Ophthalmoscopy
Binocular telescopes, 3:260
Binocular transient visual loss, 5:185–186
  monocular transient visual loss compared with, 5:171
Binocular vision
  abnormalities of, 6:52–53, 53*i*. *See also specific type*
    abnormal visual experience and, 6:49–51, 50*i*, 51*i*
  assessment of, 6:93–94
  physiology of, 6:41–44, 42*i*, 43*t*
  reduced, 5:308–309
  single
    Panum's area of, 6:42*i*, 43, 52
    testing field of, 6:89–90, 90*i*
BIO. *See* Binocular indirect ophthalmoscope
Bio-Hep-B. *See* Hepatitis B vaccine
Biofilm, microbial, 8:116
  staphylococci forming, 8:124
  virulence and, 1:4
Biologic response modifiers. *See also* Immunotherapy
  in cancer chemotherapy, 1:257–262, 260*t*
Biomechanics of cornea, 8:12–13, 13*i*, 14*i*, 13:18–28
  incisional effect and, 8:13, 14*i*
  keratorefractive surgery affecting, 13:19–28
Biometry/biometrics
  before cataract surgery, 11:87
  as factor in primary angle closure, 10:123
  in IOL selection, 3:217–218
    clear lens extraction/refractive lens exchange and, 13:160
  primary angle closure and, 10:123
Biomicroscopy
  slit-lamp, 3:279–284, 280*i*, 8:16–20
    of anterior segment, 5:258–259
    astronomical telescope in, 3:280, 281*i*
    binocular viewing system of, 3:284, 285*i*
    before cataract surgery, 11:81–83
      limitations of, 11:83
    in choroidal/ciliary body melanoma, 4:224, 244
    clinical procedure for, 8:19
    in diabetic macular edema, 12:112
    Galilean telescope in, 3:280–281, 282*i*
    in glaucoma, 10:33–36, 34*i*, 35*i*, 35*t*
      congenital/infantile, 6:275
    illumination system of, 3:281, 283*i*, 284*i*
      direct illumination methods and, 8:16–18, 17*i*, 18*i*
      indirect illumination methods and, 8:18–19
    inverting prism in, 3:280, 282*i*
    in iris nevus, 4:215–216
    lenses for, 3:285–288, 286*i*, 287*i*, 288*i*, 289*i*
    objective lens of, 3:281, 283*i*
    in ocular trauma, 12:290
    in optic disc evaluation, 10:51
    in pediatric cataract, 6:295
    in posterior vitreous detachment, 12:258, 279
    in recurrent corneal erosions, 8:99

  before refractive surgery, 13:44–45, 45*i*, 46*i*
  in retinal examination, 12:17–18
  in striae in LASIK flaps, 13:122
  ultrasound, 2:54, 55*i*, 8:37, 38*i*
Bioptic telescope lens, 3:260
Bioptics, 13:143, 155–156, 157*t*
Bioterrorism, smallpox vaccination and, ocular complications of, 8:162
Biotherapy. *See* Biologic response modifiers; Immunotherapy
Bipedicle (bucket handle) flap, 8:437–438
Bipolar cells, 2:80, 83*i*, 351–352, 5:24, 12:10–11
  cone, 2:351–352, 352*i*
  differentiation of, 2:142
Bipolar disorder, 1:265
  lithium for, 1:277
Birdshot retinochoroidopathy (vitiliginous chorioretinitis), 9:177*t*, 180–181, 180*i*, 181*i*, 12:174*t*, 177–178, 178*i*
  HLA association in, 9:94*t*, 181
Birth defects. *See specific type and* Congenital anomalies
Birth trauma
  corneal edema caused by, 8:300, 300*i*
  infantile corneal opacities and, 6:255, 256*t*
  nystagmus caused by, 6:161
Birth weight, retinopathy and, 6:325, 326, 12:125, 126. *See also* Retinopathy, of prematurity
Bisoprolol
  for heart failure, 1:131
  for hypertension, 1:88*t*, 90*t*
Bisphosphonates, for osteoporosis, 1:246
Bites, eyelid injuries caused by, 7:187
Bitolterol, 1:157*t*
Bitoric ablation, 13:26, 27*i*
Bitôt spot, 8:92, 93, 93*i*
Bjerrum (arcuate) scotoma, 10:60, 62*i*
"Black box" optical system, 3:76–77, 77*i*
Black sunburst lesions, in sickle cell disease, 12:121
Bladder (Wedl) cells, 4:99, 99*i*, 11:49, 186
BLAST protocol, 2:226
Blastula, 2:133
Blau syndrome (familial juvenile systemic granulomatosis), 6:318
Bleb, filtering. *See* Filtering bleb; Filtering procedures
Bleb-associated endophthalmitis, 9:207, 208*t*, 212–213, 12:331, 332*i*
Blebitis, 12:331
  bleb-associated endophthalmitis differentiated from, 9:212–213
  treatment of, 9:219
Bleeding/blood loss. *See* Hemorrhages
Bleeding diathesis. *See also* Coagulation, disorders of
  cataract surgery in patients with, 11:201–202
Bleeding time, 1:165
  aspirin affecting, 1:167–168
Blend zone, 13:92
Bleomycin, 1:257, 259*t*
Bleph-10/Bleph-30. *See* Sulfacetamide
Blepharitis
  cataract surgery in patients with, 11:206
  infectious, 8:119*t*, 164*t*
  in meibomian gland dysfunction, 8:83, 164*t*
  refractive surgery in patients with, 13:44, 46*i*
  in rosacea, 8:84
  seborrheic, 8:86–87, 164*t*

staphylococcal, **8:**119*t*, 163–168, 164*t*, 165*t*, 166*i*, 167*i*
  marginal infiltrates in, **8:**165, 166*i*, 168, 229
  types of, **8:**164*t*
Blepharochalasis, **7:**228–229
Blepharoconjunctivitis
  contact, **8:**205–207, 206*i*
  herpes simplex virus causing, **8:**140–141, 141*i*, 143
  marginal corneal infiltrates associated with, **8:**229
  staphylococcal, **8:**164–165
    keratitis and, **8:**165–168, 166*i*, 167*i*
Blepharophimosis syndrome, **6:**213, 213*i*, **7:**153, 154*i*, 212
  with congenital ectropion, **7:**154
  with epicanthus, **7:**156
Blepharoplasty, **7:**229–234
  complications of, **7:**232–234, 233*i*
    eyelid retraction, **7:**224, 233, 233*i*
  infraciliary incision for, for anterior orbitotomy, **7:**110–111
  laser resurfacing as adjunct to, **7:**237
  techniques for, **7:**230–232
Blepharoptosis. *See* Ptosis
Blepharospasm
  botulinum toxin for, **6:**195–196, **7:**226
  in congenital/infantile glaucoma, **6:**272–273
  essential, **5:**286–288, 287*i*, 287*t*, **7:**226
    treatment of, **5:**288
  functional (nonorganic/nonphysiologic), **5:**314–315
  reflex, **5:**290
  transient visual loss and, **5:**173
Blepharostat, McNeill-Goldmann, for penetrating keratoplasty, **8:**455
Blessig-Iwanoff cysts, **2:**88, 89*i*
Blind spot, **5:**23
  idiopathic enlargement of, **5:**107, **12:**176
  prolonged enlargement of, **9:**182
Blindness, **3:**245*t*, 252. *See also* Low vision; Visual loss/impairment
  age-related macular degeneration causing, **4:**137
  bilateral, complete, evaluation of as functional disorder, **5:**305–306, 306*i*
  after blepharoplasty, **7:**232
  cerebral/cortical, **6:**456
    occipital lobe lesion causing, **5:**170
  in childhood glaucoma, **6:**277
  color. *See* Color vision, defects in
  congenital
    anomalies causing, **8:**282
    Leber congenital amaurosis causing, **6:**334, 452, 454–455
  day, in cone dystrophy, **5:**104
  diabetic retinopathy causing, **1:**201, **4:**135, **12:**99, 102
  functional. *See* Functional visual loss
  "hysterical." *See* Functional visual loss
  legal, **3:**245
  monocular
    evaluation of, as functional disorder, **5:**306–307, 308*i*
    transient. *See* Monocular transient visual loss
  near, **3:**245*t*, 252
  night. *See* Night blindness
  ocular infections causing, **8:**51, 51*t*
  in retinitis pigmentosa, **12:**212
  retinopathy of prematurity causing, **6:**331

river (onchocerciasis), **8:**51*t*, 132, **9:**195–197
  snow, **8:**388
  trachoma causing, **8:**174
  transient. *See* Transient visual loss
  xerophthalmia causing, **8:**92
Blindsight, **5:**196
Blink-induced excursion patterns, of RGP contact lenses, **3:**194–195
Blinking (blink reflex), **8:**6–7, 55
  abnormal, illusions caused by, **5:**188
  medication absorption and, **2:**381–382
  in meibomian gland lipid release, **8:**57
  in newborn, **6:**451
  protective/defensive function of, **8:**55, 113
  tear secretion and, **2:**294
Blocadren. *See* Timolol
Bloch-Sulzberger syndrome (incontinentia pigmenti), **2:**269, **6:**402*t*, 418–419, 418*i*, 419*i*, **12:**233*t*, 237
Blocked fluorescence, **12:**19–20
Blood. *See also* Hemorrhages
  clotting pathways of, **1:**164, 164*i*. *See also* Coagulation
  composition of, **1:**159
  cornea stained by, **4:**73, 76*i*, **8:**399, 400–401, 400*i*, 401*i*
  in LASIK interface, **13:**131, 131*i*
Blood–aqueous barrier, **2:**304, 305
  breakdown of, clinical implications of, **2:**322
Blood–brain barrier, fluorescein leakage and, **12:**19
Blood cells, **1:**159
  development of, **1:**160
Blood clotting/coagulation. *See* Coagulation
Blood glucose. *See* Glucose, plasma levels of
Blood–ocular barrier, **12:**12
  fluorescein leakage and, **12:**19
  immune response and
    of anterior chamber/anterior uvea/vitreous, **9:**36
    of retina/retinal pigment epithelium/choroid, **9:**40–41
Blood oxygenation level-dependent, **5:**68
  definition of, **5:**78
Blood-pool isotope scans, **1:**119
Blood pressure. *See also* Hypertension
  ambulatory monitoring of, **1:**92, 292
  classification of, **1:**81, 82, 82*t*
  normal, **1:**81, 82, 82*t*
  phenylephrine affecting, **2:**405
  screening, **1:**292
    oral contraceptives/pregnancy and, **1:**96
  in shock, **1:**318
Blood–retina barrier, **2:**84, 304
Blood vessels. *See* Vascular system
Blowout fractures, **2:**8
  diplopia and, **5:**218–219
  of medial orbital wall, **7:**101–102
  orbital cellulitis following, **7:**42
  of orbital floor, **7:**21, 102–106, 103*i*
    in children, **6:**138–140, 139*i*
      vertical deviations and, **6:**138–140, 139*i*
  surgery for, **7:**104–106
Blue bloaters, **1:**154
Blue-cone achromatopsia, gene defects causing, **2:**350
Blue-cone monochromatism, **6:**336, **12:**198
  electroretinogram patterns in, **12:**30*i*
  ocular findings in carriers of, **2:**270*t*

Blue-dot (cerulean) cataract, 11:36, 37*i*
Blue-green laser, 12:314
Blue-green phototoxicity, 2:459
Blue-light entoptoscopy, before cataract surgery, 11:86
Blue-light phototoxicity, 2:371, 459, 463
Blue nevus, 7:171, 8:264
Blue sclera, 8:288
    in Ehlers-Danlos syndrome, 8:288
    in keratoglobus, 8:334, 335
    in Marfan syndrome, 8:354
    in osteogenesis imperfecta, 8:288
Blue-yellow color vision, deficiency in, 12:43, 195, 196*t*
    tests for, 12:44, 45*i*
Blunt trauma. *See also* Trauma
    anterior uveitis caused by, 9:107
    in children, 6:447–450, 448*i*, 449*i*
        abuse and, 6:442
        orbital fractures and, 6:138, 449, 449*i*
    corneal injury caused by, 8:396, 396*i*
    eyelid, 7:184
    glaucoma and, 4:81–84, 10:109–114, 110–113*i*
    gonioscopic findings due to, 10:44, 45*i*
    LASIK flap dislocation and, 13:126–127
    optic neuropathy caused by, 2:102
    posterior segment, 12:290–295
    ptosis caused by, 7:219
    retinal breaks/detachment caused by, 12:254, 255*i*
        in young patient, 12:254–255
Blur circles, 3:36–38, 38
    pupil size affecting, 3:109–110
Blurred retinal images, 3:328
Blurred vision/blurring, 5:213
    SSRIs causing, 1:276
    in uveitis, 9:101–102, 102*t*
    vertebrobasilar insufficiency and, 5:186
Bobbing, ocular, 5:208, 256
Body dysmorphic disorder, 1:266
Body mass index (BMI), cataract risk and, 11:73
BOLD. *See* Blood oxygenation level-dependent
Bone
    brown tumor of, orbital involvement and, 6:380
    cortical and trabecular, 1:241
    Paget disease of, angioid streaks in, 12:83
    physiology of, 1:241
    unifocal and multifocal eosinophilic granuloma of,
        7:88
Bone cyst, aneurysmal, orbital involvement and, 6:380
Bone density, measurement of, 1:242–243
Bone marrow, as lymphoid tissue, 9:16
Bone marrow transplantation
    for mucopolysaccharidoses, 6:438
    for thalassemia, 1:159, 169
Bone spicules, in cone–rod dystrophies, 12:215
Bony orbit. *See* Orbit
Bony tumors, of orbit, in children, 6:380
Borderline neoplastic proliferations, 4:16
Borrelia burgdorferi, 1:18–21, 5:284, 362, 8:128, 9:191,
    12:191. *See also* Lyme disease
Botox. *See* Botulinum toxin
Botryoid rhabdomyosarcoma, 4:198, 6:373, 7:80
Bottom-up acuity, in functional visual disorder
    evaluation, 5:308–309
Botulinum toxin, 2:449
    for acute spastic entropion, 7:202
    for blepharospasm, 5:288, 6:195–196, 7:226

for classic congenital (essential infantile) esotropia,
    6:100
complications of use of, 6:196
cosmetic uses of, 7:239
for esotropia in sixth nerve palsy, 6:107
for hemifacial spasm, 5:289, 7:226
indications/techniques/results of, 6:195–196
for overcorrection of intermittent exotropia, 6:114
pharmacology and mechanism of action of, 6:195
for ptosis, 5:286
ptosis caused by, 5:277, 6:196, 7:219
for strabismus, 6:195–196
as tarsorrhaphy alternative, 8:428
for undercorrection of intermittent exotropia, 6:111
Bourneville disease/syndrome (tuberous sclerosis),
    5:336*t*, 338–340, 339*i*, 6:402*t*, 409–412, 410*i*, 411*i*
    glaucoma associated with, 10:32
Bow zone, 2:324, 324*i*
Bowen disease, 7:173
Bowman probe, 6:243, 244*i*, 7:262, 263*i*
Bowman's layer/membrane, 2:45–46, 46*i*, 298*i*,
    299–300, 4:61–62, 61*i*, 8:9*i*, 10
    anatomy of, 2:45–46, 46*i*, 298*i*, 299
    biochemistry and metabolism of, 2:299–300
    corneal dystrophy and, 8:315, 316*i*
    refractive surgery and, 2:299–300
Bowman's zone, development of, 2:152, 152*i*
bp. *See* Base pair
Brachium conjunctivum, 5:34
Brachycephaly, 6:422
Brachydactyly, in Saethre-Chotzen syndrome, 6:426
Brachytherapy
    for choroidal hemangioma, 4:245
    for melanoma, 4:218, 237
        of iris, 4:228
    for metastatic eye disease, 4:273–275
    for retinoblastoma, 4:263
Bradyarrhythmias, 1:133–135
    sinus bradycardia, 1:133
Bradykinetic movement disorders, 1:278. *See also*
    Parkinson disease
Bradykinin, 8:198*t*, 9:76
Brain. *See specific structure and under Cerebral*
Brain lesions
    nystagmus caused by, 6:159*t*
    in Sturge-Weber syndrome, 6:414, 414*i*
    in tuberous sclerosis, 6:410, 411*i*
Brain stem lesions
    arteriovenous malformations, 5:355
    facial weakness/paralysis caused by, 5:282–283
    horizontal gaze palsy with, 5:208, 209*i*
Brain stones (calcified astrocytic hamartomas), in
    tuberous sclerosis, 5:339
Branch retinal artery occlusion, 4:133, 12:146–148,
    146*i*, 147*i*
Branch retinal vein occlusion, 4:134–135, 135*i*,
    12:136–141, 137*i*, 139*i*, 140*i*
    intravitreal triamcinolone for, 12:141
    neovascularization in, 4:130–133, 12:138
    photocoagulation for, 12:138–139, 139–140, 139*i*,
        140*i*
        wavelength selection and, 12:315*t*
    vitrectomy for, 12:140–141
Branch Vein Occlusion Study (BVOS), 12:139–140,
    140*i*

Branchial arch syndromes, **6**:431–432, 432*i*, 433*i*
BRAO. *See* Branch retinal artery occlusion
Brawny scleritis, **4**:90, 90*i*
Break, in retinal reflex, axis determination and, **3**:130, 131*i*
Breaks (retinal). *See* Retinal breaks
Breast cancer, **1**:252
    eye involvement and, **1**:262, **4**:267–268, 268*t*, 269*i*, 273–275, 279–280, **7**:95*i*, 96
    metastatic, numb chin associated with, **5**:301
    screening for, **1**:294–296, 295*t*
Breast examination, for cancer screening, **1**:295*t*, 296
Breast feeding
    fluorescein dye transmission to breast milk and, **12**:21
    glaucoma medications and, **10**:176
    refractive surgery contraindicated during, **13**:41
Breathing exercises, **1**:156
Brethaire. *See* Terbutaline
Brethine. *See* Terbutaline
Brevibloc. *See* Esmolol
Brevital. *See* Methohexital
Brewster angle, **3**:13, 13*i*
Bricanyl. *See* Terbutaline
Bridge flap, **8**:437
Bridle suture, **11**:121
Brief psychotic disorder, **1**:265
Bright-flash electroretinogram, **12**:33
Brightness (radiance), **2**:460, 460*t*, **3**:15, 16*t*. *See also* Intensity
    as image characteristic, **3**:39
    for medical lasers, **3**:18, 18*t*
Brightness acuity, evaluation of before cataract surgery, **11**:84
Brightness Acuity Test (BAT), **3**:253
Brightness discrimination, **3**:111
    minimum perceptible acuity and, **3**:111
    minimum visible acuity and, **3**:111
Brimonidine, **2**:407, 408, **10**:161*t*, 170–171
    in children, **6**:283
Brinzolamide, **2**:411*t*, 412, **10**:163*t*, 168–169
    in children, **6**:283
British antilewisite (BAL), for Wilson disease, **2**:281
Brivudine, **1**:77
Broad-beam illumination, for slit-lamp biomicroscopy, **8**:16
Broad-beam lasers, for photoablation, **13**:30
    central island formation and, **13**:101–102
Brodmann area 8, **5**:34
Brodmann area 17 (striate cortex), **5**:29, 30*i*, **6**:44, 45, 45*i*, 47*i*. *See also* Visual (calcarine/occipital) cortex
    development of, **6**:46, 48*i*
        abnormal visual experience affecting, **6**:49–52, 50*i*, 51*i*, 67–68
Brodmann area 18 (parastriate cortex), **5**:29, 31, **6**:44. *See also* Visual (calcarine/occipital) cortex
Brodmann area 19, **6**:44
Bromfenac, **1**:197
Bromides, abuse of, **1**:268*t*
Bromocriptine, for Parkinson disease, **1**:279
Bronchial lavage, **1**:155
Bronchiectasis, **1**:154
Bronchitis, **1**:154
Bronchodilators, **1**:156–157, 157*t*
Bronchogenic carcinoma, orbital metastases in, **7**:96

Bronchoscopy, **1**:155
    in cancer screening, **1**:297
Bronchospasm, in asthma, **1**:153–154
Brow and forehead lift, **7**:239–241, 240*i*
Brow lift, **7**:241
Brow ptosis, **7**:234–235, 234*i*
Brown albinism, **6**:346*t*
Brown and Brenn (B&B) stain, **4**:36*t*
Brown and Hopps (B&H) stain, **4**:36*t*
Brown-McLean syndrome, **11**:167
Brown (superior oblique tendon sheath) syndrome, **5**:219–220, 220*i*, **6**:135, 144–146, 145*i*
    iatrogenic, tucking procedure causing, **6**:175
    inferior oblique muscle paralysis compared with, **6**:137*t*
    surgery for, **6**:146, 181
Brown tumor of bone, orbital involvement and, **6**:380
Browpexy, **7**:235
Bruch's membrane, **2**:70, 71*i*, **12**:12, 13*i*, 15
    choroidal neovascularization and, **12**:63, 63*i*
        in age-related macular degeneration, **4**:139
    development of, **2**:144
    drusen affecting, **12**:55–57, 56*i*
    rupture of, **4**:26
        by choroidal melanoma, **4**:159, 160*i*
        photocoagulation causing, **12**:319
Brücke's muscle, **4**:150
Brückner test
    for pediatric cataract, **6**:292
    for strabismus and amblyopia, **6**:83
Bruits
    carotid, **1**:107, **5**:179, 354. *See also* Carotid occlusive disease
    in orbital disorders, **7**:27
Brun nystagmus, **5**:248
Brunescent cataracts, **11**:46
    lens proteins in, **11**:13
Brush marks, in meibomian gland dysfunction, **8**:82
Brushfield spots, **4**:219*t*, 220*i*, **6**:266
BRVO. *See* Branch retinal vein occlusion
Buccal mucous membrane graft
    for eyelid repair, **7**:187
    for symblepharon, **7**:207
Buccal nerve, **5**:56
Bucket handle (bipedicle) flap, **8**:437–438
Bucrylate. *See* Cyanoacrylate adhesives
Budesonide, for pulmonary diseases, **1**:157*t*
Budge-Waller, ciliospinal nucleus of, **5**:56, 58*i*
Bulbar conjunctiva, **2**:29, 32*i*, 36, **8**:8. *See also* Conjunctiva
    in superior limbic keratoconjunctivitis, **8**:96, 97, 97*i*
Bulbar vernal keratoconjunctivitis, **6**:234–235
Bulla
    of cornea, **8**:25*t*
    of eyelid, **8**:24*t*
Bullous keratopathy, **4**:68–69, 70*i*
    after cataract surgery, **11**:164*t*, 192–193, 193*i*
    disciform keratitis and, **8**:151
    flexible contact lenses for, **3**:202
Bull's-eye depigmentation, in cone dystrophy, **5**:104
Bull's-eye maculopathy
    differential diagnosis of, **12**:217, 217*t*
    hydroxychloroquine causing, **1**:198
Bull's eye optic, corneal implant correction of presbyopia and, **13**:175–176

Bumetanide
for diastolic dysfunction, 1:131
for hypertension, 1:88*t*
Bumex. *See* Bumetanide
Bundle branch block, left or right, 1:134–135
Bundle of His, 1:133, 134
Buphthalmos (megaloglobus)
in glaucoma, 6:277, 10:147
in neurofibromatosis, 6:408
Bupivacaine, 2:445*t*, 447, 448
for blepharoplasty, 7:231
maximum safe dose of, 1:322
toxic reaction to, 1:323
Bupropion, 1:276
Burkitt lymphoma
Epstein-Barr virus associated with, 1:30, 254
of orbit, 4:195, 6:375
Burns
chemical. *See* Chemical injury
corneal, in children, accidental cigarette burns, 6:445
eyelid, 7:187
thermal, 8:387–389
Burst-forming unit–erythroid, 1:160
Busacca nodules
in iridocyclitis, 4:219*t*
in sarcoidosis, 4:155, 9:105*i*, 198, 199*i*
in children, posterior synechiae and, 6:270
in uveitis, 9:105, 105*i*
Butazolidin. *See* Phenylbutazone
Butenafine, 1:65*t*, 76
Butterfly dystrophy, 12:222, 222*i*
Butylcyanoacrylate tissue adhesive, 8:441. *See also*
Cyanoacrylate adhesives
BVOS (Branch Vein Occlusion Study), 12:139–140,
140*i*
Byetta. *See* Exenatide
Bypass grafting, coronary artery, 1:121–122
troponin levels in determining need for, 1:117

C

C4 complement, in aqueous humor, 2:319
C5a complement, 8:198*t*
C5a peptidase, streptococcal production of, 8:124
C (parafollicular) cells, 1:221
C-reactive protein
in coronary artery disease, 1:111
in giant cell arteritis, 1:190, 5:122
central retinal artery occlusion and, 12:150
in immune-mediated disease, 8:202*t*
in innate immune response, 9:47
c-wave, of electroretinogram, 5:101, 12:31, 38, 39*i. See
also* Electroretinogram
Ca^{2+}-ATPase (calcium pump), in calcium homeostasis
in lens, 11:20–21
Ca^{2+}/protein kinase C–dependent signal transduction,
in tear secretion, 2:292–293, 292*i*
CABG. *See* Coronary artery bypass graft
CADASIL. *See* Cerebral autosomal dominant
arteriopathy with subcortical infarcts and
leukoencephalopathy
Café-au-lait spots
in neurofibromatosis, 5:337, 6:403, 7:75
in tuberous sclerosis, 5:338

in von Hippel–Lindau disease, 6:412
CAIs. *See* Carbonic anhydrase inhibitors
Cajal, interstitial nucleus of, 5:34, 202
skew deviation and, 5:223
Calan. *See* Verapamil
Calanolide, 1:42
Calcarine artery, 5:20, 20*i*
Calcarine cortex. *See* Occipital (primary visual/
calcarine/striate) cortex
Calcarine fissure, 5:29, 30*i*
Calcific band keratopathy (calcium hydroxyapatite
deposition), 8:356, 373–374, 374*i*
in sarcoidosis, 8:88
Calcific (calcified) drusen, 4:138, 12:58
Calcific plaques, senile, 4:91, 91*i*
Calcified astrocytic hamartomas (brain stones), in
tuberous sclerosis, 5:339
Calcinosis, in scleroderma, 1:185
Calcitonin/calcitonin nasal spray, for osteoporosis,
1:245*t*, 246
Calcitonin gene-related peptide
in iris–ciliary body, 2:308
in signal transduction, 2:311–312, 312*i*, 313*i*, 314*t*
in tear secretion, 2:290
Calcium
in aqueous humor, 2:317
for osteoporosis, 1:244
in signal transduction
in iris–ciliary body, 2:311–312, 312*i*, 313*i*
in tear secretion, 2:292–293, 292*i*
Calcium antagonists. *See* Calcium channel blockers
Calcium channel blockers, 2:310
for angina, 1:120–121
for heart failure, 1:130
for hypertension, 1:89*t*, 90*t*, 93
for non-ST-segment elevation acute coronary
syndrome, 1:122–123
ocular effects of, 1:325*t*
Calcium channels, 2:310
L-type, 2:310
mutations in, 2:349
Calcium chloride, for medical emergencies, 1:316*t*
Calcium embolus, transient visual loss and, 5:175, 176*i*,
177*t*
Calcium homeostasis, in lens, 11:20–21
Calcofluor white staining, 8:65*t*
Caldwell-Luc procedure, for thyroid-associated
orbitopathy, 5:332
Callender classification, of uveal melanomas, 4:157, 160
Calmodulin, in rods, 2:344*t*
CALT. *See* Conjunctiva-associated lymphoid tissue
Calvarium, in craniosynostosis, 6:421, 422*i*, 424
CAM. *See* Cell-adhesion molecules
cAMP, in signal transduction
in iris–ciliary body, 2:311–312, 312*i*, 313*i*
in tear secretion, 2:293, 293*i*
"Can opener" capsulotomy, 11:110, 111*i*
Canaliculi, lacrimal, 2:33*i*, 35, 6:239, 7:254, 255*i*
atresia of, 6:239–240
common, 6:239
congenital abnormalities of, 7:257–258
infection/inflammation of, 7:268*i*, 276, 276*i*
obstruction of, 7:271*i*, 275
irrigation in evaluation of, 7:270–271, 270*t*, 275
trauma to, 7:186, 276–277

Canaliculitis, 7:268*i*, 276, 276*i*, 8:119*t*
Canaliculodacryocystorhinostomy, for canalicular
    obstruction, 7:275
Canaliculotomy, for canaliculitis, 7:276
Canals. *See specific type*
Cancer, 1:251–262. *See also specific type or organ or
    structure affected and* Carcinoma; Intraocular
    tumors; Tumors
    carcinogenesis and, 1:253
    chemicals causing, 1:252–253
    chemotherapy for, 1:256–262, 258–260*t*
    corneal nerve enlargement and, 8:347, 357*i*, 358*t*
    etiology of, 1:252–255
    eyelid manifestations of, 4:176*t*
    genetic and familial factors in, 1:254–255, 2:215,
        216*i*
    in HIV infection/AIDS, 1:50–51
    hypercoagulability and, 1:171
    incidence of, 1:251
    loss of telomeric DNA and, 2:203
    oncogenesis and, 8:248–249, 248*t*
    ophthalmic considerations and, 1:262
    radiation causing, 1:253
    radiation therapy for, 1:255–256
    recent developments in, 1:251
    retinopathy associated with, 5:101, 108–109, 9:61,
        12:237–238, 238*i*
    screening for, 1:294–300, 295*t*
    therapy of, 1:255–262. *See also* Chemotherapy
        recent developments in, 1:251
    vaccines against, 1:262
    viruses causing, 1:254
Cancer checkup, 1:295*t*
Cancer chemotherapy. *See* Chemotherapy
Cancer-cluster families, 1:254
Cancer genes, 2:215, 216*i*, 8:248, 248*t*
Cancer vaccines, 1:262
Candela, 3:14, 16*t*
Candesartan, 1:88*t*, 90*t*
Candida (candidiasis)
    albicans, 1:25, 8:130, 130*i*
        adherence in virulence of, 8:116
    endogenous endophthalmitis caused by, 9:213–214,
        219–220, 223–225, 12:187–188, 188*i*
    keratitis caused by, 8:185, 186
    as normal ocular flora, 8:115, 115*t*
    postoperative endophthalmitis caused by, 9:210
    retinitis caused by, 9:163–164, 164*i*
Candidate gene screening, 2:226–227
    positional, 2:227
Candle power (luminous intensity), 3:16*t*
Candlewax drippings, in sarcoidosis, 4:155, 9:199
Cannabis use/abuse, 1:268*t*
Canthal index, Farcas, 6:207
Canthal reconstruction, 7:188–193. *See also* Eyelids,
    reconstruction of
Canthal tendons, 7:146
    lateral, 7:146
    medial, 7:146
    trauma involving, 7:186
Canthal tissues, trauma involving, 7:186
Canthal tumors, 7:277–278
Canthaxanthine, retinopathy caused by, 12:249, 250*i*,
    250*t*

Cantholysis
    for traumatic visual loss, 7:107
    for trichiasis, 7:208
Canthoplasty, for persistent corneal epithelial defects,
    8:102
Canthotomy
    lateral, for lateral orbitotomy, 7:114
    for traumatic visual loss, 7:107
CAP. *See* Chromosome arm painting
Capillary-free zone (foveal avascular zone), 2:88, 88*i*,
    12:8
Capillary hemangiomas. *See* Hemangiomas; Retinal
    angiomatosis
Capillary malformations, orbital, 6:380
Capillary nonperfusion. *See* Retinal capillary
    nonperfusion
Capillary plexus, of ciliary process, 2:66
Capillary telangiectasias, 1:106
Capoten. *See* Captopril
Capozide. *See* Captopril
Capravirine, 1:42
Capsid (viral), 8:119–120
Capsofungin, 1:76
Capsular cataracts, 11:37
Capsular fibrosis, 11:187
    Nd:YAG laser capsulotomy for, 11:187, 187–191,
        189*i*
Capsular opacification, 11:164*t*, 186–187
    in children, 11:198
    with multifocal IOLs, 13:173
    Nd:YAG laser capsulotomy for, 11:187–191, 189*i*
Capsular phimosis, 11:187
    Nd:YAG laser capsulotomy for, 11:187, 187–191,
        189*i*
Capsular rupture, during phacoemulsification, 11:164*t*,
    179–180
Capsular theory (Helmholtz hypothesis), of
    accommodation, 13:167–168
Capsulectomy/vitrectomy, for pediatric cataract, 11:197
    lensectomy without intraocular lens implantation
        and, 6:295–296, 298*i*
    lensectomy with intraocular lens implantation and,
        6:299–300, 300*i*
Capsulopalpebral fascia, 7:140–141, 145
Capsulopupillary portion of tunica vasculosa lentis,
    11:29, 29*i*
Capsulorrhexis
    in children, 11:196
    for ECCE with nucleus expression, 11:110, 111*i*
    mature cataract/poor red reflex and, 11:210–211
    for phacoemulsification, 11:126–127
    in uveitis, 9:235–236
Capsulotomy
    anterior
        "can opener," 11:110, 111*i*
        in children, 11:196
        for ECCE with nucleus expression, 11:110, 111*i*
        for phacoemulsification, 11:126–127
    Nd:YAG laser, 11:187–191, 189*i*
        in children, 11:197
        complications of, 11:190–191
        contraindications to, 11:188
        indications for, 11:188
        lens-particle glaucoma and, 11:67–68
        procedure for, 11:188–190, 189*i*

retinal detachment and, 11:175, 190, 12:334
posterior, in children, 11:197
CAPT (Complications of Age-Related Macular
Degeneration Prevention Trial), 12:62
Captopril
for heart failure, 1:130
for hypertension, 1:88t, 90t
for non-ST-segment elevation acute coronary
syndrome, 1:123
ocular effects of, 1:325t
CAR. See Cancer, retinopathy associated with
CAR antigen (recoverin), 2:344t, 5:109
cancer-associated retinopathy and, 9:61
Carbacephems, 1:59t, 69
Carbachol, 2:309, 395, 396i, 397, 398t
for glaucoma, 10:162t, 166
Carbamazepine, 1:283t
as mood stabilizer, 1:277
Carbapenems, 1:59–60t, 69–70. See also specific agent
Carbatrol. See Carbamazepine
Carbenicillin, 1:67, 2:428t, 429
Carbidopa, for Parkinson disease, 1:279
Carbocaine. See Mepivacaine
Carbohydrates
in aqueous humor, 2:316t, 318
metabolism of
in cornea, 2:297–299, 298i
disorders of, corneal changes in, 8:335–338, 337t
in lens, 2:330, 11:14–16, 15i
in retinal pigment epithelium, 2:357–358
Carbon, corneal pigmentation caused by, 8:377t
Carbon dioxide, in aqueous humor, 2:322
Carbon dioxide laser, 3:22–23. See also Lasers
for orbital lymphangioma, 7:69
for skin resurfacing, 7:237–238
Carbonic anhydrase
in aqueous humor, 2:320
dynamics and, 2:304
in ciliary epithelium, 2:411, 412
Carbonic anhydrase inhibitors, 2:305, 411–413, 411t
adverse reactions to topical use of, 8:101
for cystoid macular edema, 12:155
for glaucoma, 2:305, 411–413, 411t, 10:162–163t,
168–169
in children, 6:283
for IOP control in chemical burns, 8:392
in suppression of aqueous formation, 2:411, 10:19
Carboxypenicillins, 1:67
Carcinogenesis, 1:253
chemical, 1:252–253
genetic and familial factors in, 1:254–255
loss of telomeric DNA and, 2:203
radiation in, 1:253
viral, 1:254
Carcinoma, 4:17t, 18i. See also specific type or structure
affected and Carcinoma in situ; Adenocarcinoma
adenoid cystic (cylindroma)
of eyelid, 7:168
of lacrimal glands, 4:193–194, 194i, 7:90–91
basal cell
of eyelid, 4:179–180, 179i, 7:174–179, 175i
intraocular extension of, 4:275
medial canthal/lacrimal sac involvement and,
7:284

of conjunctiva
intraocular extension of, 4:275
staging of, 4:285t
definition of, 8:247
of eyelid, 4:177–180, 179i
metastatic, 4:267–275. See also specific type and
structure affected and Metastatic eye disease
ancillary tests in evaluation of, 4:271–273, 274i
clinical features of, 4:268–271, 269i, 270i, 271i,
272i, 272t, 273–275
diagnostic factors in, 4:273
mechanisms of spread and, 4:268–271
primary sites and, 4:267–275, 268t
prognosis for, 4:274–275
treatment of, 4:273–274
sebaceous, 4:180–182, 181i
squamous cell
of conjunctiva, 4:53, 53i
of eyelid, 4:177–179, 178i, 7:179–180, 179i
actinic keratosis and, 4:174–177
in situ (Bowen disease), 7:173
medial canthal/lacrimal sac involvement and,
7:284
of orbit, secondary, 7:92i, 93
retinoblastoma associated with, 4:265t
thyroid, retinoblastoma associated with, 4:265t
Carcinoma in situ
of conjunctiva, 8:257, 257i
of cornea, 4:76
Cardene. See Nicardipine
Cardiac arrest. See Cardiopulmonary arrest
Cardiac disease. See Heart disease
Cardiac enzymes, in ischemic heart disease, 1:116–117
Cardiac failure. See Congestive heart failure
Cardiac glycosides. See Digitalis/digitoxin/digoxin
Cardiac rhythm, disorders of, 1:132–141. See also
Arrhythmias
Cardiac-specific troponins (troponins T and I), in
myocardial infarction, 1:117, 118i
Cardiac transplantation, for heart failure, 1:132
Cardinal points, 3:76
for calculation of retinal image size, 3:106i
Cardinal positions of gaze, 5:241i, 6:28, 28i, 86
extraocular muscle action and, 6:29–30
yoke muscles and, 6:28i, 36, 86
Cardiogenic shock, 1:317. See also Shock
Cardiolite scintigraphy. See Technetium-99m Sestamibi
scintigraphy
Cardiopulmonary arrest, 1:313–317
Cardiopulmonary resuscitation, 1:313–317
medications used in, 1:316t
retinal hemorrhage in children caused by, 6:444
for ventricular fibrillation, 1:140
Cardioselective beta-blockers, 1:92
Cardiovascular disorders. See also specific type
central retinal artery occlusion and, 12:148, 149
diabetes and, 1:216–217, 218
hypertension and risk of, 1:81, 84, 86t
in Lyme disease, 1:19
ocular ischemic syndrome and, 12:151
primary open-angle glaucoma and, 10:89
screening for, 1:293–294
Cardioversion
for atrial fibrillation, 1:138
for atrial flutter, 1:137–138

for atrial tachycardia, 1:137
for torsades de pointes, 1:140
for ventricular fibrillation, 1:140
for ventricular tachycardia, 1:139
Cardizem. *See* Diltiazem
Cardura. *See* Doxazosin
Carmustine, 1:260*t*
Carney complex, eyelid manifestations of, 4:173*t*
Carotenoids (xanthophylls)
absorption spectrum for, 12:313, 314*i*
in lens, 2:369, 369*i*
in macula, 12:7–8
in retina, 2:373
structure of, 2:373*i*
Carotid arteries
common, 5:11, 178*i*
disorders of, 1:107–109. *See also specific type and*
Carotid occlusive disease
dissection of, pain caused by, 5:299, 300
external, 5:11, 11–12*i*, 178*i*, 8:7
eyelids supplied by, 7:147, 8:7
internal, 5:11, 11–12*i*, 13, 14*i*, 178*i*, 8:7
aneurysm of, 5:350–351
chiasmal syndromes caused by, 5:162
third nerve palsy and, 5:228–229, 229*i*
dissection of, 5:354–355
Horner syndrome caused by, 5:263–264, 264*i*
supraclinoid, 5:16
orbit supplied by, 7:15
stenting of, 5:182
Carotid bruits, 1:107, 5:179, 354. *See also* Carotid
occlusive disease
Carotid-cavernous fistula, 5:236, 237*i*, 7:70, 71*i*
Carotid endarterectomy
for carotid stenosis, 1:101, 107–108, 109, 5:181–182
for ocular ischemic syndrome, 9:222, 12:151–152
Carotid occlusive disease, 1:101, 107–109
central retinal artery occlusion and, 12:149
diabetic retinopathy and, 12:105
ocular ischemic syndrome and, 9:221–222,
12:150–152, 151*i*
retinopathy of, 12:145
central retinal vein occlusion and, 12:143, 145
Carotid-ophthalmic anastomosis, 5:178*i*
Carotid plexus, 2:117
Carotid siphon, 5:178*i*
cerebral ischemia/stroke and, 1:102
Carotid stenosis, 1:101, 107. *See also* Carotid occlusive
disease
evaluation of, 5:179
prognosis for, 5:180–181
Carotid territory ischemia, 5:177. *See also* Carotid
occlusive disease
evaluation of, 5:179–180
Carotid ultrasonography (duplex scanning), 5:179
Carotidynia, 5:300
Carpenter syndrome, 8:351*t*
Carrier (genetic), 2:183, 263–264, 269–273
inborn errors of metabolism and, 6:435
ocular findings in, 2:270–271*i*, 270*t*
Carrier (infection), in HIV infection/AIDS, 1:38–39
Carteolol, 2:410, 410*t*
cholesterol levels affected by, 1:150
for glaucoma, 10:160*t*, 165
in children, 6:282

Cartesian conoid, 3:53–54, 54*i*
Cartesian ellipsoid, 3:53–54, 54*i*
Cartrol. *See* Carteolol
Caruncle, 2:22*i*, 30, 4:43, 8:8
Carvedilol
for heart failure, 1:131
for hypertension, 1:89*t*
Case-control studies, 1:345*i*, 347–349, 348*i*
Case reports, 1:345–346, 345*i*
Case series, 1:345*i*, 346–347
Caseating granulomas, 4:13, 15*i*
Caspases, in Alzheimer disease, 1:286
Cat-scratch disease, 5:368, 8:127, 178, 12:184–185, 185*i*
Parinaud oculoglandular syndrome and, 6:229
Catabolism, glucose, 1:202
Cataflam. *See* Diclofenac
Catalase
in lens, 2:368, 11:17
in retina and retinal pigment epithelium, 2:372
Catapres. *See* Clonidine
Cataract, 4:97–103, 102*i*. *See also specific type*
age-related, 11:45–49, 71–74, 72*t*
amblyopia and, 6:71–72, 302
after anterior chamber phakic IOL insertion, 13:153*t*
anterior polar, 6:288, 288*i*, 292*t*
atopic dermatitis and, 11:66
brunescent, 11:46
lens proteins in, 11:13
capsular, 11:37
cerulean, 4:97, 11:36, 37*i*
hereditary factors in, 6:287*t*
chemical injuries causing, 11:57
in children, 6:285–303. *See also* Cataract, congenital
and infantile; Cataract, pediatric
"Christmas tree"
in children, 6:293*i*
in myotonic dystrophy, 5:335
complete (total), 11:38
congenital and infantile, 2:172, 4:95, 6:285, 285*t*,
287, 453, 11:33–39, 35*t*, 195–200. *See also*
Cataract, pediatric
aniridia and, 11:33
bilateral, 6:287, 295, 11:35*t*, 195–196
causes of, 6:295, 296*i*
definition of, 11:33
etiology of, 11:35*t*
morphologic classification of, 11:34–39
surgical management of, 11:195–200. *See also*
Cataract surgery, in children
unilateral, 6:287, 295, 296*i*, 11:35*t*, 196
contrast sensitivity affected by, 3:115
contusion, 11:55, 56*i*
coronary, 4:97, 11:36
cortical, 11:46–48, 48*i*, 49*i*, 50*i*, 51*i*, 52*i*
in cytomegalic inclusion disease, 6:218
degenerative ocular disorders and, 11:69
diabetic, 11:60–61, 61*i*
in children, 6:288*t*, 343
"sugar," 2:330–332
aldose reductase in development of, 2:331–332,
354, 11:14–16, 60
surgery for, 11:204–205
preoperative evaluation and, 11:83
disorders associated with premature formation of,
4:103

drug-induced, 11:50–54
electrical injury causing, 11:59, 60i
electroretinogram and, 12:36
epidemiology of, 11:71–74
evaluation of, 11:75–88
    in children, 6:292–294
exogenous agents causing, 4:103
in galactosemia, 11:61–62, 62i
glassblowers,' 11:56
glaucoma and, 11:67–68, 68i
    in children, 11:198
    management of, 11:217–221, 218i, 220i
history in, 11:75–77, 77t
    in children, 6:294
hypermature, 11:48, 51i
    phacolytic glaucoma and, 4:96, 11:67
hypocalcemia and, 11:62
intraocular lens implantation and. See Cataract
    surgery
intumescent, 11:48
    phacomorphic glaucoma and, 11:68, 68i
ischemia causing, 11:69
in juvenile idiopathic (chronic/rheumatoid) arthritis,
    9:142, 142i, 143
lamellar (zonular), 11:37–38, 39i
    in children, 6:289, 290i, 292t
    hereditary factors in, 6:287t
lens proteins and, 11:13
low vision aids for, 11:78
in Lowe syndrome, 6:288t, 348
management of, 11:75–88. See also Cataract surgery
    in children, 11:195–200
    in glaucoma patient, 11:217–221, 218i, 220i
    medical, 11:77–78
mature, 11:48, 50i
    capsulorrhexis and, 11:210–211
    phacolytic glaucoma and, 11:67
membranous, 11:38, 40i
metabolic, 11:60–63
Morgagnian, 4:101, 102i, 11:48, 52i
muscarinic therapy and, 2:398, 400
in myotonic dystrophy, 11:62–63, 63i
in neurofibromatosis type 2, 6:408, 409
nuclear, 4:102–103, 11:45–46, 47i
    in children, 6:289, 289i, 292t
    congenital, 11:37, 38i
nutritional disease and, 11:63–64
in pars planitis, 9:151–152
pediatric, 6:285–295, 285t, 293i, 453, 11:35t,
    195–200. See also Cataract, congenital and
    infantile
    abuse and, 6:442
    age at onset and, 6:287
    amblyopia and, 6:71–72, 302
    evaluation of, 6:292–294, 297t
    hereditary factors in, 6:287, 287t
    history in, 6:294
    laterality and, 6:287
    morphologic types of, 6:287–292, 288t, 292t
    ocular examination and, 6:295
    surgery for, 6:295–303
    systemic implications of, 6:286, 286t
    visual function and, 6:294, 453
    workup for, 6:295, 296i, 297t

persistent fetal vasculature (persistent hyperplastic
    primary vitreous) and, 4:106, 6:290–291, 292i,
    292t, 324, 11:42, 197, 12:282, 283i
polar, 11:34–35, 36i
    in children, 6:288, 288i
        hereditary factors in, 6:287t
    surgery for removal of, 11:212–213
after posterior chamber phakic IOL insertion,
    13:153t, 154
posterior lenticonus/lentiglobus and, 11:31
    in children, 6:289–290, 291i, 292t
quetiapine use and, 1:272
radiation-induced, 1:256, 11:55–57
after refractive surgery, 11:211
removal of. See Cataract surgery
in retinitis pigmentosa, 12:207
rosette, 11:55
rubella, 2:172–173, 4:95, 6:218, 11:38–39
scleritis and, 8:239
senescent, in diabetes, 11:61
in siderosis bulbi, 11:58
skin diseases and, 11:66
snowflake, 11:60–61, 61i
socioeconomic impact of, 11:71
starfish, 6:293i
steroid-induced, 11:50–52
    pediatric uveitis treatment and, 6:320
subcapsular
    anterior, 4:97–100, 99i
    posterior (cupuliform), 4:99, 99i, 11:48–49, 53i
        in children, 6:291, 292t
        corticosteroids causing, 11:50–52
        in myotonic dystrophy, 11:62–63
"sugar," 2:330–332
    aldose reductase in development of, 2:331–332,
        354, 11:14–16, 60
sunflower
    in chalcosis, 11:59, 12:299
    in Wilson disease, 11:62
surgery for. See Cataract surgery
sutural (stellate), 11:35–36, 37i
tetanic, 11:62
total (complete), 11:38
traumatic, 4:25–26, 11:54–60. See also specific type
    in children, 6:293i, 447
    surgery for, 11:225–228, 227i, 228i
uveitis and, 9:235–237, 11:64, 65i, 155, 223
in Vogt-Koyanagi-Harada syndrome, 9:205
in Wilson disease, 11:62
zonular (lamellar), 11:37–38, 39i
    in children, 6:289, 290i, 292t
    hereditary factors in, 6:287t
Cataract surgery, 11:89–162, 112–137. See also specific
    procedure
anesthesia for, 11:93–97, 95i, 96i
    in diabetic patient, 11:205
angle-closure glaucoma and, 10:200
anterior capsule fibrosis/phimosis and, 11:187
anticipated poor wound healing and, 11:200
in anticoagulated patient, 11:98, 168–169, 201–202
in arthritis patients, 11:203
astigmatism and
    modification of preexisting, 11:102–103
    suture-induced, 11:184
    toric IOL for, 13:161–163

biometry before, 11:87
in bleeding diathesis, 11:201–202
Brown-McLean syndrome after, 11:167
capsular opacification and contraction and, 11:164*t*, 186–191
Nd:YAG laser capsulotomy for, 11:187–191, 189*i*
capsular rupture and, 11:164*t*, 179–180
in children, 6:295–303, 298*i*, 299*i*, 300*i*, 11:195–200
amblyopia and, 6:71–72, 302
aphakia correction and, 11:199–200
complications of, 6:302–303, 11:198
glaucoma after, 6:279–280, 302–303
with intact posterior capsule, 6:297–299, 298*i*
planning, 11:195–196
postoperative care and, 11:198
prognosis for, 11:198
techniques for, 11:196–198
uveitis and, 6:322
choroidal hemorrhage and. *See* Cataract surgery, suprachoroidal hemorrhage/effusion and
in chronic obstructive pulmonary disease, 11:203–204
chronic uveitis after, 11:164*t*, 178
ciliary block (malignant) glaucoma after, 11:178, 182
in claustrophobic patient, 11:200
clear corneal incision for, 11:100–101, 123–125, 125*i*, 126*i*
minimizing bleeding risk and, 11:202
clear lens extraction, 11:138, 222
communication with patient and, 11:201
complications of, 11:162, 163–194, 164*t*. *See also specific type*
in children, 11:198
in glaucoma patient, 11:218–219, 220*i*
conjunctiva examination before, 11:81–82
corneal conditions and, 11:207–211
corneal edema and, 11:104, 166–168, 192–193, 193*i*
corneal endothelial changes caused by, 8:419–420
corneal melting after, 11:180–181
in patients with dry eye, 11:180, 206–207
corneal pachymetry before, 11:87
corneal topography before, 11:87
cyclodialysis and, 11:181–182
cystoid macular edema and, 11:104, 164*t*, 172–174, 173*i*, 12:154
in glaucoma patient, 11:218–219
after Nd:YAG capsulotomy, 11:190–191
in dementia/mentally disabled patient, 11:201
Descemet's membrane detachment and, 11:168
developmentally abnormal eye and, 11:212–215
in diabetic patients, 11:204–205, 12:118
preoperative evaluation and, 11:83
economic impact of, 11:71
elevated intraocular pressure after, 11:164*t*, 172
endophthalmitis after, 9:207–209, 208*t*, 11:164*t*, 176–178, 176*i*. *See also* Postoperative endophthalmitis
prevention of, 11:97
epithelial downgrowth and, 11:185
external eye disease and, 11:206–207
external eye examination before, 11:80–81
extracapsular cataract extraction (ECCE). *See also* Extracapsular cataract extraction
early techniques for, 11:90, 92*i*
modern techniques for, 11:92–93

with nucleus expression, 11:108–112, 111*i*
by phacoemulsification, 11:112–137. *See also* Phacoemulsification
filtering bleb and, 11:181
filtering surgery and
cataract surgery combined with, 11:220–221
cataract surgery following, 11:219–220
for open-angle glaucoma, 10:195–197
flat or shallow anterior chamber and, 11:163–166
intraoperative complications, 11:163–165
postoperative complications, 11:165–166
preoperative considerations, 11:82
for Fuchs heterochromic iridocyclitis, 9:145
fundus evaluation before, 11:83–84
in glaucoma patient, 11:217–221, 218*i*, 220*i*
complications of, 11:218–219, 220*i*
filtering surgery before, 11:219–220
filtering surgery combined with, 11:220–221
hemorrhage and, 11:164*t*, 168–171
at-risk patients and, 11:215–217
high refractive error and, 11:221–222
clear lens extraction for, 11:138, 222
high hyperopia, 11:222
high myopia, 11:222
history of development of, 11:89–93, 90*i*, 91*i*, 92*i*, 93
hyphema after, 11:171
hypotony as complication of, flat anterior chamber and, 11:165, 166
in hypotony patients, 11:223
illusions caused by, 5:188
incisions for, 11:106, 110, 121–126. *See also type of incision and type of surgery*
modification of preexisting astigmatism and, 11:102–103
indications for, 11:78–79
in children, 6:294
informed consent for, 11:88
intracapsular cataract extraction (ICCE), 11:103–108, 107*i*. *See also* Intracapsular cataract extraction
early techniques for, 11:90–91, 92*i*, 93*i*
intraocular lens implantation and. *See also* Intraocular lenses
in adults, 11:139–156, 140–142*i*
in children, 6:297–300, 299*i*, 11:156–157, 199–200
complications of, 11:191–194
intraoperative preparation for, 11:97–98
iridodialysis and, 11:181
juvenile rheumatoid arthritis–associated iridocyclitis/uveitis and, 9:143
after keratoplasty, 11:209–210
macular function evaluation before, 11:85
macular infarction after, 11:178
in nanophthalmos, 8:287, 11:213, 214*i*
nucleus removal in, 11:110–111. *See also* Extracapsular cataract extraction
chopping techniques for, 11:132–134, 133*i*
with extracapsular cataract extraction (ECCE), 11:100–101
nuclear flip techniques for, 11:135
splitting techniques for, 11:131–132, 132*i*
small capsulorrhexis and, 11:126
whole, 11:129–131, 129*i*, 130*i*
in obese patients, 11:205–206
ocular conditions and, 11:206–224

outcome of, in children, 6:303, 303*i*
outcomes of, 11:160–162
pars plana lensectomy, 11:138–139
in pars planitis, 9:151–152
patient preparation for, 11:88, 105–106, 121
in patient unable to communicate, 11:201
with penetrating keratoplasty and intraocular lens
    insertion (triple procedure), 11:208–209
in persistent fetal vasculature, 6:295, 325
phacolysis, 11:138
posterior capsule opacification and, 11:186–187
    in children, 11:186–187
    Nd:YAG laser capsulotomy for, 11:186–187,
        187–191, 189*i*
posterior infusion syndrome and, 11:164–165
postoperative care and, 11:80, 108, 112
    in children, 6:300–301, 302–303, 11:198
potential acuity estimation before, 11:85
preoperative evaluation/preparation for, 11:79–80,
    97–98
    in children, 11:195–196
pseudophakic bullous keratopathy after, 8:419–420,
    11:164*t*, 192–193, 193*i*
psychosocial considerations in, 11:200–201
pupillary capture and, 11:184–185, 185*i*
pupillary irregularity caused by, 5:259
after radial keratotomy, 13:65
refraction before, 11:87
after refractive surgery, 11:211
    intraocular lens power calculation and, 11:82,
        150–152, 211
with refractive surgery, 13:173
    planning, 11:82, 102–103
retained lens material and, 11:182–183, 12:337–339,
    338*t*, 339*i*
retinal detachment after, 11:104, 164*t*, 175–176, 175*i*,
    12:334–336, 334*i*
    in children, 11:198
    retained lens material and, 12:337, 338–339
in retinal disease, 11:224
retinal light toxicity and, 11:171–172, 12:308
in retinitis pigmentosa patient, 12:212
retrobulbar hemorrhage and, 11:169
scleral tunnel incision for, 11:99–100, 100*i*, 121–123,
    123*i*, 124*i*
    modification of preexisting astigmatism and,
        11:102
shallow anterior chamber and. *See* Cataract surgery,
    flat or shallow anterior chamber and
single-plane incisions for, 11:99
slit-lamp examination before, 11:81–83
small-incision for, topical anesthesia and, 11:94–96
specular microscopy before, 11:87
stromal/epithelial edema after, 11:166
suprachoroidal hemorrhage/effusion and,
    11:169–170
    delayed, 11:171
    expulsive, 11:170–171
        patients at risk for, 11:215–217
    flat anterior chamber and, 11:163, 166
systemic conditions and, 11:201–206
tolerance to lens crystallins and, 9:90
after trauma, 11:225–228, 227*i*, 228*i*
uveitis and, 11:164*t*, 178
in uveitis patient, 9:235–237, 11:155, 223

viscoelastics in (viscosurgery), 11:144–145, 157–160,
    161*t*
visual function evaluation after, 11:160
visual function evaluation before, 11:84–85
vitreal complications of, 11:164*t*, 183–184
    in glaucoma patient, 11:219
    with ICCE, 11:104–105
vitreocorneal adherence after, 11:167
vitreous abnormalities and, 12:288
    posterior vitreous detachment, 12:257, 279
wound closure for
    after ECCE with nucleus expression, 11:112
    scleral tunnel incisions and, 11:99–100, 100*i*
    single-plane incisions and, 11:99
wound construction for, 11:98–103
    modification of preexisting astigmatism and,
        11:102–103
wound leak and, 11:181
    flat anterior chamber and, 11:165–166
in zonular dehiscence/lens subluxation or
    dislocation, 11:226–227, 227*i*, 228*t*
Catarrhal (marginal corneal) infiltrates
    blepharoconjunctivitis and, 8:229
    staphylococcal blepharitis and, 8:165, 166*i*, 168, 229
Catastrophic antiphospholipid antibody syndrome,
    1:183
Catenary (hydraulic support) theory, of
    accommodation, 13:171
Caterpillar hairs, ocular inflammation caused by, 8:395
Cathepsin D, in aqueous humor, 2:317, 319
Cathepsin O, in aqueous humor, 2:317, 319
Catheter angiography, 5:66
Catheter-based reperfusion. *See* Percutaneous
    transluminal coronary angioplasty
Cation balance, in lens, maintenance of, 11:19–21, 21*i*
Cationic protein, 8:200*t*
Cats, *Bartonella henselae* transmitted by, 8:127, 178
Caudal basilar artery, 5:18
Caudal pons, 2:116
Causal risk factors, 1:361, 362. *See also* Risk factor
Cause and effect diagram, 1:370, 371*i*
Cautery, thermal
    for involutional ectropion, 7:197
    for involutional entropion, 7:204
    for punctal occlusion, 8:77, 77*i*
Cavernous-carotid fistula, 7:70, 71*i*
Cavernous hemangioma, 4:12. *See also* Vascular
    malformations
    of orbit, 4:196, 197*i*, 7:67, 68*i*
    of retina, 4:247, 248*i*, 12:163–164, 164*i*
Cavernous optic atrophy of Schnabel, 4:206, 207*i*
Cavernous sinus, 2:117, 119, 120*i*, 5:10, 23
    eyelids drained by, 8:7
    lesions of, MR imaging of, 5:74, 74*i*
    ophthalmoplegia and, 5:235–236
Cavernous sinus thrombosis, 5:357–358, 6:231–232
    aseptic, 5:357
    septic, 5:357
        orbital infections causing, 7:42, 44
Cavitation, 11:116–117, 118*i*
    definition of, 11:114
CBD. *See* Corneal dystrophies, of Bowman's layer
CCAAT box, 2:183
CCR5/CCR5 receptor, in HIV infection/AIDS, 1:44,
    9:242

CCR5 receptor antagonists, for HIV infection/AIDS, 1:42
CCTV. See Closed circuit television
CD4/CD8 ratio, in HIV infection/AIDS, 1:37
CD4+ T cells. See also T cells
 class II MHC molecules as antigen-presenting platform for, 9:19–20, 20i
 in delayed hypersensitivity, 8:201, 9:25, 63–66, 65i
 differentiation of, 9:22–24, 23i
 in external eye defense, 8:114
 in HIV infection/AIDS, 1:37, 40, 9:242–243, 244t, 246–248
 in immune processing, 9:22–24, 23i
 in SARS, 1:34
CD8+ T cells. See also T cells
 class I MHC molecules as antigen-presenting platform for, 9:19–22, 21i
 cytotoxic, 9:24, 25, 66–70, 69i
  in viral conjunctivitis, 9:35
 in external eye defense, 8:114
 in immune processing, 9:23i, 24
 in SARS, 1:34
 suppressor, 9:23i, 24
CD11b, identification of macrophages/monocytes and, 8:68
CD40, in Sjögren syndrome, 8:78
CD40 ligand, in Sjögren syndrome, 8:78
CD95 ligand. See Fas ligand
CD163, identification of macrophages/monocytes and, 8:68
CDKs. See Cyclin-dependent kinases
cDNA, 2:184, 200
 from ciliary body–encoding plasma proteins, 2:319
 sequencing, in mutation screening, 2:231
cDNA clone, 2:183
cDNA library, 2:189, 227
CEA. See Carotid endarterectomy
Ceclor. See Cefaclor
Cedax. See Ceftibuten
CeeNU. See Lomustine
Cefaclor, 1:57t
 ocular effects of, 1:324t
Cefadroxil, 1:57t, 2:430
 for endocarditis prophylaxis, 1:10t
Cefamandole, 1:57t, 2:430
Cefazolin, 1:57t, 2:428t, 429–430
 for bacterial keratitis, 8:182t
 for endocarditis prophylaxis, 1:10t
Cefdinir, 1:59t
Cefditoren, 1:59t
Cefepime, 1:59t, 68, 2:430
Cefixime, 1:58t
Cefizox. See Ceftizoxime
Cefmetazole, 1:59t
Cefobid. See Cefoperazone
Cefonicid, 1:57t
Cefoperazone, 1:58t, 2:430
Cefotan. See Cefotetan
Cefotaxime, 1:58t, 2:430
Cefotetan, 1:58t
Cefoxitin, 1:57t, 69, 2:430
Cefozopran, 1:68
Cefpirome, 1:59t, 68, 2:430
Cefpodoxime, 1:58t
Cefprozil, 1:58t

Ceftazidime, 1:58t, 2:428t, 430
 for bacterial keratitis, 8:182t
 for endophthalmitis, 9:217, 218t, 12:300, 329
Ceftibuten, 1:59t
Ceftin. See Cefuroxime
Ceftizoxime, 1:58t, 2:430
Ceftriaxone, 1:58t, 2:430
 for bacterial keratitis, 8:182t
 for endophthalmitis, 9:218t
 for gonococcal conjunctivitis, 8:172
  in neonates, 6:222, 8:173
 for Lyme disease, 5:364
Cefuroxime, 1:58t, 2:430
 for Lyme disease, 5:364
 ocular effects of, 1:324t
Cefzil. See Cefprozil
"Ceiling effect," 1:364
Celebrex. See Celecoxib
Celecoxib, 1:173, 196, 197t, 2:307
Celestone. See Betamethasone
Cell-adhesion molecules, 8:198t
 in homing, 9:27–28
 in neutrophil recruitment and activation, 9:48, 49i
Cell death, programmed (PCD/apoptosis), 2:125, 181, 182, 6:206, 8:247t, 248
 by cytotoxic T lymphocytes, 9:68–70, 69i
 in DNA repair, 2:213
 Fas ligand in, 9:38, 68, 69i
Cell lysis
 complement-mediated, 9:59, 60i
 by cytotoxic lymphocytes, 9:68, 69i
Cell-mediated immunity. See Cellular immunity
Cell surface markers
 identification of macrophages/monocytes and, 8:68
 lymphocyte, 9:15
Cell turnover, eyelid skin and ocular surface, 8:246
Cell wall, bacterial, 8:123
 innate immune response and, 9:44
CellCept. See Mycophenolate mofetil
Cellophane maculopathy, 5:105, 12:87
Cellular atypia
 definition of, 8:247t
 in primary acquired melanosis, 4:57–58, 57i, 58i
Cellular immunity (cell-mediated immunity), 1:4, 8:199i, 199t, 201. See also Lymphocyte-mediated immune effector responses
 deficient, in HIV infection/AIDS, 1:37
Cellular retinaldehyde-binding protein/cytoplasmic retinal-binding protein (CRALBP), 2:361t
 in aqueous humor, 2:317
 mutations in, 2:351
Cellular retinoic acid-binding protein, 2:361t
Cellular retinoid-binding protein, 2:361t
Cellulitis, 4:170, 170i, 7:41–44
 orbital, 7:20, 42–44, 43i, 44t, 45i
  in children, 6:231–233, 232i
   fungal (mucormycosis), 6:233, 233i, 7:45–46
    exenteration in management of, 7:45–46, 128
   after strabismus surgery, 6:185–186, 186i
 preseptal, 7:41–42
  in children, 6:230–231, 7:41
   Haemophilus causing, 6:230, 7:41
   after strabismus surgery, 6:185–186
Cellulose acetate butyrate (CAB), 3:183
CEN, 2:205

Center of rotation, 6:27–28, 27*i*
Centering procedures
  for LASIK, 13:114
  for PRK/LASEK, 13:95–96, 96*i*
    decentered ablation and, 13:102–103, 102*i*
    radial keratotomy outcome affected by, 13:61
Centimorgan, 2:183
Central areolar choroidal dystrophy, 12:226, 227*i*
Central areolar pigment epithelial atrophy, 4:139
Central caudal nucleus, in ptosis, 5:226
Central cloudy dystrophy of François, 8:310*t*, 323, 324*i*
  in megalocornea, 8:290, 290*i*
Central corneal thickness, in applanation tonometry
    measurements, 10:27–28
Central (pupillary) cysts, 6:265
Central fusional disruption (horror fusionis), 6:53, 115
Central islands, after PRK, 13:101–102, 101*i*
Central nervous system
  disorders of. *See* Neurologic disorders
  infection of, papilledema caused by, 5:116
  lymphoma of, in HIV infection/AIDS, 5:359
  metabolic abnormalities of, retinal degeneration and,
    12:240–244
  mucormycosis of, 5:367
  systemic lupus erythematosus affecting, 1:180, 181*t*,
    182
Central neurofibromatosis, 6:408. *See also*
    Neurofibromatosis, bilateral acoustic (type 2)
  developmental glaucoma and, 10:156
Central posterior keratoconus (posterior corneal
    depression), 6:254
Central posterior surface. *See* Base curve
Central ray
  for mirrors, 3:91, 91*i*
  through convex spherical lens, 3:71
Central retinal artery, 2:84, 102, 103, 104, 104*i*, 105*i*,
    5:11–12*i*, 15, 16*i*, 12:12
  occlusion of, 4:133–134, 5:105–106, 106*i*,
    12:148–150, 148*i*, 149*i*
    in sickle cell hemoglobinopathies, 12:121
Central retinal vein, 2:104, 104*i*, 5:16*i*, 20, 21–22*i*
  occlusion of, 4:133–134, 134*i*, 5:106–107, 106*i*,
    12:141–145, 142*i*
    electroretinogram in, 12:34*i*, 35, 35*i*
    evaluation and management of, 12:143–144
    iris neovascularization in, 12:142, 144–145
    ischemic, 12:141, 141–142
    nonischemic, 12:141
    papillophlebitis and, 12:141
    primary open-angle glaucoma and, 10:90
    secondary angle-closure glaucoma and, 10:144
Central scotoma, in low vision, 3:247*i*, 253
Central serous chorioretinopathy/retinopathy/
    choroidopathy, 5:105, 12:51–54
  age-related macular degeneration differentiated
    from, 12:53, 59, 68–69, 69*i*
  fluorescein angiography in, 12:22*i*, 52
Central suppression, 6:53–54
Central surgical space (intraconal fat/surgical space),
    7:12–13, 109, 110*i*
Central Vein Occlusion Study Group (CVOS), 12:144
  iris neovascularization in central retinal vein
    occlusion and, 12:144–145
Central vestibular nystagmus, 5:246*t*, 247–248

Central vision loss. *See also* Visual loss/impairment
  in leukemia, 6:344
Central zone, 2:74, 8:38, 39*i*
  in radial keratotomy, 13:59, 60
Centromere, 2:183
Cephalexin, 1:57*t*, 2:429–430
  for endocarditis prophylaxis, 1:10*t*
Cephalosporins, 1:57–59*t*, 68–69, 2:427–428, 427*i*, 428*t*,
    429–430. *See also specific agent*
  allergic reaction to, 2:428
  for endophthalmitis, 9:217
  structure of, 2:427, 427*i*
Cephalothin, 2:429–430
Cephamycins, 1:59*t*
Cephradine, 1:57*t*, 2:429–430
Ceramide trihexoside accumulation, in Fabry disease,
    8:340, 12:244
  plasma infusions for, 2:281
Ceratoxin A and B, 2:457
Cerebellar angioma, 5:340
Cerebellar arteries
  anterior inferior, 2:117, 5:18, 19*i*
  posterior inferior, 5:18, 19*i*
  superior, 5:18
Cerebellar hemangioblastoma, in retinal angiomatosis,
    5:340
Cerebellopontine angle, 2:116
  tumors of, 5:234, 283, 284, 285*i*
Cerebellum, 5:39
  dysfunction of, in multiple sclerosis, 5:320
Cerebral achromatopsia, 5:194
Cerebral akinetopsia, in Alzheimer disease, 1:288
Cerebral aneurysm, 5:350–354, 350*i*
  clinical presentation of, 5:351, 352*i*
  laboratory investigation of, 5:351–352, 353*i*
  prognosis of, 5:352–353
  ruptured, 1:105, 106, 5:351, 352*i*
  treatment of, 5:353–354
Cerebral (intracerebral) angiography/arteriography. *See*
    Angiography
Cerebral artery
  anterior, 5:16
  middle, 5:16, 17, 20*i*
  posterior, 5:11, 16, 18, 20*i*
Cerebral autosomal dominant arteriopathy with
    subcortical infarcts and leukoencephalopathy
  headache in, 5:298
  transient visual loss and, 5:179
Cerebral/cortical blindness, 6:456
  occipital lobe lesion causing, 5:170
Cerebral ischemia, 1:101–105. *See also* Stroke
Cerebral ptosis, 5:277
Cerebral venous thrombosis, 5:357–358
Cerebrofacial/encephalotrigeminal angiomatosis. *See*
    Sturge-Weber disease/syndrome
Cerebrohepatorenal (Zellweger) syndrome, 12:233*t*,
    234, 236, 242
Cerebrospinal fluid, in syphilitic serology, 5:362
Cerebrovascular accident. *See* Stroke
Cerebrovascular circulation, 5:178*i*
Cerebrovascular disease, 1:101–109. *See also specific*
    type and Stroke
  in diabetes, 1:218
  hypertension management and, 1:91*t*, 95
  neuro-ophthalmic signs of, 5:345–358

in pregnancy, **5:**344
transient visual loss caused by, **5:**345–346
Cerebyx. *See* Fosphenytoin
Ceroid lipofuscinosis, **6:**437*t,* 438, **12:**233*t,* 234, 236, 241, 241*i*
Cerulean cataract, **4:**97, **11:**36, 37*i*
hereditary factors in, **6:**287*t*
Cervical cancer
screening for, **1:**294
viral carcinogenesis and, **1:**254, 291
Cervical ganglion, superior, **5:**57
dilator muscle innervation and, **2:**65
Cervicofacial trunk, of cranial nerve VII, **5:**56
Cetamide. *See* Sulfacetamide
Cethromycin (ABT-773), **1:**75
Cevimeline, for dry eye, **8:**75
C₃F₈. *See* Perfluoropropane
CFEOM1 (congenital fibrosis of extraocular muscles type 1) syndrome, **5:**220
cGMP
in cone phototransduction, **2:**345
in rod phototransduction, **2:**342–343, 343*i,* 344*t*
cGMP-gated channel
cone, **2:**345
mutations in, **2:**350
rod, **2:**342
mutations in, **2:**349
CGRP. *See* Calcitonin gene-related peptide
Chalasis, **8:**24*t*
Chalazion, **4:**171, 171*i,* **7:**158–159, 160*i,* **8:**87–88, 87*i*
in children, **6:**388
internal hordeolum and, **8:**168
irregular astigmatism caused by, **3:**170
in rosacea, **8:**84
Chalcosis, **12:**299
cataracts in, **11:**59
corneal pigmentation in, **8:**377*t*
Chamber angle. *See* Anterior chamber angle
Chamber deepening. *See also* Anterior chamber, flat or shallow
for angle-closure glaucoma, **10:**200
CHAMPS (Controlled High-Risk Subjects Avonex Multiple Sclerosis Prevention Study), **5:**324
Chancre, syphilitic, **1:**16
Chandler syndrome, **4:**79, **8:**301
Charcot-Marie-Tooth disease, retinal degeneration and, **12:**232*t,* 235
CHARGE association, **6:**263, 360
Charged-particle radiation
for choroidal hemangioma, **4:**245
for melanoma, **4:**237
for retinal capillary hemangioma, **4:**247
Charles Bonnet syndrome, **5:**191
Chart review, monitoring systems and, **1:**365–366
Chatter, definition of, **11:**114
Checklist (system of care), **1:**370, 371*i*
CHED. *See* Congenital hereditary endothelial dystrophy
CHED1/CHED2 genes, **8:**298
Chédiak-Higashi syndrome, **4:**120, **6:**347*t,* 348, **12:**240
Cheek advancement flap (Mustardé flap), for eyelid repair, **7:**191*i,* 192
Cheek elevation, in eyelid repair, **7:**192
Chelation therapy, for band keratopathy, **2:**394, **8:**374
Chemical carcinogenesis, **1:**252–253
Chemical conjunctivitis, in neonates, **6:**223

Chemical injury (burns), **8:**389–393
acid burns, **8:**391
alkali burns, **8:**389–391, 390*i*
cataracts caused by, **11:**57
in children, **6:**445
limbal transplantation for, **8:**392, 393
management of, **8:**391–393
mucous membrane grafting for, **8:**439
Chemodenervation. *See also* Botulinum toxin
for strabismus and blepharospasm, **6:**195–196
Chemokines, **8:**197, 198*t,* **9:**80, 81*t*
Chemoreduction, for retinoblastoma, **4:**261, 261*i,* **6:**397, 398*i*
Chemosis, **8:**23, 24*t*
extraocular surgery causing, **8:**420
ionizing radiation causing, **8:**388
Chemotaxis, **9:**7
in neutrophil recruitment and activation, **9:**48, 49*i*
Chemotherapy (cancer), **1:**256–262, 258–260*t. See also specific agent*
for lacrimal gland tumors, **7:**91
for lymphoma, **4:**278
for melanoma, **4:**238
for metastatic eye disease, **4:**273–275
for optic nerve glioma, **5:**151, **7:**75
recent developments in, **1:**251
for retinoblastoma, **4:**261, 261*i,* **6:**397, 398*i*
for rhabdomyosarcoma, **7:**80
Cherry-red spot, **6:**349–350
in central retinal artery occlusion, **5:**105, 106*i,* **12:**148, 148*i,* 149*i*
in gangliosidoses, **6:**350, 437*t*
in inborn errors of metabolism, **6:**436–437*t*
in lysosomal metabolism disorders, **12:**243–244, 244*i*
myoclonus and, **6:**436*t,* **12:**243
Cherry-red spot myoclonus syndrome, **6:**436*t,* **12:**243
Chest compressions, in CPR, **1:**314–315
Chest pain, in angina pectoris, **1:**113
Chest physiotherapy, postoperative, **1:**156
Chest x-ray
in cancer screening, **1:**295*t,* 296
in congestive heart failure, **1:**127
in pulmonary diseases, **1:**155
CHF. *See* Congestive heart failure
Chi-square tests, **1:**344
Chiasm (optic), **2:**104
anterior, lesions of, **5:**158, 159*i*
gliomas involving, **5:**149, 150, 163
in neurofibromatosis, **6:**406–407, 406*i*
lesions of, **5:**158–163
in multiple sclerosis, **5:**321
parasellar, **5:**160–163, 162*i*
treatment of, **5:**160–163, 162*i,* 163
visual field patterns in, **5:**158, 159*i,* 160*i,* 161*i*
mid, lesions of, **5:**158, 160*i*
ocular development and, **2:**145
posterior, lesions of, **5:**158, 161*i*
Chibroxin. *See* Norfloxacin
Chickenpox. *See* Varicella
Chievitz, transient nerve fiber layer of, **2:**140, 144
Childhood glaucoma. *See* Glaucoma, childhood
Children. *See also specific topic*
abuse of
cataract and, **6:**442
gonococcal conjunctivitis and, **6:**225

ocular trauma and, **6:**442–445, 443*i*, 444*i*,
   12:301–302, 302*i*
ametropia correction in, **3:**145–146
anisometropia in, **3:**118, 147
  amblyopia caused by. *See* Amblyopia,
    anisometropic
bacterial conjunctivitis in, **8:**169–172, 170*t*, 172*i*
cancer in, **1:**251
cataract in. *See* Cataract, congenital and infantile;
  Cataract, pediatric
cataract surgery in, **6:**295–303, 298*i*, 299*i*, 300*i*,
   11:195–200. *See also* Cataract surgery, in children
clinical refraction in, **3:**144–147
Coats disease in, **12:**156
corneal transplantation in, **8:**470–471, 470*t*
decreased/low vision in, **6:**451–459
drusen in, **5:**133–134
electroretinogram in, **12:**35, 35*i*
emmetropia in, **3:**120
enucleation in, **7:**121
examination of, **6:**3–5, 4*i*
  preparation for, **6:**3
  rapport and, **6:**3–5
eye development in, **6:**199–203
glaucoma in. *See* Glaucoma, childhood
hyperopia in, **3:**119–120, 146–147
hypertension in, **1:**81
immunization schedule for, **1:**303, 304*t*
intraocular lens implantation in, **6:**297–300, 299*i*,
   11:156–157, 199–200
low vision in, **3:**266–267, **6:**451–459
mydriasis in epilepsy and, **1:**283–284
myopia in, **3:**120, 146
nystagmus in, **5:**241–243, **6:**159–171, 333–334, 334*t*.
   See also Nystagmus
  types of, **6:**162–168
ocular trauma in, **6:**441–450, 457*t*, **12:**254–255
  abuse and, **6:**442–445, 443*i*, 444*i*, **12:**301–302, 302*i*
optic nerve sheath meningioma in, **5:**148
orbital cellulitis in, **6:**231–233, 232*i*, **7:**42
orbital fractures in, **6:**138–140, 139*i*, 449–450, 449*i*
orbital metastatic disease in, **6:**374–376, **7:**94, 94*i*
preoperative assessment in, **1:**328–329
preoperative sedation for, **1:**335
preseptal cellulitis in, **6:**230–231, **7:**41
refractive surgery in, amblyopia and, **13:**195
retinal degeneration onset in, **12:**233–234
staphylomas in, **4:**65, 92
third nerve palsy in, **5:**231
Chip and flip technique, for nucleus removal,
  11:130–131
Chlamydia, **8:**128
conjunctivitis caused by, **4:**46–47, 48*i*, **8:**119*t*,
  174–178, 175*i*, 176*i*
  in adults, **8:**177
  in neonates, **6:**222–223, **8:**174
cytoplasmic inclusions formed by, **8:**69, 69*i*
isolation of, **8:**136
ocular infection/inflammation caused by, **8:**119*t*,
  128, 174–178, 175*i*, 176*i*
persistence and, **8:**117
psittaci, **1:**22, **8:**174
specimen collection for diagnosis of, **8:**135*t*
trachoma caused by, **8:**174–177, 175*i*, 176*i*

trachomatis, **1:**21–22, **4:**46–47, 48*i*, **6:**222, **8:**69, 174
  gonococcal coinfection and, **1:**13, 14, 22
Chloasma, of eyelids, **7:**170
Chlorambucil, **1:**200, 258*t*
  for Behçet syndrome, **1:**194
  in cancer chemotherapy, **1:**258*t*
  for uveitis, **9:**119, 119*t*
  in children, **6:**321–322
Chloramphenicol, **1:**62*t*, 74, **2:**431*t*, 434
  for endophthalmitis, **9:**218*t*
  intravenous administration of, **2:**389
Chlorhexidine, for *Acanthamoeba* keratitis, **8:**189
Chloride
  in aqueous humor, **2:**316*t*, 317
  in tear film, **2:**290
  in vitreous, **2:**337
Chloroma (granulocytic sarcoma), **6:**375, **7:**94–95
Chloromycetin. *See* Chloramphenicol
Chloroprocaine, maximum safe dose of, **1:**322*t*
Chloroptic. *See* Chloramphenicol
Chloroquine, **1:**198
Chloroquine toxicity, **12:**247–248, 248*i*
  cornea verticillata caused by, **8:**375
  electroretinogram in, **12:**36
Chlorothiazide, **1:**88*t*, 90*t*
Chlorpromazine, **1:**271
  cornea verticillata caused by, **8:**375
  lens changes caused by, **11:**53
  retinal degeneration caused by, **12:**248
Chlorpropamide, **1:**212*t*
Chlortetracycline, **2:**433–434
Chlorthalidone, **1:**88*t*, 90*t*
CHM (Rab escort protein 1/*REP 1*) gene mutation,
  2:351
  in choroideremia, **2:**351, **12:**224
Chocolate cyst, **7:**68, **8:**273
Cholesterol emboli (Hollenhorst plaques)
  in branch retinal artery occlusion, **4:**133, **12:**146,
   147*i*
  in central retinal artery occlusion, **12:**149
  transient visual loss and, **5:**173, 173*i*, 177*t*
Cholesterol levels
  classification of, **1:**144, 144*t*
  drugs for modification of. *See* Lipid-lowering
   therapy
  elevated. *See* Hypercholesterolemia
  goals for, hypercholesterolemia management and,
   1:145, 146, 147*t*
  risk assessment and, **1:**144, 144*t*, 145, 145*t*, 146*i*,
   147*t*
  screening, **1:**293
Cholesterolosis, vitreous involvement in, **12:**286
Cholestyramine, for hypercholesterolemia, **1:**149*t*
Choline magnesium trisalicylate, **1:**197*t*
Cholinergic agents, **2:**394–403, 395*i*, 396*i*. *See also*
  specific agent and Muscarinic agents; Nicotinic
  agents
  antagonists, **2:**394, 396*i*, 400–402, 401*t*, 402*i*, 403
   as mydriatics, **2:**310, 400, 401*t*
  direct-acting agonists, **2:**394, 394–398, 396*i*, 397*i*,
   398*t*, 399*i*
  indirect-acting agonists, **2:**394, 396*i*, 398–400, 398*t*,
   399*i*, 403
  as miotics, **2:**309, 394–400, 398*t*, 399*i*
Cholinergic neurons, **2:**308

Cholinergic receptors
cholinergic drug action and, 2:394, 395*i*, 396*i*
in iris–ciliary body, 2:308, 308*t*
signal transduction and, 2:311–312, 312*i*, 314*i*, 314*t*
Cholinesterase/acetylcholinesterase
in acetylcholine degradation, 2:395, 397*i*
defective, succinylcholine effects and, 2:279
Cholinesterase/acetylcholinesterase inhibitors,
2:398–400, 399*i*, 403
cataracts caused by, 11:53–54
for high accommodative convergence/
accommodative esotropia, 6:102–103
miotic action of, 2:309, 398–400, 398*t*, 399*i*
Chondritis, auricular or nasal, in relapsing
polychondritis, 1:187
Chondroitin sulfate
in cornea, 2:300
in corneal storage medium, 2:454, 8:449
as viscoelastic, 2:452, 11:159, 160, 161*t*
Chondrosarcoma, of orbit, 6:374, 7:81
Chopping techniques, 11:132–134, 133*i*
Chord diameter, of contact lens, 3:174, 174*i*. See also
Diameter
Chorda tympani, 2:119, 5:55
Choriocapillaris, 2:71–73, 71*i*, 72*i*, 73*i*, 4:151, 151*i*,
12:15
in choroideremia, 12:224, 225*i*
differentiation of, 2:149
in gyrate atrophy, 12:225
Chorionic villus sampling, 2:183, 278
Chorioretinal biopsy, in uveitis, 9:113
Chorioretinal inflammation, 12:173–193. See also
specific disorder and Chorioretinitis;
Chorioretinopathy
Chorioretinal scar
juxtapapillary, in ocular histoplasmosis syndrome,
12:79
toxoplasmic chorioretinitis adjacent to, 12:186, 186*i*
Chorioretinitis, 5:299, 333, 9:107
in coccidioidomycosis, 9:163, 226
differential diagnosis of, 9:111*t*
fungal, 4:124, 125*i*
in ocular histoplasmosis syndrome, 9:160–163, 160*i*,
161*i*, 162*i*
in onchocerciasis, 9:195–197
sclopetaria, 4:164–165
in syphilis, 9:187, 189*i*, 190, 12:190–191, 190*i*
HIV infection/AIDS and, 9:189, 255–256
in infants and children, 6:220
posterior placoid, 9:255
toxoplasmic, 1:26, 12:186–187, 186*i*, 187*t*
vitiliginous (birdshot retinochoroidopathy), 9:177*t*,
180–181, 181*i*, 12:174*t*, 177–178, 178*i*
HLA association in, 9:94*t*, 181
Chorioretinopathy. See also *specific type and*
Retinopathy
central serous, 5:105, 12:51–54
age-related macular degeneration differentiated
from, 12:53, 59, 68–69, 69*i*
fluorescein angiography in, 12:22*i*, 52
infectious, 12:183–193
noninfectious, 12:173–183
Choristomas, 2:125, 4:12, 5:337, 8:275, 277, 278*i*. See
also Dermoids
complex, 4:44, 8:277, 278*i*

conjunctival, 4:43–44, 44*i*
definition of, 4:12, 8:275
epibulbar, 8:275–277, 276*i*, 277*i*, 278*i*
episcleral osseous, 4:88
neuroglial, 8:277
of orbit, 6:381, 7:63. See also *specific type*
osseous, 8:277
phakomatous (Zimmerman tumor), 4:169, 8:277
scleral, 4:88
Choroid, 5:24, 12:15
amelanotic tumors of, differential diagnosis of,
4:240*t*
anatomy of, 2:69–73, 69*i*, 70*i*, 12:15
dark, in Stargardt disease, 6:338, 12:216, 216*i*
detachment of, 4:166
development of, 2:149–150
diseases of
inflammatory, 12:173–193. See also
Chorioretinitis; Chorioretinopathy;
Choroidopathy
pain caused by, 5:298
noninflammatory, 12:165–172
Th1 delayed hypersensitivity and, 9:68*t*
dystrophies of, 12:224–229
fluorescein angiography in study of, 12:18–22, 20*i*,
22*i*
granulomatous inflammation of, 4:27–28, 28*i*
gyrate atrophy of, 2:262*t*, 12:225–226
hemangiomas of, 4:164, 243–246, 243*i*, 244*i*, 12:170,
171*i*
age-related macular degeneration differentiated
form, 12:70
in children, 6:390
in Sturge-Weber syndrome, 4:164
immune response in, 9:34*t*, 40–41
ischemia of, 12:166–167, 167*i*, 168*i*, 169*i*
in leukemia, 4:281–282, 6:343
melanocytoma of, 4:158, 209*i*, 217, 227
melanoma of, 4:159–163, 222–241, 223*i*. See also
Choroidal/ciliary body melanoma
enucleation for, 7:120
nevus differentiated from, 4:216–217, 229–230
spindle cell, 4:160, 160*i*
spread of, 4:161–163, 161*i*
staging of, 4:289–290*t*
metastatic disease of, 4:163–164, 163*i*, 269–271, 269*i*,
270*i*, 271*i*, 272*i*
neoplastic disease of, 4:157–163
neovascularization of. See Choroidal
neovascularization
in neurofibromatosis, 6:404, 407
nevus of, 4:157–158, 159*i*, 216–217, 216*i*, 6:390
melanoma differentiated from, 4:216–217,
229–230
osteoma of, 4:164–165, 6:390
melanoma differentiated from, 4:230–233, 233*i*
photocoagulation causing lesions/detachment of,
12:319, 320, 321*i*
photocoagulation for disorders of, wavelength
selection and, 12:313–317, 315–316*t*
rupture of, 4:27–28, 28*i*, 164–165, 12:292, 293*i*
in Sturge-Weber syndrome, 6:415–416, 415*i*
topography of, 4:151, 151*i*

tumors of
　age-related macular degeneration differentiated
　　from, **12**:70
　in children, **6**:390
　in uveitis, **9**:103*t*
vasculature of, **2**:71–73, 71*i*, 72*i*, 73*i*, **4**:118–119
　development of, **2**:149
　insufficiency of, central retinal artery occlusion
　　and, **12**:148, 149*i*
　perfusion abnormalities and, **12**:166–167, 167*i*,
　　168*i*, 169*i*
Choroidal artery
　anterior, **5**:16
　lateral, **5**:18
Choroidal/ciliary body melanoma (posterior uveal
　melanoma), **4**:159–163, 222–241, 223*i*, 224*t*
　classification of, **4**:233, 234*t*
　diagnosis of, **4**:224–227, 225*i*, 227*i*, 228*i*
　　differential, **4**:228–233, 229*t*, 231*i*, 232*i*, 233*i*
　　dilemmas in, **4**:228–229
　incidence of, **4**:229
　metastatic evaluation and, **4**:233–237, 234*t*, 235*t*
　open-angle glaucoma caused by, **10**:106
　prognosis for, **4**:239–242
　spindle cell, **4**:160, 160*i*
　spread of, **4**:161–163, 161*i*
　staging of, **4**:289–290*t*
　treatment of, **4**:234*t*, 235–240
Choroidal fissure. *See* Embryonic fissure
Choroidal hemorrhage. *See* Choroidal/suprachoroidal
　hemorrhage
Choroidal neovascularization, **4**:156, 157*i*, **12**:63,
　64–67, 65*i*
　in age-related macular degeneration, **4**:139–140,
　　12:20*i*, 63, 64–67, 65*i*
　　prophylactic photocoagulation and, **12**:61–62
　　treatment of, **12**:70–78, 71–72*t*, 77*t*
　　　photocoagulation, **12**:70–73, 71–72*t*, 73*i*, 74*i*
　　　photodynamic therapy, **12**:71–72*t*, 73–76,
　　　　320–322
　angioid streaks and, **12**:83–84
　central serous chorioretinopathy and, **12**:53
　choroidal rupture and, **12**:292, 293*i*
　classic, **12**:20*i*, 64, 65*i*, 66
　conditions associated with, **12**:86–87, 86*t*
　fellow eye considerations and, **12**:76–78
　fluorescein angiography in, **12**:20*i*, 63, 64–67, 65*i*
　in histoplasmosis, **9**:162*i*, 163
　idiopathic, **12**:82–83
　indocyanine green angiography in, **12**:63
　in myopia, **12**:71–72*t*, 85–86
　occult, **12**:20*i*, 64–66, 65*i*
　in ocular histoplasmosis syndrome, **12**:72*t*, 79–82,
　　80*i*
　　management of, **12**:72*t*, 80–82
　pathologic (high/degenerative) myopia and,
　　12:71–72*t*, 85–86
　photocoagulation for, **12**:70–73, 71–72*t*, 73*i*, 74*i*
　　wavelength selection and, **12**:73, 316*t*
　photodynamic therapy for, **12**:71–72*t*, 73–76,
　　320–322
　poorly defined/demarcated, **12**:66–67
　in Sorsby macular dystrophy, **12**:223, 223*i*
　subfoveal, **12**:327, 328*i*
　transpupillary therapy for, **12**:320
　treatment of, **12**:70–78, 71–72*t*, 73*i*, 74*i*, 77*t*
　in uveitis, **9**:240
　vitrectomy for, **12**:327, 328*i*
　in Vogt-Koyanagi-Harada syndrome, **9**:205, 240
　well-defined/demarcated, **12**:66–67
Choroidal Neovascularization Prevention Trial
　(CNVPT), **12**:61
Choroidal/suprachoroidal hemorrhage
　cataract surgery and, **11**:164*t*, 169–170
　　delayed, **11**:171
　　expulsive, **11**:170–171
　　　patients at risk for, **11**:215–217
　flat or shallow anterior chamber and, **11**:163, 166
　expulsive, **4**:25, 26*i*
Choroidal vasculopathy, polypoidal (posterior uveal
　bleeding syndrome), age-related macular
　degeneration differentiated from, **12**:67–68, 69*i*
Choroidal vein, **5**:20, 21–22*i*
Choroideremia, **12**:224–225
　electroretinogram in, **12**:35
　ocular findings in carriers of, **2**:270*t*, 271*i*
　REP 1 (Rab escort protein 1/*CHM*) gene mutations
　　in, **2**:351, **12**:224
　retinal pigment epithelium in, **2**:363
Choroiditis, **9**:107. *See also* Choroidopathy
　geographic (serpiginous/helicoid peripapillary
　　choroidopathy), **9**:177*t*, 182–183, 184*i*
　in HIV infection/AIDS
　　Cryptococcus neoformans causing, **9**:257
　　multifocal, **9**:257–258
　　Pneumocystis carinii causing, **9**:256–257, 256*i*, 257*i*
　multifocal
　　in HIV infection/AIDS, **9**:257–258
　　and panuveitis (MCP), **9**:177*t*, 185, 185*i*, **12**:174*t*,
　　　178–179, 179*i*
　in ocular histoplasmosis, **9**:160–161, 161*i*
　punctate inner (PIC), **9**:177*t*, 182, 183*i*
Choroidopathy. *See also* Choroiditis
　central serous, **5**:105, **12**:51–54
　　age-related macular degeneration differentiated
　　　from, **12**:53, 59, 68–69, 69*i*
　　fluorescein angiography in, **12**:22*i*, 52
　hypertensive, **12**:98, 98*i*, 99*i*
　punctate inner (PIC), **12**:174*t*, 179, 179*i*
　serpiginous/helicoid peripapillary (geographic
　　choroiditis), **9**:177*t*, 182–183, 184*i*, **12**:174*t*,
　　176–177, 177*i*
Choyce Mark intraocular lenses, **11**:141*i*, 143
"Christmas tree" cataracts
　in children, **6**:293*i*
　in myotonic dystrophy, **5**:335
Chromatic aberration, **3**:40, 102–103, 104*i*
　duochrome test and, **3**:140
　prisms producing, **3**:89
Chromatid, **2**:183, 205
Chromatin, **2**:183, 204
Chromosomal aneuploidy. *See also specific disorder*
　autosome, **2**:249–251
　sex chromosome, **2**:249
Chromosome arm painting, **2**:247–249, 248*i*, 249*i*
Chromosomes, **2**:199–205, 241–242. *See also*
　Autosomes
　abnormalities of. *See also specific type*
　　congenital anomalies and, **2**:159–160
　　etiology of, **2**:253–255

identification of, 2:246–255. *See also* Cytogenetics
acrocentric, 2:182
analysis of, 2:246–255. *See also* Cytogenetics
bacterial artificial (BAC), 2:183
histones forming, 2:204
homologous, 2:188
human artificial, for glaucoma, 10:177
morphologically variant (cytogenetic markers), 2:221
sex, 2:242. *See also* X chromosome; Y chromosome
aneuploidy of, 2:249
mosaicism and, 2:252
structure of, 2:199, 204–205
translocation of, 2:197
Down syndrome caused by, 2:250
yeast artificial (YAC), 2:198
Chronic bronchitis, 1:154
Chronic cyclitis. *See* Intermediate uveitis; Pars planitis
Chronic disease, anemia of, 1:161
iron deficiency differentiated from, 1:159
Chronic lymphocytic leukemia (CLL) type lymphoma, of orbit, 4:195
Chronic obstructive pulmonary disease, 1:154
ocular surgery in patient with, 1:329
ocular surgery in patients with, 11:203–204
recent developments in, 1:153
Chronic progressive external ophthalmoplegia, 5:334, 334i, 6:150–151, 153t, 12:236, 245, 246t, 247i
mitochondrial DNA deletions and, 2:218
Chronic progressive external ophthalmoplegia (CPEO)-plus syndromes, 2:218
CHRPE. *See* Congenital hypertrophy of retinal pigment epithelium
Chrysiasis, corneal pigmentation in, 8:377t
CHSD. *See* Congenital hereditary stromal dystrophy
Churg-Strauss syndrome, 1:189t, 193
Chymotrypsin (alpha-chymotrypsin), for ICCE, 11:105
Cialis. *See* Tadalafil
Cicatricial ectropion, 7:196i, 200–201
after blepharoplasty, 7:233
Cicatricial entropion, 7:205–207, 205i, 206i
Cicatricial pemphigoid, 8:200, 217t, 219–223, 221i, 222i
cataract surgery in patients with, 11:207
drug-induced (pseudopemphigoid), 8:219–220, 394, 395
mucous membrane grafting for, 8:439
CID. *See* Cytomegalic inclusion disease
Cidofovir, 1:48, 65t, 77, 2:440t, 443–444
for cytomegalovirus retinitis, 1:29, 48, 9:252, 12:193
for herpes simplex virus infection, 1:28
iritis/hypotony caused by, 9:252
uveitis caused by, 9:141, 252
Cigarette burns of cornea, in children, 6:445
Cigarette smoking
cancer and, 1:252, 296, 297
cataract development and, 11:64, 73–74
cessation of, 1:155–156
heart disease and, 1:111
hypertension and, 1:85
thyroid disease and, 1:201, 225, 5:331, 7:53–54
Cilastin, with imipenem, 1:59t, 69
Cilia. *See* Eyelashes
Ciliary arteries, 2:36, 38–40, 39i, 40i, 67
anterior, 2:36, 38–40, 39i, 40i, 5:15, 6:16
anterior segment ischemia after strabismus surgery and, 6:189, 189i

choroid supplied by, 12:15
extraocular muscles supplied by, 2:38, 6:16
optic nerve supplied by, 2:102, 103
posterior, 2:38–40, 39i, 40i, 5:15, 16i
Ciliary band, gonioscopic visualization of, 2:61
Ciliary block, after cataract surgery, flat anterior chamber and, 11:166
Ciliary block glaucoma. *See* Aqueous misdirection
Ciliary body
ablation of, 10:204–206, 204t, 205i, 206i
anatomy of, 2:53i, 55i, 56i, 66–69
biochemistry and metabolism of, 2:303–314
development of, 2:154
hyalinization of, 4:156
immunologic microenvironment of, 9:36–37
melanocytoma of, 4:158, 217
melanoma of, 4:159–163, 222–241, 223i. *See also* Choroidal/ciliary body melanoma
staging of, 4:289–290t
metastatic disease of, 4:163–164, 269–271
neoplastic disorders of, 4:157–164
in children, 6:388–389, 389i
nevus of, 4:216–217
signal transduction in, 2:308–310, 310–312, 312i, 313i
stroma of, 2:66–67
tear in (angle recession), 4:25, 25i
glaucoma and, 4:83, 83i
topography of, 4:150, 150i
uveal portion of, 2:67
in uveitis, 9:105
Ciliary body ablation procedures, 10:204–206, 204t, 205i, 206i
Ciliary epithelium, 2:66–67, 68i
aqueous humor composition and, 2:315–317
benign adenomas and cysts of, 4:242
development of, 2:154
medulloepithelioma (diktyoma) of, 4:144–146, 147i, 283
nonpigmented, 2:66, 68i
pigmented, 2:67, 68i
acquired hyperplasia of, 4:241–242
Ciliary flush, 8:59
in uveitis, 9:102, 103
Ciliary ganglion, 2:13–15, 14i, 110, 5:49
branches of, 2:15
Ciliary margin, 7:146
Ciliary muscle, 2:67–69, 68i
in accommodation, 2:73, 11:22, 22t, 13:167–171, 168i, 169i
development of, 2:154
miotics affecting, 2:309
muscarinic drugs affecting, 2:394, 398, 400–401, 401t
Ciliary muscle spasm (spasm of accommodation), 5:314
accommodative excess caused by, 3:148
Ciliary nerves
long, 2:38, 297, 7:15
short, 2:15, 38, 110, 7:15
ciliary muscle supplied by, 2:69
iris sphincter supplied by, 2:66
posterior, 2:38
Ciliary processes, 2:55i, 66
in aqueous humor formation, 10:17, 19i
development of, 2:154

Cilioretinal artery, **2:**84, 103, **5:**15, **12:**12
  macular preservation in central retinal artery
    occlusion and, **12:**148, 149*i*
Ciliospinal nucleus, of Budge-Waller, **5:**56, 58*i*
Cilium, photoreceptor, **2:**79, 82*i*
Ciloxan. *See* Ciprofloxacin
CIN. *See* Conjunctival intraepithelial neoplasia
Cingulate gyrus, **5:**56
Cipro. *See* Ciprofloxacin
Ciprofloxacin, **1:**62*t*, 73, **2:**430–433, 431*t*
  for bacterial keratitis, **8:**183
  corneal deposits caused by, **8:**376
  for endophthalmitis, **9:**218*t*
  for gonococcal conjunctivitis, **8:**172
  ocular effects of, **1:**324*t*
Circle of least confusion, **3:**94, 94*i*
Circle of Willis, **2:**102, 103*i*, 119–121, 121*i*, **5:**16
  intracranial aneurysm on, **5:**350*i*
Circle of Zinn-Haller (circle of Haller and Zinn),
    2:103, **5:**15, **10:**48, 49
Circularly polarized light, **3:**10
Circulatory failure, **1:**126
Cirrhosis, from hepatitis C, **1:**31
11-*cis* retinaldehyde, **2:**359, 360*i*, **12:**14
11-*cis* retinol dehydrogenase, mutations in, **2:**351
Cisapride, perioperative, **1:**331, 332*t*
Cisplatin, **1:**260*t*
Citrate, in tear film, **2:**290
Citrobacter, **8:**126
CJDCR. *See* Conjunctivodacryocystorhinostomy
CK. *See* Conductive keratoplasty; Creatine kinase
CK-MB, in myocardial infarction, **1:**117
Cl. *See* Chloride
Claforan. *See* Cefotaxime
CLAP diseases, **6:**215. *See also specific disorder*
CLAPIKS (contact lens assisted, pharmacologically
    induced keratosteepening), **13:**207–208
Clarin-1, in Usher syndrome, **12:**235
Clarithromycin, **1:**49, 60*t*, 71, **2:**436
  for bacterial keratitis, **8:**182*t*
  for endocarditis prophylaxis, **1:**10*t*
Class I major histocompatibility complex molecules,
    9:20–22, 21*i*, 90, 92*t*
Class II major histocompatibility complex molecules,
    9:19, 20*i*, 90, 92*t*
  primed macrophages as, **9:**51*i*, 52
Class III major histocompatibility complex molecules,
    9:91
Classic congenital esotropia, **6:**97–100, 98*t*, 99*i*
Claude syndrome, **5:**227
Claustrophobia, cataract surgery in patients with,
    11:200
Clavulanic acid, **1:**69–70. *See also specific antibiotic
    combination*
Clear cell hidradenoma (eccrine acrospiroma), **7:**167
Clear corneal incision, for cataract surgery, **11:**100–101,
    123–125, 125*i*, 126*i*
  minimizing bleeding risk and, **11:**202
Clear lens extraction, **11:**138, 222
  refractive (refractive lens exchange), **13:**156–161
    advantages of, **13:**161
    complications of, **13:**160–161
    disadvantages of, **13:**161
    indications for, **13:**156
    informed consent for, **13:**158

IOL calculations for, **13:**160
    patient selection for, **13:**156–158
    retinal detachment and, **13:**158, 160, 161, 192
    surgical planning/techniques for, **13:**158–160
Cleft syndromes, **7:**38–39, 38*i*, 39*i*
  lacrimal outflow disorders and, **7:**258, 258*i*
Cleocin. *See* Clindamycin
Climatic droplet keratopathy, **8:**368–369. *See also*
    Spheroidal degeneration
Climatotherapy, for vernal keratoconjunctivitis, **8:**211
Clinafloxacin, **1:**62*t*
Clindamycin, **1:**60*t*, 71
  for endocarditis prophylaxis, **1:**10*t*
  for endophthalmitis, **12:**300
  for *Pneumocystis carinii* (*Pneumocystis jiroveci*)
    pneumonia, **1:**45
  for toxoplasmosis, **6:**216, **9:**168
Clinical heterogeneity, **2:**184, 241
"Clinical history method," for IOL power calculation
    after refractive surgery, **13:**200–201, 201*t*
Clinical refraction. *See* Refraction, clinical
Clinical research/studies
  application to clinical practice and, **1:**362–370
    data presentation and, **1:**368–370, 369*i*, 370*i*, 371*i*
    measurement system design and, **1:**363–364
    monitoring system implementation and,
      1:364–366
    quality improvement and, **1:**370, 371*i*
    results analysis and, **1:**366–368
  designs for, **1:**345–360, 345*i*
  evaluation of, **1:**339–344
    clinical relevance and, **1:**344
    intervention issues and, **1:**342
    outcome issues and, **1:**342–343
    participants and setting and, **1:**341
    sample size and, **1:**342
    validity and, **1:**343, 363
  interpreting results for patients and, **1:**360–362
Clinical trials (experimental/interventional studies),
    1:345, 351–352, 351*i*. *See also* Clinical research
  for new drug, **2:**393
  systematic reviews/meta-analyses of, **1:**352
Clinoid process
  anterior, **5:**13, 15, 26
  posterior, **2:**117
Clinoril. *See* Sulindac
Clip-on lenses
  for overrefraction, **3:**142, 164–165
  for prism correction, **3:**170
Clivus, **2:**117, **5:**5, **12:**9*t*
CLL type lymphoma. *See* Chronic lymphocytic
    leukemia (CLL) type lymphoma
Clobetasol, for orbital hemangiomas in children, **6:**378
Clofazimine, **1:**49
Clofibrate, for hypercholesterolemia, **1:**149*t*
Clomid. *See* Clomiphene
Clomiphene, ocular effects of, **1:**325*t*
Clonal deletion, **9:**88
Clonal inactivation, **9:**88
Clonazepam, for nystagmus, **5:**255
Clone
  cDNA, **2:**183
  genomic, **2:**186
  positional, **2:**225–226

Clonidine
for heart failure, 1:130
for hypertension, 1:89t
in perioperative setting, 1:333
Cloning, bacterial, for DNA amplification, 2:227, 229i
Cloning vector, 2:184
Clopidogrel
for carotid disease, 1:107
cataract surgery in patient taking, 11:202
for cerebral ischemia/stroke, 1:104
Cloquet's canal, 2:91, 147
Close-focus telescopes, 3:260
Closed circuit television, 3:261
Closed-loop trackers, 13:98
Clostridium
botulinum, toxin derived from, 6:195. *See also*
Botulinum toxin
difficile, 1:8–10
Clotrimazole, 1:64t
Clotting. *See* Coagulation
Cloudy cornea, in inborn errors of metabolism,
6:436–437t
Cloverleaf field, 10:70, 71i
Cloxacillin, 1:55t, 67, 2:429
Clozapine, 1:271, 272
Clozaril. *See* Clozapine
CLSLK. *See* Contact lens superior limbic
keratoconjunctivitis
Club-shaped endings, in scleral spur, 2:54
Clump cells, in iris, 4:149
Cluster headache, 5:297
Clusters A, B, and C personality disorders, 1:166
cM. *See* Centimorgan
CME. *See* Cystoid macular edema
CMV. *See* Cytomegaloviruses
CN. *See* Congenital nystagmus
CNBG3 gene, in achromatopsia, 6:336
CNGA3 gene, in achromatopsia, 6:336
CNS. *See* Central nervous system
CNV. *See* Choroidal neovascularization
CNVPT (Choroidal Neovascularization Prevention
Trial), 12:61
CO_2 laser. *See* Carbon dioxide laser
Coactinon. *See* Emivirine
Coagulation. *See also* Hemostasis
disorders of, 1:168–172
acquired, 1:168–170
cataract surgery in patients with, 11:201–202
hereditary, 1:168
laboratory evaluation of, 1:165
before cataract surgery, 11:202
pathways of, 1:164, 164i
Coagulation factors, 1:164, 164i
abnormalities/deficiencies of, 1:168
vitamin K and, 1:168
Coating properties, of viscoelastics, 11:159
Coats disease, 4:121–122, 122i, 6:332–333, 333i,
12:156–157, 157i
in children, 6:332–333, 333i
photocoagulation for, 12:157
wavelength selection and, 12:316t
retinoblastoma differentiated from, 4:256, 256t, 257i,
6:394
Coats reaction, 12:156, 157i
Coats white ring, 8:368, 368i

Coaxial illumination, for operating microscope, 3:297
Cobblestone (paving-stone) degeneration, 4:128, 129i,
12:263, 264i
Cobo irrigating keratoprosthesis, 8:471
Cocaine
abuse of, 1:270–271
anisocoria and, 5:262
in Horner syndrome diagnosis, 5:262, 7:212, 212i
norepinephrine uptake affected by, 2:310, 406
as topical anesthetic, 2:446t
Cocaine abstinence syndrome, 1:270
Coccidioides immitis (coccidioidomycosis), 9:163,
226–227, 227i
optic nerve infection caused by, 4:205
Cochlear artery, 5:18
Cochlear nerve, 5:32, 54
Cochlin, in vitreous, 2:337
Cockayne syndrome, 8:351t
childhood glaucoma and, 10:155t
Coding strand of DNA (sense DNA), 2:195, 201–202
Codominance (codominant inheritance), 2:184, 260
Codon, 2:184, 200, 201, 201i, 8:306
amber, 2:182
initiator, 2:189
stop/termination, 2:196, 201, 201i
frameshift mutation and, 2:186
Coefficient of variation, specular photomicroscopy in
evaluation of, 8:37
Coenzyme Q_{10}, for Leber hereditary optic neuropathy,
5:136
Cogan microcystic dystrophy, 4:70–71, 72i, 8:311, 312
Cogan-Reese (iris nevus) syndrome, 4:79, 219t, 8:301
Cogan syndrome, 1:192, 8:228–229
Cogan's lid twitch, 5:275, 325, 6:151
Cogentin. *See* Benztropine
Cogwheel pursuit, 5:210
Coherence, 3:7–9, 8i, 9i
applications of, 3:8–9, 9i
of laser light, 3:8, 18, 20t
spatial (lateral), 3:7–8, 8i
temporal (longitudinal), 3:8, 8i
Coherence tomography, optical. *See* Optical coherence
tomography
Cohesive viscoelastics, 11:158
Cohort studies (follow-up studies), 1:345i, 348i,
350–351
Coil embolization, of aneurysm, 5:353–354
COL1A1/COL1A2 genes, in osteogenesis imperfecta,
8:288
Cold (temperature), anterior segment injuries caused
by, 8:388
Cold mirror, 3:9
Colesevelam, for hypercholesterolemia, 1:149t
Colestipol, for hypercholesterolemia, 1:149t
Colistimethate, 2:428t
Colistin, 1:54
Colitis
granulomatous (Crohn disease), 1:177, 9:131–132
ulcerative, 1:177, 9:131–132
Collaborative Initial Glaucoma Treatment Study
(CIGTS), 10:86, 89t, 158
Collaborative Normal-Tension Glaucoma Study
(CNTGS), 10:92
Collaborative Ocular Melanoma Study (COMS), 4:213,
236, 239–241

Collagen, **8**:10–11
  corneal, **2**:46–47
  in lens capsule, **2**:323
  scleral, **2**:50, 51, **8**:14
  stromal, **2**:46–47, 300
    corneal haze after PRK and, **13**:103
  types and tissue distribution of, **2**:333–335, 334*t*
  in vitreous, **2**:89, 147, 333–335, 334*t*, 335*i*, **12**:7, 279
Collagen cornea shields, for drug administration,
    2:390–391
Collagen plugs, for dry eye, **7**:274, **8**:76–77
Collagen shrinkage, **13**:22*t*, 137–142. *See also*
    Thermokeratoplasty
  corneal biomechanics affected by, **13**:27–28, 28*i*
Collagen-vascular diseases. *See also* Connective tissue
    disorders
  Purtscher-like retinopathy and, **12**:95
  uveitis in, **9**:173–175
Collagenase inhibitors, for peripheral ulcerative
    keratitis, **8**:231
Collagenases, **8**:198*t*, **9**:86
  in ocular infections, **8**:117
Collagenoma, in tuberous sclerosis, **6**:410
Collagenous layer, posterior (retrocorneal fibrous
    membrane), **2**:301–302, **8**:33–34
Collarette, iris, **2**:64, 155
Collateral vessels, retinochoroidal, in papilledema,
    5:116–117
Collector channels, **2**:58–59, 60*i*
Colliculus
  facial, **2**:116, 117, **5**:227
  superior, **5**:27, 31, 54
    superficial, **5**:34
Collier's sign, **5**:254, 270, 279
Collimating keratoscope, **8**:41
Colloid bodies. *See* Optic disc (optic nerve head),
    drusen of
Colloidal iron stain, **4**:36, 36*t*
Colobomas, **2**:125, 170–172, 171*i*, **5**:259
  cystic, **2**:165–166
  definition of, **2**:125
  embryonic fissure closure and, **2**:138, 143*i*, 165–166,
    171
  eyelid, **6**:210, **7**:157–158, 157*i*
    in mandibulofacial dysostosis (Treacher Collins
      syndrome), **6**:432
  Fuchs (tilted disc syndrome), **5**:139–140, 140*i*,
    6:360–361, 361*i*
  in Goldenhar syndrome, **6**:431
  iris, **2**:171, 171*i*, **6**:262–264, 263*i*
    cataract surgery in patients with, **11**:212, 213*i*
  lens, **2**:171–172, **6**:304, 304*i*, **11**:31, 31*i*
  macular, **2**:173
  optic nerve/optic disc, **2**:171*i*, 175, **4**:204–205,
    6:359–360, 360*i*
  retinal, **2**:171
  uveal, **4**:152
Colobomatous cyst (microphthalmos with cyst), **6**:383,
    383*i*, **7**:37–38
Colon cancer. *See* Colorectal cancer
Colonoscopy, in cancer screening, **1**:298–299
  virtual, **1**:291, 299
Colony-forming unit–culture, **1**:160
Colony-forming unit–erythroid, **1**:160
Colony-forming unit–spleen, **1**:160

Colony-stimulating factors, in cancer therapy, **1**:261
Color blindness. *See* Color vision, defects in
Color contrast, sunglasses affecting, **3**:165, 166*i*
Color flow Doppler imaging, in ischemic heart disease,
    1:118
Color plate testing, pseudoisochromatic, in low vision
    evaluation, **5**:96
Color vision, **12**:43
  defects in, **5**:96, **12**:195–198, 196*t*, 197*i*. *See also*
    specific type
    achromatopsia, **6**:336, 455, **12**:196–198
    acquired, **12**:195, 196*t*
    assessment of, **12**:43–44, 44*i*, 45*i*
    blue-cone monochromatism, **6**:336
    in cone dystrophies, **12**:213–214
    congenital, **12**:195–196, 196*t*
    in dominant optic atrophy, **5**:136, **6**:364
    genetic basis of, **2**:346–347, 346*i*, **12**:195–196, 197*i*
    ocular findings in carriers of, **2**:270*t*
    vision rehabilitation and, **3**:254
  evaluation of, **12**:43–44, 44*i*, 45*i*
  nuclear cataract affecting, **11**:45–46
  testing, in low vision evaluation, **5**:96
  trivariant, **2**:345–347
Colorectal cancer, **1**:252, 297–299
  in Gardner syndrome, fundus findings and, **4**:230
  incidence of, **1**:297
  screening for, **1**:298–299
Coma, **5**:256
  eye movements in patients in, **5**:256
  myxedema, **1**:226
  nonketotic hyperglycemic-hyperosmolar, **1**:216
Coma (wavefront aberration), **3**:93, 233*i*, 239, **13**:16,
    17*i*
Combined hamartoma, of retina and retinal pigment
    epithelium, **4**:147, 242, 242*i*
Combined sutures, for penetrating keratoplasty, **8**:459,
    459*i*
Combipres. *See* Clonidine
Combivent. *See* Albuterol, with ipratropium
Combivir. *See* Lamivudine (3TC), with zidovudine
Comitant (concomitant) deviations, **5**:213, 216–217,
    6:10
  vertical, **6**:127
Comma sign, in sickle cell hemoglobinopathies, **12**:122
Commissure, posterior, **2**:110, **5**:39
Common canaliculus, **6**:239
Common carotid artery, **5**:11, 178*i*
Common cause factors, **1**:368–370
Common migraine, **5**:294. *See also* Migraine headache
Commotio retinae (Berlin disease/edema), **4**:28,
    12:291, 292*i*
Communicating artery
  anterior, **5**:16
  posterior, **5**:20
Communication
  between clinician and pathologist, **4**:31–32
  between clinician and patient, cataract surgery and,
    11:201
Compartment syndrome, visual loss after orbital
    trauma and, **7**:104
Complement, **8**:198*t*, **9**:7, 74–76, 76*i*
  in adaptive immune response, **9**:74–76
  in aqueous humor, **2**:319
  cell lysis mediated by, **9**:59, 60*i*

in innate immune response, **9:**46–47, 75
receptors for, in phagocytosis, **9:**50
Complementary DNA (cDNA), **2:**184, 200
from ciliary body–encoding plasma proteins, **2:**319
sequencing, in mutation screening, **2:**231
Complementary DNA clone (cDNA clone), **2:**183
Complementary DNA library (cDNA library), **2:**189, 227
Complete (third-degree) atrioventricular block, **1:**134
Complete blood count, in immune-mediated disease, **8:**202*t*
Complete cataract, **11:**38
Completed stroke, **1:**102
Complex cells, **5:**29
Complex choristomas, **4:**44, **8:**277, 278*i*
Complex partial seizures, **1:**281, 320
Compliance with therapy, for amblyopia, **6:**74
Complications of Age-Related Macular Degeneration
Prevention Trial (CAPT), **12:**62
Compound heterozygote, **2:**184, 261
Compound nevi, **7:**170–171
of conjunctiva, **4:**55–56, 56*i*
in children, **6:**387
of eyelid, **4:**183, 183*i*
Compression sutures, for corneal astigmatism after
penetrating keratoplasty, **8:**466
Compressive optic neuropathy
intraorbital/intracanalicular, **5:**145–151
in thyroid-associated orbitopathy, **5:**330, 330*i*
Compromised host. *See* Immunocompromised host
Computed tomography (CT scan), **5:**61–62
in acquired tearing evaluation, **7:**272
in cerebral ischemia/stroke, **1:**103
in choroidal/ciliary body melanoma, **4:**227, 228*i*
dual-energy quantitative, in osteoporosis, **1:**243
in foreign-body identification, **12:**290, 297, 297*i*
indications for, **5:**75–78, 75*t*, 76*i*
in intracranial hemorrhage, **1:**106
in intraparenchymal hemorrhage, **5:**77*t*
limitations of, **5:**77*t*
in orbital evaluation, **7:**29
MRI compared with, **7:**31–33, 32*i*, 33*t*
in pulmonary diseases, **1:**155
in retinoblastoma, **4:**254–255
Computerized corneal topography, **8:**41–46, 42*i*, 43*i*,
44*i*, 45*i*, 46*i*, **13:**6–12, 47
Computerized tomographic angiography (CTA),
5:67–68
definition of, **5:**78
limitations of, **5:**77*t*
Computerized videokeratoscopy. *See* Videokeratoscopy
Computers, as low vision devices, **3:**262–263
Comtan. *See* Entacapone
Concave (minus) lenses, anophthalmic socket
camouflage and, **7:**127
Concave mirror
retinoscopy settings and, **3:**125, 126*i*
vergence calculations for, **3:**92–93
Conchae (turbinates), nasal, **7:**20
inferior, **5:**10
infracture of, for congenital tearing/nasolacrimal
duct obstruction, **6:**245–246, **7:**263, 265*i*
Concomitant (comitant) deviation, **5:**213, 216–217,
6:10
vertical, **6:**127

Concretions, conjunctival, **8:**366–367
Concussive trauma. *See also* Trauma
anterior segment, **8:**396–403
Condensing lens
in fundus camera, **3:**275, 278*i*
in indirect ophthalmoscopy, **3:**273*i*, 274–275
conjugacy of pupils and, **3:**274*i*
fundus illumination and, **3:**275*i*
illumination source and, **3:**279*i*
Conductive keratoplasty, **13:**27–28, 28*i*, 50*t*, 139–142,
140*i*, 141*i*, 141*t*, 142*i*
penetrating keratoplasty after, **13:**204
for presbyopia, **13:**173
risks/benefits of, **13:**50*t*, 139, 141–142
Cone dystrophies/degeneration, **5:**104, **12:**213–214,
215*i*
electroretinogram patterns in, **12:**30*i*, 214
Cone inner segments, **2:**82*i*. *See also* Cones
Cone outer segments, **2:**79, 80, 82*i*, 87–88. *See also*
Cones
differentiation of, **2:**141
Cone response, **2:**354–355, 355*i*
single-flash (photopic/light-adapted
electroretinogram), **12:**28*i*, 29, 206*t*
in hereditary retinal/choroidal degenerations,
12:205, 206*t*
Cone–rod dystrophies/degenerations, **12:**214–215
electroretinogram patterns in, **12:**30*i*, 214
Stargardt disease differentiated from, **6:**338
Cone–rod homeobox-containing *(CRX)* gene, **12:**204
cone–rod dystrophy and, **12:**215
Cones, **2:**79–80, 82*i*, **12:**10. *See also* Cone outer
segments
abnormalities of, **12:**195–198, 196*t*, 197*i*. *See also*
Color vision, defects in
amacrine cells for, **2:**352
bipolar cells for, **2:**351–352, 352*i*
electrophysiologic responses of, **2:**354–355, 355*i*
extrafoveal, **2:**79–80
foveal, **2:**80, 87–88
gene defects in, photoreceptor dysfunction/
degeneration and, **2:**349–350
horizontal cells for, **2:**352, 352*i*
phototransduction in, **2:**345
Confluent drusen, **12:**57
Confocal microscopy, **8:**37–38
in fleck dystrophy, **8:**323
in lattice dystrophy, **8:**318
in posterior polymorphous dystrophy, **8:**328
Confocal scanning laser ophthalmoscopy
in optic nerve head evaluation, **10:**55
in retinal examination, **12:**24–25
Confoscan, **8:**38
Confounding factor, **1:**350, 367
Confrontation testing, **5:**89–90
before cataract surgery, **11:**85
in functional visual disorder evaluation, **5:**310
before refractive surgery, **13:**44
Confusion, **1:**284
in elderly patients, **1:**237–238
visual, **6:**52, 53*i*
Confusion tests, in functional visual disorder
evaluation, **5:**307, 308*i*
monocular reduced vision and, **5:**308

Congenital, definition of, 2:184, 239–240. *See also*
Genetics
Congenital anomalies, 2:159–178, 160*i*, 4:12,
6:205–206, 457*t. See also specific type*
of anterior chamber, 2:168–169, 168*i*, 169*i*, 170*i*
cataract surgery in patients with, 11:212–215
chromosomal analysis and, 2:247*t*
of conjunctiva, 4:43–45, 44*i*
of cornea, 2:167–168, 167*i*, 4:62–65, 6:250–255, 251*i*,
252*i*, 254*i*, 8:281–283, 285–302
craniofacial malformations, 6:421–434, 7:38–39, 38*i*,
39*i*
definition of, 6:206
diagnostic approach to, 8:282–283
of eyelid, 4:169, 6:209–214, 7:153–158
genetic influences and, 2:159–160
of iris, 2:169–170
of lens, 2:172–173, 4:94–95, 95*i*, 95*t*, 11:30–39
nongenetic teratogens causing, 2:159, 160–162, 160*i*,
161*i*, 162*i*, 163*i*
of optic disc and nerve, 2:173–175, 174*i*, 176*i*, 177*i*,
4:204–205, 5:138–141
of orbit, 4:188, 188*i*, 7:38–39, 38*i*, 39*i*
of pigmentation, 2:175–178, 177*i*, 178*i*
of retina, 2:173, 4:119–122, 121*i*, 122*i*, 123*i*
of sclera, 4:88–89, 8:281–283, 285–288
of trabecular meshwork, 4:78–79, 78*i*, 79*i*
of uveal tract, 4:151–152
of vitreous, 4:106–107, 106*i*
Congenital aphakia, 6:304, 11:30
Congenital bilateral mydriasis, 6:268
Congenital cataract. *See specific type and* Cataract,
congenital and infantile
Congenital (infantile) esotropia, 6:97–101, 98*t*, 99*i*
classic (essential), 6:97–100, 98*t*, 99*i*
Congenital exotropia, 6:114–115, 115*i*
Congenital fibrosis of extraocular muscles type I
(CFEOM1) syndrome, 5:220
Congenital fibrosis syndrome, 5:220–221, 221*i*,
6:152–154
Congenital glaucoma, 6:271, 272–277, 273*i*, 274*t*, 275*i*,
276*i*, 277*i*, 8:299–300, 10:6*t. See also* Glaucoma,
childhood
genetics of, 6:271
Congenital hereditary endothelial dystrophy, 4:62–63,
63*i*, 6:256*t*, 257, 8:297–298, 298*i*, 309*t*
Congenital hereditary stromal dystrophy, 6:256*t*, 257,
8:297
Congenital hypertrophy of retinal pigment epithelium
(CHRPE), 2:173, 178, 178*i*, 4:122–123, 123*i*, 6:390,
391*i*, 12:14, 264
melanoma differentiated from, 4:230, 231*i*, 232*i*
Congenital infection syndrome/TORCH syndrome,
6:215. *See also specific disorder*
reduced vision and, 6:455–456
Congenital iris ectropion syndrome, 6:269–270, 270*i*
glaucoma in neurofibromatosis and, 6:408
Congenital lacrimal fistula, 6:240
Congenital miosis (microcoria), 6:268
Congenital mydriasis, 6:268
Congenital myopia, 3:121, 146
Congenital nevocellular nevi of skin, 6:387, 388*i*
Congenital night blindness
with normal fundi, 12:198–200, 199*i*, 200*i*

with prominent fundus abnormality, 12:200–202,
201*i*, 202*i*
stationary, 6:336–337, 12:198–200, 199*i*, 200*i*
electroretinogram patterns in, 12:30*i*, 198–200,
199*i*, 200*i*
with myopia, ocular findings in carriers of, 2:270*t*
Congenital nystagmus, 5:241–242, 6:162–165, 164*t*
characteristic signs of, 5:242
latent, 6:165, 166*i*
motor, 6:160, 161, 162–164, 163*i*, 164*t*, 452
periodic alternating, 6:165
sensory defect, 6:164
Congenital ocular motor apraxia, 5:207, 6:156
Congenital ptosis. *See* Ptosis
Congenital retinal arteriovenous malformations,
12:164. *See also* Racemose angioma
Congenital rubella syndrome, 6:217–218, 218*i*, 8:163,
9:158–159, 159*i*
cataracts and, 2:172–173, 4:95, 6:218, 11:38–39
Congenital strabismus, 6:11
Congenital syphilis, 1:15, 302, 6:220–221, 9:187–188,
188*i*
corneal manifestations of/interstitial keratitis, 4:67,
6:220, 260, 260*i*, 8:226–227, 227*i*, 299, 9:187–188,
188*i*
Congenital tarsal kink, 6:211, 211*i*
Congenital tilted disc syndrome (Fuchs coloboma),
5:139–140, 140*i*, 6:360–361, 361*i*
Congestive heart failure, 1:111, 125–132
atrial fibrillation and, 1:131, 132
classification of, 1:126, 126*t*
clinical course of, 1:128–129
clinical signs of, 1:126
compensated, 1:126
decompensated, 1:126
diagnosis of, 1:127
epidemiology of, 1:127
etiology of, 1:128
high-output, 1:128
hypertension management and, 1:91*t*, 95, 130
ischemic heart disease causing, 1:127, 128
management of
invasive or surgical, 1:132
medical and nonsurgical, 1:130–132
after myocardial infarction, 1:128
pathophysiology of, 1:128–129
refractory, 1:126
symptoms of, 1:126
Congo red stain, 4:36, 36*t*
Conidia, 8:129
Conidiophores, 8:129
Conjugacy
in indirect ophthalmoscopy, 3:272–275, 274*i*
in saccades testing, 5:202–203
Conjugate, in geometrical optics, 3:26
Conjugate eye movements (versions), 6:36–38, 37*i*. *See
also specific type*
Conjugate points, in geometrical optics, 3:26
Conjunctiva, 2:29, 32*i*, 36, 7:140*i*, 141*i*, 142*i*, 145
aging of, 8:361
amyloid deposits in, 4:50, 51*i*, 8:348, 348*i*. *See also*
Amyloidosis/amyloid deposits
anatomy of, 2:29, 32*i*, 36, 8:8
biopsy of, 8:427–428
in cicatricial pemphigoid, 8:221–222, 222*i*

for ocular microbiology, **8:**135

blood under, **8:**90, 91*t*, 396

blood vessels of, **2:**36, **8:**8, 59

bulbar, **2:**29, 32*i*, 36, **8:**8

  in superior limbic keratoconjunctivitis, **8:**96, 97, 97*i*

carcinoma of. *See also* Conjunctiva, tumors of

  intraocular extension of, **4:**275

  squamous cell, **4:**53, 53*i*, **8:**255*t*, 257*i*, 260–261, 260*i*

  staging of, **4:**285*t*

concretions of, **8:**366–367

congenital anomalies of, **4:**43–45, 44*i*

contact lenses causing injury to, **8:**214–216, 215*i*

cysts of, **4:**45, 46*i*, **6:**386, **8:**254, 254*i*

  nevi and, **4:**55–56, 56*i*

  after strabismus surgery, **6:**187, 188*i*

degenerations of, **4:**49–50, 49*i*, 50*i*, **8:**365–367

development of, **8:**6

discharge from, **8:**24*t*

disorders of, **4:**43–59, 44*i*, **8:**24*t*. *See also specific type and* Conjunctivitis; Keratoconjunctivitis

  immune-mediated, **8:**201, 207–224

  ionizing radiation causing, **8:**388–389

  neoplastic, **4:**51–59, **8:**253–278, 253*t*. *See also* Conjunctiva, tumors of

  Th1 delayed hypersensitivity and, **9:**68*t*

drug absorption and, **2:**383

dysplasia of, **4:**51–52, 52*i*

epibulbar, **4:**43

epithelium of, **2:**36, **8:**8, 58

  cysts of, **4:**45, 46*i*, **8:**254, 254*i*

    nevi and, **4:**55–56, 56*i*

  cytologic identification of, **8:**64, 66*i*

  evaluation of, in pseudoepiphora, **7:**273

  physiology of, **8:**58

  tumors of, **4:**51–53, 52*i*, 53*i*, **8:**255–261, 255*t*

  wound healing/repair and, **8:**383, 424

erosions of, **8:**25*t*

  punctate epithelial, **8:**24*t*

examination of

  in glaucoma, **10:**33

  slit-lamp, before cataract surgery, **11:**81

in external eye defense, **8:**114

extraocular surgery affecting, **8:**420

follicles of, **8:**24*t*, 25*t*, 26, 28*i*

  in external eye defense, **8:**114

foreign body on, **8:**404, 404*i*, 405*i*

forniceal, **2:**29, 32*i*, 36, **4:**43, **8:**8

goblet cells in. *See* Goblet cells

granuloma of, **8:**24*t*, 25*t*, 169

  in sarcoidosis, **8:**88

hemangiomas of, **8:**270, 270*t*

hemorrhage of, **8:**396

  in hereditary hemorrhagic telangiectasia, **8:**91

hypersensitivity reactions of, **8:**198–201, 199*i*, 199*t*

immune response/immunologic features of, **8:**195, 196*t*, 201, **9:**33–36, 34*t*

incisions in, for extraocular muscle surgery, **6:**183–184

infection/inflammation of, **4:**45–49, **8:**23–26, 24*t*, 25*t*, 26*i*, 27*i*, 28*i*, 169–174, 170*t*, 172*i*. *See also* Conjunctivitis; Keratoconjunctivitis

intraepithelial neoplasia of, **4:**51–52, 52*i*, **8:**255*t*, 257–259, 257*i*, 258*i*

laceration of, **8:**403

lithiasis of, **8:**367

lymphoid tissue associated with (CALT). *See* Conjunctiva-associated lymphoid tissue

lymphoma of, **8:**274–275, 274*i*

mast cells in, **9:**13–14

mechanical functions of, **8:**59–60

melanocytic lesions of, **4:**55–59, 56*i*, 56*t*, 57*i*, 58*i*

melanoma of, **4:**58–59, 58*i*, **8:**268–269, 268*i*

  intraocular extension of, **4:**275

  primary acquired melanosis and, **4:**58–59, 58*i*

  staging of, **4:**286*t*

membrane of, **8:**24*t*, 25*t*

  in epidemic keratoconjunctivitis, **8:**159

  in ligneous conjunctivitis, **8:**213

nevus of, **4:**55–56, 56*i*, 56*t*, **8:**265–266, 266*i*, 267*t*

  in children, **6:**387, 387*i*

normal flora of, **8:**114–115, 115*t*

palpebral, **2:**29, 30*i*, 32*i*, 36, **4:**43, 168, **8:**8

papillae of, **8:**23–26, 24*t*, 25*t*, 26*i*, 27*i*

papillomas of, **8:**162, 255–256, 255*t*, 256*i*

pH of, chemical injury management and, **8:**391

pigmented lesions of, **8:**267*t*

  benign, **8:**263–265, 263*t*

  malignant, **8:**263*t*, 268–269, 268*i*

  preinvasive, **8:**263*t*, 266–268, 267*t*

pseudomembrane of, **8:**24*t*, 25*t*

scarring of after strabismus surgery, **6:**187–188, 188*i*

scrapings/swabbings from, **8:**63–64

specimen collection from

  for ocular cytology, **8:**63–64

  for ocular microbiology, **8:**134–135

stem cells of, **8:**59, 108, 246

stroma of, **4:**43

subepithelial lesions of, **4:**53–55, 54*i*, 55*i*

tarsal, **8:**8

telangiectasia of, **5:**342, 342*i*

  in ataxia-telangiectasia, **6:**417

topography of, **4:**43, 44*i*

transplantation of, **8:**423*t*, 424–425, 429–433

  for chemical burns, **8:**392

  indications for, **8:**423*t*, 432

  for wound closure after pterygium excision, **8:**429, 430*i*, 431–432

tumors of, **4:**51–59, **8:**253–278, 253*t*

  epithelial, **8:**255–261, 255*t*

  glandular, **8:**261–263, 262*i*

  human papillomaviruses causing, **8:**162, 255–256, 255*t*, 256*i*

  inflammatory, **8:**270*t*, 271, 271*i*

  intraocular extension of, **4:**275

  lymphatic and lymphocytic, **8:**273–275, 273*i*, 274*i*

  malignant, **8:**263*t*, 268–269, 268*i*, 270, 270*t*

  metastatic, **8:**275

  neuroectodermal, **8:**263–269, 263*t*

  neurogenic and smooth muscle, **8:**269

  staging of, **4:**285*t*, 286*t*

  vascular and mesenchymal, **8:**269–272, 270*i*

  viral, **8:**162

ulceration of, **8:**25*t*

in uveitis, **9:**103*t*

vascular anomalies of, noninflammatory, **8:**90–92, 91*t*

wound healing/repair of, **8:**383, 424

Conjunctiva-associated lymphoid tissue (CALT/ conjunctival MALT), 2:36, 8:5, 8, 59, 201, 9:34t, 36
Conjunctival arteries, posterior, 2:36
Conjunctival autograft, 8:423t, 429–433. See also Conjunctiva, transplantation of
    indications for, 8:423t
    for wound closure after pterygium excision, 8:430i, 431–432
Conjunctival flaps, 8:436–438, 437i
    for corneal edema after cataract surgery, 11:193
    for ICCE, 11:106
    for neurotrophic keratopathy, 8:104
    in scleral-tunnel incision for cataract surgery, 11:121–122
    for symblepharon, 7:207
    for wound closure after pterygium excision, 8:429, 430i
Conjunctival inclusion cysts, 4:45, 46i, 6:386, 8:254, 254i
    nevi and, 4:55–56, 56i
    after strabismus surgery, 6:187, 188i
Conjunctival intraepithelial neoplasia (CIN), 4:51–52, 52i, 8:255t, 257–259, 257i, 258i
Conjunctivalization of cornea, 8:58
Conjunctivitis, 4:45–49, 8:23–26, 24t, 25t, 26i, 27i, 28t. See also Keratoconjunctivitis
    acute, 4:45
        hemorrhagic, 8:163
        purulent, 8:170–171
    adenoviruses causing, in children, 6:225–226
    allergic, 8:207–209, 9:74
        drugs for, 2:423–425, 424t
        seasonal, 6:234, 8:207–209
    bacterial, 4:46–47, 48i, 8:169–174, 170t, 172i
        in children, 6:224–225, 8:169–172, 170t, 172i
        in neonates, 6:222–223, 222i, 8:172–174
    chemical, in neonates, 6:223
    in children, 6:224–229, 224t, 8:169–172, 170t, 172i
        preseptal cellulitis caused by, 6:230
    chlamydial, 8:119t, 174–178, 175i, 176i
        in adults, 8:177
        in neonates, 6:222–223, 8:174
    chronic, 4:45
        in staphylococcal blepharitis, 8:164–165. See also Blepharoconjunctivitis
    contact lens–induced, 3:210, 4:45, 8:214–216, 215i
    coxsackievirus, 8:163
    enterovirus, 8:163
    Epstein-Barr virus causing, 8:156–157
    follicular, 4:46, 47i, 8:24t, 25t, 26, 28i
        adenoviral, 8:157, 158
        in Lyme disease, 12:191
        medication toxicity causing, 8:394
    giant papillary (contact lens–induced), 3:210, 4:45, 8:214–216, 215i
    gonococcal, 8:119t, 171–172, 172i
        in children, 6:225
        in neonates, 6:222, 222i, 8:172, 173
    Haemophilus causing, 8:119t, 170–171
        in children, 6:224–225
    hay fever, 8:207–209
    hemorrhagic, acute, 8:163
    herpes simplex virus causing
        in children, 6:226, 227i
        in neonates, 6:219–220, 223

herpes zoster causing, in children, 6:226–227, 228i
    in HIV infection/AIDS, 9:261
    infectious, 4:46–47, 48i, 8:119t. See also specific causative agent
        in children, 6:224–229
    in infectious mononucleosis, 6:228
    influenza virus causing, 6:228
    ligneous, 8:213–214
        in children, 6:388
    in Lyme disease, 9:191, 192
    measles virus causing, 8:162
    microsporidial, 8:190
    in molluscum contagiosum, 6:228–229, 229i
    mumps virus causing, 6:228
    neonatal. See Ophthalmia, neonatorum
    noninfectious, 4:47–49
    papillary, 4:45–46, 47i, 8:23–26, 24t, 25t, 26i, 27i
    in Parinaud oculoglandular syndrome, 4:49, 6:229, 230i, 8:178, 12:184–185
    in pharyngoconjunctival fever, 6:226
    in reactive arthritis/Reiter syndrome, 1:177, 8:228, 9:131
    in rubeola, 6:228
    seasonal allergic, 6:234, 8:207–209
    staphylococcal, 8:119t
    in Stevens-Johnson syndrome, 6:237–238, 238i, 8:217
    after strabismus surgery, 6:185
    streptococcal, 8:119t, 170–171
        in children, 6:224–225
    toxic
        contact lens solutions causing, 8:107
        medications causing, 8:393–395
    in trachoma, 6:229
    trachoma-inclusion, in neonates, 6:222–223
    varicella-zoster virus causing, 6:226–227, 228i, 8:151–156
    vernal, 6:234–235, 235i, 8:209–211, 209i, 210i, 9:13
    viral, 4:46–47, 48i
        in children, 6:225–229
        immune response to, 9:35
Conjunctivochalasis, 8:361, 367, 367i
Conjunctivodacryocystorhinostomy
    for canalicular obstruction, 7:275–276
    after canthal repair, 7:193
    for punctal agenesis and dysgenesis, 7:265
Connective tissue
    eyelid, 2:23
    orbital, 2:20, 20i
    pericanalicular, 2:57, 58i
Connective tissue disorders
    corneal changes in, 8:350–354, 351–353t
    mixed, 1:185
    peripheral ulcerative keratitis in, 8:229–232, 230t, 232i
    refractive surgery contraindicated in, 13:198
    scleritis in, 8:234–241
    uveitis in, 9:173–175
    vasculitis associated with, 7:60
Connective tissue mast cells, 9:13–14
Connective tissue tumors, of orbit, in children, 6:380
Conoid
    Cartesian, 3:53–54, 54i
    of Sturm, 3:93–94, 94i, 95i
        astigmatic dial refraction and, 3:134–136, 135i

Consanguinity, 2:184, 264
Consecutive esodeviation, 6:98t, 106–107
Consecutive exotropia, 6:115
Consensual response, in pupillary reaction to light, 5:258
Consensus sequence, 2:184
Consent, informed
    for cataract surgery, 11:88
    for refractive surgery, 13:49–50
        clear lens extraction/refractive lens exchange and, 13:158
        model forms for, 13:51–56
        phakic intraocular lens insertion and, 13:146
Conservation (genetic), 2:184
Conserved base-pair mutations, 2:214
CONSORT (Consolidated Standards of Reporting Trials) guidelines, 1:352
Constant exotropia, 6:114–115
Construct validity, 1:363
Constructive interference, 3:7, 8i
Consultand, 2:275
Contact, arc of, 6:28
Contact dermatoblepharitis, 8:205–207, 206i
Contact hypersensitivity, 9:66
    response to poison ivy as, 9:29–30
Contact inhibition, in corneal wound repair, 4:19
Contact lens electrode, corneal, for electroretinogram, 12:29
Contact lens method, for IOL power calculation after refractive surgery, 11:151, 13:201–202
Contact lens solutions
    allergic reactions to, 8:107, 107i
    toxic conjunctivitis caused by, 8:107
Contact lens superior limbic keratoconjunctivitis (CLSLK), 3:208
Contact lenses, 3:173–212. See also specific type and Flexible (soft) contact lenses; Rigid gas-permeable contact lenses
    Acanthamoeba keratitis associated with, 3:207, 4:66, 67i, 8:187
    accommodation affected by, 3:149–150, 179–180
    alternating vision bifocal
        concentric, 3:198–199, 198i
        segmented, 3:198–199, 198i
    for aphakia in children, 6:300, 11:199
    astigmatism correction and, 3:181–182
    bacterial keratitis associated with, 8:179
        after radial keratotomy, 13:206
    bandage, 3:202, 8:441
        for chemical burns, 8:392
        contraindications to in exposure keratopathy, 8:95
        for corneal abrasion, 8:407
        with cyanoacrylate adhesives, 8:442
        for dry eye, 8:75t
        after LASIK, 13:122
        for perforating injury, 8:410
        for peripheral ulcerative keratitis, 8:231
        after PRK/LASEK, 13:96, 97, 206
            overcorrection and, 13:100
            sterile infiltrates associated with, 13:104, 104i
        for recurrent corneal erosions, 8:99
        after LASIK, 13:122
        for Thygeson superficial punctate keratitis, 8:225
    base curve of, 3:174i, 177

bifocal
    alternating, 3:182–183, 198–199, 198i
    simultaneous vision, 3:182–183
care of, 3:206–207
conjunctivitis caused by (giant papillary conjunctivitis), 3:210, 4:45, 8:214–216, 215i
convergence affected by, 3:149–150, 180
design of, 3:174i, 193i
diameter of, 3:174i, 176i, 177
discontinuing use of, before refractive surgery, 13:41
distortion reduction and, 3:181
in dry eye patients, 8:76
federal regulations for, 3:211–212
field of vision and, 3:177
fitting parameters for, 3:192–195. See also Fitting
flexible. See Flexible (soft) contact lenses
for fundus biomicroscopy, 3:285–289, 285i, 286i, 289i
fungal keratitis associated with, 8:185
gas-permeable scleral, 3:200–202
gas transmissibility of, 3:183–185. See also Flexible (soft) contact lenses; Rigid gas-permeable contact lenses; Scleral contact lenses
    rigid contact lenses and, 3:185
glossary of terms related to, 3:174–176
HIV transmission and, 3:211
image size with, anisometropia and, 3:177–179
for induced anisophoria, 3:162
for keratoconus, 3:199–200, 200i, 202, 8:332
after keratorefractive surgery, 3:202
keratosteepening and (contact lens assisted, pharmacologically induced keratosteepening/ CLAPIKS), 13:207–208
after LASIK, 13:207
lenticular, 3:175
manufacturing of, 3:185–186
materials for, 3:183–185, 183t, 184t
monovision and, 3:183
for myopia reduction (orthokeratology), 3:203–205, 204i, 205i, 13:84–85
optics of, clinically important features of, 3:177–183
parameters of, 3:174i, 176i, 192–195, 193i
parts of, 3:174–176, 174i
for pellucid marginal degeneration, 8:333
polymers for rigid (hard) lenses and, 3:183–184
power curve of, 3:177
power of, 3:177, 194
presbyopia in wearers of, correcting, 3:182–183
after PRK, 13:206
problems/complications with, 3:207–211
    ocular surface, 8:106–108
after radial keratotomy, 3:202, 13:205–206
in reducing meridional magnification, 3:181
after refractive surgery, 13:204–208
rehabilitative use of, 3:202–203
for retinal examination, 12:17
rigid (hard) corneal. See Rigid corneal contact lenses; Rigid gas-permeable contact lenses
scleral, 3:185–186, 200–202, 201i
selecting, 3:186–189, 187t, 188i, 190i, 192t
simultaneous vision bifocal
    aspheric, 3:199, 199i
    multifocal, 3:199, 199i
for slit-lamp delivery of photocoagulation, 12:317, 318t

soft. *See* Flexible (soft) contact lenses
tear (fluid) lens and, **3:**180–181, 181*i*
therapeutic use of, **3:**202–203. *See also* Contact
lenses, bandage
toric soft, **3:**195–197, 197*i*, 197*t*
for trial fitting
disinfection of, **1:**51, **8:**50, **9:**262
fluorescein patterns in, **3:**195
use of, overtime, **3:**173, 173*i*
wavefront technology and, **3:**205–206
Contig, **2:**184, 225
Contiguous gene deletion syndrome, **2:**255
Continuous outcome, in screening/diagnostic test,
1:355
Continuous positive airway pressure (CPAP), **1:**156
Continuous subcutaneous insulin infusion (CSII),
1:210–211
Continuous sutures, for penetrating keratoplasty,
8:457–459, 458*i*
Continuous-tear circular capsulorrhexis, for
phacoemulsification, **11:**126–127
Contour interaction (crowding phenomenon), **6:**68
Contour interaction (crowding) bars, for amblyopia
evaluation, **6:**71, 71*i*, 79
Contour stereopsis tests, **6:**93
Contraceptives, oral
central retinal vein occlusion and, **12:**143
hypercoagulability associated with, **1:**171
hypertension and, **1:**96
ocular effects of, **1:**325*t*
tetracycline use and, **2:**433–434
Contracted fornices, anophthalmic socket and, **7:**125
Contracted socket, **7:**125–126, 126*i*
Contractility, myocardial, **1:**129
enhancement of in heart failure management,
1:130–131
reduction of in angina management, **1:**120–121
Contraction, wound, **4:**19
Contralateral antagonist, **6:**37
Contralateral corneal autograft, **8:**472
Contralateral thalamus, **5:**50, 50*i*
Contrast
definition of, **3:**112
enhancing, for low vision patients, **3:**263, 263*i*
Contrast angiography, **5:**66, 68*i*
Contrast sensitivity, **3:**112–115, 114*i*, **12:**45–47
definition of, **3:**114
in glaucoma, **10:**59
loss of, with multifocal IOLs, **11:**146, **13:**164, 173
Snellen acuity and, **3:**112–113
sunglasses affecting, **3:**165
testing, **12:**45–47, 46*i*
in cataract patient, **11:**76, 84–85
spatial, in low vision evaluation, **5:**97
in vision rehabilitation, **3:**251–252
Contrast sensitivity curve, **3:**114, 114*i*
Contrast sensitivity function (CSF), **3:**112–115, 114*i*,
5:97
Contrast threshold, **3:**114, **5:**97
Contrecoup mechanism, in blunt trauma, retinal
breaks caused by, **12:**254
Control charts, **1:**368, 371*i*
Controlled High-Risk Subjects Avonex Multiple
Sclerosis Prevention Study (CHAMPS), **5:**324
Contusion cataract, **11:**55, 56*i*

Contusion injury. *See also* Trauma
lens damage caused by, **11:**55, 56*i*
retinal breaks caused by, **12:**254, 255*i*
Convergence, **6:**38
assessment of, **5:**203–204, **6:**87–88
disorders of, **5:**210–211
fusional, **6:**38, 43, 88
near point of, **6:**87
in near reflex, **2:**111
in refractive accommodative esotropia, **6:**101
spectacle and contact lens correction affecting,
3:149–150, 180
Convergence insufficiency, exotropia and, **6:**112, 117
Convergence paralysis, exotropia and, **6:**117
Convergence-retraction nystagmus, **5:**254, **6:**167
Convergence spasm, **5:**211
Convergent strabismus, **6:**9
Converging lens, **3:**143
Converse bobbing, **5:**256
Conversion disorders, **1:**266
Convex (plus) lenses, anophthalmic socket camouflage
and, **7:**127
Convex mirror, vergence calculations for, **3:**93
COPD. *See* Chronic obstructive pulmonary disease
Copeland intraocular lens, **11:**140*i*, 141*i*, 143
Copeland retinoscope, **3:**125, 125*i*
Copper
in aqueous humor, **2:**317
corneal deposition of, **6:**260, **8:**355–356, 377*t*, **11:**62
Kayser-Fleischer ring caused by, **4:**74, **8:**356, 356*i*,
377*t*
foreign body of, **11:**59, **12:**299
Cor pulmonale, **1:**154
Cordarone. *See* Amiodarone
Corectopia, **2:**170, **6:**269
midbrain, **5:**260
Coreg. *See* Carvedilol
Corgard. *See* Nadolol
Cornea
abnormal, keratoconus and, **3:**199–200, 200*i*
abrasions of, **4:**19–20, **8:**406–407
cataract surgery in diabetic patients and, **11:**205
in children, **6:**445
with contact lenses, **3:**208
aging of, **8:**362
amyloid deposits in. *See* Cornea, deposits in,
amyloid
anatomy of, **2:**43*i*, 44, 45–49, 46*i*, 48*i*, 49*i*, **8:**8–13, 9*i*
refractive surgery and, **3:**231–234, 235*i*, **13:**5–6
anesthesia of
congenital, **8:**299
herpes simplex epithelial keratitis and, **8:**144
neurotrophic keratopathy and, **8:**102, 151
apex of, **3:**175, 205, **8:**39, 40*i*
apical zone of, **3:**174, 205, **8:**38
basal lamina of, **2:**45, 46*i*
biochemistry and metabolism of, **2:**297–302, 298*i*
biomechanics of, **8:**12–13, 13*i*, 14*i*, **13:**18–28
incisional effect and, **8:**13, 14*i*
keratorefractive surgery affecting, **13:**19–28
biopsy of, **8:**440
for ocular microbiology, **8:**135
blood staining of, **4:**73, 76*i*, **8:**399, 400–401, 400*i*,
401*i*, **10:**110, 110*i*

Bowman's layer/membrane of, 2:45–46, 46*i*, 298*i*, 299–300, 4:61–62, 61*i*, 8:9*i*, 10
  anatomy of, 2:45–46, 46*i*, 298*i*, 299
  biochemistry and metabolism of, 2:299–300
  dystrophy of, 8:315, 316*i*
  refractive surgery and, 2:299–300
central, 2:45, 46*i*
childhood systemic diseases affecting, 6:259, 259*i*
congenital/developmental anomalies of, 2:167–168, 167*i*, 4:62–65, 6:250–255, 251*i*, 252*i*, 254*i*, 8:285–302
  basic concepts of, 8:281–283
  causes of, 8:281–282
  central, 6:254–255, 254*i*
  diagnostic approach to, 8:282–283
  opacities, 8:297–298
  peripheral, 6:251–253, 251*i*, 253*i*
  secondary abnormalities causing, 8:298–302
  of size and shape, 6:250–251, 251*i*, 8:288–291
  of structure and/or clarity, 8:291–298
conjunctival mechanical functions and, 8:59–60
conjunctivalization of, 8:58
curvature of, 8:39–40
  in infants and children, 6:199, 200*t*, 201*i*
  keratometry in measurement of, 3:298–302, 299*i*, 300*i*
  keratoscopy in measurement of, 3:302, 8:41, 41*i*
  mean, 8:43, 45*i*, 13:7
  power and, 8:39–40, 13:6–7, 7*i*
  radius of, 8:9, 41
    instantaneous (tangential power), 8:43, 43*i*, 44*i*, 13:7, 7*i*
    keratometry in measurement of, 8:40–41
    in schematic eye, 3:106*i*
degenerations of. *See* Corneal degenerations; Keratopathy
deposits in, 8:346*t*
  amyloid, 8:345–349, 347*t*, 348*i*, 372. *See also* Amyloidosis/amyloid deposits
    in Avellino dystrophy, 4:72–73
    in gelatinous droplike dystrophy, 8:321, 321*i*, 347*t*, 348–349
    in lattice dystrophy, 4:71–72, 75*i*, 8:318, 349
  differential diagnosis of, 8:346*t*, 350
  drug-induced, 8:375–376, 376*t*
  immunoglobulin synthesis disorders and, 8:349–350
Descemet's membrane of. *See* Descemet's membrane/layer
development of, 2:150–152, 150*i*, 151*i*, 152*i*, 6:199, 200*t*, 201*i*, 249, 8:6
diameter of, in infants and children, 6:199, 200*t*, 201*i*, 250
  abnormalities of, 6:250–251, 251*i*
disorders of, 4:61–76, 8:24–25*t*. *See also specific type and* Keratitis; Keratoconjunctivitis; Keratopathy
  blunt trauma causing, 8:396, 396*i*
  cataract surgery in patients with, 11:207–211
  contact lens–related, 3:207–209, 208*i*, 8:108
  contrast sensitivity affected by, 3:115
  decreased vision and, 5:103
  degenerations. *See* Corneal degenerations; Keratopathy
  dystrophies. *See* Corneal dystrophies
  ectatic, 8:329–355

illusions caused by, 5:188
immune-mediated, 8:201–202, 224–234
in infants and children, 6:249–260
inherited, 8:309–310*t*
ionizing radiation causing, 8:388–389
metabolic disorders and, 6:436–437*i*, 8:309–310*t*, 335–357, 337*t*, 339*t*, 346*t*, 347*t*, 351–353*t*, 358*t*. *See also specific disorder*
neoplastic, 4:76, 8:253–278. *See also specific tumor type*
NSAID use and, 1:197–198
in rosacea, 8:84–85, 84*i*, 85*i*
Th1 delayed hypersensitivity and, 9:68*t*
thermal burns causing, 8:387
ultraviolet radiation causing, 8:388
donor. *See* Donor cornea
drug absorption and, 2:383–386, 385*i*
dysplasia of, 4:76
dystrophies of. *See* Corneal dystrophies
edema of, 8:33–34, 34*t*
  birth trauma causing, 8:300, 300*i*
  after cataract surgery, 11:104, 166–168, 192–193, 193*i*
    persistent, with vitreocorneal adherence, 11:167
  cold-induced, 8:388
  in congenital/infantile glaucoma, 6:272, 273*i*
  in Fuchs endothelial dystrophy, 8:324, 325, 325*i*, 326*i*, 327
  intraocular lenses and, 11:104, 192–193, 193*i*
  intraocular surgery causing, 8:418–420
  in keratoconus, 8:330
  after keratotomy, 13:59, 60*i*
  management of, 8:441–442
  orthokeratology causing, 13:85
  pathophysiology of, 8:385–386
endothelium of, 4:61–62, 61*i*, 8:9*i*, 12
  anatomy of, 2:47–49, 49*i*, 298*i*
  anterior chamber phakic IOLs affecting, 13:151, 153*t*
  biochemistry and metabolism of, 2:301–302
  development of, 8:6
  dysfunction of, corneal edema and, 8:33–34, 34*t*, 385–386
  glucose metabolism in, 2:297–299, 298*i*
  intraocular surgery causing changes in, 8:419–420
  iris-fixated phakic IOLs affecting, 13:153*t*, 154
  posterior chamber phakic IOLs affecting, 13:153*t*, 154
  PRK/LASEK and, 13:105
  wound healing/repair of, 4:21–22, 21*i*, 8:384–386
enlargement of, in congenital/infantile glaucoma, 6:273
epithelium of, 4:61–62, 61*i*, 8:9–10, 9*i*, 58
  anatomy of, 2:45, 46*i*, 298*i*, 299
  biochemistry and metabolism of, 2:299
  cytologic identification of, 8:64
  defects of, 8:25*t*
    persistent, 8:101–104, 103*i*
    after penetrating keratoplasty, 8:461
  evaluation of in pseudoepiphora, 7:273
  intraocular surgery causing changes in, 8:418–419
  physiology of, 8:58
  preservation of in LASEK, 13:94–95, 94*i*
  protection of during cataract surgery in diabetic patients, 11:205

removal of for PRK, **13**:93–94, 93*i*
tumors of, **8**:255–261, 255*t*
wound healing/repair of, **4**:21–22, 21*i*, **8**:383–384, 424
  after PRK/LASEK, **13**:97
erosions of
  in herpetic keratitis, **8**:151
  after LASIK, **13**:122
    in diabetic patients, **13**:197
  punctate epithelial, **8**:24*t*, 30*i*
  recurrent, **8**:98–100, 100*i*
    eye pain and, **5**:298, **8**:98
    posttraumatic, **8**:407
examination of, **8**:15–51. *See also* Examination, ophthalmic
  before cataract surgery, **11**:81–82, 207–208
  in glaucoma, **10**:33–34
    in children, **6**:274
exposure of, in craniosynostosis-induced proptosis, **6**:427–428
in external eye defense, **8**:114
extraocular surgery affecting, **8**:420
farinata, **8**:370
fetal, secondary abnormalities affecting, **8**:298–302
flat (cornea plana), **8**:290–291, 309*t*
  sclerocornea and, **8**:290, 291, 295, 295*i*
foreign body in, **8**:404–406, 406*i*
  in children, **6**:445–446
function of, **8**:5
guttata/guttae, **8**:34
  Brown-McLean syndrome and, **11**:167
  cataract surgery and, **11**:81, 82
  central, **2**:47, 49*i*
  in Fuchs dystrophy, **2**:49*i*, **4**:73, **8**:324, 325, 325*i*, 326*i*
  peripheral (Hassall-Henle bodies/warts), **2**:47, **8**:362, 375
hydration of, **8**:11–12
hypersensitivity reactions of, **8**:198–201, 199*i*, 199*t*
immune response/immunologic features of, **8**:195–196, 196*t*, 201–202, **9**:34*t*, 39, 40*i*
infection/inflammation of, **4**:65–67, **8**:24–25*t*, 26–29, 30*i*, 31*i*, 32*i*, 32*t*, 179–192. *See also* Keratitis; Keratoconjunctivitis
innervation of, **2**:297, **8**:9
intraepithelial neoplasia of, **4**:76, **8**:255*t*, 259, 259*i*
keloids of, **8**:373
  congenital, **8**:299
lacerations of, **12**:295
  in children, **6**:447
  Seidel test in identification of, **8**:22, 22*i*
layers of, **2**:297, 298*i*
limbal mechanical functions and, **8**:59–60
marginal infiltrates of
  blepharoconjunctivitis and, **8**:229
  staphylococcal blepharitis and, **8**:165, 166*i*, 168, 229
melting of (keratolysis)
  cataract surgery and, **11**:180–181
    in patients with dry eye, **11**:180, 206–207
  peripheral ulcerative keratitis and, **8**:231
mucin tear secretion affecting, **8**:57
multifocal, retinoscopy in detection of, **8**:49
neovascularization of
  contact lens wear causing, **8**:108

inflammation and, **8**:29
  in stem cell deficiency, **8**:109
nonepithelial cells in, **2**:45
oblate shape of, **13**:6
opacification of
  in central cloudy dystrophy of François, **8**:323, 324*i*
  chromosomal aberrations and, **8**:298
  congenital, **8**:297–298
  in hereditary syndromes, **8**:298
  infantile, **6**:255–259, 256*i*, 256*t*, 258*i*
  inflammation causing, **8**:29
  after lamellar keratoplasty, **8**:474
  penetrating keratoplasty for, **8**:453
  in Peters anomaly, **11**:32
  in Schnyder crystalline dystrophy, **8**:322, 322*i*
oxygen supply of, **3**:185
perforation of. *See also* Corneoscleral laceration; Perforating injuries
  in children, **6**:447
  LASIK and, **13**:121
  management of, **8**:441–442
    steps in surgical repair and, **8**:411–412, 413*i*, 414*i*
  NSAID use and, **1**:197–198
  radial keratotomy and, **13**:64
  wound healing/repair and, **8**:385
peripheral, **2**:45, 46*i*
phacoemulsification affecting, **11**:167–168
pigmentation/pigment deposits in, **4**:73–74, 76*i*, **8**:375
  drug-induced, **8**:376–378, 377*t*
plana, **8**:290–291, 309*t*
  sclerocornea and, **8**:290, 291, 295, 295*i*
posterior depression of (central posterior keratoconus), **6**:254
prolate shape of, **13**:6
  intrastromal corneal ring segments and, **13**:77
refractive index of, **3**:40*t*, **8**:8, 40
refractive power of, **8**:39–40
  keratometry in measurement of, **8**:40–41
reshaping, orthokeratology and, **3**:203–205, 204*i*, 205*i*
in schematic eye, **3**:106*i*
scleralization of, **4**:64
sensation in
  measurement of (esthesiometry), **8**:35
  reduction of
    in herpes simplex epithelial keratitis, **8**:144
    in neurotrophic keratopathy, **8**:102–103, 151
shape of, **8**:8–9, 39–40, **13**:5–6, 8
  curvature and power and, **8**:39–40, **13**:6–7, 7*i*
  disorders of, **6**:250–251, **8**:288–291
  orthokeratology and, **3**:203–205, 204*i*, 205*i*
  refractive surgery and, **3**:231–234, 235*i*, **13**:5–6, 47
size of, disorders of, **6**:250–251, 251*i*, **8**:288–291
specimen collection from, **8**:135, 136*i*
staphyloma of, congenital, **4**:65
stem cells of, **8**:8, 108, 246, 424
stroma of, **4**:61–62, 61*i*, **8**:9*i*, 10–12, 10*i*, 11*i*
  anatomy of, **2**:46–47, 298*i*, 300–301
  biochemistry and metabolism of, **2**:300–301
  development of, **2**:151, 151*i*, 152*i*, **8**:6
  inflammation of, **8**:29, 31*i*, 32*t*
    in systemic infections, **8**:189–190

neovascularization of, contact lenses causing,
    8:108
wound healing/repair of, 4:20, 8:384
surgery affecting
    extraocular procedures and, 8:420
    intraocular procedures and, 8:418–420
thickness of, 8:31, 33*i*
    intraocular pressure and, 8:11, 34
    measurement of, 3:293–294, 294*i*, 8:31–34, 33*i*.
        See also Pachymetry
        before refractive surgery, 13:47–48
    minimum requirements for LASIK and, 13:111
    primary open-angle glaucoma and, 10:10
topography of, 2:43*i*, 44, 3:302–303, 303*i*, 304*i*,
    4:61–62, 61*i*, 8:38–49, 9:39, 40*i*, 13:6–12
    after arcuate keratotomy, 13:69
    astigmatism detection/management and, 8:46, 48
    cataract surgery and, 11:82, 87
    central islands after PRK and, 13:101, 101*i*
    computerized, 8:41–46, 42*i*, 43*i*, 44*i*, 45*i*, 46*i*,
        13:6–12, 47
    elevation-based, 13:6, 8
    indications for, 8:46–48, 47*i*, 48*i*
    in IOL selection, 3:218
    keratorefractive surgery and, 8:46–48, 47*i*, 48*i*
    before LASIK, 13:111
    after limbal relaxing incisions, 13:69
    limitations of, 8:48–49, 13:11
    measurement of, 8:38–49
    after penetrating keratoplasty, 13:12
    placido-based, 3:302–303, 303*i*, 304*i*, 8:41, 13:6, 7,
        8, 47
        computerized, 8:41–46, 42*i*, 43*i*, 44*i*, 45*i*, 46*i*,
            13:6
        in keratoconus, 8:331, 331*i*
    after radial keratotomy, 13:10, 10*i*, 63
    refractive surgery and, 13:6–12, 47, 48*i*
        indications for, 13:9–10, 9*i*
transparency of, 8:11–12
transplantation of, 8:447–451, 453–476. *See also*
    Donor cornea; Keratoplasty, penetrating
    autograft procedures for, 8:453, 471–472
    basic concepts of, 8:447–451
    for chemical burns, 8:393
    clinical approach to, 8:453–476
    donor selection and, 8:449–451, 451*t*
    eye banking and, 8:449–451, 451*t*
    histocompatibility antigens and, 8:447
    immune privilege and, 8:195–196, 447–448
    immunobiology of, 8:447–448
    lamellar keratoplasty (allograft procedure) and,
        8:472–476, 473*i*
    pediatric, 8:470–471, 470*t*
    rabies virus transmission and, 8:163
    after refractive surgery, 13:203–204
tumors of, 4:76, 8:253–278. *See also specific type*
in uveitis, 9:103*t*
vascularization of
    in atopic keratoconjunctivitis, 8:212, 213*i*
    after lamellar keratoplasty, 8:474
vertex of, 8:39, 40*i*
verticillata, 8:340, 341*i*, 375–376, 376*t*
    in Fabry disease, 12:244, 246*i*
wound healing/repair of, 4:19–24, 8:383–386, 424
    keratorefractive surgery and, 13:28–29

zones of, 8:38–39, 39*i*, 40*i*
Cornea–air interface, reflection at, 3:13
Cornea–aqueous interface, reflection at, 3:13
Cornea Donor Study, 8:469
Cornea shields, collagen, for drug administration,
    2:390–391
Corneal allografts. *See* Corneal grafts
Corneal arcus
    in dyslipoproteinemia/hyperlipoproteinemia, 1:151,
        293, 8:338, 339*t*, 369
    juvenilis, 2:127, 8:302, 338, 339*t*, 369
    in Schnyder crystalline dystrophy, 8:322, 322*i*
    senilis, 8:369
Corneal autografts. *See* Corneal grafts
Corneal bandage lenses. *See* Bandage contact lenses
Corneal buttons, 4:68–69
Corneal cap, 8:9
Corneal contact lens electrode, for electroretinogram,
    12:29
Corneal contact lenses, rigid. *See* Rigid corneal contact
    lenses
Corneal degenerations, 4:67–70, 8:361*t*, 362, 368–375.
    See also specific type and Keratopathy
    dystrophies differentiated from, 8:361*t*
    endothelial, 8:375
    epithelial/subepithelial, 8:368–369
    stromal
        age-related (involutional) changes and, 8:369–370
        peripheral, 8:370–371
        postinflammatory changes and, 8:372–374
Corneal dystrophies, 4:70–73, 72*i*, 73*i*, 74*i*, 75*i*,
    8:311–328. *See also specific type*
    anterior, 8:311–315
    of Bowman's layer, 8:315, 316*i*
    definition of, 8:311
    degenerations differentiated from, 8:361*t*
    diagnostic approach to, 8:308
    endothelial, 8:324–329
        cataract surgery in patients with, 11:208, 210*i*
        congenital hereditary, 6:256*t*, 257, 8:297–298, 298*i*,
            309*t*
        Fuchs, 2:49, 49*i*, 4:73, 75*i*, 8:310*t*, 324–327, 325*i*,
            326*i*
    epithelial
        basement membrane (map-dot-fingerprint/
            anterior membrane), 4:70, 72*i*, 8:310*t*,
            311–313, 312*i*
            cataract surgery in patients with, 11:208, 209*i*
            refractive surgery in patients with, 13:44, 46*i*
        juvenile (Meesmann), 8:310*t*, 313, 314*i*
    gene linkage of, 8:308, 309–310*t*
    Lisch, 8:310*t*, 313–315, 314*i*
    metabolic disorders and, 8:309–310*t*, 335–357
    molecular genetics of, 8:305–308, 309–310*t*
    stromal, 8:316–323, 316*t*
        congenital hereditary, 6:256*t*, 257, 8:297
        posterior amorphous, 8:297
Corneal elastosis, 8:368–369. *See also* Spheroidal
    degeneration
Corneal endothelial rings, traumatic, 8:396, 397*i*
Corneal flap folds, after LASIK, 13:122–126, 124*i*, 125*i*
Corneal grafts. *See also* Donor cornea; Keratoplasty,
    penetrating
    allografts, 8:453
    autografts, 8:453, 471–472

disease recurrence in, 8:461, 462*i*
endothelial failure of
    late nonimmune, 8:464
    primary, 8:461, 461*i*
inflammatory necrosis of, after lamellar keratoplasty,
    8:475
prior LASIK affecting, 13:204
rejection of, 8:448, 449, 466–470, 468*i*, 469*i*, 9:39,
    40*i*, 41. *See also* Rejection (graft)
Corneal haze. *See* Haze formation
Corneal incision, clear, for cataract surgery,
    11:100–101, 123–125, 125*i*, 126*i*
    minimizing bleeding risk and, 11:202
Corneal inlays, 13:71–85
    alloplastic, 13:72–73, 73*i*, 175
    homoplastic, 13:71–72
    for keratophakia, 13:71–72, 72–73, 73*i*
    for presbyopia, 13:175–176
Corneal intraepithelial neoplasia, 4:76, 8:255*t*, 259, 259*i*
Corneal light reflex tests, 6:82–84, 84*i*
"Corneal light shield," 13:95
Corneal melting (keratolysis)
    cataract surgery and, 11:180–181
        in patients with dry eye, 11:180, 206–207
    peripheral ulcerative keratitis and, 8:231
Corneal nerves, 2:297, 8:9
    enlarged, 8:357, 357*i*, 358*t*
        in multiple endocrine neoplasia, 1:230–231, 231*i*,
        8:357, 357*i*, 358*t*
Corneal nodules, Salzmann, 8:372, 372*i*
Corneal onlays, 13:71–85
    alloplastic, for epikeratoplasty (epikeratophakia),
    13:77
Corneal power maps, 13:6–7, 47
Corneal refractive therapy, 13:84–85
Corneal ring segments, intrastromal, 13:23–24, 26*i*,
    77–84, 78*i*, 79*t*
    complications of, 13:81–82, 82*i*
    corneal transplantation after, 13:204
    expulsion of, 13:81, 82*i*
    instrumentation for, 13:79–80, 79*t*
    for keratoconus, 13:83, 186
    outcomes of, 13:80–81
    patient selection for, 13:78–79
    penetrating keratoplasty after, 13:204
    risks/benefits of, 13:50*t*
    technique for, 13:80, 80*i*
Corneal storage medium, 2:454, 8:449
Corneal stress model, 8:11, 12*i*, 13:23, 24*i*
Corneal surgery
    incisional, 13:59–70. *See also* Keratotomy
        for astigmatism correction, 13:66–69, 67*i*, 69*t*
        biomechanics affected by, 8:13, 14*i*
        for hyperopia, 13:66
        for myopia, 13:59–66. *See also* Radial keratotomy
    refractive. *See* Keratorefractive surgery
Corneal tattoo, 8:377*t*, 442–443
Corneal transplant. *See* Cornea, transplantation of;
    Donor cornea; Keratoplasty, penetrating
Corneal ulcers, 8:25*t*. *See also* Keratitis
    in herpes simplex keratitis, 8:143, 143*i*, 144*i*, 151
    Mooren, 8:231, 232–234, 233*i*, 234*i*
    neurotrophic, herpetic keratitis and, 8:103, 103*i*, 151
    in vernal conjunctivitis/keratoconjunctivitis, 6:235,
        8:210

von Hippel internal. *See* Keratoconus, posterior
Corneal wedge resection, for corneal astigmatism after
    penetrating keratoplasty, 13:67*i*, 187
Corneoretinal dystrophy, Bietti crystalline, 8:342–343
Corneoscleral junction, 2:51, 55*i*, 58*i*
Corneoscleral laceration. *See also* Anterior segment,
    trauma to; Perforating injuries
    repair of, 8:410–416, 411*i*
        anesthesia for, 8:411
        in children, 6:447
        postoperative management and, 8:416–417
        secondary repair measures and, 8:415–416, 417*i*,
            418*i*
        steps in, 8:411–414, 412*t*, 413*i*, 414*i*, 415*i*
    Seidel test in identification of, 8:22, 22*i*
Corneoscleral meshwork, 2:56–57, 57*i*, 4:77–78
Coronal scalp flap, for anterior orbitotomy, 7:110
Coronary angiography/arteriography, 1:115, 119–120,
    123–124
Coronary angioplasty, percutaneous transluminal
    (PTCA/balloon angioplasty)
    for angina, 1:121
    for ST-segment elevation acute coronary syndrome,
        1:125
    troponin levels in determining need for, 1:117
Coronary artery bypass graft (CABG), 1:121–122
    troponin levels in determining need for, 1:117
Coronary artery stenosis, hemodynamically significant,
    1:120
Coronary cataract, 4:97, 11:36
Coronary heart disease (coronary artery
    atherosclerosis), 1:111. *See also* Ischemic heart
    disease
    in diabetes, 1:218
    hypercholesterolemia and, 1:143, 143–144
    hypertension management and, 1:91*t*, 94
    risk factors for, 1:112–113
    screening for, 1:293–294
Coronary syndrome, acute. *See* Acute coronary
    syndrome; Myocardial infarction
Coronary vasospasm, angina pectoris caused by, 1:113
Coronavirus, SARS caused by, 1:33
Corpuscular theory of light, 3:3
Corrected loss variance, 10:69
Corrected pattern standard deviation, 10:69
Correcting lenses, in retinoscopy, 3:128–129, 129*i*
Correspondence, 6:41–43, 42*i*
Corrugator muscle, 7:140, 143*i*
Cortex
    lens, 2:75*i*, 76, 324–325, 324*i*, 4:94, 11:9
        degenerations of, 4:100–101, 101*i*, 102*i*
    occipital/visual. *See* Occipital (primary visual/
        calcarine/striate) cortex
    vitreous, 4:105, 12:279
Cortical blindness. *See* Cerebral blindness
Cortical bone, 1:241
Cortical cataracts, 11:46–48, 48*i*, 49*i*, 50*i*, 51*i*, 52*i*
Cortical potentials, 12:39–41
    electrically evoked, 12:41
    visually evoked. *See* Visually evoked cortical
        potentials
Cortical spokes, 11:47–48, 49*i*
Cortical visual impairment (cortical blindness). *See*
    Cerebral blindness

Corticosteroids (steroids), 1:194–196, 2:416–420, 417*t*,
  419*t*
  for *Acanthamoeba* keratitis, 8:188
  for adenovirus infection, 8:159
  adverse effects of, 2:418–420
  for allergic conjunctivitis, 8:209
  for anaphylaxis, 1:319
  anti-inflammatory/pressure-elevating potency of,
    2:419–420, 419*t*
  for bacterial keratitis, 8:183–184
  for Behçet syndrome, 1:193–194
  for Bell's palsy, 5:284
  after cataract surgery in children, 6:302
  cataracts caused by, 11:50–52
  for central retinal vein occlusion, 12:144
  for chalazion, 8:87–88
  for chemical burns, 8:392
  for cicatricial pemphigoid, 8:222, 223
  for Cogan syndrome, 8:229
  for corneal graft rejection, 8:469
  corneal wound healing and, 13:28
  for cystoid macular edema, 12:155
  for dry eye, 8:75, 75*t*
  for endophthalmitis, 9:217, 218*t*, 219
  for eyelid hemangioma, 7:158
  fungal keratitis associated with use of, 8:185
  for giant cell arteritis, 1:190
    central retinal artery occlusion and, 12:150
  for giant papillary conjunctivitis, 8:216
  glaucoma induced by, 10:116–117
  herpes simplex keratitis and, 8:146, 148
  for herpes zoster, 8:155
  for hyphema, 6:448, 8:401, 402
  for idiopathic intracranial hypertension, 5:119
  for idiopathic orbital inflammation, 4:190, 7:58
  intraocular pressure affected by, 2:419–420, 419*t*,
    10:116–117
  for juvenile rheumatoid arthritis, 9:143
  after LASIK, 13:115
    elevated IOP/glaucoma and, 13:189, 190*i*, 208
  for meibomian gland dysfunction, 8:83
  for multifocal choroiditis and panuveitis syndrome,
    12:178
  for ocular allergy, 6:236, 236*t*, 8:209
  ocular side effects of, 1:325*t*
  for orbital hemangiomas in children, 6:377–378
  in orbital surgery, 7:114–115
  for pars planitis, 9:149–150, 12:182
  in perioperative setting, 1:334
  for peripheral ulcerative keratitis, 8:231
  after PRK/LASEK, 13:96, 97
    complications associated with, 13:105, 189, 208
    myopic regression in overcorrection and, 13:100
  ptosis caused by eyedrops containing, 5:278
  for pulmonary diseases, 1:157*t*, 158
  for punctate inner choroidopathy, 12:179
  for rheumatic disorders, 1:194–196
  for rosacea, 8:86
  route of administration of in ocular inflammation,
    2:420, 421*t*
  for scleritis, 8:240–241
  for seborrheic blepharitis, 8:86
  for shock, 1:319
  for staphylococcal eye infection, 8:167
  for Stevens-Johnson syndrome, 6:237, 8:218
  for stromal keratitis, 8:148, 149*t*
  in tear secretion, 2:293–294
  for Thygeson superficial punctate keratitis, 8:225
  for thyroid-associated orbitopathy, 5:331
  for toxocariasis, 6:317–318, 12:191
  for toxoplasmosis, 6:217, 9:169
  for traumatic visual loss, 7:104, 108
  for tuberculous ocular disease, 9:195, 196*i*
  for uveal lymphoid infiltration, 4:280
  for uveitis, 9:96, 114, 114*t*, 115–118, 115*t*, 117*i*, 128
    before cataract surgery, 9:235
    in children, 6:319
    intraocular pressure elevation and, 9:238
    tuberculous, 9:195, 196*i*
    viral, 9:140
  for vernal keratoconjunctivitis, 8:211
  for Vogt-Koyanagi-Harada syndrome, 9:205, 12:181
  withdrawal from, 1:195
  wound healing affected by, 8:383
Corticotroph adenomas, 1:228
Corvert. *See* Ibutilide
Corynebacterium, 8:125
  diphtheriae, 8:125
    invasive capability of, 8:117
    as normal ocular flora, 8:115*t*
    ocular infection caused by, 8:125
  xerosis, 8:92, 125
Corzide. *See* Nadolol
Cosmetic facial surgery, 7:235–248. *See also specific
  procedure and* Facial surgery
Cosmetic optics, for anophthalmic socket, 7:127
Cosmid vector, 2:184
Cosopt, 2:411*t*, 414–415, 10:164*t*, 173
  for childhood glaucoma, 6:283
Cottage cheese pattern, in treated retinoblastoma,
  6:398
Cotton-wool spots, 4:129, 12:145–146, 146*i*
  in branch retinal vein occlusion, 12:136
  in central retinal vein occlusion, 5:106, 106*i*, 107,
    12:141, 142*i*
  in diabetic retinopathy, 12:104
  in HIV retinopathy, 5:361, 9:248, 249*i*
  precapillary retinal arteriole obstruction causing,
    12:145–146, 146*i*
  in radiation retinopathy, 1:256
  in systemic lupus erythematosus, 1:182, 9:173, 173*i*
Couching, 11:89, 90*i*, 91*i*
Cough, 1:153
  in COPD, cataract surgery and, 11:204
Coumadin. *See* Warfarin
Counseling, genetic. *See* Genetic testing/counseling
Coup mechanism, in blunt trauma, retinal breaks
  caused by, 12:254
Coupling, 8:13, 13:19, 66, 67*i*
Cover tests, 6:80–82, 81*i*
  ARC testing and, 6:57
  for intermittent exotropia evaluation, 6:111
Cover-uncover test, 6:80–81, 81*i*
Covera. *See* Verapamil
Coviracil. *See* Emtricitabine
Cowden disease, eyelid manifestations of, 4:176*t*
Cowdry type I inclusion bodies, 8:69
Cow's eye, 10:147
COX-1/COX-2. *See* Cyclooxygenase
COX-2 inhibitors, 1:173, 196, 197*t*, 2:307, 9:96

Coxsackievirus conjunctivitis, **8:**163

Cozaar. *See* Losartan

CP. *See* Cicatricial pemphigoid

CPAP. *See* Continuous positive airway pressure

CPEO. *See* Chronic progressive external ophthalmoplegia

CPEO-plus syndromes, **2:**218

CPK. *See* Creatine kinase

CPR. *See* Cardiopulmonary resuscitation

CRA. *See* Central retinal artery

Crab louse *(Phthirus pubis),* **8:**133, 133*i*
  ocular infection caused by, **8:**133, 169
    cholinesterase inhibitors for, **2:**400

CRABP. *See* Cellular retinoic acid-binding protein

"Crack babies," **1:**271

CRALBP. *See* Cellular retinaldehyde-binding protein/ cytoplasmic retinal-binding protein

Cranial fossa
  anterior, **5:**9, 10
  middle, **7:**21

Cranial nerve I (olfactory nerve), anatomy of, **2:**93, 94*i*, 95*i*

Cranial nerve II. *See* Optic nerve

Cranial nerve III (oculomotor nerve), **7:**13, 14
  aberrant regeneration of, **5:**232, 232*i*, 270
    synkinesis in, **7:**211, 215–217
  in accommodation, **11:**22
  anatomy of, **2:**94*i*, 108–110, 109*i*, 110*i*, **5:**43, 44*i*, 45–49, 45–49*i*
  aneurysms affecting, **2:**109
  congenital palsy of, ptosis caused by, **7:**215–217
  extraocular muscles innervated by, **2:**18–19, 108–110, 109*i*
  inferior division of, **2:**110
  motor root of, **2:**14, 14*i*
  palsy of. *See* Third nerve (oculomotor) palsy
  superior division of, **2:**110

Cranial nerve IV (trochlear nerve), **7:**13, 14
  aberrant regeneration of, superior oblique myokymia and, **6:**156
  anatomy of, **2:**94*i*, 111, 112*i*, **5:**43, 44*i*, 45–49*i*
  extraocular muscles innervated by, **2:**18
  palsy of. *See* Fourth nerve (trochlear) palsy

Cranial nerve V (trigeminal nerve)
  anatomy of, **2:**94*i*, 112–116, 113*i*, **5:**50, 50*i*, 51*i*, 52, 53*i*, 54
  divisions of, **2:**113*i*, 114–116
  eyelids supplied by, **8:**6
  in herpes simplex infection, **8:**140
  in herpes zoster, **8:**152, 153–154
  neurotrophic keratopathy caused by damage to, **8:**102
  in reflex tear arc, **8:**57
  V₁ (ophthalmic nerve), **2:**94*i*, 113, 113*i*, 114–115, **5:**52, 53*i*, **7:**14, 15
    facial innervation and, **7:**137
    in reflex tear arc, **7:**253
    sensory root of, **2:**13, 14*i*, 113
  V₂ (maxillary nerve), **2:**94*i*, 113, 113*i*, 116, **5:**52, 52*i*, **7:**15
    facial innervation and, **7:**137
  V₃ (mandibular nerve), **2:**94*i*, 113, 113*i*, 116, **5:**52, 53*i*

Cranial nerve VI (abducens nerve), **7:**13, 14
  anatomy of, **2:**94*i*, 116–117, 116*i*, **5:**43, 44*i*

extraocular muscles innervated by, **2:**18

palsy of. *See* Sixth nerve (abducens) palsy

Cranial nerve VII (facial nerve), **2:**117–119, 118*i*, **7:**15, 136, 136*i*, 137–139, 138*i*
  aberrant regeneration of, synkinesis in, **7:**211, 227–228
  anatomy of, **2:**117–119, 118*i*, **5:**54–56, 55*i*
  brain stem lesions involving, **5:**282–283
  cervicofacial division of, **2:**118
  disorders of, **5:**281–290
    diagnosis of, **5:**281, 282*i*
    overactivity, **5:**286–290, 287*t*
    treatment of, **5:**286
    underactivity, **5:**281–286, 283*t*
  distribution of, **5:**282*i*
  essential blepharospasm and, **5:**286–288, 287*i*, **7:**227
  facial myokymia and, **5:**289
  habit spasm and, **5:**290
  hemifacial spasm and, **5:**288–289, 288*i*, **7:**227–228
  labyrinthine segment of, **2:**118
  mastoid segment of, **2:**118
  palsy/paralysis/weakness of. *See* Facial paralysis/ weakness
  peripheral lesions involving, **5:**283–285, 284*i*
  reflex blepharospasm and, **5:**290
  in reflex tear arc, **7:**253
  spastic paretic facial contracture and, **5:**289
  supranuclear lesions involving, **5:**281
  surgical ablation of, for benign essential blepharospasm, **7:**227
  synkinesis of, **5:**280, 280*i*, 284
  temporofacial division of, **2:**118
  tympanic segment of, **2:**118

Cranial nerve VIII (auditory nerve), **5:**54, 55*i*

Cranial nerves, **5:**42–49. *See also specific nerve*
  anatomy of, **2:**13, 93–121, 94*i*
  eyelids supplied by, **7:**147
  orbit supplied by, **7:**14*i*, 15, 19*i*
  palsy/paralysis of
    isolated, **5:**235
    multiple, **5:**235
    neuroimaging of, **5:**74, 74*i*

Craniofacial cleft syndromes, **7:**38–39, 38*i*, 39*i*. *See also specific type*
  lacrimal outflow disorders and, **7:**257–258, 258*i*

Craniofacial dysostosis (Crouzon syndrome), **6:**425, 425*i*, 426*i*, **7:**38, 39*i*, **8:**351*t*
  V-pattern deviations associated with, **6:**119–121, 429

Craniofacial malformations, **6:**421–434, **7:**38–39, 38*i*, 39*i*. *See also specific type*
  approach to child with, **6:**421
  congenital exotropia and, **6:**114
  craniosynostotic, **6:**421–431, 422*i*, 423*i*, **7:**38
  Crouzon, **6:**425, 425*i*, 426*i*, **7:**38, 39*i*
  management of, **6:**430–431
  nonsynostotic, **6:**431–434
  ocular complications of, **6:**426–430

Craniopharyngiomas
  chiasmal syndromes caused by, **5:**161*i*, 162
  nystagmus caused by, **5:**251, **6:**159*t*, 167

Craniosynostosis, **6:**421–424, 422*i*, 423*i*, **7:**38
  etiology of, **6:**424
  syndromes associated with, **6:**425–431. *See also specific type*

CRAO. *See* Central retinal artery, occlusion of

CRBP. *See* Cellular retinoid-binding protein
Creases, eyelid. *See* Eyelids, creases of
Creatine kinase (CK)/creatine kinase isoenzymes, in myocardial infarction, **1**:117
Crede (silver nitrate) prophylaxis, **6**:223
Creeping angle closure, **10**:126
Crest cells. *See* Neural crest cells
CREST syndrome, **1**:185
Cretinism, **1**:221
Creutzfeldt-Jakob disease, corneal transplant in transmission of, **8**:134
Cribriform plate, **2**:93
Cricothyrotomy, **1**:316
    for anaphylaxis, **1**:319
Crigler massage, for nasolacrimal duct obstruction, **7**:261
Crigler-Najjar syndrome, **2**:262*t*
Critical angle, **3**:47–48, 48*i*
Crixivan. *See* Indinavir
Crocodile shagreen, **8**:370
Crocodile tears, **5**:281
Croconazole, **1**:64*t*, 76
Crohn disease (granulomatous ileocolitis), **1**:177, **9**:131–132
Crolom. *See* Cromolyn
Cromolyn, **2**:424, 424*t*
    for allergic conjunctivitis, **8**:208
    for giant papillary conjunctivitis, **8**:216
    for ocular allergy, **6**:236, 236*t*, **8**:208
    for pulmonary diseases, **1**:157*t*, 158
Cross-cylinder refraction, **3**:136–139, 138*i*
Cross-fixation, in classic congenital (essential infantile) esotropia, **6**:98
Cross-over test, alternating, for ocular misalignment, **5**:214
Cross-sectional studies, **1**:349–350
Cross syndrome (oculocerebral hypopigmentation), **6**:346*t*
Crossed diplopia, **6**:59*i*, 60
Crossing over (genetic), **2**:184, 204, 244–245, **8**:307. *See also* Recombination
    unequal, **2**:197
        color vision abnormalities and, **2**:346, 346*i*
Crouzon syndrome (craniofacial dysostosis), **6**:425, 425*i*, 426*i*, **7**:38, 39*i*, **8**:351*t*
    V-pattern deviations associated with, **6**:119–121, 429
Crowding (contour interaction) bars, for amblyopia evaluation, **6**:71, 71*i*, 79
Crowding phenomenon (contour interaction), **6**:68
CRT contact lens, **3**:204, 204*i*, 205*i*
CRV. *See* Central retinal vein
CRVO. *See* Central retinal vein, occlusion of
CRX gene, **12**:204
    cone–rod dystrophy and, **12**:215
    in Leber congenital amaurosis, **6**:335
CRYO-ROP study, **4**:137, **6**:325, 326, 329–330, 351–352
Cryoglobulinemic vasculitis, essential, **1**:189*t*
Cryoglobulins, precipitation of, ophthalmic findings and, **8**:350
Cryolathe, **13**:106
Cryoprobe, for lens extraction, **11**:105
Cryoretinopexy, for retinal detachment in uveitis, **9**:240
Cryotherapy
    for basal cell carcinoma of eyelid, **7**:179
    for branch retinal vein occlusion, **12**:140

    for Coats disease, **12**:157
    for congenital distichiasis, **7**:157
    for conjunctival intraepithelial neoplasia, **8**:258
    for conjunctival papillomas, **8**:256
    for corneal intraepithelial neoplasia, **8**:259
    for melanoma, **4**:238
    for pars planitis, **9**:150
    for retinal angiomas/hemangiomas, **4**:247, **6**:413
    for retinal breaks, **12**:265
    for retinoblastoma, **4**:262
    for retinopathy of prematurity, **4**:137, **6**:329–330, 331*i*, **12**:132–134, 133*i*
    for squamous cell carcinoma of conjunctiva, **8**:260
    for trichiasis, **7**:208, **8**:104
    for von Hippel syndrome/disease, **12**:163
Cryotherapy for Retinopathy of Prematurity (CRYO-ROP) Study, **4**:137, **6**:325, 326, 329–330, 351–352
Cryptococcus neoformans (cryptococcosis), **5**:367–368, **8**:130, **9**:163
    in HIV infection/AIDS, **9**:257
    optic nerve infection caused by, **4**:205
Cryptophthalmos, **2**:125, 166, 166*i*, **6**:209, 209*i*, **7**:158, 159*i*, **8**:285–286, 285*i*
Cryptophthalmos-syndactyly (Fraser syndrome), **6**:209, **8**:286
    eyelid manifestations of, **4**:173*t*, **6**:209
Cryptosporidium parvum (cryptosporidiosis), in HIV infection/AIDS, **1**:48
Crystal violet stain, **4**:36*t*
CrystaLens, **13**:165, 178–179, 179*i*
Crystalline dystrophy
    Bietti corneoretinal, **8**:342–343
    Schnyder, **8**:310*t*, 321–323, 322*i*, 338
Crystalline keratopathy, infectious, **8**:180, 181*i*
    after penetrating keratoplasty, **8**:464, 464*i*
Crystalline lens. *See* Lens
Crystalline maculopathy/retinopathy, drug toxicity causing, **12**:249, 250*i*, 250*t*
Crystallins, **2**:76, 323, 325–327, 326*t*, **11**:11–12, 11*i*. *See also* Lens proteins
    alpha (α), **2**:326, 326*t*, **11**:11–12, 11*i*
    beta (β), **2**:326–327, 326*t*, **11**:11, 11*i*, 12
    betagamma (β,γ), **2**:326–327, 326*t*, **11**:11, 11*i*, 12
    delta (δ), **2**:326*t*, 327
    development of, **2**:140
    epsilon (ε), **2**:326*t*, 327
    evolution and molecular biology of, **11**:13
    gamma (γ), **2**:326*t*, 327, **11**:11, 11*i*, 12
    taxon-specific, **2**:326*t*, 327
Crystalloids, for shock, **1**:318
CS. *See* Cockayne syndrome
CSCR. *See* Central serous chorioretinopathy
CSD. *See* Cat-scratch disease
CSF. *See* Cerebrospinal fluid; Contrast sensitivity function
CSII. *See* Continuous subcutaneous insulin infusion
CSM method, for visual acuity assessment in children, **6**:78–79, 78*t*
CSME (clinically significant macular edema). *See* Macular edema
CSNB. *See* Congenital night blindness, stationary
CSR (central serous retinopathy). *See* Central serous chorioretinopathy
CSS. *See* Churg-Strauss syndrome
CST. *See* Cavernous sinus thrombosis

CT/CT scan. *See* Computed tomography
CTA. *See* Computerized tomographic angiography
CTLs. *See* Cytotoxic T lymphocytes
CTNS gene, in cystinosis, 8:343
Cu-Zn SOD, 2:372
Cultured limbal epithelium, for transplantation, 8:425, 433. *See also* Limbal transplantation
Cupping of optic disc, 2:96, 98
    glaucomatous, 10:51–53, 52*t*, 53*i*
        in infants and children, 6:276, 10:49–50
        physiologic cupping compared with, 10:52, 52*t*
    in megalopapilla, 6:361
    physiologic, glaucomatous cupping compared with, 10:52, 52*t*
    vertical, 10:52
Cupric oxide, antioxidant effect of, oral supplements and, 2:374, 374*t*, 454
Cupuliform (posterior subcapsular) cataract, 4:99, 99*i*, 11:48–49, 53*i*
    in children, 6:291, 292*t*
    corticosteroids causing, 11:50–52
    in myotonic dystrophy, 11:62–63
Curvature (corneal), 8:39–40
    axial, 8:43, 13:6–7, 7*i*
        in infants and children, 6:199, 200*t*, 201*i*
    keratometry in measurement of, 3:298–302, 299*i*, 300*i*
    keratoscopy in measurement of, 3:302, 8:41, 41*i*
    mean, 8:43, 45*i*, 13:7
    power and, 8:39–40, 13:6–7, 7*i*
    radius of, 8:9, 41
        instantaneous (tangential power), 8:43, 43*i*, 44*i*, 13:7, 7*i*
        keratometry in measurement of, 8:40–41
    in schematic eye, 3:106*i*
Curvularia, ocular infection caused by, 8:130
Cushing syndrome
    corticotroph adenoma causing, 1:228–229
    hypertension in, 1:83, 84*t*
Cutaneous basophil hypersensitivity, 9:66
Cutaneous horn, 7:164
Cutaneous leishmaniasis, ocular involvement in, 8:132
Cutaneous leukocytoclastic angiitis, 1:189*t*
Cuticular (basal laminar) drusen, 4:138, 12:221
    age-related macular degeneration differentiated from, 12:59, 67
    vitelliform exudative macular detachment and, 12:220, 220*i*
Cutler-Beard procedure, 7:189, 190*i*
CVOS (Central Vein Occlusion Study Group), 12:144
    iris neovascularization in central retinal vein occlusion and, 12:144–145
CVS. *See* Chorionic villus sampling
CXCR4, in HIV infection/AIDS, 9:242
CXCR4 receptor antagonists, for HIV infection/AIDS, 1:42
Cyanoacrylate adhesives, 8:441–442
    in corneoscleral laceration repair, 8:412
    for perforating injury, 8:410, 441–442
    for peripheral ulcerative keratitis, 8:231
    as tarsorrhaphy alternative, 8:428–429
Cyclic adenosine monophosphate (cAMP), in signal transduction
    in iris–ciliary body, 2:311–312, 312*i*, 313*i*
    in tear secretion, 2:293, 293*i*

Cyclic esotropia, 6:98*t*, 105
Cyclic guanosine monophosphate (cGMP)
    in cone phototransduction, 2:345
    mutations in, 2:226
    in rod phototransduction, 2:342–343, 343*i*
Cyclic guanosine monophosphate (cGMP)-gated channel
    cone, 2:345
        mutations in, 2:350
    rod, 2:342
        mutations in, 2:349
Cyclin-dependent kinases, in carcinogenesis, 1:253
Cyclitic membrane formation, after penetrating injury, 12:296
Cyclitis, chronic. *See* Intermediate uveitis; Pars planitis
Cycloablation, for childhood glaucoma, 6:281–282
Cyclocryotherapy, for childhood glaucoma, 6:281–282
Cyclodeviations, double Maddox rod test for evaluation of, 6:85
Cyclodialysis, 4:24–25, 25*i*, 83, 8:398, 10:44
    after cataract surgery, 11:181–182
    in lowering intraocular pressure, 10:206
Cyclogyl. *See* Cyclopentolate
Cyclomydril. *See* Cyclopentolate
Cyclooxygenase (COX-1/COX-2), 1:196, 9:79
    aspirin affecting, 1:331, 2:422
    in free radical generation, 2:366
    nonsteroidal anti-inflammatory drugs and, 1:196, 2:306, 422, 9:96. *See also* Cyclooxygenase-2 (COX-2) inhibitors
    in prostaglandin synthesis, 2:305–306, 306*i*
Cyclooxygenase-2 (COX-2) inhibitors, 1:173, 196, 197*t*, 2:307, 9:96
Cyclopentolate, 2:310, 401*t*
    for cycloplegia/cycloplegic refraction, 3:142*t*, 6:94, 94*t*
        in premature infant, 6:326
    for uveitis, 9:114, 128
Cyclophosphamide, 1:200, 258*t*
    for Behçet syndrome, 1:194
    in cancer chemotherapy, 1:258*t*
    for cicatricial pemphigoid, 8:222–223
    for peripheral ulcerative keratitis, 8:231
    for rheumatoid arthritis, 1:174
    for scleritis, 8:241
    for uveitis, 9:119, 119*t*
        in children, 6:321–322
    for Wegener granulomatosis, 1:192
Cyclophotocoagulation, endoscopic, for childhood glaucoma, 6:282
Cyclopia, 2:125, 163–165, 164*i*
    sonic hedgehog mutations causing, 2:165
Cycloplegia/cycloplegics, 2:310, 3:141–142, 142*t*, 11:22
    for amblyopia, 6:73
    anticholinergic agents and, 2:310
    binocular balance testing and, 3:141
    for chemical burns, 8:392
    for hyphema, 6:448, 8:401
    intraocular pressure affected by, 10:117
    muscarinic antagonists and, 2:400–401, 401*t*
    refraction with. *See* Cycloplegic refraction
    side effects of, 3:142, 6:95
    for traumatic iritis, 8:397
    for uveitis, 9:114–115, 114*t*, 128

Cycloplegic refraction, 3:141–142
  in children, 3:146, 6:94–95, 94*t*
  before refractive surgery, 13:42–43
    PRK/LASEK, 13:91, 92
Cyclospora cayatanensis (cyclosporiasis), in HIV
    infection/AIDS, 1:48, 49
Cyclosporine, 2:393–394, 9:97
  for allergic conjunctivitis, 8:208
  for atopic keratoconjunctivitis, 8:213
  for Behçet syndrome, 1:194
  for corneal graft rejection, 8:469
  for dry eye, 2:295, 393, 450, 8:75, 75*t*
  for peripheral ulcerative keratitis, 8:231
  for rheumatoid arthritis, 1:174
  for scleritis, 8:241
  for Thygeson superficial punctate keratitis, 8:225
  for uveitis, 9:97, 119*t*, 120
    in children, 6:320
  for vernal keratoconjunctivitis, 8:211
  for Vogt-Koyanagi-Harada syndrome, 9:205
Cyclosporine A, topical, for dry eye/
    keratoconjunctivitis sicca, 2:295, 393, 450, 8:75, 75*t*
Cyclothymic disorder, 1:265
Cyclovertical muscle palsies, 3-step test in, 6:90–92, 91*i*
Cyclovertical strabismus, surgery planning and, 6:178
Cyklokapron. *See* Tranexamic acid
Cylinder axis
  locating, 3:130–132, 130*i*, 131*i*, 132*i*
  refinement of, cross-cylinder refraction for,
    3:136–139
Cylinder power, 3:95–98
  combined lenses and, 3:99–101, 101*i*
  finding, 3:132–133
  refinement of, cross-cylinder refraction for,
    3:136–139, 138*i*
Cylinders (cylindrical lenses), 3:94–95, 97*i*. *See also*
    Spherocylindrical lenses
  combining, at oblique axes, 3:100–101, 101*i*
  correcting, 3:145
  distortion and, 3:145. *See also* Meridional
    magnification
  guidelines for prescribing, 3:337–338
  location effect of, 3:329–330
  power of. *See* Cylinder power
  prescribing guidelines for, 3:325–339
    revised, 3:337–338
Cylindroma (adenoid cystic carcinoma)
  of eyelid, 7:168
  of lacrimal glands, 4:193–194, 194*i*, 7:90–91
Cymbalta. *See* Duloxetine
CYP1B1 gene
  in glaucoma, 6:271, 10:13*t*
  in Peters anomaly, 8:294
Cyst. *See specific type*
Cystadenoma (apocrine hidrocystoma), of eyelid,
    7:167–168, 169*i*
Cystathionine β-synthase, abnormality of in
    homocystinuria, 6:307, 437*t*, 438
Cysteamine, for cystinosis, 6:259, 8:343–344,
    12:244–245
Cystic carcinoma, adenoid (cylindroma)
  of eyelid, 7:168
  of lacrimal glands, 4:193–194, 194*i*, 7:90–91
Cystic eye, 2:165
Cystic fibrosis, 1:154

Cystic retinal tufts, 12:259, 260, 261*i*
Cysticercosis, 8:133
Cysticercus cellulosae (cysticercosis), 9:171, 172*i*
  orbital involvement and, 7:47
Cystinosis, 6:259, 437*t*, 8:309*t*, 343–344, 344*i*
  corneal changes in, 6:259, 259*i*, 8:309*t*, 343–344, 344*i*
  cysteamine for, 6:259, 8:343–344
  retinal degeneration in, 12:244–245
Cystoid degeneration, peripheral, 4:126, 126*i*, 12:264
  reticular, 4:126, 126*i*, 12:264, 275, 275*i*
  typical, 4:126, 126*i*, 12:264, 275, 275*i*
Cystoid macular edema, 5:104–105, 12:154–156, 155*i*
  angiographic, 12:154
  cataract surgery and, 11:104, 164*t*, 172–174, 173*i*
    in glaucoma patient, 11:218–219
    after Nd:YAG capsulotomy, 11:190–191
  in pars planitis, 9:148, 151, 12:154
  postoperative, 12:332, 333*i*
  prostaglandins and, 9:79
  in retinitis pigmentosa, 12:154, 212, 213*i*
  in sarcoidosis, 8:88
  in uveitis, 9:239
Cystotome, for anterior capsulotomy, 11:109, 126
Cytarabine, 1:258*t*
Cytochrome-b gene, in Leber hereditary optic
    neuropathy, 2:219, 219*i*
Cytogenetics, 2:246–255
  indications for, 2:246, 247*t*
  markers in, 2:221
  preparation for, 2:247–249, 248*i*, 249*i*
Cytoid bodies, 4:128–129, 130*i*
Cytokeratins, in immunohistochemistry, 4:37
Cytokines, 8:197, 198*t*, 9:7, 80–83, 81–82*t*. *See also*
    specific type
  in cancer therapy, 1:261
  in delayed hypersensitivity, 9:63–66, 65*i*
  in external eye defense, 8:113, 114
  in immune processing, 9:22, 23*i*
  in immunotherapy, 9:66–70
  in inflammation/rheumatic disorders, 1:199
  in Sjögren syndrome, 8:78
  in tear film, 2:291
Cytology (ocular), 8:63–70. *See also specific cell type*
  in immune-mediated keratoconjunctivitis, 8:203,
    203*t*
  impression, 8:64, 70*i*
  interpretation of, 8:64–70, 65*t*
  specimen collection for, 8:63–64
  staining procedures in, 8:65*t*
Cytolysin, enterococci producing, 8:125
Cytolysis, immune, 9:59, 60*i*
Cytomegalic inclusion disease, 6:218, 219*i*, 9:157
Cytomegaloviruses, 1:29–30, 9:156–157, 157*i*, 249–250
  cancer association and, 1:254
  congenital infection caused by, 1:29, 6:218, 219*i*,
    9:157
  in HIV infection/AIDS, 1:3, 29, 5:359, 360*i*
    treatment of, 1:47–48
  infection in children caused by, 6:218–219, 219*i*
  retinitis caused by, 1:3, 29, 4:123, 124*i*, 9:156–157,
    157*i*, 12:192–193, 192*i*
    antiviral immunity in, 9:71
    cidofovir for, 1:29, 48, 2:443–444, 9:252
    fomivirsen for, 1:48
    foscarnet for, 1:29, 48, 2:443, 9:251

ganciclovir for, **1:**29, **2:**443, **9:**155, 250–251
in HIV infection/AIDS, **1:**3, 29, 47–48, **9:**71,
156–157, 249–253, 251*i*
Cytoplasmic genes, **2:**217
Cytoplasmic inclusions
in chlamydial infection, **8:**69, 69*i*
cytologic identification of, **8:**65*t*, 69, 69*i*
Cytoplasmic retinal-binding protein/cellular
retinaldehyde-binding protein (CRALBP), **2:**361*t*
in aqueous humor, **2:**317
mutations in, **2:**351
Cytoskeletal (urea-soluble) lens proteins, **2:**327–328,
11:11*i*, 12
Cytotoxic drugs, **9:**96
for Wegener granulomatosis, **1:**192
Cytotoxic hypersensitivity (type II) reaction, **8:**199*i*,
199*t*, 200, **9:**54*t*. See also Cytotoxic T lymphocytes
Cytotoxic T lymphocytes, **9:**24, 25, 66–70, 69*i*
in external eye defense, **8:**114
in viral conjunctivitis, **9:**35
Cytotoxicity, antibody-dependent, **8:**200, **9:**70–72
Cytovene. See Ganciclovir
Cytoxan. See Cyclophosphamide

D

d4T. See Stavudine
D-15 test, for color vision, **12:**44, 45*i*
D-penicillamine, for Wilson disease, **2:**281, **8:**356
Daclizumab, for uveitis in children, **6:**322
Dacryoadenitis, **8:**119*t*
Epstein-Barr virus causing, **8:**119*t*, 156–157
mumps virus causing, **8:**119*t*, 163
sclerosing, **4:**190
Dacryoadenoma, **8:**261
Dacryocele. See Dacryocystocele
Dacryocystectomy, for lacrimal sac tumors, **7:**284
Dacryocystitis, **7:**278–283, **8:**119*t*
acute, **7:**278–279, 279*i*
chronic, **7:**279
tumor associated with, **7:**283–284
Dacryocystocele/dacryocele, **6:**240–241, 240*i*,
7:260–261, 260*i*
Dacryocystography
for acquired tearing evaluation, **7:**272, 273*i*
for dacryolith evaluation, **7:**284
for lacrimal sac tumor evaluation, **7:**284
Dacryocystorhinostomy, **7:**279–283, 281*i*, 282*i*
for congenital tearing/nasolacrimal duct obstruction,
6:247, **7:**266–267
for dacryocystitis, **7:**279–283, 281*i*, 282*i*
Dacryoliths, **7:**283
Dacryoplasty, balloon (balloon catheter dilation), for
congenital tearing/nasolacrimal duct obstruction,
6:246, **7:**264–265
Dactinomycin, **1:**257, 259*t*
DADP. See Amdoxovir
DAG. See Diacylglycerol
Dalen-Fuchs nodules/spots
in sympathetic ophthalmia, **4:**153, 154*i*, **9:**202
in Vogt-Koyanagi-Harada syndrome, **9:**203, 204*i*
Dalfopristin/quinupristin, **1:**63*t*, 74
DALK. See Deep anterior lamellar keratoplasty
Danazol, ocular effects of, **1:**325*t*

Dannheim intraocular lens, **11:**143
Danocrine. See Danazol
Dantrolene, for malignant hyperthermia, **1:**337*t*, **6:**192,
193*t*
Dapiprazole, **2:**309, 408
Dapsone
for cicatricial pemphigoid, **8:**222
for *Pneumocystis carinii (Pneumocystis jiroveci)*
pneumonia, **1:**45
Daptomycin, **1:**63*t*, 75
Daranide. See Dichlorphenamide
Daraprim. See Pyrimethamine
Darier disease, **8:**309*t*
Dark adaptation, sunglasses affecting, **3:**165
Dark adaptation testing, **12:**41–42, 42*i*
in congenital night blindness with fundus
abnormality, **12:**200–201
in congenital stationary night blindness, **12:**198, 199*i*
Dark-adapted electroretinogram, **12:**27, 28*i*, 29, 206*t*.
See also Dark adaptation testing
Dark choroid, in Stargardt disease, **6:**338, **12:**216, 216*i*
Dark-field illumination, for *Treponema pallidum*
visualization, **8:**128
Darkschewitsch, nucleus of, **5:**39
Data presentation, **1:**368–370, 369*i*, 370*i*, 371*i*
Database, monitoring systems and, **1:**364–365
Dawn phenomenon, **1:**210
Day blindness (hemeralopia), in cone/cone–rod
dystrophies, **5:**104, **12:**214
Daypro. See Oxaprozin
DC. See Dendritic cells
DCCT (Diabetes Control and Complications Trial),
1:210, 214–215, **12:**105, 106
DCR. See Dacryocystorhinostomy
ddC (dideoxycytidine). See Zalcitabine
ddI. See Didanosine
DDT. See Dye disappearance test
de Morsier syndrome (septo-optic dysplasia), **2:**175,
176*i*, **5:**139, **6:**362, 454
Deafness
albinism and, **6:**347*t*
cataract surgery in patients with, **11:**201
mitochondrial DNA mutations and, **2:**218, 220
in peripheral vestibular nystagmus, **5:**246
and retinal degeneration, **12:**235. See also Usher
syndrome
Death, sudden, **1:**115–116
Debridement
for *Acanthamoeba* keratitis, **8:**189
for chemical burns, **8:**392
epithelial, for PRK, **13:**93–94, 93*i*
for fungal keratitis, **8:**187
for herpes simplex epithelial keratitis, **8:**145
for recurrent corneal erosions, **8:**100
Decadron. See Dexamethasone
Decamethonium, **2:**403
Decentered ablation, **13:**102–103, 102*i*
Decentration
bifocal segment, **3:**163–164, 170
of intraocular lenses, **11:**164*t*, 191–192, 192*i*
of phakic intraocular lenses, **13:**151, 154–155, 155*i*
for prism correction, **3:**170
Decibel, **5:**92, **10:**60
Decompression
optic canal, for traumatic visual loss, **7:**108

orbital, **7:**115, 116*i*
  complications of, **7:**117
  for lymphangioma, **7:**69
  for thyroid/Graves ophthalmopathy/orbitopathy,
    5:331–332, **7:**54, 115
  for traumatic visual loss, **7:**107, 108
Decongestants
  ocular, **2:**451
  tear production affected by, **8:**81*t*
Decorin, **8:**10, 14
Decosanoids, for glaucoma, **10:**164*t*, 171–172
Decreased vision. *See* Low vision; Visual loss/
    impairment
Deep anterior lamellar keratoplasty (DALK), **8:**472, 475
Deep brain stimulation, for Parkinson disease, **1:**280
Deep lamellar endothelial keratoplasty (DLEK), **8:**472,
    475
Deep mimetic muscles, **7:**135–137, 138–139
Deep plane rhytidectomy, **7:**241*i*, 245
Deep superior sulcus deformity, anophthalmic socket
    and, **7:**124, 124*i*
Deep temporalis fascia, **7:**138
De-epithelialization, for PRK, **13:**93–94, 93*i*
Defense mechanisms, host
  impaired, **8:**117–118. *See also* Immunocompromised
    host
  of outer eye, **8:**113–114
Defensins, in tear film, **2:**290
Defibrillator-cardioverters, implantable (ICDs), **1:**111,
    139–140
  for heart failure, **1:**131
  laser surgery in patient with, **13:**41
  for tachyarrhythmias, **1:**139–140
Defibrillators, portable, public availability of, **1:**313,
    316
Defocus, positive and negative, **13:**15, 15*i*
Defocus aberrations, **3:**238
Defogging, before PRK/LASEK, **13:**91
Deformation, **6:**206
Defy. *See* Tobramycin
Degeneracy, of genetic code, **2:**185
Degenerated epithelial cells. *See* Keratinization
    (keratinized/degenerated epithelial cells)
Degenerations
  anterior chamber/trabecular network, **4:**79–84
  cataracts associated with, **11:**69
  chorioretinal, generalized, **4:**139–140
  choroidal, diffuse, **12:**224–226
  conjunctival, **4:**49–50, 49*i*, 50*i*, **8:**365–367
  corneal, **4:**67–70, **8:**361*t*, 362, 368–375
  definition of, **4:**15–16, **8:**361
  dystrophies differentiated from, **8:**361*t*
  elastotic/elastoid (elastosis), **4:**49*i*, 50
    conjunctival, **8:**365
    corneal, **8:**368–369. *See also* Spheroidal
      degeneration
    solar, of eyelid, **4:**177, 177*i*
  eyelid, **4:**171–174, 173*i*, 173*t*, 174*i*
  lens, **4:**97–102, 102*i*, **10:**102*i*. *See also* Cataract
  macular. *See* Macular degeneration
  optic nerve, **4:**206–208, 207*i*, 208*i*
  orbital, **4:**191, 192*i*
  peripheral and reticular cystoid, **4:**126, 126*i*

retinal, **4:**126–140. *See also specific type and*
    Dystrophies, retinal
    hearing loss and, **12:**235. *See also* Usher syndrome
    systemic disease and, **12:**231–251
  retinal pigment epithelium, **12:**58
  scleral, **4:**90*i*, 91–92, 91*i*, **8:**378, 378*i*
  uveal tract, **4:**155–156
  vitreous, **4:**108–114
Degenerative myopia. *See* High (pathologic/
    degenerative) myopia
Degenerative retinoschisis, typical and reticular, **4:**126,
    12:276, 276*i*
Degradation, optical, for amblyopia, **6:**73
Dehydration, preoperative fasting and, **1:**331
Dehydrogenase, in rods, **2:**344*t*
Deiters tract, ascending, **5:**34
Delavirdine, **1:**41
  for postexposure HIV prophylaxis, **1:**46–47*t*
Delayed hypersensitivity (type IV) reaction, **8:**199, 199*t*,
    201, **9:**25, 54*t*, 63–66, 65*i*, 68*t*
  in chronic mast cell degranulation, **9:**73
  contact dermatoblepharitis as, **8:**205–207, 206*i*
  contact lenses and, **8:**107, 107*i*
  in graft rejection, **8:**448
  response to poison ivy as, **9:**30
  topical medication and, **8:**205–207, 206*i*
  tuberculin form of, **9:**31, 66
Delayed hypersensitivity (DH) T cells, **9:**25, 63–66, 65*i*,
    68*t*. *See also* T cells
Delayed suprachoroidal hemorrhage, after cataract
    surgery, **11:**171
Delirium, **1:**284
Delivery (birth), difficult. *See also* Obstetric history
  corneal edema caused by, **8:**300, 300*i*
  infantile corneal opacities and, **6:**255, 256*t*
  nystagmus caused by, **6:**161
Dellen, **8:**106
  after strabismus surgery, **6:**188–189, 188*i*
Delta (δ)-crystallins, **2:**326*t*, 327
Delta hepatitis, **1:**31–32
Delusions, **1:**264
Demadex. *See* Torsemide
Demecarium, **2:**400
Demeclocycline, **2:**433–434
Dementia, **1:**284–289
  AIDS-associated (HIV encephalopathy), **1:**37, **5:**361.
    See also HIV infection/AIDS
  Alzheimer, **1:**240, 284–289
  cataract surgery in patients with, **11:**201
  in elderly, **1:**240, 284
  hypertension and, **1:**96
  Lewy body, **1:**285
  mixed, **1:**285
  multi-infarct, **1:**284
  toxic, **1:**285
  vascular, **1:**285
Demi-Regroton. *See* Reserpine
Demodex
  brevis, **8:**115, 133, 168
  folliculorum, **8:**115, 133, 168
  as normal ocular flora, **8:**115, 115*t*, 133, 168
  ocular infection caused by, **8:**133, 168
de Morsier syndrome (septo-optic dysplasia), **2:**175,
    176*i*, **5:**139, **6:**362, 454
Demulcents, **2:**449–450, **8:**75

Demyelinating disease, MR imaging of, **5:**66*i*
Demyelinating plaques, in multiple sclerosis, **5:**318, 319*i*
Denaturing gradient gel electrophoresis, **2:**230
Dendrites, **8:**25*t*
  in amebic keratitis, **8:**187
  in herpes simplex virus keratitis, **4:**65–66, **8:**143, 143*i*, 144*i*, 145*i*
  in herpes zoster ophthalmicus, **8:**154
Dendritic cells, **8:**195, 196*i*, 196*t*, **9:**15
Dendritic keratitis
  contact lens wear and, **3:**208
  herpes simplex virus causing, **8:**143, 143*i*, 144*i*, 145*i*, 146
  herpes zoster causing, **8:**154
Dendritic melanocytes, **8:**245
Denervation
  with botulinum toxin, **6:**195–196
  and extirpation, **6:**175*t*
Dentate nucleus, **5:**40
Dentate processes, **12:**8
  enclosed ora bays and, **12:**8–9
  meridional folds and, **12:**9, 262, 263*i*
Deorsumduction/deorsumversion. *See* Depression of eye
Deoxyribonucleic acid. *See* DNA
Depacon. *See* Valproate/valproic acid
Depakote. *See* Valproate/valproic acid
Dependence (drug), **1:**267
Depigmentation, bull's-eye, in cone dystrophy, **5:**104
Depo-Medrol. *See* Methylprednisolone
Depot injections, corticosteroid, for uveitis, **9:**115*t*, 116–117, 117*i*
Deprenyl. *See* Selegiline
Depression of eye (downgaze), **6:**34, 36
  disorders of, in blowout fractures, **7:**102–104
    surgery and, **7:**104
  extraocular muscles controlling
    inferior rectus, **6:**14, 30, 30*t*, 33*i*
    superior oblique, **6:**15, 30*t*, 31, 34*i*
  ptosis exacerbation in, **7:**208–209
  ptotic eyelid position in, **7:**211
Depression (mood disorder), **1:**265
  drugs for (antidepressants), **1:**274–276, 275*t*
    ocular effects of, **1:**324*t*
  in elderly, **1:**239, 265
    pseudodementia and, **1:**240
Depression (perimetric term), definition of, **10:**60
Deprivation amblyopia, **6:**70
  eye trauma and, **6:**441–442
  visual development affected by, **6:**49–52, 50*i*, 51*i*, 67–68
Depth of field, **3:**36, 36*i*
Depth of focus, **3:**35–36, 35*i*
Depth perception
  stereo acuity testing of, **6:**93–94
  stereopsis differentiated from, **6:**44
Dermal melanocytosis, **7:**171–172. *See also* Nevus, of Ota
Dermal ridges/papillae, **8:**245, 246*i*
Dermatan sulfate
  in cornea, **2:**300, **8:**10
  in mucopolysaccharidoses, **8:**335–336
Dermatan sulfate–proteoglycan, in cornea, macular dystrophy and, **8:**320

Dermatitis
  atopic, **8:**207
    cataracts associated with, **11:**66
    keratoconjunctivitis and, **8:**211–213, 212*i*, 213*i*
  zoster, **8:**153
Dermatoblepharitis, **8:**119*t*
  contact, **8:**205–207, 206*i*
  herpes simplex virus causing, **8:**119*t*, 140–141, 141*i*, 143
  varicella-zoster virus causing, **8:**119*t*, 151–156
Dermatochalasis, **7:**228, 228*i*
  pseudoptosis and, **7:**219, 220*i*
Dermatographism, in Behçet syndrome, **1:**193
Dermatologic disorders. *See* Skin, disorders of
Dermatomyositis, **1:**186–187, 188*i*
  eyelid manifestations of, **4:**173*t*
Dermis, eyelid, **4:**167*i*, 168, **8:**245, 246*i*
  neoplasms of, **4:**180
Dermis-fat grafts
  for anophthalmos, **7:**37, 121
  for exposure and extrusion of orbital implant, **7:**125
  for superior sulcus deformity, **7:**124
Dermoids (dermoid cysts/tumors), **2:**125, **4:**12, **8:**275, 276*i*, 309*t*
  conjunctival, **4:**43
  corneal, **2:**168, **4:**64*i*, **6:**257, 258*i*
    infantile opacities and, **6:**256*t*, 257
  epibulbar, **6:**386, 386*i*, **8:**275–276, 276*i*
  of eyelid, **4:**169
  Goldenhar syndrome and, **2:**168, **4:**43–44, **6:**257, 431, 432*i*, **8:**276
  limbal, **4:**43–44, **6:**257, 258*i*, 386, 386*i*
    Goldenhar syndrome and, **6:**257, 431
  orbital, **2:**178, **4:**188, 188*i*, **7:**63–64, 65*i*
    in children, **6:**381, 382*i*
Dermolipomas (lipodermoids), **2:**168, **4:**43–44, 44*i*, **8:**277, 277*i*
  in children, **6:**386–387, 386*i*
  Goldenhar syndrome and, **4:**43–44, **6:**386, 386*i*, 431
  of orbit, **7:**64, 65*i*
Dermopathy, in hyperthyroidism/Graves ophthalmopathy, **1:**224, **7:**53
Derry disease (GM_1 gangliosidosis type II), **6:**350, 437*t*
Desaturated 15-hue test, Lanthony, in low vision evaluation, **5:**96
Descemet membrane–stripping keratoplasty (DSEK), **8:**476
Descemetocele, management of, **8:**441–442
  lamellar keratoplasty and, **8:**473, 473*i*
Descemet's membrane/layer, **4:**61–62, 61*i*, **8:**9*i*, 12
  anatomy of, **2:**47, 48*i*, 298*i*
  biochemistry and metabolism of, **2:**301–302
  detachment of
    after cataract surgery, **11:**168
    during intraocular surgery, **8:**419
  development of, **2:**151–152, 151*i*
  guttae in, **2:**47, 49*i*
    in Fuchs dystrophy, **2:**49, 49*i*, **4:**73, 75*i*
  injuries to, infantile corneal opacities and, **6:**255, 256*t*
  intraocular surgery causing changes in, **8:**419
  rupture of, **4:**26, 27*i*
    birth trauma and, **8:**300, 300*i*
    in keratoconus, **4:**27*i*, 70, 71*i*, **8:**330
Descending optic atrophy, **4:**206

Desferroxamine, retinopathy caused by, 12:249
Desmin, in immunohistochemistry, 4:37, 37*i*
Desmoid tumors, of orbit, 6:380
Desmosomes, epithelial, 2:45
Desquamating skin conditions, ocular surface involved in, 8:89
Destructive interference, 3:7, 8*i*
Desyrel. *See* Trazodone
Deutan defects, 12:43, 195, 196*t*
   ocular findings in carriers of, 2:270*t*
Developmental anomalies. *See specific type and* Congenital anomalies
Developmental field, definition of, 6:206
Developmental glaucoma, 10:147. *See also* Glaucoma
Developmental (juvenile-onset) myopia, 3:120–122, 146
Deviations. *See also specific type and* Esodeviations; Exodeviations; Horizontal deviations; Strabismus; Vertical deviations
   comitant (concomitant), 5:213, 216–217, 6:10
      vertical, 6:127
   incomitant (noncomitant), 5:213, 217, 218*i*, 6:10
      esodeviations, 6:98*t*, 107–108
         strabismus surgery planning and, 6:176–177
      vertical, 6:127
         strabismus surgery planning and, 6:177
   in infants, 6:451
   primary, 6:36
   prisms producing, 3:84–85, 84*i*
      prism diopter and, 3:85–86, 86*i*
   secondary, 6:36
   seizures causing, 1:284
   skew, in infants, 6:451
   terminology in description of, 6:9–11
Dexamethasone, 2:417*t*
   anti-inflammatory/pressure-elevating potency of, 2:419*t*
   cataracts caused by, 11:51–52
   in combination preparations, 2:432*t*
   for corneal graft rejection, 8:469
   for endophthalmitis, 9:218*t*, 12:329
   intravenous administration of, 2:389
   after PRK/LASEK, glaucoma associated with, 13:105
   supratarsal injection of, for vernal keratoconjunctivitis, 8:211
   for uveitis, 9:115*t*
Dextran
   in corneal storage medium, 2:454, 8:449
   in demulcents, 2:450
Dextrocycloversion, 6:36
Dextroversion (right gaze), 6:36
DFP. *See* Diisopropyl phosphorofluoridate
DGGE. *See* Denaturing gradient gel electrophoresis
DH. *See* Delayed hypersensitivity (type IV) reaction
DHA. *See* Docosahexaenoic acid
DHD. *See* Dissociated horizontal deviation
DHPG. *See* Ganciclovir
DiaBeta. *See* Glyburide
Diabetes Control and Complications Trial (DCCT), 1:210, 214–215, 12:105, 106
Diabetes mellitus, 1:201–221
   cataracts associated with, 11:60–61, 61*i*
      in children, 6:288*t*, 343

"sugar," 2:330–332
   aldose reductase in development of, 2:331–332, 354, 11:14–16, 60
   surgery for, 11:204–205, 12:118
      preoperative evaluation and, 11:83
   in children, 6:343
   classification of, 1:203–206, 204–205*t*
   clinical presentations of, 1:206–207
   complications of
      acute, 1:216
      long-term, 1:216–218
      ocular, 1:218–219. *See also* Diabetes mellitus, cataracts associated with; Diabetic macular edema; Diabetic retinopathy
      tight glucose control affecting, 1:215
   corneal changes in, 8:336–338
      neurotrophic keratopathy/persistent corneal epithelial defect, 8:102
   definition of, 1:202, 203*t*
   diagnosis of, 1:203*t*, 207, 208*t*
   diet in management of, 1:207–209
   dyslipidemia and, 1:150
   exercise in management of, 1:207–209
   gestational, 1:203*t*, 205*t*, 206
   glucose metabolism and, 1:202
   glucose surveillance (glycemic control) and, 1:215–216
      importance of glucose control and, 1:214–215, 215*i*
      retinopathy incidence and progression affected by, 1:215, 215*i*, 12:105
         Diabetes Control and Complications Trial, 12:105, 106
         United Kingdom Prospective Diabetes Study, 12:105, 107
   hypertension management and, 1:91*t*, 95
   insulin therapy for, 1:208–211, 209*t*
   latent, in adults (LADA), 1:206
   management of, 1:207–216
      recent developments in, 1:201
   metabolic syndrome and, 1:206
   ophthalmic examination timetables and, 12:119, 119*t*
   ophthalmologic considerations and, 1:218–220
   oral agents for, 1:211–214, 212*t*
   prediabetic disorders and, 1:206
   prevention of, 1:207, 208*t*
   primary open-angle glaucoma and, 10:10–11, 88–89
   refractive surgery in patient with, 13:197–198
   retinopathy of. *See* Diabetic retinopathy
   screening for, 1:207, 208*t*, 300–301
   surgical considerations in patients with, 1:220–221, 332–333
   terminology used in, 12:100
   type 1 (insulin-dependent/IDDM/juvenile-onset), 1:203–205, 204*t*, 6:343, 12:100
   type 2 (non–insulin-dependent/NIDDM/adult-onset), 1:204*t*, 205–206, 12:100
      approach to treatment of, 1:214
Diabetic ketoacidosis, 1:216
Diabetic macular edema, 12:112–116, 113*i*
   laser treatment of, 12:113–116, 114*i*, 115*i*, 116*t*
      wavelength selection and, 12:315*t*
   surgical treatment of, 12:116
Diabetic macular ischemia, 12:116
Diabetic nephropathy, 1:217–218

Diabetic neuropathy, 1:218
  neurotrophic keratopathy/persistent corneal
    epithelial defect and, 8:102
Diabetic papillopathy, 5:127, 127i
Diabetic retinopathy, 1:215, 4:132i, 135–136, 136i,
    12:99–119
  anterior chamber angle neovascularization and,
    12:111
  cataract surgery and, 12:118
  in children, 6:343
  classification of, 12:102
  cotton-wool spots in, 12:104
  diabetic keratopathy/persistent corneal epithelial
    defect and, 8:102
  epidemiology of, 12:100–101
  glycemic control affecting, 1:215, 215i, 12:105
    Diabetes Control and Complications Trial, 12:105,
      106
    United Kingdom Prospective Diabetes Study,
      12:105, 107
  iris neovascularization and, 12:111
  macular edema and, 12:112–116, 113i
  medical management of, 12:105–106
  nonproliferative, 12:102, 104i
    in children, 6:343
    progression to PDR and, 12:102–105, 104i
  ophthalmic examination timetables and, 12:119, 119t
  pathogenesis of, 12:101
  photocoagulation for, 12:106–111, 108i, 110i,
    117–118
    wavelength selection and, 12:315t
  preproliferative, 12:104
  proliferative, 12:102
    cataract surgery and, 11:205
    high-risk, 12:109
      photocoagulation and, 12:117–118
  stages/progression of, 12:102–105, 104i
  surgical management of, 12:111–112
  tractional retinal detachment and, 12:112, 273, 341
  vitrectomy for, 12:111–112, 112t, 116–117
  vitreous hemorrhage in, 12:111–112, 116–117, 287
Diabetic Retinopathy Study (DRS), 12:108, 108i,
    109–110, 110i
Diabetic Retinopathy Vitrectomy Study (DRVS),
    12:111–112, 112t, 117
Diabinese. See Chlorpropamide
Diacylglycerol (DAG), in signal transduction, in tear
    secretion, 2:292, 292i, 293
Diagnostic agents, 2:451–452
Diagnostic electron microscopy, 4:40
Diagnostic positions of gaze, 6:87, 88i
Diagnostic tests. See Screening/diagnostic tests
Diagnostic ultrasonography. See Ultrasonography/
    ultrasound
Dialyses, 12:253, 254, 255i
  treatment of, 12:266t, 267t
Diameter, contact lens, 3:174, 174i, 177
Diamidines, for Acanthamoeba keratitis, 8:189
Diamox. See Acetazolamide
Diaphragm pump, for phacoemulsification aspiration,
    11:119, 119i
  vacuum rise time for, 11:120i, 121
Diarrhea, in HIV infection/AIDS, 1:48–49
Diastole (diastolic phase), 1:128

Diastolic dysfunction, 1:129
  causes of, 1:128
  management of, 1:131
Diathermy
  for retinal capillary hemangioma, 4:247
  for thermokeratoplasty, 13:27, 137
  transscleral, for melanoma, 4:238
Diazepam, 1:273
  for medical emergencies, 1:316t
  perioperative, 1:332t, 335
Diazoxide, for hypertensive emergency, 1:94
Dibenamine, 2:309
DIC. See Disseminated intravascular coagulation
Dichlorphenamide, 2:413
Dichromats, 12:195, 196t, 197i
Diclofenac, 1:196, 197t, 2:306–307, 417t, 422
  corneal problems associated with, 1:197–198
  with misoprostol, 1:197t
Dicloxacillin, 1:55t, 2:429
Didanosine, 1:41
  for postexposure HIV prophylaxis, 1:46–47t
Dideoxycytidine. See Zalcitabine
DIDMOAD syndrome
  in children, 6:343
  pleiotropism in, 2:259
Diet/diet therapy
  cancer and, 1:252
  coronary artery disease and, 1:111
  in diabetes management/prevention, 1:207, 207–209
    surgery and, 1:220, 333
  in hypercholesterolemia, 1:146, 148t
  in inborn errors of metabolism, 2:280–281
Diethylcarbamazine, for loiasis, 8:191
Difference map, after keratorefractive surgery, 13:9–10,
    10i
Differential membrane filtration (Rheopheresis), for
    nonneovascular AMD, 12:62
Diffraction, 3:11–12, 12i
Diffractive multifocal intraocular lenses, 3:228, 228i,
    13:163, 173
Diffuse anterior scleritis, 8:236, 236t, 237i
Diffuse episcleritis, 8:29
Diffuse illumination, for slit-lamp biomicroscopy, 8:16
Diffuse iris nodular nevi (iris mamillations),
    6:264–265, 265i
  central (pupillary) cyst rupture and, 6:265
Diffuse lamellar (interface) keratitis (DLK), after
    LASIK, 13:127, 128i, 129t
Diffuse reflection, 3:41–42, 43i
Diffuse soft-tissue histiocytosis. See Histiocytosis
Diffuse toxic goiter, 1:224. See also Graves
    hyperthyroidism
Diffuse transmission, 3:41–42, 43i
Diffuse unilateral subacute neuroretinitis (DUSN),
    6:318, 9:172–173, 172i, 173i, 12:189–190, 189i
Diffuse uveitis. See Panuveitis
Diffusion, in aqueous humor dynamics/formation,
    2:304, 10:18
Diffusion-weighted magnetic resonance imaging
    (DWI), 5:78
  in cerebral ischemia/stroke, 1:104
Diflucan. See Fluconazole
Diflunisal, 1:197t
Digenic inheritance, 2:185

Digital pressure, for intraocular pressure estimation, 10:29
Digital rectal exam, in cancer screening, 1:295*t*
Digitalis/digitoxin/digoxin
  for heart failure, 1:130
  ocular effects of, 1:142, 325*t*
  in perioperative setting, 1:333
  retinopathy caused by, 12:250
Dihydropyridines
  contraindications to in non-ST-segment elevation
    acute coronary syndrome, 1:122–123
  for hypertension, 1:89*t*, 93
Dihydroxy propoxymethyl guanine. *See* Ganciclovir
Diisopropyl phosphorofluoridate, 2:309, 399
Diktyoma (medulloepithelioma), 4:144–146, 147*i*, 283, 6:369
  teratoid, 4:146
Dilacor. *See* Diltiazem
Dilantin. *See* Phenytoin
Dilated fundus examination, before refractive surgery, 13:46
Dilator muscle, 2:62*i*, 64–65, 65*i*
  α-adrenergic agents affecting, 2:405, 408
  development of, 2:154
  miotics affecting, 2:309
  mydriatics affecting, 2:309–310, 400
Diltiazem
  for angina, 1:120
  for heart failure, mortality increases and, 1:130
  for hypertension, 1:89*t*
  for non-ST-segment elevation acute coronary
    syndrome, 1:122
Dimorphic fungi, 8:129
Dinucleotide repeats, 2:190
Diode laser. *See also* Lasers
  cycloablation with, for childhood glaucoma, 6:281, 282
  hyperthermia with
    for melanoma, 4:238
    for retinoblastoma, 4:262
  semiconductor, 3:23
Diopter, 3:63, 8:39
  prism, 3:85–86, 86*i*
Dioptric mean, 3:93
Dioptric power, of bifocal segment, occupation and, 3:163
Diovan. *See* Valsartan
Diphenhydramine, for allergic reactions/medical
    emergencies, 1:316*t*, 319
Diphtheria, immunization against, 1:307–308
Diphtheria-tetanus-pertussis vaccine (DTP), 1:291, 307
Diphtheria and tetanus toxoid with acellular pertussis
    vaccine (DTaP), 1:291, 304*t*, 307
  in combination vaccines, 1:309
Diphtheroids, 8:125
  as normal ocular flora, 8:115, 115*t*, 125
Dipivefrin (dipivalyl epinephrine), 2:389, 407*t*, 409
  for glaucoma, 10:161*t*, 169–170
    in children, 6:283
Diploid, definition of, 2:185
Diplopia, 5:213–237
  with bifocals, progressive addition lenses and, 3:152
  after blepharoplasty, 7:233
  in blowout fractures, 7:102–104
    surgery and, 7:104

  in children, 6:42, 42*i*, 43, 52–53
  comitant deviations with, 5:213, 216–217
  crossed, 6:59*i*, 60
  divergence insufficiency and, 5:216
  in epiretinal membrane, 12:88
  heteronymous, 6:59*i*, 60
  history of, 5:213
  homonymous, 6:58–60, 59*i*
  incomitant deviations with, 5:213, 217, 218*i*
  after LASIK, 13:132
    in amblyopia patient, 13:194
  monocular, 3:170–171, 5:216
    in cataracts, 11:45, 47, 77
    multifocal IOLs and, 3:228–229
  in multiple sclerosis, 5:321
  in myasthenia gravis, 5:326
  ocular motor cranial nerve lesions and
    central, 5:221–227, 223*t*
    peripheral, 5:227–237
  Panum's area and, 6:43, 52
  paradoxical, 6:56, 56*i*
  paretic syndromes causing, 5:221, 222*i*
    restrictive syndromes compared with, 5:217, 218*i*
  physical examination of, 5:213–214, 214*i*, 215*i*
  restrictive syndromes causing, 5:217–221
    paretic syndromes compared with, 5:217, 218*i*
    posttraumatic, 5:218–219
  skew deviation and, 5:223–224
  after strabismus surgery, 6:56, 184–185
  strabismus surgery for elimination of, 6:173–174
  testing for, 6:58–60, 59*i*
  after third nerve (oculomotor) palsy surgery, 6:147
  uncrossed, 6:58–60, 59*i*
Dipping, ocular, 5:256
Diprivan. *See* Propofol
Dipyridamole
  cataract surgery in patient taking, 11:202
  for central retinal vein occlusion, 12:144
Direct ophthalmoscopy. *See* Ophthalmoscopy
Direct response, in pupillary reaction to light, 5:258
Direct sequencing, for mutation screening, 2:231, 232*i*
Directionality, of laser light, 3:18, 20*i*
Dirithromycin, 1:60*t*, 71
Disalcid. *See* Salsalate
Disc edema. *See* Optic disc (optic nerve head), edema
    of
Disc sign, in sickle cell hemoglobinopathies, 12:123
Disciform keratitis, herpes simplex virus causing,
    8:147, 147*i*
Disciform scar
  in choroidal neovascularization, 12:63*i*, 64
  in Coats disease, 12:156
Discoid rash, in systemic lupus erythematosus, 1:179,
    181*t*, 182
Disconjugate eye movements (vergences), 6:38. *See also
    specific type*
  in infants, 6:451
Disconnection syndrome, 5:192
Discontinuity, zones of, 2:76
Disease-modifying (slow-acting) antirheumatic drugs,
    1:174
Dislocated lens, 4:94, 95*i*, 11:40. *See also* Ectopia lentis
  cataract surgery and, 11:226–227, 227*i*, 228*i*
  in children, 6:304–309, 305*t*
    abuse and, 6:442

Disodium ethylenediaminetetraacetic acid (EDTA), for band keratopathy, 2:394, 8:374

Disomy, uniparental, 2:197

Dispersed repetitive DNA, 2:185

Dispersion, 3:40, 49–50, 51*i*

Dispersive viscoelastics, 11:158

Disruption, definition of, 6:206

Dissection, gross, for pathologic examination, 4:33–34, 34*i*

Dissections (arterial), 5:354–355, 354*i. See also specific type or artery affected*

Disseminated intravascular coagulation, 1:169–170 choroidal perfusion abnormalities and, 12:166–167

Dissimilar image tests, 6:84–85

Dissimilar segments, for induced anisophoria, 3:162, 162*i*

Dissimilar target tests, 6:85–86

Dissociated horizontal deviation, 6:116, 116*i*, 131

Dissociated/disconjugate/disjunctive nystagmus, 5:240, 6:168

Dissociated vertical deviation, 6:116, 116*i*, 130–132, 131*i* surgery for, 6:131, 181–182

Distaclor. *See* Cefaclor

Distance spectacles, 3:254

Distance visual acuity magnification for in low vision (telescopes), 3:82–84 testing in children, 6:78–80 nystagmus and, 6:161–162 distance for, 3:111–112 in low vision, 3:251

Distichiasis, 2:28, 4:169, 8:104 acquired, 7:147 congenital, 6:211, 212*i*, 7:147, 157

Distortion, cylinders in spectacle lenses causing, 3:145. *See also* Meridional magnification contact lenses for reduction/elimination of, 3:181

Distribution, normal, clinical relevance of research and, 1:344

Distributive shock, 1:317. *See also* Shock

Disuse anopsia. *See* Deprivation amblyopia

Diupres. *See* Reserpine

Diuretics central retinal vein occlusion and, 12:143 for diastolic dysfunction, 1:131 for hypertension, 1:81, 86, 87–92, 88*t*, 90*t* ocular effects of, 1:325*t* in perioperative setting, 1:334

Diuril. *See* Chlorothiazide

Diurnal variation in intraocular pressure, 10:25 in vision, after radial keratotomy, 13:63

Divergence, 6:38 fusional, 6:38, 88

Divergence excess exotropia, 6:112

Divergence insufficiency/paralysis, 5:211, 216 esodeviation and, 6:98*t*, 106

Divergent strabismus, 6:9

Diverging lens, 3:143, 144*i*

Dix-Hallpike maneuver, 5:247

Dk (gas permeability constant). *See also* Gas transmissibility definition of, for contact lenses, 3:175 for flexible contact lenses, 3:184–185

for rigid contact lenses, 3:183–184

Dk/L, of contact lenses, 3:75

DKA. *See* Diabetic ketoacidosis

DLEK. *See* Deep lamellar endothelial keratoplasty

DLK. *See* Diffuse lamellar (interface) keratitis

DM. *See* Diabetes mellitus

DMARDs. *See* Disease-modifying (slow-acting) antirheumatic drugs

DME. *See* Diabetic macular edema

DNA, 2:185, 199–205, 200*i*, 200*t*, 201*i*, 202*i*, 8:306 amplification of, in polymerase chain reaction, 2:193 analysis of, 2:227–231, 228*i*, 229*i*, 232*i*, 233*i* antisense, 2:182, 202 complementary (cDNA), 2:184, 200 from ciliary body–encoding plasma proteins, 2:319 sequencing, in mutation screening, 2:231 dispersed repetitive, 2:185 fecal, testing in cancer screening, 1:298 junk, 2:203 methylation of, 2:210 mitochondrial, 2:215–220, 219*i* diseases associated with deletions/mutations of, 2:217–220 galtonian inheritance of, 2:186, 257 Leber hereditary optic neuropathy, 2:218–220, 219*i*, 5:134–135, 6:365 maternal inheritance/transmission and, 2:217, 257, 269 retinal degeneration and, 12:233*t*, 245 genetic code for translation of, 2:215–217 genomic structure of, 2:217 in replicative segregation, 2:195 molecular manipulation of, 2:227–231, 228*i*, 229*i*, 232*i*, 233*i* recombinant, 2:194, 227, 229*i* repair of, 2:212–213 replication of, 2:194, 212 origin, 2:192, 212 segregation and, 2:195 slippage, 2:195 RNA creation from, 2:209 satellite, 2:195, 203, 223 sense, 2:195, 201–202 sequencing of, 2:231, 232*i* database for, 2:226 structure of, 2:199, 200*i* telomeric (telomeres), 2:197, 203, 205

DNA libraries, 2:189, 227, 228*i* cDNA, 2:189, 227 genomic, 2:189, 227, 228*i*

DNA polymerase, for mitochondrial DNA synthesis, 2:217

DNA probes, in infection diagnosis, 1:3

DNA viruses, 8:119 cancer association of, 1:254 ocular infection caused by, 8:120–121

Do not resuscitate orders, surgery in elderly patients and, 1:238

DOA (OPA1) gene, 5:136

Dobutamine, for heart failure, 1:130–131

Dobutrex. *See* Dobutamine

Docosahexaenoic acid, in retinal pigment epithelium, 2:358

Dog bites, eyelid injuries caused by, 7:187

Dog tapeworm *(Echinococcus granulosus)*, orbital infection caused by, **7:**47
Dolichocephaly, **6:**424
Doll's head maneuver/phenomenon, **5:**313
 in saccadic dysfunction, **5:**206
Dolobid. *See* Diflunisal
Domains, immunoglobulin, **9:**55, 56*i*
Dominance columns, ocular, **5:**29
Dominant (familial) drusen, **6:**340, **12:**220–221, 221*i*
Dominant inheritance (dominant gene/trait), **2:**185, 260–261, **8:**307
 autosomal, **2:**265–266, 267*i*
 disorders associated with, **2:**185
  gene therapy for, **2:**237–238, 238*i*
  X-linked, **2:**268–269
 X-linked, **2:**268, 268*t*
Dominant negative mutation, **2:**185
 gene therapy for disorders caused by, **2:**238, 238*i*
Donepezil, for Alzheimer disease, **1:**288
Donor cornea, **8:**449–451
 disease transmission from, **8:**451*t*
 preparation of
  for lamellar keratoplasty, **8:**474
  for penetrating keratoplasty, **8:**455
 prior LASIK affecting, **13:**204
 rejection of. *See* Rejection (graft)
 selection/screening of, **8:**449–451
  HIV infection transmission and, **1:**51
 storage of, **2:**454, **8:**449
Donor splice site, **2:**185
L-Dopa, for Parkinson disease, **1:**279
Dopamine
 antipsychotic mechanism of action and, **1:**271
 for heart failure, **1:**130–131
 in Parkinson disease, **1:**278
Doppler imaging
 in cerebral ischemia/stroke, **1:**103
 in ischemic heart disease, **1:**118
 in orbital evaluation, **7:**34
Dorello's canal, **2:**117, **5:**23, 234
Doripenem, **1:**69
Dorsal midbrain (Parinaud) syndrome, **5:**208–209, 210*i*
 eyelid retraction in, **5:**279, **7:**224
 nystagmus in, **6:**167
Dorsal subnucleus, of cranial nerve VII, **5:**54
Dorsal vermis, **5:**41
Dorsal visual processing stream, in pursuit system, **5:**203
Dorsolateral pontine nuclei, **5:**34
Dorzolamide, **2:**411*t*, 412, **10:**163*t*, 168
 for childhood glaucoma, **6:**283
 in combination preparations, **2:**411*t*, 414
Dot-and-blot hemorrhages, **5:**183, 184*i*
 ischemia causing, **4:**131, 132*i*
"Double-click-stop technique," **3:**136
Double convexity deformity, **7:**236
Double elevator palsy/paresis (monocular elevation deficiency), **6:**137–138, 138*i*, **7:**214
Double heterozygotes, **2:**243
Double Maddox rod testing, **6:**85
 in superior oblique muscle palsy, **6:**132
Double ring sign, in optic nerve hypoplasia, **5:**139, 139*i*, **6:**362, 362*i*, 453
Double simultaneous stimulation, in confrontation testing, **5:**90

Double vision. *See* Diplopia
Doubling principle, **3:**299
"Dowager's hump," **1:**242
Down syndrome (trisomy 21/trisomy G syndrome), **2:**250–251, 251*t*
 Brushfield spots in, **4:**219*t*, 220*i*, **6:**266
 childhood glaucoma and, **10:**155*t*
 mosaicism in, **2:**252
 pharmacogenetics and, **2:**279
Downbeat nystagmus, **5:**248–249, 248*i*, **6:**167
 differential diagnosis of, **5:**249
Downgaze. *See* Depression of eye
Downregulatory T cells, in suppression, **9:**88
Doxazosin
 for heart failure, **1:**130
 for hypertension, **1:**89*t*
Doxorubicin, **1:**257, 259*t*
Doxycycline, **1:**61*t*, **2:**433
 for chalazia in children, **6:**388
 for chemical burns, **8:**392
 for chlamydial conjunctivitis, **8:**177
 for Lyme disease, **5:**364
 for meibomian gland dysfunction, **8:**83
 ocular effects of, **1:**324*t*
 for rosacea, **2:**394, **8:**86
 for seborrheic blepharitis, **8:**86–87
 for syphilis, **9:**190
 for toxoplasmosis, **9:**169
Doyne's honeycombed dystrophy, **12:**220. *See also* Drusen
 EFEMP1 defects causing, **2:**351, **12:**220–221
DPE. *See* Dipivefrin
Dressler syndrome, **1:**115
DRS (Diabetic Retinopathy Study), **12:**108, 108*i*, 109–110, 110*i*
Drug dependence, **1:**267
Drug-induced uveitis, **9:**141
Drug resistance. *See also specific agent and specific organism*
 antibiotic, **1:**3, 66
  new drug classes and, **1:**74–75
 antiretroviral, **1:**41, 43, 44
Drug tolerance, **1:**267
Drugs. *See also specific drug or drug group*
 allergic reaction to, **1:**319–320
  penicillins, **1:**67–68
 antibiotic, **1:**53–78, 55–65*t*, **2:**427–437, 428*t*, 431*t*
 cytotoxic, **9:**96
  for Wegener granulomatosis, **1:**192
 diabetes mellitus associated with, **1:**204*t*
 dry eye caused by, **8:**76, 80, 81*t*
 genetics affecting (pharmacogenetics), **2:**278–279
 glaucoma caused by, **10:**116–117, 145–146
 keratopathy caused by, **4:**70
 lens changes caused by, **11:**50–54
 medication use by elderly and, **1:**235–236
 mydriasis caused by, **5:**266
 ocular, **2:**393–458. *See also specific agent*
  absorption of, **2:**382–386, 382*i*, 383*i*, 385*i*
  adrenergic, **2:**404–411, 404*i*
  age/aging and, **1:**235–236
  anti-inflammatory, **2:**416–427
  antibiotic, **2:**427–437, 428*t*, 431*t*, 432*t*
   new, **2:**457
  antifibrinolytic, **2:**453

antifungal, **2:**437–439, 438*t*
antioxidant/vitamin supplements, **2:**454–455
antiviral, **2:**439–444, 440*t*, 441*i*
carbonic anhydrase inhibitors, **2:**411–413, 411*t*
cholinergic, **2:**394–403, 395*i*, 396*i*
cicatricial pemphigoid (pseudopemphigoid)
    caused by, **8:**219–220, 394, 395
combined agents, **2:**414–415
concentration of, absorption affected by, **2:**384
corneal deposits and pigmentation caused by,
    8:375–378, 376*t*, 377*t*
for corneal storage medium, **2:**454
decongestants, **2:**451
diagnostic agents, **2:**451–452
for dry eye, **2:**449–450
in eyedrops, **2:**381–384, 382*i*, 383*i*, 385*i*
fibrinolytic, **2:**452
growth factors, **2:**456–457
hyperosmolar, **2:**451
interferons, **2:**455
intraocular injection of, **2:**386–387
intraocular pressure affected by. *See* Antiglaucoma
    agents
intravenous administration of, **2:**388–389
investigational/clinical testing of, **2:**393
for irrigation, **2:**451
legal aspects of use of, **2:**393–394
local administration of, **2:**386–388
local anesthetics, **2:**445–449, 445*t*, 446*t*
methods of design and delivery of, **2:**389–391
new, **2:**455–457
off-label usage of, **2:**393–394
in ointments, **2:**386
    lubricating, **5:**286
oral preparations of, sustained-release, **2:**388
osmotic agents, **2:**415–416, 415*t*
partition coefficients of, **2:**384
periocular injection of, **2:**386
pharmacodynamics of, **2:**380, 392
pharmacokinetics of, **2:**380, 381–391
pharmacologic principles and, **2:**379–392
pharmacotherapeutics of, **2:**380
prostaglandin analogs, **2:**413–414, 414*t*
purified neurotoxin complex, **2:**449
receptor interactions and, **2:**392
solubility of, absorption affected by, **2:**384
systemic absorption of, **2:**380, 382, 383, 383*i*
systemic administration and, **2:**388–389
thrombin, **2:**453
tissue binding of, **2:**385–386
topical, **2:**381–386, 382*i*, 383*i*, 385*i*. *See also*
    Eyedrops
    sustained-release devices for, **2:**390
toxicity of, **2:**379, 380–381, **8:**101–102
    aging and, **2:**381
    keratoconjunctivitis and, **8:**393–395
    tissue binding and, **2:**385–386
    ulcerative keratopathy and, **8:**101–102, 375–376
viscoelastics, **2:**452
viscosity of, absorption affected by, **2:**384
vitamin/antioxidant supplements, **2:**454–455
ocular toxicity and, **1:**323–326, 324–325*t*
    age-related macular degeneration differentiated
        from, **12:**59
    electroretinogram in, **12:**36

optic neuropathy caused by, **5:**152
retinal degenerations caused by, **12:**247–251
for parasellar tumors, **5:**163
platelet dysfunction caused by, **1:**167–168, 331–332
thrombocytopenia caused by, **1:**167
Drusen, **2:**79
in age-related macular degeneration, **4:**137–139,
    137*i*, 138*i*, **12:**55–57, 56*i*
calcific (calcified), **4:**138, **12:**58
in children, **5:**133–134, **6:**368, 368*i*
confluent, **12:**57
cuticular (basal laminar), **4:**138, **12:**221
    age-related macular degeneration differentiated
        from, **12:**59, 67
    vitelliform exudative macular detachment and,
        12:220, 220*i*
diffuse, **4:**137, 137*i*
dominant (familial), **6:**340, **12:**220–221, 221*i*
extruded, **5:**129
giant, **4:**257–259, **5:**132
    in tuberous sclerosis, **6:**411
hard, **4:**138, 138*i*, **12:**57
optic disc/nerve, **4:**206–208, 208*i*, **5:**115, 115*i*,
    129–134, 131*i*
    astrocytic hamartoma differentiated from,
        5:132–134, 133*i*
    papilledema differentiated from, **5:**130–132, 132*i*,
        133*i*
    pseudopapilledema and, **5:**115, 115*i*, **6:**368, 368*i*
regressed, **12:**58
soft, **4:**138, 138*i*, **12:**56*i*, 57
Drusenoid retinal pigment epithelial detachment,
    12:220, 221*i*
DRVS (Diabetic Retinopathy Vitrectomy Study),
    12:111–112, 112*t*, 117
Dry eye syndrome, **5:**188, 298, **8:**71–109. *See also*
    specific causative factor
    aqueous tear deficiency causing, **8:**56, 57, 71–80, 72*t*.
        See also Aqueous tear deficiency
    in blepharospasm, **7:**226, 227
    cataract surgery in patients with, **11:**11, 206–207
        corneal melting and, **11:**180, 206–207
    classification of, **8:**71, 72*t*
    conjunctival noninflammatory vascular anomalies
        causing, **8:**90–92, 91*t*
    contact lens wear and, **3:**210
    epithelial defect after PRK and, **13:**104
    evaporative tear dysfunction causing, **8:**72*t*, 80–90
    glaucoma and, **8:**76
    after LASIK, **8:**80, **13:**110, 127, 184
    limbal stem cell deficiency causing, **8:**108–109
    medications causing, **8:**76, 80, 81*t*
    non–Sjögren syndrome, **8:**72*t*, 80
    nutritional/physiologic disorders causing, **8:**92–94
    after PRK/LASEK, **8:**80, **13:**105
        epithelial defect and, **13:**104
    punctal occlusion for, **7:**274
    radiation causing, **1:**256
    refractive surgery and, **8:**80, **13:**44, 184–185
    rose bengal in diagnosis of, **8:**22
    sarcoidosis and, **8:**88
    Sjögren syndrome, **1:**186, 187*t*, **8:**72*t*, 78–80, 79*t*
    structural/exogenous disorders causing, **8:**94–108
    surface inflammation and, **2:**295, 295*i*
    systemic diseases associated with, **8:**74*t*

tear film abnormalities and, 2:294
tests for, 8:61–63, 62i, 62t
treatment of
    medical management, 2:295–296, 295i, 449–450, 8:74–76, 75t
    surgical management, 8:75t, 76–77, 76i, 77i
DSEK. See Descemet membrane stripping keratoplasty
DTacP-IPV-Hib vaccine, 1:309
DTacP-IPV vaccine, 1:309
DTaP (diphtheria and tetanus toxoid with acellular pertussis vaccine), 1:291, 304t, 307
    in combination vaccines, 1:309
DTP (diphtheria-tetanus-pertussis) vaccine, 1:291, 307
DTPa-HBV-IPV/Hib vaccine, 1:309
Dual-energy quantitative computed tomography, for bone density measurement, 1:243
Dual-photon x-ray absorptiometry, for bone density measurement, 1:243
Duane syndrome, 5:220, 221i, 6:141–144, 142i, 143i
    esotropic, 6:142–143, 142i
    exotropic (retraction), 5:220, 221i, 6:116, 142, 142i
    Goldenhar syndrome and, 6:141, 431
    synkinesis in, 7:211, 217
    variants of, 5:220–221
Duchenne muscular dystrophy
    mutation rate of, 2:256
    retinal degeneration and, 12:236
Ductions, 6:34–35. See also specific type
    forced. See Forced ductions
Dulcitol (galactitol)
    in cataract formation, 2:331–332, 11:16, 61
    in lens glucose/carbohydrate metabolism, 2:331i, 11:16
Duloxetine, 1:276
Duochrome (red-green/bichrome) test, 3:140
    before refractive surgery, 13:43
        PRK/LASEK, 13:91
Duplex ultrasonography. See also Ultrasonography
    in carotid evaluation, 5:179
    in cerebral ischemia/stroke, 1:103
Duplication mapping, 2:221
Dura mater, optic nerve, 2:101i, 102, 4:203, 204i
Duracef. See Cefadroxil
Dural sheath, of optic disc, 5:26
Dural sinus fistula, 5:236–237, 7:70
Dural sinus thrombosis, 5:357–358
Duranest. See Etidocaine
DUSN. See Diffuse unilateral subacute neuroretinitis
DVD. See Dissociated vertical deviation
DWI. See Diffusion-weighted magnetic resonance imaging
DXA. See Dual-photon x-ray absorptiometry
Dyazide. See Triamterene
Dye disappearance test, 7:268, 269i, 8:20
Dye laser, 3:23. See also Lasers
Dynabac. See Dirithromycin
Dynacin. See Minocycline
DynaCirc. See Isradipine
Dynamic imbalance, of vestibulo-ocular reflex, 5:200
Dynapen. See Dicloxacillin
Dyrenium. See Triamterene
Dysautonomia, familial (Riley-Day syndrome), 2:262t, 6:260
    neurotrophic keratopathy in, 8:103
    racial and ethnic concentration of, 2:259

Dyscephalic mandibulo-oculofacial syndrome. See Hallermann-Streiff syndrome
Dyschromatopsia. See Color vision, defects in
Dyscoria, 6:261
Dysgenesis
    definition of, 2:125
    mesodermal. See Axenfeld-Rieger syndrome; Leukomas
Dysgeusia, Horner syndrome and, 5:265
Dyskeratosis, 4:177, 177i
    benign hereditary intraepithelial, 8:255t, 309t
    definition of, 4:169, 8:247t
Dyskinesia, tardive, 5:286
Dyslexia, surface, in Alzheimer disease, 1:288
Dyslipoproteinemia/dyslipidemia, 1:150. See also Hyperlipidemia; Hyperlipoproteinemia
    diabetic, 1:150
    screening for, 1:293
Dysmorphic sialidosis, 8:342
Dysphotopsias, 3:222–223, 223i, 224i
Dysplasia
    of conjunctival epithelium, 4:51, 52i
    of corneal epithelium, 4:76
    definition of, 2:125, 6:206, 8:246–247, 247t
    squamous, of conjunctiva, 8:257, 257i
Dysplastic nevus, 4:184
Dyspnea, 1:153
Dysraphia, definition of, 6:205
Dysthymic disorder, 1:265
Dysthyroid ophthalmopathy/orbitopathy. See Thyroid ophthalmopathy
Dystonia, facial, 7:226–228
Dystopia canthorum, 6:209, 209i
Dystrophies. See also specific type
    choroidal, 12:224–229. See also specific type
    corneal, 4:70–73, 72i, 73i, 74i, 75i. See also specific type and Corneal dystrophies
        anterior, 8:311–315
        cataract surgery in patients with, 11:208, 209i
        endothelial, 8:324–329
        metabolic disorders and, 8:309–310t, 335–357
        refractive surgery in patients with, 13:44, 46i
        stromal, 8:316–323, 316t
    definition of, 4:16, 8:311
    degenerations differentiated from, 8:361t
    foveomacular, 12:219–220, 219i
    hereditary, 12:203–229. See also specific type
    macular. See Macular dystrophy
    pattern, 12:222–223, 222i
        age-related macular degeneration differentiated from, 12:59, 67
    retinal. See also specific type and Degenerations, retinal
        electroretinogram in evaluation of, 12:33–34, 34i
        hereditary, 12:203–229. See also specific type
        inner, 12:228–229
        photoreceptor, 12:205–215
    vitreoretinal, 12:228–229
Dystrophin, mutations in gene for, in Duchenne muscular dystrophy, 12:236

E

E-game, for visual acuity testing in children, 6:78t, 79
E-selectin, in neutrophil rolling, 9:48, 49i

Eales disease, 12:153
Early Manifest Glaucoma Trial, 10:88t
Early-onset Alzheimer disease, 1:286
Early-onset (childhood) nystagmus, 5:241–243,
    6:159–171, 333–334, 334t. See also Nystagmus
    types of, 6:162–168
Early receptor potential, 12:31, 31i
Early Treatment Diabetic Retinopathy Study (ETDRS),
    12:103–104. See also ETDRS visual acuity chart
    diabetic macular edema and, 12:113–116, 114i, 115i
    scatter laser tretment and, 12:108, 108i
Early Treatment for Retinopathy of Prematurity
    (ETROP) study, 6:329
Early Treatment for Retinopathy of Prematurity
    Randomized Trial, 12:133–134
EB. See Elementary body
EBAA. See Eye Bank Association of America
Eberconazole, 1:76
EBMB. See Epithelial dystrophies, basement membrane
Ebola virus/Ebola hemorrhagic fever, 1:35
EBV. See Epstein-Barr virus
EBV-associated hemophagocytic lymphohistiocytosis/
    syndrome (EBV-HLH), 1:30
ECCE. See Extracapsular cataract extraction
Eccentric fixation, 6:69
    ARC testing and, 6:57
Ecchymoses, 1:166. See also Purpura
    periorbital
        in child abuse, 6:442
        in neuroblastoma, 6:374, 374i
Eccrine sweat glands, of eyelid, 4:168t, 7:167
    tumors arising in, 7:167, 168i
ECG. See Electrocardiography
Echinocandins, 1:76
        for Pneumocystis carinii (Pneumocystis jiroveci)
            pneumonia, 1:45
Echinococcus granulosus (echinococcosis), orbital
    infection caused by, 7:47
Echocardiography, 5:179–180
    in cerebral ischemia/stroke, 1:103
    in congestive heart failure, 1:127
    exercise (stress), 1:118
    in ischemic heart disease, 1:118
    transesophageal Doppler
        in amaurosis fugax, 1:107
        in cerebral ischemia/stroke, 1:103
Echography. See Ultrasonography
Echothiophate, 2:309, 398t, 399, 400
    cataracts caused by, 11:53–54
    in Down syndrome patients, pharmacogenetics and,
        2:279
    for glaucoma, 10:166
        in children, 6:283
    for high accommodative convergence/
        accommodative esotropia, 6:102–103
    for refractive accommodative esotropia, 6:102
    succinylcholine and, 1:334
Eclampsia, 1:96, 5:343. See also Preeclampsia
    choroidal perfusion abnormalities and, 12:166, 168i
Eclipse (solar) retinopathy, 12:307–308
Econopred. See Prednisolone
ECP. See Endoscopic cyclophotocoagulation
Ecstasy (MDMA/3,4-
    methylenedioxymethamphetamine), 1:270

Ectasia/ectatic disorders
    corneal, 8:329–355. See also specific type
        after LASIK, 13:131–132
            intrastromal corneal ring segments for, 13:84
    retinal, 12:157–158. See also Retinal telangiectasia/
        telangiectasis
Ectodactyly-ectodermal dysplasial–clefting (EEC)
    syndrome, 8:89
Ectoderm, 2:126, 133, 135i, 137i
    in lens development, 2:145
    ocular structures derived from, 2:133t, 8:6
Ectodermal dysplasia, 8:89, 309t
    anhidrotic, 8:89
Ectopia (displaced pupil), 2:170
Ectopia lentis, 4:94, 95i, 95t, 10:130, 131i, 131t, 11:40
    causes of, 10:131t
    in children, 6:305, 305–306, 305i
    et pupillae, 6:269, 305–306, 305i, 11:40, 42
    in homocystinuria, 6:307, 307i, 11:42
    in hyperlysinemia, 6:308, 11:42
    in Marfan syndrome, 6:306–307, 306i, 11:41, 41i
    secondary angle-closure glaucoma and, 10:130, 131i,
        131t
    simple, 4:94, 6:305, 11:40
    in sulfite oxidase deficiency, 6:308, 11:42
    systemic conditions associated with, 4:105t
    traumatic, 11:40, 55, 56i
        cataract surgery in patients with, 11:226–227,
            227i, 228i
    treatment of, 6:308–309
    in Weill-Marchesani syndrome, 6:308
Ectopic lacrimal gland, 6:382, 8:277
Ectopic tissue masses, orbital, in children, 6:381–384
Ectropion, 2:64, 7:195–201, 196i
    anophthalmic, 7:126–127
    cicatricial, 7:196i, 200–201
        after blepharoplasty, 7:233
    congenital, 6:210, 7:154, 155i
        iris, 6:269–270, 270i
            glaucoma in neurofibromatosis and, 6:408
    involutional, 7:195–198, 196i, 197i
    mechanical, 7:196i, 201
    paralytic, 7:196i, 199–200, 200i
    tarsal, 7:198
    uveae, 2:64, 4:156, 6:269
        iris nevus causing, 4:215–216
Eczema, of eyelid, 8:24t
Edema
    corneal. See Cornea, edema of
    epithelial, 8:24t
        cataract surgery and, 11:166
        central (Sattler's veil), 8:106
        intraocular surgery causing, 8:418–419
    eyelid, 7:160
    in hypothyroidism, 1:225
    macular. See Macular edema
    optic disc. See Optic disc (optic nerve head), edema
        of
    retinal, 4:130–131, 130i, 131i
        in branch retinal vein occlusion, 12:136
        in central retinal artery occlusion, 12:148, 148i
        in central retinal vein occlusion, 12:141, 142i
        in clinically significant macular edema, 12:114,
            114i

stromal, **8**:33
  cataract surgery and, **11**:166
Edetate disodium, for band keratopathy, **2**:394, **8**:374
Edge lift, of contact lens, **3**:175
Edinger-Westphal complex/nucleus, **2**:108, 109*i*, **5**:45,
    57, 59*i*
Edrophonium, **2**:396*i*, 403, **5**:224
  in myasthenia gravis diagnosis, **2**:403, **5**:326–327,
    6:151, 151*i*, 153*t*, **7**:213
  toxic reaction to, **1**:323
EDS. *See* Ehlers-Danlos syndrome
EDTA, for band keratopathy, **2**:394, **8**:374
EEC syndrome. *See* Ectodactyly-ectodermal
    dysplasial–clefting (EEC) syndrome
EEG. *See* Electroencephalography
EF. *See* Ejection fraction
Efavirenz, **1**:41–42
  for postexposure HIV prophylaxis, **1**:46–47*t*
EFEMP1 protein (EGF-containing fibrillin-like
    extracellular matrix protein) mutations, **2**:351
  familial (dominant) drusen and, **12**:220–221
Effective irradiance, **2**:462
Effective radiant exposure, **2**:462
Effector blockade, **9**:38
Effector cells, **9**:11, 25, 26*i*
  locations of, **9**:34*t*
  lymphocytes as, **9**:11, 15, 25, 26*i*
  macrophages as, **9**:14–15
  neutrophils as, **9**:13, 48–50, 49*i*
Effector phase of immune response arc, **9**:17–19, 18*i*,
    25, 26*i*, 43–86
  adaptive immunity and, **9**:27, 54–75, 55*t*
  antibody-mediated, **9**:54–63, 55*t*
  blockade of, in anterior chamber–associated immune
    deviation, **9**:38
  cells in. *See* Effector cells
  combined antibody and cellular, **9**:55*t*, 70–74
  innate immunity and, **9**:43–54
  lymphocyte-mediated, **9**:55*t*, 63–70
  mediator systems and, **9**:74–86
  response to poison ivy and, **9**:30
  response to tuberculosis and, **9**:31
  in viral conjunctivitis, **9**:35
Efferent fibers, visceral, **2**:117
Efferent lymphatic channels, **9**:8
Efferent pupillary pathway, **2**:110
Efferent visual pathways/efferent visual system,
    5:32–49. *See also* Ocular motor pathways
  ocular motility and, **5**:197
Effexor. *See* Venlafaxine
Effusion
  suprachoroidal, cataract surgery and, **11**:169–170
    flat or shallow anterior chamber and, **11**:163, 166
  uveal, secondary angle-closure glaucoma and, **10**:141
Eflone. *See* Fluorometholone
EGF-containing fibrillin-like extracellular matrix
    protein (EFEMP1) mutations, **2**:351
  familial (dominant) drusen and, **12**:220–221
Ehlers-Danlos syndrome, **1**:166, **2**:262*t*, **8**:288, 309*t*,
    350–354, 351*t*
  angioid streaks in, **12**:83
  blue sclera in, **8**:288
  keratoglobus in, **6**:250, **8**:334
Ehrlichiosis, human granulocytic, **1**:19
Eicosanoids, **2**:305–308, 306*i*, **8**:198*t*, **9**:78–79, 78*i*

Ejection fraction, in congestive heart failure, **1**:127
EKC. *See* Epidemic keratoconjunctivitis
Elastases, in ocular infections, **8**:117
Elastic tendons, anterior, **2**:67
Elastin, **8**:14
Elastoid (elastotic) degeneration/elastosis, **4**:49*i*, 50
  conjunctival, **8**:365
  corneal, **8**:368–369. *See also* Spheroidal degeneration
    solar, of eyelid, **4**:177, 177*i*
Eldepryl. *See* Selegiline
Elder abuse, **1**:236–237
Elderly patients. *See* Age/aging; Geriatrics
Electric field, of light wave, **3**:3, 4*i*
Electrical injury, lens damage/cataracts caused by,
    11:59, 60*i*
Electrically evoked potentials, **12**:41
Electrocardiography (ECG)
  in atrial flutter, **1**:137
  in atrial tachycardia, **1**:136
  in congestive heart failure, **1**:127
  exercise, **1**:119
  in ischemic heart disease, **1**:114, 116, 119
  in junctional tachycardia, **1**:137
  in sinus tachycardia, **1**:136
  in stroke evaluation, **1**:103
  in torsades de pointes, **1**:140
  in ventricular fibrillation, **1**:140
  in ventricular tachycardia, **1**:138
Electroencephalography (EEG), in epilepsy diagnosis,
    1:282
Electrolysis, for trichiasis, **7**:207, **8**:104
Electrolytes
  in lens, maintenance of balance of, **11**:19–21, 21*i*
  in tear film, **2**:290
Electromagnetic energy/radiation, adverse effects of on
    retina, **12**:305–309, 306*i*
Electromagnetic wave spectrum, **3**:4, 6*i*
Electromyography, **6**:32
  in myasthenia gravis, **5**:328, **6**:152
Electron microscopy, diagnostic, **4**:40
Electrooculogram, **12**:36–38, 37*i*, 38*i*. *See also specific
    disorder*
  trans-RPE potential as basis for, **2**:362
Electrophoresis
  denaturing gradient gel, **2**:230
  hemoglobin, in sickling disorders, **12**:120
Electrophysiologic testing. *See also specific test*
  of retina, **2**:354–355, 355*i*, **12**:27–41
    in functional visual disorders, **5**:306
    in Leber congenital amaurosis, **12**:211–212
    in low vision evaluation, **5**:99–102
Electroretinogram, **2**:354, **12**:27–36
  in achromatopsia, **12**:30*i*, 196
  aging affecting, **12**:31
  applications and cautions for, **12**:33–36, 34*i*, 35*i*
  bright-flash, **12**:33
  before cataract surgery, **11**:86
  in choroideremia, **12**:35
  in cone dystrophies, **12**:30*i*, 214
  in cone–rod dystrophies, **12**:30*i*, 214
  in congenital night blindness with fundus
    abnormality, **12**:200–201
  in congenital stationary night blindness, **12**:30*i*,
    198–200, 199*i*, 200*i*
  dark-adapted. *See* Electroretinogram, scotopic

in Duchenne muscular dystrophy, 12:236
in elderly patients, 12:31
focal, 12:31–32
foveal, 12:31–32
in fundus albipunctatus, 12:200
in glaucoma, 10:59
in hereditary retinal/choroidal degenerations,
    12:204–205, 206*t*
interpretation of, 12:30–31, 30*i*, 206*t*
in Leber congenital amaurosis, 6:335, 452, 455,
    12:211–212
in low vision evaluation, 5:101–102, 102*i*
    in infant, 6:452
macular, 12:33–34, 34*i*
multifocal, 12:32, 32*i*
in newborns, 12:31
in ocular ischemic syndrome, 12:151
pattern, 12:33, 33*i*
pediatric, 12:35, 35*i*
photopic/light-adapted, 12:28*i*, 29, 205, 206*t*
    in hereditary retinal/choroidal degenerations,
        12:205, 206*t*
recording, 12:27–29, 28*i*
in retinal disease, 12:30–31, 30*i*, 33–36, 34*i*, 35*i*,
    205–206, 206*t*
in retinitis pigmentosa, 12:34*i*, 208–209
scotopic/dark-adapted, 12:27, 28*i*, 29, 206*t*. See also
    Dark adaptation testing
in siderosis, 12:26, 299
specialized types of, 12:31–33
Elementary body, *Chlamydia,* 8:128
Elestat. *See* Epinastine
Elevated intraocular pressure, 10:96
after anterior chamber phakic IOL insertion, 13:153*t*
after cataract surgery, 11:164*t*, 172
    flat anterior chamber and, 11:166
    in glaucoma patient, 11:218
    stromal/epithelial corneal edema and, 11:166
cataract surgery in patients with, 11:212
central retinal vein occlusion and, 12:143
corticosteroids causing, 2:419–420, 419*t*, 10:116–117
cycloplegics causing, 2:401
drugs for. *See specific agent and* Antiglaucoma agents;
    Glaucoma, management of
in glaucoma, 10:3, 10, 83–84
    congenital/childhood glaucoma and, 6:274–275
    uveitis and, 9:237
in hyphema, 8:400, 401–402
    in children, 6:447
    surgery and, 8:402, 403*t*
after iris-fixated phakic IOL insertion, 13:153*t*, 154
after LASIK, 13:189, 190*i*, 208–209
lens epithelium affected by, 4:98
open-angle glaucoma without, 10:92–96, 94*t*. See
    also Glaucoma, normal-tension
orbital trauma and, 7:107, 107–108
after penetrating keratoplasty, 8:460–461
after posterior chamber phakic IOL insertion,
    13:153*t*
after PRK, 13:105, 189, 208
after refractive surgery, 13:208–209
refractive surgery in patients with, 13:189–191, 190*i*
in Terson syndrome, 12:95
in Valsalva retinopathy, 12:93
Elevation-based topography, 13:6, 8

Elevation of eye (upgaze), 6:34, 36
in Brown syndrome, 5:219, 220*i*, 6:144, 145*i*
conjugate paresis of, 5:211
disorders of
    in blowout fractures, 7:102–104, 103*i*
        surgery and, 7:104
    conjugate limitation, 5:207
extraocular muscles controlling
    inferior oblique, 6:16, 30*t*, 31
    superior rectus, 6:14, 30, 30*t*, 32*i*
monocular deficiency of (double elevator palsy),
    6:137–138, 138*i*, 7:214
11p13 syndrome (short arm 11 deletion syndrome),
    2:254–255
ELISA. *See* Enzyme-linked immunosorbent assay
ELK. *See* Endothelial lamellar keratoplasty
Ellipsoid
Cartesian, 3:53–54, 54*i*
of cone, 2:79, 82*i*
of rod, 2:79, 82*i*
Elliptically polarized light, 3:10
ELM. *See* External limiting membrane
ELOVL4 gene, in Stargardt disease, 12:216
Elschnig pearls, 4:100, 100*i*, 11:186
Elschnig spots, 12:98, 98*i*
Elspar. *See* Asparaginase
Emadine. *See* Emedastine
Emboli
branch retinal artery occlusion and, 12:146
calcium, transient visual loss and, 5:175, 176*i*, 177*t*
central retinal artery occlusion and, 12:146–147
cholesterol (Hollenhorst plaques)
    in branch retinal artery occlusion, 4:133, 12:146,
        147*i*
    in central retinal artery occlusion, 12:149
    transient visual loss and, 5:173, 173*i*, 177*t*
choroidal perfusion abnormalities and, 12:166–167
fat, retinal findings in, 12:95
platelet-fibrin, transient visual loss and, 5:175, 176*i*,
    177*t*
retinal vasculitis and, 12:153
stroke caused by, 1:102
transient visual loss caused by, 5:174*t*, 175–183, 176*i*,
    178*i*
    clinical aspects of, 5:177*t*
    clinical and laboratory evaluation of, 5:179–180
    prognosis for, 5:180–181, 180*t*
    treatment of, 5:181–182, 182*t*
Embolization, coil, of aneurysm, 5:353–354
Embryogenesis, 2:126, 133–136, 134*i*, 135*i*, 137*i*, 138*i*.
    See also Eye, development of
Embryology. *See also* Congenital anomalies; Eye,
    development of
terms used in, 2:125–128
Embryonal rhabdomyosarcoma, 4:198, 199*i*, 6:373, 7:80
Embryonic fissure, 2:137–138, 137*i*
closure of, 2:138, 143*i*
    colobomas and, 2:138, 143*i*, 165–166, 171
    persistence of, in fetal alcohol syndrome, 2:161
Embryonic nucleus, 2:146, 11:9, 26–27, 27*i*
    opacification of (congenital nuclear cataract), 11:37,
        38*i*
Embryotoxon, posterior, 2:127, 168, 168*i*, 4:78, 78*i*,
    6:251–252, 251*i*, 8:291, 292*i*. *See also*
    Neurocristopathy
    in Axenfeld-Rieger syndrome, 6:251*i*, 252, 253, 8:292

Emedastine, 2:423, 424*t*
Emergencies, 1:313–326. *See also specific type*
  cardiopulmonary arrest, 1:313–317
  medications used in, 1:316*t*
  ocular side effects of systemic medications,
    1:323–326, 324–325*t*
  recent developments and, 1:313
  seizures, 1:320–321
  shock, 1:317–320
  status epilepticus, 1:320–321
  toxic overdose, 1:321–323, 322*t*
Emissaria/emissarial channels, 2:50, 4:88, 88*i*
  melanoma spread via, 4:159–161, 162*i*
Emission, spontaneous and stimulated, in lasers,
    3:19–21, 21*i*
Emivirine, 1:42
Emmetropia, 3:115–116, 115*i*
  in infants and children, 3:120
  retinal reflex in, 3:127–128
Emmetropization, 3:120
  developmental model of, 3:121
Emollients, ocular, 2:450
Emphysema, 1:154
Emphysema (ocular), of orbit and eyelids, in blowout
    fractures, 7:101–102, 104
Empirical horopter, 6:42, 42*i*, 43
Emtricitabine, 1:41
Emtriva. *See* Emtricitabine
Emulsification. *See also* Phacoemulsification
  instrument settings for, 11:135*t*, 136–137
Enalapril/enalaprilat
  for heart failure, 1:130
  for hypertension, 1:88*t*, 90*t*, 94
  ocular effects of, 1:325*t*
Enbrel. *See* Etanercept
Encapsulation, polysaccharide, as microbial virulence
    factor, 1:4
Encephalitis, herpes, 1:27, 5:360, 361*i*
Encephalitozoon, keratoconjunctivitis caused by, 8:190
Encephaloceles, 2:166, 7:38
  of orbit, 6:384
Encephalofacial angiomatosis. *See* Sturge-Weber
    disease/syndrome
Encephalopathy
  HIV, 1:37, 5:361
  inherited, resembling migraine, 5:297–298
  Leigh necrotizing (Leigh syndrome), 2:262*t*
    mitochondrial DNA mutation and, 2:219*i*, 220
Encephalotrigeminal/cerebrofacial angiomatosis. *See*
    Sturge-Weber disease/syndrome
Enchondromas, of orbit, in Maffucci syndrome, 6:377
Encopred. *See* Prednisolone
End-replication problems, telomeres in prevention of,
    2:205
End-stopped cells, 5:29
Endarterectomy, carotid
  for carotid stenosis, 1:101, 107–108, 109, 5:181–182
  for ocular ischemic syndrome, 9:223, 12:151–152
Endarteritis, in syphilis, 1:16
Endemic Kaposi sarcoma, 9:258
Endocanalicular laser dacryocystorhinostomy,
    7:281–282
Endocapsular tension ring, 11:227, 228*i*
Endocarditis prophylaxis, 1:7, 8–11*t*
  ocular surgery and, 1:334

Endocrine disorders, 1:201–231. *See also specific type*
  diabetes mellitus, 1:201–221
  hypothalamic-pituitary axis and, 1:227–230
  multiple endocrine neoplasia syndromes, 1:230–231
  recent developments in, 1:201
  thyroid disease, 1:221–227
Endocrinopathies. *See* Endocrine disorders
Endoderm, 2:134, 135*i*, 137*i*
Endoflagella, of spirochetes, 8:128
Endogenous antigens, 8:447. *See also* Human leukocyte
    (HLA) antigens
Endogenous endophthalmitis, 9:207, 209*i*, 213–214,
    214*i*. *See also* Endophthalmitis
Endolenticular phacoemulsification, 11:129
Endometrial tissue sampling, for cancer screening,
    1:295*t*
Endonucleases, 2:185. *See also* Restriction
    endonucleases
Endophthalmitis, 9:207–220
  bacterial
    toxins affecting severity of, 9:46
    vitreous affected in, 4:107
  bleb-associated, 9:208*t*, 209, 212–213
  diagnosis/differential diagnosis of, 9:215–216
  endogenous, 9:207, 209*i*, 213–214, 214*i*
    bacterial, 12:183–184, 183*i*
    fungal, 9:223–227
    molds/*Aspergillus* causing, 9:225–226, 225*i*,
      12:188–189, 189*i*
    nocardial, 9:223, 223*i*
    yeasts/*Candida* causing, 9:163–164, 213–214, 219,
      223–225, 12:187–188, 188*i*
  evisceration for, 7:123
  exogenous, 9:207, 208*t*, 209–213, 209*i*
  fungal, 9:208*t*, 210, 212, 213–214, 214*i*, 219, 223–227
    iris nodule in, 4:219*t*
    vitreous affected in, 4:107
  infectious, 9:207–214, 208*t*. *See also specific causative
    agent*
    differential diagnosis of, 9:215
  intraocular specimens for diagnosis of
    collection of, 9:215–216
    cultures and laboratory evaluation of, 9:216
  after penetrating keratoplasty, 8:461
  after perforating injury, 8:410
  phacoantigenic (lens-induced/phacoanaphylaxis),
    4:96, 96*i*, 97*i*, 9:64, 135–136, 135*i*, 136*i*,
    10:105–106, 11:64, 67
  postoperative, 9:207, 208*t*, 209–211, 12:328–331
    acute-onset, 9:210–211, 210*i*, 211*i*, 12:329, 330*i*
    bleb-associated, 9:207, 208*t*, 212–213, 12:331, 332*i*
    after cataract surgery, 9:207, 208*t*, 209, 11:164*t*,
      176–178, 176*i*
      prevention of, 11:97
    chronic (delayed-onset), 9:211, 212*i*, 12:329–331,
      331*i*
    after strabismus surgery, 6:186, 186*i*
      scleral perforation and, 6:185, 186*i*
    vitrectomy for, 12:328–331
  posttraumatic, 9:207, 208*t*, 211–212, 12:300
  prophylaxis of, 9:214–215
  Propionibacterium acnes causing, 4:97, 98*i*, 9:53,
    208*t*, 209, 211, 212*i*
  signs and symptoms of, 9:207

sterile, **9:**207
    after cataract surgery, **11:**176
    in toxocariasis, **9:**170, 171*t*
    treatment of, **9:**217–220
        medical, **9:**217–219, 218*t*
        outcomes of, **9:**219–220
        surgical, **9:**217
Endophthalmitis Vitrectomy Study (EVS), **9:**217, 220, **11:**177, **12:**329, 330
Endoscopic brow and forehead lift, **7:**239–241, 240*i*
Endoscopic brow lift, **7:**241
Endoscopic cyclophotocoagulation, for childhood glaucoma, **6:**282
Endoscopic dacryocystorhinostomy, **7:**282–283, 282*i*
Endoscopic laser delivery system, in lowering intraocular pressure, **10:**205
Endoscopic midface lift, **7:**243*i*, 248–249
Endoscopy, nasal, for acquired tearing evaluation, **7:**271
Endothelial cell density, specular photomicroscopy in evaluation of, **8:**36, 36*i*
Endothelial degenerations, **8:**375
Endothelial dystrophies, **8:**324–329
    cataract surgery in patients with, **11:**208, 210*i*
    congenital hereditary, **4:**62–63, 63*i*, **6:**256*t*, 257, **8:**297–298, 298*i*, 309*t*
    Fuchs, **2:**49, 49*i*, **4:**73, 75*i*, **8:**310*t*, 324–327, 325*i*, 326*i*
Endothelial failure, after penetrating keratoplasty
    late nonimmune, **8:**464
    primary, **8:**461, 461*i*
Endothelial graft rejection, **8:**468–469, 469*i*. *See also* Rejection (graft)
Endothelial lamellar keratoplasty (ELK), **8:**475
Endothelial meshwork, **2:**57, 58*i*, 59*i*
Endothelial rings, corneal, traumatic, **8:**396, 397*i*
Endotheliitis (disciform keratitis), herpes simplex virus causing, **8:**147, 147*i*
Endothelin receptors, in signal transduction in iris–ciliary body, **2:**314*t*
Endothelium
    corneal, **4:**61–62, 61*i*, **8:**9*i*, 12
        anatomy of, **2:**47–49, 49*i*, 298*i*
        anterior chamber phakic IOLs affecting, **13:**151, 153*t*
        biochemistry and metabolism of, **2:**301–302
        development of, **8:**6
        dysfunction of, corneal edema and, **8:**33–34, 34*t*, 385–386
        glucose metabolism in, **2:**297–299, 298*i*
        intraocular surgery causing changes in, **8:**419–420
        iris-fixated phakic IOLs affecting, **13:**153*t*, 154
        posterior chamber phakic IOLs affecting, **13:**153*t*, 154
        PRK/LASEK and, **13:**105
        wound healing/repair of, **4:**21–22, 21*i*, **8:**384–386
    retinal blood vessel, **2:**84
Endotoxins, microbial, **8:**123
    in innate immune response, **9:**43–44, 46
    virulence and, **1:**4
Energix-B. *See* Hepatitis B vaccine
Energy, for medical lasers, **3:**18, 18*t*
Energy production
    in lens, **2:**330
    in rods, **2:**344

Enfuvirtide, **1:**42
Engerix-B. *See* Hepatitis B vaccine
Enhanced S cone/blue cone syndrome (Goldmann-Favre syndrome), **6:**342, **12:**201, 202*i*, 229
Enhancer region, **2:**185–186, 202, 202*i*
Enophthalmos, **7:**24, 25
    in blowout fractures, **7:**102, 103
        surgery and, **7:**105
    orbital varices and, **7:**70
Enoxacin, **1:**62*t*, 73
Enoxaparin, for non-ST-segment elevation acute coronary syndrome, **1:**123
Entacapone, for Parkinson disease, **1:**279
Enteritis, regional (Crohn disease), **1:**177, **9:**131–132
Enterobacter, **8:**126
Enterobacteriaceae, **8:**126–127
Enterococcus, **8:**125
    bleb-associated endophthalmitis caused by, **9:**213
    endocarditis caused by, **1:**7
    faecalis, **8:**125
    vancomycin-resistant, **1:**3, 5, 71, 72
Enterocolitis, pseudomembranous, *Clostridium difficile* causing, **1:**8
Enteropathic arthritis, **1:**177
Enteroviruses, **8:**121
    conjunctivitis caused by, **8:**163
Enthesitis
    in juvenile idiopathic (chronic/rheumatoid) arthritis, uveitis and, **6:**313, 314*i*
    in spondyloarthropathies, **1:**175
        ankylosing spondylitis, **1:**175
Entoptic images/phenomena, Purkinje's, evaluation of before cataract surgery, **11:**86
Entoptoscopy, blue-light, before cataract surgery, **11:**86
Entrance pupil, **3:**110
Entropion, **7:**201–207
    acute spastic, **7:**201–202, 202*i*
    cicatricial, **7:**205–207, 205*i*, 206*i*
    congenital, **6:**210, **7:**156–157
    involutional, **7:**202–205, 203*i*
    lash margin, in anophthalmic socket, **7:**127
Enucleation, **7:**119–122
    for blind eyes in retinopathy of prematurity, **6:**332
    in childhood, **7:**121
    complications of, **7:**123
    for corneoscleral laceration, **8:**410–411
    definition of, **7:**119
    guidelines for, **7:**120–121
    for melanoma, **4:**237
    for metastatic eye disease, **4:**273–275
    ocular prostheses after, **7:**122
    orbital implants after, **7:**121–122
    for prevention of sympathetic ophthalmia, **8:**410–411
    removal of wrong eye and, **7:**123
    for retinoblastoma, **4:**260, **6:**396–397
    rubeosis iridis and, **4:**155–156
    for sympathetic ophthalmia prevention, **7:**119–120, **9:**200, **12:**300–301
    for uveal lymphoid infiltration, **4:**280
Envelope
    nuclear, **2:**203
    viral, **8:**120
Environmental factors
    in glaucoma, **10:**15

in migraine, 5:296
Enzymatic method, for DNA sequencing, 2:231, 232*i*
Enzymatic vitreolysis, 2:339
Enzyme defects, disorders associated with, 2:261, 262*t*
  in children, 6:435–439, 436–437*t*
  management of, 2:281, 6:438
  recessive inheritance of, 2:261–263
Enzyme-linked immunosorbent assay (ELISA)
  in HIV infection/AIDS, 1:39, 9:245–246
  in Lyme disease, 1:20
  in toxoplasmosis, 9:167
EOG. *See* Electrooculogram
EOMs. *See* Extraocular muscles
Eosinophil chemotactic factor, 8:200*t*
Eosinophilic granuloma, of orbit, 6:276*i*, 375, 7:88
Eosinophils, 9:13
  cytologic identification of, 8:65*t*, 66, 67*i*
    in immune-mediated keratoconjunctivitis, 8:203*t*
    in external eye, 8:196*t*
  in inflammation, 4:13, 14*i*
  mediators released by, 8:200*t*
Eotaxin, 8:200*t*
Ependymoma, nystagmus caused by, 6:159*t*
Eperezolid, 1:63*t*, 75
Ephelis. *See also* Freckle
  conjunctival, 4:56*t*, 8:263
  of eyelid, 7:171
Epiblast, 2:134, 134*i*, 136
Epiblepharon, 6:211, 7:155*i*, 156
Epibulbar conjunctiva, 4:43
Epibulbar tumors
  in children, 6:385–388
  choristomas, 8:275–277, 276*i*, 277*i*, 278*i*
  dermoids, 6:386, 386*i*, 8:275–276, 276*i*
  Goldenhar syndrome and, 6:431
Epicanthus, 6:212, 212*i*, 7:155*i*, 156
  inversus, 6:212, 7:156
    in blepharophimosis syndrome, 6:213, 213*i*
  palpebralis, 6:212, 212*i*, 7:156
  supraciliaris, 6:212, 7:156
  tarsalis, 6:212, 212*i*, 7:156
Epicapsular star (tunica vasculosa lentis remnant), 11:32, 32*i*
Epidemic Kaposi sarcoma, 9:258
Epidemic keratoconjunctivitis, 8:158, 158*i*, 159, 159*i*, 160*i*
  in children, 6:225–226
    preseptal cellulitis caused by, 6:230
Epidermal cysts
  of eyelid, 7:164–166, 165*i*
  of orbit, 4:188
Epidermal growth factor, 2:456
Epidermal growth factor–containing fibrillin-like extracellular matrix protein (EFEMP1) mutations, 2:351
  familial (dominant) drusen and, 12:220–221
Epidermal necrolysis, toxic, 8:216–217, 217*t*
Epidermis, eyelid, 4:167*i*, 168, 8:245, 246*i*
  neoplasms of, 4:174–185
    benign, 7:164–166, 165*i*
    premalignant, 7:172–173, 172*i*, 173*i*
Epidermoid cysts, 8:275
  of orbit, 6:381, 7:63
Epifrin. *See* Epinephrine

Epikeratoplasty (epikeratophakia), 13:20*t*, 23, 25*i*, 73–77
  for keratoconus, 13:75–76, 186
Epilation, mechanical, for trichiasis, 7:207, 8:104
Epilepsy, 1:280–284. *See also* Seizures
  hallucinations and, 5:190
  ocular deviation with, 5:211
Epimerase deficiency, galactosemia caused by, 11:62
Epimyoepithelial islands, 7:92
Epinastine, 2:424*t*
Epinephrine, 2:407*t*, 409
  adrenochrome deposition caused by, 8:376–378, 377*i*, 377*t*
  for anaphylaxis, 1:319, 320
  dipivalyl. *See* Dipivefrin
  for glaucoma, 10:160*t*, 165, 169, 170, 170*i*
    in children, 6:283
  with local anesthetic
    for blepharoplasty, 7:231
    for eyelid surgery, 7:150
    maximum safe dosage and, 1:322*t*
    toxic reaction to, 1:322
  for medical emergencies, 1:316*t*
  in personal emergency kits, 1:320
  for pulmonary diseases, 1:157
Epinucleus, 11:131
EpiPen/EpiPen Jr, 1:320
Epiphora. *See* Tearing
Epiretinal membrane, 5:105, 12:87–89, 88*i*, 324–325, 325*i*
  vitrectomy for, 12:88, 323–324, 325*i*
  vitreomacular traction syndrome differentiated from, 12:91*t*
Episclera, 2:50, 4:87
  disorders of. *See also specific type and* Episcleritis
    immune-mediated, 8:234–235, 235*i*
    examination of, in glaucoma, 10:33
    melanosis of, 8:264–265, 265*i*
    nodular fasciitis causing tumor of, 4:92
    in scleral wound healing, 8:386
Episcleral osseous choristoma, 4:88
Episcleral plexus, ciliary body, 2:67
Episcleral surgical space, 7:109
Episcleral venous pressure, 10:22–23
  elevated, open-angle glaucoma caused by, 10:108–109, 108*t*, 109*i*
Episcleritis, 4:89, 8:25*t*, 29–31, 234–235, 235*i*
  in herpes zoster, 8:154
  immune-mediated, 8:234–235, 235*i*
  nodular, in children, 6:388
  in reactive arthritis/Reiter syndrome, 8:228
  in Stevens-Johnson syndrome, 8:217
Epithelial cells. *See also* Epithelium
  keratinization of (keratinized/degenerated), 8:23
    cytologic identification of, 8:64, 65*t*, 67*i*
      in immune-mediated keratoconjunctivitis, 8:203*t*
    in meibomian gland dysfunction, 8:80
    in vitamin A deficiency, 8:93
Epithelial cysts, of eyelids, benign, 7:164–166, 165*i*
Epithelial debridement. *See* Debridement
Epithelial defects
  conjunctival, 8:24*t*
  corneal, 8:25*t*

after LASIK, **13**:122
in diabetic patients, **13**:197
persistent, **8**:101–104, 103*i*
after penetrating keratoplasty, **8**:461
after PRK/LASEK, **13**:104
Epithelial degenerations, **8**:368–369
Epithelial downgrowth (ingrowth)
cataract surgery and, **11**:185
after LASIK, **13**:129–131, 130*i*
secondary angle-closure glaucoma and, **10**:141–143
Epithelial dystrophies, **4**:70–71, 72*i*
basement membrane, **8**:310*t*, 311–313, 312*i*
cataract surgery in patients with, **11**:208, 209*i*
refractive surgery in patients with, **13**:44, 46*i*
juvenile (Meesmann), **8**:310*t*, 313, 314*i*
map-dot-fingerprint (basement membrane/anterior
membrane), **4**:70, 72*i*, **8**:310*t*, 311–313, 312*i*
cataract surgery in patients with, **11**:208, 209*i*
refractive surgery in patients with, **13**:44, 46*i*
Epithelial edema, **8**:24*t*. See also Cornea, edema of
after cataract surgery, **11**:166
central (Sattler's veil), **8**:106
intraocular surgery causing, **8**:418–419
Epithelial erosions
herpetic keratitis and, **8**:151
after LASIK, **13**:122
in diabetic patients, **13**:197
punctate
of conjunctiva, **8**:24*t*
of cornea, **8**:24*t*, 30*i*, 32*t*
refractive surgery and, **13**:44, 45*i*
Epithelial graft rejection, **8**:467, 468*i*. See also Rejection
(graft)
Epithelial hyperplasias, of eyelids, **7**:163–164, 164–165*i*
Epithelial inclusion cysts, **8**:254, 254*i*
conjunctival, **4**:45, 46*i*, **6**:386
nevi and, **4**:55–56, 56*i*
after strabismus surgery, **6**:187, 188*i*
orbital, **4**:188
Epithelial ingrowth/implantation. See Epithelial
downgrowth
Epithelial invasion of iris, **4**:219*t*
Epithelial keratitis/keratopathy
adenoviral, **8**:158, 160*i*
dry eye and, **8**:72
herpes simplex virus causing, **8**:143–146, 143*i*, 144*i*,
145*i*
in herpes zoster ophthalmicus, **8**:154
measles virus causing, **8**:162
punctate, **8**:24*t*, 29, 30*i*, 32*t*
exposure causing, **8**:95
microsporidial, **8**:190
staphylococcal blepharoconjunctivitis and, **8**:165,
166*i*, 168
superficial Thygeson, **8**:224–225, 225*i*
Epithelial tumors, of lacrimal glands, **7**:89–91, 90*i*
exenteration for, **7**:128
Epithelial ulcer, geographic, in herpes simplex keratitis,
8:143, 144*i*, 146
Epitheliitis, acute retinal pigment (ARPE/Krill disease),
9:177*t*, 178, 179*i*
Epithelioid (Leber) cells, **8**:68, **9**:15, 52–53. See also
Macrophages
Epithelioid histiocytes, **4**:13, 14*i*

Epitheliopathy
acute posterior multifocal placoid pigment
(APMPPE), **9**:177*t*, 178, 179*i*, **12**:173–175, 174*t*,
175*i*
in herpetic keratitis, **8**:151
microcystic, **8**:107
Epithelium. See also under Epithelial and Ocular surface
ciliary, **2**:66–67, 68*i*
aqueous humor composition and, **2**:315–317
benign adenomas and cysts of, **4**:241–242
development of, **2**:154
nonpigmented, **2**:66, 68*i*
pigmented, **2**:67, 68*i*
acquired hyperplasia of, **4**:241–242
conjunctival, **2**:36, **8**:8, 59
cysts of, **4**:45, 46*i*, **8**:254, 254*i*
nevi and, **4**:55–56, 56*i*
cytologic identification of, **8**:64, 66*i*
dysplasia of, **4**:51, 52*i*
evaluation of, in pseudoepiphora, **7**:273
lesions of, **4**:51–53, 52*i*, 53*i*
physiology of, **8**:59
wound healing/repair and, **8**:383, 424
corneal, **4**:61–62, 61*i*, **8**:9–10, 9*i*, 58
anatomy of, **2**:45, 46*i*, 298*i*, 299
biochemistry and metabolism of, **2**:299
cytologic identification of, **8**:64
defects of, **8**:25*t*
persistent, **8**:101–104, 103*i*
after penetrating keratoplasty, **8**:461
dysplasia of, **4**:76
evaluation of, in pseudoepiphora, **7**:273
glucose metabolism in, **2**:297–299, 298*i*
healing of, after PRK/LASEK, **13**:97
intraocular surgery causing changes in, **8**:418–419
metabolic damage in contact lens overwear
syndromes and, **8**:106–107
physiology of, **8**:58
preservation of in LASEK, **13**:94–95, 94*i*
removal of for PRK, **13**:93–94, 93*i*
wound healing/repair of, **4**:21–22, 21*i*, **8**:383–384,
424
development of, **8**:6
in external eye defense, **8**:114
eyelid, hyperplasia of, **7**:163–164, 164*i*, 165*i*
immune and inflammatory cells in, **8**:196*t*
lens, **2**:74–76, 74*i*, 324, 324*i*, **4**:93–94, **11**:6–9, 8*i*
abnormalities of, **4**:98–100, 99*i*, 100*i*
active transport and, **11**:19–20
development of, **11**:27*i*, 28
opacification of (capsular cataract), **11**:37
limbal, **8**:58
physiology of, **8**:58–59
retinal pigment. See Retinal pigment epithelium
tumors of, **8**:255–261, 255*t*
benign, **8**:255–257, 255*t*, 256*i*
malignant, **8**:260–261
preinvasive, **8**:255*t*, 257–259
pigmented, **8**:263*t*, 266–268, 267*t*
Epitopes, **9**:7, 11, 19, 56
Epivir. See Lamivudine
Eplerenone, **1**:88*t*
Eprosartan, **1**:88*t*, 90*t*
Epsilon (ε)-crystallins, **2**:326*t*, 327

Epstein-Barr virus, **1:**30, 254
    ocular infection caused by, **8:**156–157, 156*i*
    posterior uveitis caused by, **9:**157–158
Epstein intraocular lens, **11:**140*i*, 143
Eptifibatide, for non-ST-segment elevation acute
    coronary syndrome, **1:**123
Equator, **11:**5, 8
Equatorial retina, **12:**8
Equatorial streaks, in histoplasmosis, **9:**160, 161*i*
Erbium:YAG (Er:YAG) laser
    for phacolysis, **11:**138
    for scleral expansion, **13:**177
Erdheim-Chester disease, eyelid manifestations of,
    4:173*t*
ERG. *See* Electroretinogram
ERM. *See* Epiretinal membrane
Erosions
    conjunctival, **8:**25*t*
        punctate epithelial, **8:**24*t*
    corneal
        in herpetic keratitis, **8:**151
        punctate epithelial, **8:**24*t*, 30*i*, 32*t*
            refractive surgery and, **13:**44, 45*i*
        recurrent, **8:**98–100, 100*i*
            eye pain in, **5:**298, **8:**98
            posttraumatic, **8:**407
    eyelid, **8:**24*t*
ERP. *See* Early receptor potential
Ertapenem, **1:**60*t*, 69
Erysiphakes, **11:**91, 93
Erythema chronicum migrans, in Lyme disease, **1:**19,
    5:363, 364*i*, **9:**191, 192*i*
Erythema multiforme, **8:**217
    major (Stevens-Johnson syndrome), **8:**216–219, 217*t*,
        218*i*, 219*i*
        in children, **6:**237–238, 238*i*
        mucous membrane grafting for, **8:**439
        scleral contact lenses in management of, **3:**202
    minor, **8:**217
Erythrocyte sedimentation rate
    in giant cell arteritis, **1:**190, **5:**121–122
        central retinal artery occlusion and, **12:**149–150
    in immune-mediated disease, **8:**202*t*
Erythrocytes, **1:**159
    cytologic identification of, **8:**68
    development of, **1:**160
Erythromycin, **1:**60*t*, 70, **2:**428*t*, 431*t*, 436
    for chlamydial conjunctivitis, **8:**177
        in neonates, **6:**223, **8:**174
    intravenous administration of, **2:**389
    for Lyme disease, **5:**364
    for meibomian gland dysfunction, **8:**83
    for ophthalmia neonatorum prophylaxis, **6:**223
    for syphilis, **9:**190
    for trachoma, **8:**177
Erythropoiesis, **1:**160
Erythropoietin, **1:**160
    for HIV infection/AIDS, **1:**44
Escape rhythm, idioventricular, **1:**134
Escherichia coli (E coli), **8:**126
    as normal ocular flora, **8:**115
    ocular infection caused by, **8:**126
ESCS. *See* Enhanced S cone/blue cone syndrome
Eserine. *See* Physostigmine
Esidrix. *See* Hydrochlorothiazide

Esimil. *See* Guanethidine
Eskalith. *See* Lithium
Esmolol, for hypertensive emergency, **1:**94
Eso- (prefix), definition of, **6:**9
Esodeviations, **6:**97–108, 98*t*. *See also specific type and*
    Esotropia
    divergence insufficiency/paralysis, **6:**98*t*, 106
    incomitant, **6:**98*t*, 107–108
    medial rectus muscle restriction causing, **6:**98*t*, 108
    negative angle kappa and, **6:**86, 87*i*
    sensory deprivation, **6:**98*t*, 105–106
    sixth nerve (abducens) palsy causing, **6:**98*t*, 107–108
    surgery for, **6:**178–179, 179*t*
    thalamic, **5:**224
Esophageal cancer, screening for, **1:**297
Esophageal dysmotility, in scleroderma, **1:**185
Esophoria, **6:**97
Esotropia, **6:**97. *See also* Esodeviations
    A-pattern, **6:**87, 121*i*, 122
        treatment of, **6:**124–125
    accommodative, **6:**98*t*, 101–104
        muscarinic agents for management of, **2:**398
        refractive surgery in patient with, **13:**195–196
    acute, **6:**98*t*, 105
    basic (acquired), **6:**98*t*, 104–105
    in child with decreased vision, **6:**452
    cyclic, **6:**98*t*, 105
    divergence insufficiency/paralysis, **6:**98*t*, 106
    in Duane syndrome, **6:**142–143, 142*i*
    in Graves eye disease, **6:**149
    with high myopia, **6:**155
    incomitant, **6:**98*t*, 107–108
    infantile (congenital), **6:**97–101, 98*t*, 99*i*
        essential (classic), **6:**97–100, 98*t*, 99*i*
    intermittent, **6:**97
    medial rectus muscle restriction causing, **6:**98*t*, 108
    in Möbius syndrome, **6:**98*t*, 154, 154*i*
    nonaccommodative, **6:**104–107
    with nystagmus, **6:**98*t*, 101, 164. *See also* Nystagmus
    sensory deprivation, **6:**98*t*, 105–106
    sixth nerve (abducens) palsy causing, **6:**98*t*, 107–108
    spasm of near synkinetic reflex and, **6:**98*t*, 106
    surgical (consecutive), **6:**98*t*, 106–107
    V-pattern, **6:**87, 120*i*, 122
        treatment of, **6:**124
Essen classification of retinoblastoma, **4:**257–259, 259*t*
Essential blepharospasm, **5:**286–288, 287*i*, 287*t*, **7:**226
    treatment of, **5:**288
Essential cryoglobulinemic vasculitis, **1:**189*t*
Essential hypertension, **1:**82–83, 83*i*
Essential infantile esotropia, **6:**97–100, 98*t*, 99*i*
Essential iris atrophy, **4:**79
EST. *See* Expressed-sequence tags
Estazolam, **1:**273
Esthesiometry, **8:**35
Estradiol, ocular effects of, **1:**325*t*
Estrogen/estrogen replacement therapy
    breast cancer risk and, **1:**295
    cholesterol levels and, **1:**143
    osteoporosis and, **1:**241, 245*t*, 246
Etanercept, **1:**173, 199
    for uveitis, **9:**120
        in children, **6:**322
ETD. *See* Evaporative tear dysfunction

ETDRS (Early Treatment Diabetic Retinopathy Study), 12:102–104
  diabetic macular edema and, 12:113–116, 114i, 115i
  scatter laser treatment and, 12:108, 108i
ETDRS visual acuity chart, 3:112, 113i
  in low vision, 3:250
Ethambutol, 1:24, 49
Ethanol. See Alcohol
Ethmoid air cells/ethmoid sinus, 5:9, 9i, 7:20, 20i
Ethmoidal artery, 2:39i, 41i, 5:13, 15
Ethmoidal bone (lamina papyracea), 2:6, 5:10, 7:7, 8i, 9, 9i, 11
Ethmoidal foramina, anterior/posterior, 2:9–10, 5:10, 7:9i, 11
Ethmoidal suture, frontal, 5:9
Ethmoidectomy, for thyroid-associated orbitopathy, 5:332
Ethnic differences
  cancer and, 1:252, 253, 254
  genetic disorders and, 2:259–260
  hypertension and, 1:97
Ethosuximide, 1:283t
Ethylene glycol
  crystalline maculopathy caused by, 12:249, 250t
  optic neuropathy caused by, 5:152
Etidocaine, 2:447
Etodolac, 1:197t
Etoposide, 1:257, 259t
Etravirine, 1:42
ETROP study, 6:329
Euchromatin, 2:204
Eukaryotes/eukaryotic cells, 2:186, 8:122
Eulexin. See Flutamide
European Carotid Surgery Trial, 1:108
Euryblepharon, 6:211, 7:154, 155i
Euthyroid Graves ophthalmopathy, 1:224–225. See also Thyroid ophthalmopathy
Evagination, 2:126
Evaporative tear dysfunction, 8:72t, 80–90
  chalazion and, 8:87–88, 87i
  desquamating skin conditions and, 8:89
  ectodermal dysplasia and, 8:89
  ichthyosis and, 8:89
  meibomian gland dysfunction and, 8:80–84, 82i
  rosacea and, 8:84–86, 84i, 85i
  sarcoidosis and, 8:88
  seborrheic blepharitis and, 8:86–87
  xeroderma pigmentosum and, 8:90
Evasion, as microbial virulence factor, 8:116
Evernimicin, 1:63t, 75
Everninomicins, 1:63t, 75
Evisceration, 7:123–124
  definition of, 7:119, 123
Evoked cortical potentials, 12:39–41
  electrical, 12:41
  visual. See Visually evoked cortical potentials
Evolving stroke, 1:102
EVS (Endophthalmitis Vitrectomy Study), 9:217, 220, 11:177, 12:329, 330
EW complex. See Edinger-Westphal complex
Ewing sarcoma
  of orbit, 6:375
  retinoblastoma associated with, 4:265t
Exact ray tracing, 3:55–56, 55i. See also Raytracing

Examination
  ophthalmic, 8:15–51. See also specific method used and Refraction
    anterior segment photography in, 8:35–38, 36i, 38i
    in children, 6:3–5, 4i
    in congenital/infantile glaucoma, 6:273–276, 275i, 276i, 277i
    corneal pachymetry in, 8:31–34, 33i
    corneal topography measurement in, 8:38–49
    in diabetic patients, timetables for, 12:119, 119t
    esthesiometry in, 8:35
    HIV infection precautions and, 1:51–52, 9:261–262
    infection prevention and, 8:50–51
    in inflammatory disorders, 8:22–31, 24–25t, 32t
    for nystagmus, 6:161–162, 162t, 163i
    before penetrating keratoplasty, 8:454
    in perforating injury, 8:408, 409t
    physical examination, 8:15–16
    before refractive surgery, 13:42–46
    for retinoblastoma, 4:254–255, 6:398
    for retinopathy of prematurity, 6:328–329, 329t, 330i, 331i, 351–356, 354i, 12:125
    slit-lamp biomicroscopy in, 8:16–20
    stains used in, 8:20–22, 21i
    vision testing, 8:15
  slit-lamp. See Biomicroscopy, slit-lamp
  under anesthesia
    for eye trauma, 6:441
    for retinoblastoma, 4:254–255, 6:398
    for Sturge-Weber syndrome, 6:416
Excimer laser, 3:23. See also Lasers
  for coronary revascularization, 1:122
  for LASIK, 13:107
    ablation technique with, 13:114, 115i
    preoperative inspection of, 13:110
    preoperative programming of, 13:112
  for photoablation, 13:29, 87, 88–89i. See also Photoablation
  for presbyopia, 13:174–175, 174i
  for photorefractive keratectomy (PRK)
    ablation technique with, 13:95–96, 96i
    calibration of, 13:91
    preoperative programming of, 13:92
  for phototherapeutic keratectomy (PTK), 8:440, 13:21t
  for recurrent corneal erosions, 8:100
  wavefront-guided, 13:134
Excision repair, 2:213
Excisional biopsy, 7:176i, 177, 8:251, 252i, 427
Exclusion criteria, 1:364
Excretory lacrimal system, 2:30i, 34–36, 35i, 7:253–256, 255i, 256i. See also Lacrimal drainage system
Excyclo- (prefix), definition of, 6:10
Excycloduction. See Extorsion
Excyclotorsion, in superior oblique muscle paralysis, 6:133
Excyclovergence, 6:38
Executive function deficit, 1:264
Exelon. See Rivastigmine
Exenatide, for diabetes, 1:214
Exenteration, 7:127–129, 128i
  definition of, 7:119, 127
  histopathology findings and, 7:114

for lacrimal gland tumors, 7:90, 128, 284
for melanoma, 4:239
Exercise
    diabetes management/prevention and, 1:201, 207,
        207–209
    hypertension management and, 1:87*t*
Exercise stress tests, in ischemic heart disease, 1:119
    echocardiography, 1:118
Exfoliation, true, 4:80, 11:65
Exfoliation syndrome (pseudoexfoliation), 4:80, 81*i*,
        97–98, 98*i*, 10:42, 99–101, 99*i*, 100*i*, 11:65–66, 66*i*
    zonular incompetence and, cataract surgery in
        patient with, 11:226–227, 227*i*, 228*i*
Exo (previx), definition of, 6:9
Exodeviations, 6:109–117. *See also specific type and
    Exotropia*
    esodeviation following surgery for (surgical/
        consecutive esodeviation), 6:98*t*, 106–107
    overcorrection in, value of, 6:113, 179–180
    positive angle kappa and, 6:86, 87*i*
    surgery for, 6:179–180, 180*t*, 181*t*
    in third nerve (oculomotor) palsy, 6:146
Exogenous endophthalmitis, 9:207, 208*t*, 209–213, 209*i*
Exon, 2:186, 202, 202*i*, 203
Exon shuffling, 2:203
Exophoria, 6:109
Exophthalmometry, 7:25
Exophthalmos. *See* Proptosis
Exorbitism. *See* Proptosis
Exotoxins, microbial, 8:117
    in innate immune response, 9:45–46
    virulence and, 1:4
Exotropia
    A-pattern, 6:121*i*, 122
        treatment of, 6:125
    congenital, 6:114–115, 115*i*
    consecutive, 6:115
    constant, 6:114–115
    convergence insufficiency and, 6:112, 117
    convergence paralysis and, 6:117
    in craniosynostosis, 6:429
    dissociated horizontal deviation and, 6:116, 116*i*
    in Duane syndrome, 6:116, 142, 142*i*
    in infant with decreased vision, 6:452
    intermittent, 6:109–114, 110*i*
    neuromuscular abnormalities causing, 6:116
    sensory, 6:115
    V-pattern, 6:120*i*, 122
        treatment of, 6:124
Expansile dot pattern, in central serous
        chorioretinopathy, 12:52
Experimental (interventional) studies (clinical trials),
        1:345, 351–352, 351*i*. *See also* Clinical research
    for new drug, 2:393
    systematic reviews/meta-analyses of, 1:352
Exposure keratitis/keratopathy, 8:94–95
    in craniosynostosis-induced proptosis, 6:427–428
Exposure staining, 8:72, 73*i*
Expressed-sequence tags, 2:186
Expression, of genes. *See* Transcription (gene)
Expressivity (genetic), 2:186, 258–259
Expulsive choroidal/suprachoroidal hemorrhage, 4:25,
        26*i*
    cataract surgery and, 11:170–171
        patients at risk for, 11:215–217

External adnexa. *See* Ocular adnexa
External-beam radiation
    for choroidal hemangioma, 4:245
    for lymphoma, 4:278
    for melanoma, 4:237–238
    for metastatic eye disease, 4:273–275
    for retinal capillary hemangioma, 4:247
    for retinoblastoma, 4:262, 6:396
    retinopathy caused by, 12:305, 306*i*
    for uveal lymphoid infiltration, 4:280
External carotid artery, 5:11, 11–12*i*, 178*i*
    eyelids supplied by, 8:7
External dacryocystorhinostomy, 7:280–281, 281*i*
External (outer) eye. *See also specific structure*
    anatomy of, 8:6–14
    cataract surgery in patients with disease of,
        11:206–207
    defense mechanisms of, 8:113–114
        compromise of, 8:117–118
    development of, 8:6
    examination of, 8:15–51. *See also* Examination,
        ophthalmic
        before cataract surgery, 11:80–81
    function of, 8:5
    HIV infection/AIDS affecting, 9:258–260
    infections of. *See* Infection (ocular)
    photography in evaluation of, 8:35
External hordeolum (stye), 4:170, 7:160, 8:168
External jugular vein, 5:23
External limiting membrane, 2:80–81*i*, 82*i*, 83, 84,
        12:11*i*, 12
    development of, 2:141
Extirpation and denervation, 6:175*t*
Extorsion (excycloduction), 6:28
    extraocular muscles in
        inferior oblique, 6:16, 30*t*, 31
        inferior rectus, 6:14, 28, 30, 30*t*, 33*i*
Extorsional strabismus, 6:10
Extracapsular cataract extraction (ECCE), 10:132. *See
    also* Cataract surgery; Phacoemulsification
    capsular opacification and contraction and, 11:164*t*,
        186–191
        Nd:YAG laser capsulotomy for, 11:187–191, 189*i*
    cystoid macular edema and, 12:154
    early techniques for, 11:90
    lens-particle glaucoma and, 11:67–68
    modern techniques for, 11:92–93
    with nucleus expression, 11:108–112, 111*i*
        advantages of, 11:108–109
        contraindications to, 11:109
        flat or shallow anterior chamber and, 11:163–166
            intraoperative complications, 11:163–165
            postoperative complications, 11:165–166
            preoperative considerations, 11:82
        indications for, 11:108–109
        instrumentation for, 11:109
        postoperative course for, 11:112
        procedure for, 11:110–112, 111*i*
        retinal detachment and, 11:175
    by phacoemulsification, 11:112–137. *See also*
        Phacoemulsification
    posterior vitreous detachment and, 12:257
    in uveitis, 9:235
Extraconal fat/surgical space (peripheral surgical
    space), 7:12–13, 109, 110*i*

Extracranial trunk, of cranial nerve VII, 5:56
Extraction restriction, post-cataract, 5:219
Extrafoveal cones, 2:79–80
Extraocular muscle surgery, 6:173–192, 193*t. See also*
    Strabismus surgery
    for A-pattern deviations, 6:122–124, 123*i*, 124–125
    adjustable suture techniques for, 6:175–176
    anatomical considerations and, 6:23–26, 24*i*, 25*i*, 173
    anesthesia for, 6:183
    for classic congenital (essential infantile) esotropia,
        6:100
    complications of, 6:184–192, 193*t*
    conjunctival incisions for, 6:183–184
    for constant exotropia, 6:114
    for dissociated vertical deviation, 6:131, 181–182
    esodeviation after, 6:98*t*, 106–107
    for esodeviations, 6:178–179, 179*t*
    for esotropia in sixth nerve palsy, 6:107–108
    for exodeviations, 6:179–180, 180*t*, 181*t*
    exotropia after, 6:115
    in Graves/thyroid ophthalmopathy, 6:149–150
    guidelines for, 6:178–183
    for high accommodative convergence/
        accommodative esotropia, 6:103
    indications for, 6:173–174
    infections after, 6:185–186, 186*i*
    for inferior oblique muscle palsy, 6:136
    for intermittent exotropia, 6:113–114
    for monocular elevation deficiency (double elevator
        palsy), 6:137–138
    for nystagmus, 6:168–171, 170*i*, 170*t*
    oblique muscle-weakening procedures in, 6:180–181
    for overcorrection of intermittent exotropia,
        6:113–114
    for partially accommodative esotropia, 6:104
    planning, 6:176–178
    prior surgery and, 6:177
    rectus muscle procedures in, 6:181–183
    for refractive accommodative esotropia, 6:102
    strengthening procedures in, 6:174–175
    for superior oblique muscle palsy, 6:134–135, 180
    techniques for, 6:174–176, 175*t*
    for third nerve (oculomotor) palsy, 6:147–148
    transposition procedures in, 6:176
    for undercorrection of intermittent exotropia, 6:114
    for V-pattern deviations, 6:122–124, 123*i*, 124
    weakening procedures in, 6:174, 175*t*
Extraocular muscles, 2:15–21, 15*i*, 16*i*, 17*i*, 18*t*, 21*t*,
    6:13–26, 17*t*, 7:12–13. See also *specific muscle and*
    Eye movements; Ocular motility
    actions of, 6:13–16, 17*t*
        gaze position and, 6:23*i*, 29–30, 31*i*, 32*i*, 33*i*, 35*i*
        primary/secondary/tertiary, 6:13, 28–29, 30*t*
    anatomy of, 2:20–21, 5:41–42, 42*i*, 6:13–26, 14*i*, 17*t*
        in infants, 6:202
        surgery and, 6:23–26, 24*i*, 25*i*
    arterial system of, 6:16
        surgery and, 6:23–25
    blood supply of, 2:16–18, 18*t*, 6:16
        surgery and, 6:23–25
    congenital fibrosis type I syndrome of, 5:220
    connective tissue relationships of, 2:20–21
    damage to
        during blepharoplasty, 7:233
        in blowout fractures, 7:102–104
            surgery and, 7:104–105
        during enucleation, 7:123
    development of, 2:157
    fascial relationships of, 6:19–23, 19*i*
    fibers types in, 2:20–21, 21*t*
    in Graves ophthalmopathy, 7:48, 50*i*, 53
    innervation of, 2:18–20, 108–110, 109*i*, 6:13–16,
        18–19, 7:12–13
        surgery and, 6:23–26, 24*i*, 25*i*
    insertions of, 2:15–16, 18*t*, 6:13–16, 17*t*
        advancing, as strengthening procedure, 6:174
    lost, during surgery, 6:190
    orbital relationships of, 6:19–23, 19*i*
    origins of, 2:16, 18*t*, 6:13–16, 17*t*
    paralysis/paresis of
        in myasthenia gravis, 6:151
        3-step test in evaluation of, 6:90–92, 91*i*
    physiology of, in infants and children, 6:202
    in ptosis, 7:211–212
    slipped, surgery and, 6:23, 191, 191*i*
        esodeviations and, 6:98*t*, 106–107
    structure of, 6:18–19
    surgery of. See Extraocular muscle surgery;
        Strabismus surgery
    tumors of, eye movements affected by, 7:26
    venous system of, 6:16
    within orbit, 2:16, 17*i*, 19*i*
Extraocular myopathy, in thyroid ophthalmopathy,
    5:329*i*, 330, 6:149, 7:48, 53
Extraperiosteal route
    for inferior anterior orbitotomy, 7:111
    for superior anterior orbitotomy, 7:109–110
Extruded drusen, 5:129
Exuberant hyperkeratosis (cutaneous horn), 7:164
Exudates
    hard, 4:131, 131*i*
        in diabetic macular edema, 12:113, 114, 114*i*
    soft. See Cotton-wool spots
Exudative retinal detachment. See Retinal detachment
Exudative retinopathy, retinopathy of prematurity and,
    12:131
Exudative vitreoretinopathy, familial, 12:284–285, 285*i*
Eye
    aging affecting, 1:235
    anatomy of, 2:43–92. See also *specific structure*
    antipsychotic drugs affecting, 1:272–273
    axial length of, in infants and children, 6:199, 200*i*
        in congenital glaucoma, 6:276
    cataract surgery in patients with disorders of,
        11:206–224
    color of, age affecting, 6:200
    congenital anomalies of, 2:159–178, 160*i*, 4:12,
        6:205–206, 457*t*. See also *specific type and*
        Congenital anomalies
    cystic, 2:165
    depression of (downgaze). See Depression of eye
    development of, 2:129–158, 6:199–203, 8:6. See also
        specific structure
        abnormalities of, 2:159–178, 160*i*, 4:12. See also
            specific type and Congenital anomalies
        cataract surgery in patients with, 11:212–215
        chronology of, 2:139*t*
        embryogenesis, 2:133–136, 134*i*, 135*i*, 137*i*, 138*i*
        growth factors in, 2:129–130

homeobox genes and, 2:130–131
neural crest cells and, 2:131–132, 133*t*
organogenesis, 2:136–158, 139*t*
dimensions of, in children, 6:199, 200*i*, 200*t*, 201*i*
dry. *See* Dry eye syndrome
elevation of (upgaze). *See* Elevation of eye
external. *See* External (outer) eye
glands of, 2:29*t*
infection of. *See* Infection (ocular)
injury to. *See* Trauma
normal flora of, 8:114–115, 115*t*
as optical system, 3:105–123
phthisical (phthisis bulbi), 4:28, 29, 29*i*
after penetrating injury, 12:295
preparation of
for lamellar keratoplasty, 8:474
for penetrating keratoplasty, 8:455–456
radiation affecting, 1:255–256
refractive states of, 3:115–119. *See also* Refractive
errors
emmetropization and, 3:120
removal of. *See* Anophthalmic socket; Enucleation;
Evisceration; Exenteration
schematic, 3:105–108, 106*i*
optical constants of, 3:106*i*
reduced, 3:106–108, 108*i*
systemic drugs affecting, 1:323–326, 324–325*t*
in systemic malignancies, 1:262
traumatic injury of. *See* Trauma
vascular system of, development of, 2:155–156
Eye Bank Association of America (EBAA), 8:449
Eye banking, 8:449–451, 451*t*. *See also* Cornea,
transplantation of
screening for prior LASIK and, 13:204
Eye Disease Case-Control Study
in branch retinal vein occlusion, 12:137
in central retinal vein occlusion, 12:142–143
Eye drops. *See* Eyedrops (topical medications)
Eye examination. *See* Examination
Eye fields, frontal, 5:202, 208, 211
Eye movements, 6:34–38. *See also specific type and*
Ocular motility
assessment of, 5:199–204, 6:80–95, 452
in diplopia, 5:213–214, 214*i*, 215*i*
in infants and children, 6:80–95, 452
binocular, 6:36–38. *See also specific type*
conjugate (versions), 6:36–38, 37*i*
disconjugate (vergences), 6:38
in infants, 6:451
control of
extraocular muscles in, 7:12–13
fundamental principles in, 5:197–199
supranuclear, 5:33–34, 35–38*i*, 39
disorders of
in blowout fractures, 7:102–104, 103*i*
surgery and, 7:104–105
in comatose patients, 5:256
conditions causing, 7:26
in Graves ophthalmopathy, 7:26
nystagmus/spontaneous, 5:239–256, 6:162. *See also*
Nystagmus
ocular bobbing and, 5:256
after orbital surgery, 7:117
in Parkinson disease, 1:280
monocular (ductions), 6:34–35

supranuclear control of, 6:39
vergence, 5:203–204
disorders of, 5:210–211
Eye muscles. *See* Extraocular muscles
Eye pain. *See* Pain
Eye patches. *See* Patching
"Eye strain," 5:298
Eyeball. *See* Globe
Eyebrows
direct elevation of, 7:235
drooping of (brow ptosis), 7:234–235, 234*i*
Eyedrops (topical medications), 2:381–384, 382*i*, 383*i*,
385*i*
administration of in children, 6:5
for allergic eye disease, 6:235, 236*t*
for childhood glaucoma, 6:282–283
corticosteroid. *See also* Corticosteroids
ptosis caused by, 5:278
for uveitis, 9:115–116, 115*t*
for mydriasis, 5:265
sustained release devices for, 2:390
Eyeglasses. *See* Spectacle lenses (spectacles)
Eyelashes (cilia), 2:22, 24*i*, 7:146–147, 8:6, 7*i*
accessory. *See* Distichiasis
development of, 2:157, 157*i*
disorders of, 8:104
entropion/ptosis of, in anophthalmic socket, 7:127
in epiblepharon, 7:155*i*, 156
follicles of, 7:142*i*
tumors arising in, 7:168–169, 169*i*
lice infestation of, 8:169
misdirection of. *See* Trichiasis
Eyelid crutches, for ptosis, 7:220
Eyelid droop. *See* Ptosis
Eyelid–globe incongruity, in tear deficiency, 2:294
Eyelid hygiene
in blepharitis/meibomian gland dysfunction, 8:83, 86
in staphylococcal eye infection, 8:167
Eyelid imbrication syndrome, 7:161
Eyelid-sharing techniques, in eyelid repair, 7:189–192
Eyelid splints, as tarsorrhaphy alternative, 8:439
Eyelid springs, for paralytic ectropion, 7:199–200
Eyelid weights, 5:286
for exposure keratopathy, 8:95
for paralytic ectropion, 7:199
Eyelids, 2:21–31, 22*i*
absence of (ablepharon), 8:285
accessory structures of, 2:30–31
aging affecting, 1:235
amyloid deposits in, 4:171–174, 173*t*, 174*i*
anatomy of, 2:21–29, 7:139–147, 140*i*, 142*i*, 144*i*,
8:6–8, 7*i*
anterior fascial support system of, 2:38*i*
basal cell carcinoma of, 4:179–180, 179*i*, 7:174–179,
175*i*
intraocular extension of, 4:275
biopsy of, 7:176–177, 176*i*, 8:250, 251*i*
in sebaceous adenocarcinoma, 8:262–263
canthal tendons and, 7:146
coloboma of, 6:210, 7:157–158, 157*i*
congenital anomalies of, 4:169, 6:209–214, 7:153–158
conjunctiva of, 2:29, 32*i*, 7:140*i*, 141*i*, 142*i*, 145. *See*
also Conjunctiva
creases of, 7:139, 143
in ptosis, 7:210, 210*i*

degenerations of, **4**:171–174, 173*i*, 173*t*, 174*i*
development of, **2**:157, 157*i*, **8**:6
disorders of, **4**:167–185, **5**:273–279, **7**:153–193, **8**:24*t*.
   See also specific type
  acquired, **7**:158–161
  congenital, **4**:169, **6**:209–214, **7**:153–158
  evaluation of, **5**:273–276, 274*i*, 275*i*, 276*i*
  function affected by, **5**:314–315
  in Graves ophthalmopathy, **7**:26, 48–51, 48*i*, 53.
    See also Thyroid ophthalmopathy
  immune-mediated, **8**:205–207, 206*i*
  lice infestation, **8**:169
  neoplastic, **4**:174–185, **7**:162–184, **8**:239*t*. *See also*
    Eyelids, tumors of
    diagnostic approaches to, **8**:250, 251*i*
    histopathologic processes and conditions and,
      8:246–247, 247*t*
    management of, **8**:252
    oncogenesis and, **8**:248–249, 248*t*
  in Parkinson disease, **1**:280
  traumatic, **7**:184–188
drooping. *See* Ptosis
dyskeratosis of, **4**:177, 177*i*
ectropion of, **7**:195–201, 196*i*. *See also* Ectropion
edema of, **7**:160
  in preseptal cellulitis, **6**:230
emphysema of, in blowout fractures, **7**:101–102, 104
entropion of, **7**:201–207. *See also* Entropion
examination of, **5**:273–276, 274*i*, 275*i*, 276*i*
  before refractive surgery, **13**:44
excursion of, **5**:273–274, 275*i*
in external eye defense, **8**:113
fissure of, **2**:21, 22*i*, 23*i*
floppy, **7**:160–161, 161*i*, **8**:95–96, 96*i*
fusion of (ankyloblepharon), **6**:210, 210*i*, **7**:154–156,
  155*i*, **8**:285
glands of, **4**:168, 168*t*. *See also specific type*
  benign tumors of, **7**:167
in herpes simplex dermatoblepharitis, **8**:140, 141*i*,
  143
in herpes zoster ophthalmicus, **8**:154
horizontal shortening/tightening of
  for cicatricial ectropion, **7**:200–201
  for involutional ectropion, **7**:198
  for involutional entropion, **7**:204
infection/inflammation of, **4**:169–171, 170*i*, 172*i*,
  8:23, 24*t*, 163–179
  in children, **6**:388
  fungal and parasitic, **8**:168–169
  staphylococcal, **8**:119*t*, 163–168, 164*t*, 165*t*, 166*i*,
    167*i*
keratosis of, **8**:24*t*
  actinic (solar), **4**:174–177, 177*i*, **7**:172–173, 172*i*
  inverted follicular, **7**:163
  seborrheic, **4**:174–175, 175*i*, **7**:163, 165*i*
lacerations of
  lid margin involved in, **7**:185, 185*i*
  lid margin not involved in, **7**:184–185
  ptosis caused by, **7**:219
  repair of, **7**:184–187, 185*i*
    secondary, **7**:186–187
lower
  blepharoplasty on, **7**:229–230, 231–232
    laser resurfacing as adjunct to, **7**:237–238
    visual loss after, **7**:232–233

crease of, **7**:139
development of, **2**:157, 157*i*
ectropion of, **6**:210. *See also* Ectropion
entropion of, **6**:210, **7**:200–202. *See also* Entropion
horizontal laxity of, in involutional ectropion,
  7:197–198
reconstruction of, **7**:189–192, 191*i*
retraction of, treatment of, **7**:224–225
retractors of, **7**:141*i*, 144*i*, 145
  in involutional ectropion, repair of, **7**:198,
    202–203
  in involutional entropion, **7**:202–203
    repair of, **7**:203*i*, 204–205
  vertical elevation of, for paralytic ectropion,
    7:199–200
lymphatics of, **2**:29, 33*i*
malpositions of, **5**:314–315, **7**:195–234. *See also*
  specific type
margin of, **2**:22, 28*i*, **7**:142*i*, 146
  contact lens edge and, **3**:194–195
  eversion of. *See* Ectropion
  infections of, **8**:163–179
  inversion of. *See* Entropion
  lacerations of, **7**:185, 185*i*
  repair of defects in, **7**:189–192, 190*i*, 191*i*
  vascular and mesenchymal tumors of, **8**:269–272,
    270*i*
movement of, in tear film renewal and distribution,
  2:294
muscles of, **5**:56
nerve supply of, **7**:147
normal flora of, **8**:114–115, 115*t*
opening of, apraxia of, **5**:278–279
orbital septum and, **2**:24–26, 24*i*, 27*i*, **7**:140–141,
  140*i*, 141*i*
orbital tumors originating in, **7**:92
papillomas of, **4**:170–171
physiology of, **8**:55
plexiform neurofibroma involving, **6**:405, 405*i*
protractors of, **7**:139–140, 143*i*
reconstruction of, **7**:188–193
  after basal cell carcinoma surgery, **7**:178–179
  for blepharophimosis syndrome, **7**:153
  for defects involving eyelid margin, **7**:189–192,
    190*i*, 191*i*
  for defects not involving eyelid margin, **7**:188–189
  for epicanthus, **7**:156
  for euryblepharon, **7**:154
  general principles of, **7**:188
  after Mohs' micrographic surgery, **7**:178–179
retraction of, **4**:168, **5**:145, 279, 279*t*, **7**:223–225, 224*i*
  after blepharoplasty, **7**:224, 233, 233*i*
  in Graves ophthalmopathy, **5**:274–275, 276*i*, 329,
    329*i*, **7**:26, 48, 48–51, 48*i*, 53, 223–224, 224*i*
    proptosis differentiated from, **7**:223–224
  seizures causing, **1**:284
  after strabismus surgery, **7**:224
  treatment of, **7**:224–225
retractors of, **7**:141*i*, 142–145, 144*i*
  in involutional ectropion, repair of, **7**:198,
    202–203, 204–205
  in involutional entropion, **7**:202–203
    repair of, **7**:203*i*, 204–205
in scleroderma, **1**:186
shape and appearance of, **5**:273, 274*i*

skin of, **2**:22, **4**:167–168, 167*i*, **7**:139, 140*i*, 141*i*, **8**:6,
   245–246
   microanatomy of, **8**:245, 245*i*
specimen collection from, **8**:134
squamous cell carcinoma of, **4**:187, 187*i*
   actinic keratosis and, **4**:176–177
strabismus surgery affecting position of, **6**:189–190,
   190*i*
in Sturge-Weber syndrome, **6**:415, 415*i*
subcutaneous tissue of, **2**:23, **7**:139
suborbicularis fat pads and, **7**:141*i*, 145–146
   midface rejuvenation surgery and (SOOF lift),
      7:241–242, 242*i*
surgery of
   anesthesia for, **7**:150–151
   for basal cell carcinoma, **7**:177–179
   for blepharophimosis syndrome, **7**:153
   blepharoplasty, **7**:229–230
   for epicanthus, **7**:156
   for euryblepharon, **7**:154
   for eyelid retraction, **7**:54, 225
   for Graves ophthalmopathy, **7**:54
   patient preparation for, **7**:149
   principles of, **7**:149–151
   for ptosis repair, **7**:220–223, 221*i*
symblepharon and, **7**:207
systemic diseases manifesting in, **4**:174*i*
in systemic lupus erythematosus, **1**:182
tarsus of, **2**:26–28, 26*i*, 30*i*, 31*i*, **7**:140*i*, 141*i*, 145
topography of, **4**:167–169, 167*i*, 168*t*
trauma to, **7**:184–188
   blunt, **7**:184
   penetrating, **7**:184–186
   ptosis caused by, **7**:219
   repair of, **7**:184–187, 185*i*
tumors of, **4**:174–185, **7**:162–184, **8**:239*t*
   appendage neoplasms, **4**:180–182, 181*i*
   basal cell carcinoma, **4**:179–180, 179*i*, **7**:174–179,
      175*i*
      intraocular extension of, **4**:275
   benign, **7**:163–166
   biopsy in evaluation of, **7**:176–177, 176*i*, **8**:250,
      251*i*
   in children, **6**:385–388
   clinical evaluation/diagnostic approaches to,
      7:162–163, **8**:250, 251*i*
   epidermal
      benign, **7**:164–166, 165*i*
      premalignant, **7**:172–173, 172*i*, 173*i*
   histopathologic processes and conditions and,
      8:246–247, 247*t*
   malignant, **7**:174–184, **8**:270*t*, 272
      staging of, **4**:291*t*
   management of, **8**:252
   masquerading neoplasms and, **7**:184
   mechanical ptosis caused by, **7**:219
   melanocytic, **4**:182–185, 182*i*, 183*i*, **7**:169–172
      benign, **7**:169–170, 170*i*, 172*i*
      malignant (melanoma), **4**:185, **7**:182–183
      premalignant, **7**:174
   in multiple endocrine neoplasia, **1**:230, 230*i*
   oncogenesis and, **8**:248–249, 248*t*
   papillomas, **4**:170–171, **6**:385
   sebaceous gland carcinoma, **8**:261–263, 262*i*

squamous cell carcinoma, **4**:177–179, 178*i*
   actinic keratosis and, **4**:176–177
   systemic malignancies and, **4**:176*i*
   vascular and mesenchymal, **8**:269–272, 270*i*
   viral, **8**:162
upper
   anatomy of, **2**:21–29, 24*i*, 25*i*, 26*i*, 27*i*
   blepharoplasty on, **7**:229–230, 231
   coloboma of, **6**:210
   congenital eversion of, **7**:154, 155*i*
   crease of, **7**:139, 140*i*, 143
      in ptosis, **7**:210, 210*i*
   development of, **2**:157, 157*i*
   entropion of, **6**:210, **7**:200–201. *See also* Entropion
   reconstruction of, **7**:188–189, 190*i*
   retractors of, **7**:142–144, 144*i*
in uveitis, **9**:103*t*
vascular supply of, **2**:29, 32*i*, **7**:147, **8**:7
   superficial venous structures, **5**:22*i*
vertical splitting of, for anterior orbitotomy, **7**:110
wound healing/repair and, **4**:24
Eyepiece (ocular), of telescope, **3**:82, 82*i*, 83*i*

F

F₃. *See* Trifluridine
F-MRI. *See* Functional magnetic resonance imaging
F (flutter) waves, **1**:137
Fab region (antibody molecule), **9**:55, 56*i*
Fabry disease (angiokeratoma corporis diffusum
      universale), **2**:262*t*, **6**:436*t*, 438, **8**:340–341, 341*i*
   cataract and, **6**:288*t*
   ocular findings in carriers of, **2**:270*t*
   plasma infusions in management of, **2**:281
   retinal degeneration and, **12**:244, 246*i*
Face. *See also under* Facial
   aging affecting, cosmetic/rejuvenation surgery and,
      7:235–248. *See also* Facial surgery
   anatomy of, **7**:135–139, 136*i*, 137*i*, 138*i*
Facelift, **7**:244–245, 245*i*, 246*i*
Facial angiofibromas, in tuberous sclerosis, **6**:410, 410*i*
Facial angioma. *See* Nevus, flammeus
Facial artery, **5**:11, 13
   eyelids supplied by, **2**:29, 32*i*, **8**:7
   orbit supplied by, **2**:29*i*, **7**:15
Facial clefts, **7**:38–39, 38*i*, 39*i*
   lacrimal outflow disorders and, **7**:258, 258*i*
Facial colliculus, **2**:116, 117, **5**:227
Facial contracture, spastic paretic, **5**:289
Facial defects. *See* Craniofacial malformations
Facial diplegia, in Guillain-Barré syndrome, **5**:285
Facial dystonia, **7**:226–228
Facial fasciculations, benign, **5**:289
Facial grimacing, blepharospasm associated with, **5**:286
Facial hemiatrophy, progressive, **8**:353*t*
Facial motor and sensory anatomy, **5**:49–56
Facial movement abnormalities, **5**:280–290, 280*i*, 282*i*
   evaluation of, **5**:273–276, 274*i*, 275*i*, 276*i*
Facial muscles, **7**:135–137, 137*i*, 138*i*
Facial myokymia, **5**:287*t*, 289
Facial nerve. *See* Cranial nerve VII
Facial numbness, pain associated with, **5**:301
Facial pain, **5**:299–301. *See also* Headache; Pain
   atypical, **5**:299

Facial paralysis/weakness, 5:280–281, 280*i*
  etiology of, 5:283*t*
  eyelid fissure changes in, 2:23*i*
  in head trauma, 5:285
  in HIV infection/AIDS, 5:284
  paralytic ectropion and, 7:199
  peripheral lesions causing, 5:227–237, 283–285, 284*i*
  progressive, 5:285
  recurrent, 5:285
  in sarcoidosis, 5:333
  supranuclear lesions causing, 5:281
Facial surgery, 7:235–248. *See also specific procedure*
  anesthesia for, 7:150–151
  cosmetic, 7:235–248
  lower face and neck surgery, 7:244–247, 245*i*, 246*i*,
    247*i*
  midface surgery (suborbicularis oculi fat/midface
    lift), 7:241–242, 242*i*, 243*i*
  patient preparation for, 7:149
  principles of, 7:149–151
  upper face surgery (brow and forehead lift),
    7:239–241, 240*i*
Facial synkinesis, 5:280, 280*i*, 284
Facial tic (habit spasm), 5:290
Facial vein, 5:20, 22*i*, 23
  eyelids drained by, 7:147
Factitious disorders, 1:266
  ocular surface, 8:105–106, 106*i*
Factive. *See* Gemifloxacin
Factor V Leiden, 1:170
Factor VIII deficiency (hemophilia A/classic
    hemophilia), 1:168
Factor VIII transfusions, 1:168
Factor Q, corneal shape and, 3:231–232
Facultative suppression, 6:55
Fadenoperation (posterior fixation suture), 6:175*t*
Falciform ligament, 5:26
Fallopian canal, 5:54
Falls, in elderly, 1:247, 248*t*
False-negative responses, in perimetry, 5:93, 10:71
False passage, probing of nasolacrimal duct obstruction
    and, 6:245
False-positive responses, in perimetry, 5:93, 10:71, 73*i*
Famciclovir, 1:65*t*, 77, 2:440*t*, 442
  for herpes simplex virus infections, 1:28, 77, 8:142*t*
  for herpes zoster, 1:28, 77, 8:155
  for herpetic retinitis (acute retinal necrosis), 12:186
Familial. *See also* Family history/familial factors;
    Genetics
  definition of, 2:239
Familial adenomatous polyposis (Gardner syndrome),
    retinal manifestations of, 2:173, 4:122–123, 230,
    6:390, 12:236–237, 237*i*
Familial Alzheimer disease, 1:286
Familial amyloid polyneuropathy, vitreous involvement
    in, 4:111, 111*i*
Familial (dominant) drusen, 6:340, 12:220–221, 221*i*
Familial dysautonomia (Riley-Day syndrome), 2:262*t*,
    6:260
  neurotrophic keratopathy in, 8:103
  racial and ethnic concentration of, 2:259
Familial exudative vitreoretinopathy, 6:324, 341–342,
    12:284–285, 285*i*
  glaucoma and, 6:279

Familial glaucoma iridogoniodysplasia. *See* Axenfeld-
    Rieger syndrome
Familial iridoplegia, 6:268
Familial juvenile nephronophthisis, retinal
    degeneration and, 12:236
Familial juvenile systemic granulomatosis (Blau
    syndrome), 6:318
Familial oculorenal syndromes, 6:348–349
Familial penetrance, 2:264–265
Familial renal–retinal dysplasia/dystrophy, 6:349,
    12:236
Family history/familial factors. *See also* Genetic/
    hereditary factors; Genetics, clinical
  congenital anomalies and, 8:282–283
  in genetic counseling, 2:276–277
  in human carcinogenesis, 1:254–255
  in nystagmus, 6:160–161, 161*t*
  pedigree analysis and, 2:275–276, 275*i*, 8:308
  in primary angle closure, 10:123–124
  in primary open-angle glaucoma, 10:10, 87
  in uveitis, 9:122
Famotidine, preoperative, 1:331
Famvir. *See* Famciclovir
Fanconi syndrome, corneal manifestations of, 6:259,
    259*i*
FAP. *See* Familial amyloid polyneuropathy
Far lines, in astigmatic eye, 3:116
Far points/far point concept, 3:115
  in astigmatic eye, 3:115–116
  cylindrical correcting lenses and, 3:145
  spherical correcting lenses and, 3:143, 144*i*
Farcas canthal index, 6:207
Farnsworth-Munsell 100-hue test, 12:43
  in low vision evaluation, 5:96
Farnsworth Panel D-15 test (Farnsworth Dichotomous
    Test for Color Blindness), 3:254, 12:44, 45*i*
  in low vision evaluation, 5:96
Faropenem, 1:60*t*, 69
FAS. *See* Fetal alcohol syndrome
Fas ligand, 9:38, 68, 69*i*
Fasanella-Servat procedure (tarsoconjunctival
    müllerectomy), for ptosis correction, 7:222
Fascia bulbi. *See* Tenon's capsule
Fascia lata, autogenous and banked, for frontalis
    suspension, 7:222
Fascia lata sling, for paralytic ectropion, 7:199
Fascicles
  cranial nerve IV, 2:111
  optic nerve, 2:98
Fascicular block (cardiology), 1:134
Fascicular lesions, diplopia and, 5:227
Fasciculations, facial, 5:289
Fasciculus, medial longitudinal, 5:34
  disruption of, 5:224
  rostral interstitial nucleus of, 5:34, 37*i*
Fasciitis
  necrotizing, of orbit, 7:44–45
  nodular, 8:271
    episcleral tumor caused by, 4:92
FasL. *See* Fas ligand
Fast hemoglobin (glycosylated hemoglobin/HbA$_1$/
    HbA$_{1c}$), in glucose control/surveillance, 1:215, 215*i*,
    216
Fast oscillation, 12:38–39, 39*i*
Fast-twitch fibers, 2:20, 21, 21*t*, 5:41

Fastigial nucleus, 5:40

Fasting, preoperative, 1:331

Fasting glucose
  in diabetes diagnosis/screening, 1:301
  impaired, 1:203*t*, 206

Fasting plasma glucose test, 1:207

FASTPAC, 10:66

Fat
  orbital, 6:19*i*, 23, 7:12, 141
  sub-brow, 7:146
  suborbicularis oculi (SOOF/suborbicularis fat pads),
    7:135, 141*i*, 145–146
    midface rejuvenation surgery and (SOOF lift),
      7:241–242, 242*i*

Fat embolism, posttraumatic, retinal findings in, 12:95

Fat-suppression techniques, in magnetic resonance
  imaging, 7:31

Fatty acid supplements, for meibomian gland
  dysfunction, 8:83

Fatty acids
  peroxidation of, 2:366–367
    in retina, 2:370
  in retinal pigment epithelium, 2:358
  in vitreous, 2:337

FAZ. *See* Foveal avascular zone

Fc receptors, 9:7, 55, 56*i*
  in antibody-dependent cellular cytotoxicity, 9:70
  on mast cells, 9:13–14
  in phagocytosis, 9:50

FDA. *See* Food and Drug Administration

Fecal DNA testing, in cancer screening, 1:298

Fecal occult blood testing, in cancer screening, 1:295*t*,
  298

Feedback, optical, in lasers, 3:22, 22*i*

Felbamate, 1:283*t*

Felbatol. *See* Felbamate

Feldene. *See* Piroxicam

Felderstruktur muscle fibers, 2:20

Fellow eye. *See also* Sympathetic ophthalmia
  in patient with choroidal neovascularization,
    12:76–78
    ocular histoplasmosis and, 12:82
  in patient with macular hole, 12:91–93
  in patient with retinal detachment, 12:267

Fellow Eye Study Group, 12:61

Felodipine, 1:89*t*, 90*t*

Felty syndrome, 1:174

Femtosecond laser
  in lamellar keratoplasty, 8:472, 474, 475
  for LASIK flap creation, 13:109–110
  for photodisruption, 13:29

Fenofibrate, for hypercholesterolemia, 1:149*t*

Fenoprofen, 1:197*t*, 2:421*t*

Fenoterol, 1:157
  with ipratropium, 1:157*t*

Fentanyl, perioperative, 1:332*t*, 335, 338

Fenton reaction, oxygen radicals produced by, 9:84

Fermat's principle, 3:51–53, 52*i*, 54*i*
  wavefront analysis and, 13:13–14

Ferric gluconate, 1:159, 161

Ferritin levels, in iron deficiency anemia, 1:161

Ferrous sulfate, for iron deficiency anemia, 1:161

Ferry lines, 4:74, 8:377*t*

Fetal alcohol syndrome, 1:270, 2:160–161, 161*i*, 162*i*,
  6:433–434, 434*i*
  childhood glaucoma and, 10:155*t*

Fetal fissure. *See* Embryonic fissure

Fetal hydantoin syndrome, 1:284

Fetal nucleus, 11:9, 27*i*, 28
  opacification of (congenital nuclear cataract), 11:37,
    38*i*

Fetal radiation, effects/ocular manifestations of, 1:255

Fetal vasculature, persistent. *See* Persistent fetal
  vasculature

FEV_1 (forced expiratory volume in 1 second), 1:155

FEVR. *See* Familial exudative vitreoretinopathy

FEVR1 gene, in familial exudative vitreoretinopathy,
  6:342

FGF. *See* Fibroblast growth factor

FGFR2 gene
  in Apert syndrome, 6:426
  in Crouzon syndrome, 6:425

FHS. *See* Fetal hydantoin syndrome

Fiber layer of Henle, 2:84, 85, 4:119

Fiberoptics
  delivery system for, in operating microscope, 3:297
  total reflection in, 3:14

Fibric acid derivatives, for hypercholesterolemia, 1:149*t*

Fibril-associated proteins, in vitreous, 2:337

Fibrillation
  atrial, 1:138
    heart failure and, 1:131, 132
    stroke and, 1:102
  ventricular, 1:140

Fibrillenstruktur muscle fibers, 2:20

Fibrillin, 2:76, 337
  defects in, in Marfan syndrome, 8:354, 11:40

Fibrin, 8:198*t*, 9:76–77

Fibrin clots, after penetrating trauma in children, 6:447

Fibrin tissue adhesive, for corneal autograft fixation,
  8:432

Fibrinogen, 9:76

Fibrinolytic agents, 2:452

Fibrinolytic system, 1:164

Fibroblast growth factor (FGF), 2:456
  in aqueous humor, 2:320
  homeobox gene expression affected by, 2:131
  in ocular development, 2:130

Fibroblast growth factor receptor-2 gene
  in Apert syndrome, 6:426
  in Crouzon syndrome, 6:425

Fibrocellular proliferation, intraocular, 4:26–27

Fibroma
  molluscum, 6:404
  ossifying, of orbit, 4:200, 6:380
  in tuberous sclerosis, 5:338, 6:410, 410*i*

Fibromatosis, juvenile, of orbit, 4:200, 6:380

Fibronectin, 8:14
  in vitreous, 2:333

Fibroplasia, retrolental. *See* Retinopathy, of prematurity

Fibrosarcoma
  eyelid manifestations of, 4:176*t*
  of orbit, 6:374, 7:81
  retinoblastoma associated with, 4:265*t*

Fibrosing (morpheaform) basal cell carcinoma, 7:175,
  175*i*

Fibrosis
  congenital, 5:220–221, 221*i*, 6:152–154

corneal wound healing/repair and, **8**:384
Fibrotic pulmonary disease, **1**:154
Fibrous astrocytes, **2**:84
Fibrous downgrowth (stromal ingrowth), secondary
    angle-closure glaucoma and, **10**:141–143
Fibrous dysplasia of orbit, **4**:200, **6**:380, **7**:81, 82*i*
    secondary, **7**:93
Fibrous histiocytoma (fibroxanthoma), **8**:271
    orbital, **4**:199, 199*i*, **7**:81
    scleral, **4**:92
Fibrovascular pigment epithelial detachment, **12**:64–66
Fibulin-1, in vitreous, **2**:333
Fick, axes of, **6**:27–28, 27*i*
Field of action/field of activation, **6**:29
Field defects. *See* Visual field defects
Field depth, **3**:36, 36*i*
Field (standard) lens, in manual lensmeter, **3**:304, 305*i*
Field of vision. *See* Visual field
15-hue test, Lanthony desaturated, in low vision
    evaluation, **5**:96
Fifth cranial nerve. *See* Cranial nerve V
Filamentary keratopathy, **8**:72*i*, 73*i*, 75–76
Filamentous fungi, **8**:129*i*, 129*t*, 130–131
    as normal ocular flora, **8**:115*t*
    ocular infection caused by, **8**:130–131
        keratitis, **8**:185–187, 186*i*
Filaments, corneal, **8**:25*t*
    in dry eye states, **8**:72
Filariae
    loa loa, **8**:191
    onchocercal, **8**:132
        in anterior chamber, **9**:196
Filensin, **2**:327
Filling defect, vascular, **12**:19
Filtering bleb
    after cataract surgery, **11**:181
    endophthalmitis associated with, **9**:207–209, 208*t*,
        212–213
    for uveitic glaucoma, **9**:237
Filtering procedures
    cataract surgery after, **11**:219–220
    cataract surgery combined with, **10**:195–197,
        11:220–221
    LASIK and, **13**:191
Fimbriae, bacterial, **8**:123
Fine-needle aspiration biopsy (FNAB), **4**:40–41, 213
    in iris melanoma, **4**:218
    in metastatic eye disease, **4**:273
    of orbit, **7**:35, 116–117
    of thyroid gland, **1**:223
    in uveal lymphoid infiltration, **4**:280
First cranial nerve. *See* Cranial nerve I
First-degree relatives, **2**:194
First-order neuron
    dilator muscle innervation and, **2**:65
    lesions of, Horner syndrome caused by, **5**:263, 264
First-order optics, **3**:55–62
    afocal systems and, **3**:81–84, 82*i*, 83*i*
    Badal principle in, **3**:80–81
    exact ray tracing in, **3**:55–56, 55*i*, 56*i*
    first approximation in, **3**:55–56
    focal length and, **3**:79
    focal points and focal planes and, **3**:69–71, 70*i*
    Gaussian reduction and, **3**:80
    graphical image analysis and, **3**:76–78, 77*i*, 77–78*i*

Knapp's law in, **3**:80–81, 81*i*
    lens combinations and, **3**:67
    lens maker's equation (LME) in, **3**:60–62, 61*i*
    negative thin lenses and, **3**:72–74, 73*i*
    objects and images at infinity and, **3**:74–75
    paraxial approximation in, **3**:56, 56*i*, 57*i*, 58*i*
    principal planes and principal points and, **3**:75–76
    small-angle approximation in, **3**:58–60
    thick lenses and, **3**:78–79, 78*i*
    thin lens approximation and, **3**:66–67
    transverse magnification in, **3**:65–66, 66*i*
    vergence and reduced vergence in, **3**:62–65, 63*i*, 64*i*
    virtual images and virtual objects in, **3**:67–69, 68*i*,
        69*i*
FISH. *See* Fluorescence in situ hybridization
Fish eye disease, **8**:309*t*, 339–340
Fish flesh pattern, in treated retinoblastoma, **6**:398
Fishbone diagram, **1**:370, 371*i*
Fissures
    calcarine, **5**:29, 30*i*
    embryonic, **2**:126, 137–138, 137*i*
        closure of, **2**:138, 143*i*
            colobomas and, **2**:138, 143*i*, 165–166
            persistence of, in fetal alcohol syndrome, **2**:161
    orbital, **2**:10–12, **5**:10, **7**:10*i*, 11, 21–22
        inferior, **2**:12, **5**:8*i*, 10, **7**:10*i*, 11, 22
        superior, **2**:10–12, 11*i*, 12*i*, **5**:8*i*, **7**:11, 21
            cranial nerve VI in, **5**:43, 45–49*i*
            lesions of, **5**:236
    palpebral
        congenital widening of (euryblepharon), **7**:154,
            155*i*
        in infants and children, **6**:200
            congenital widening of (euryblepharon), **6**:211
            slanting of, **6**:212–213
            A- and V-pattern deviations and, **6**:119, 122*i*
            surgery affecting, **6**:23, 25*i*
        vertical height of, in ptosis, **7**:206*i*, 209
Fistulas
    arteriovenous
        glaucoma associated with, **10**:32
        of orbit, **7**:70, 71*i*
    carotid-cavernous, **5**:236, 237*i*, **7**:70, 71*i*
    dural sinus, **5**:236–237, **7**:70
    lacrimal, congenital, **6**:240, **7**:258, 258*i*, 266–267
Fitting (contact lens), **3**:189–202, 190*i*
    after refractive surgery, **3**:202, 203*i*, **13**:205–208
    rigid gas-permeable lenses, **3**:191–195, 193*i*, 193*t*
    soft lenses, **3**:189–191, 190*i*, 192*t*, 195
    trial
        disinfection and, **1**:51, **8**:50, **9**:262
        fluorescein patterns and, **3**:195
Fixation (visual)
    alternating, **6**:11
    in assessment of infant with decreased vision, **6**:452,
        456
    distance acuity assessment in children and, **6**:78–79,
        78*t*
    eccentric, **6**:69
        ARC testing and, **6**:57
    monocular, **6**:11
    pediatric cataract and, **6**:294
    perimetry affected by, **10**:62–63
    recruitment during, **6**:32
    for retinoscopy, **3**:126

spasm of, **5:**194
strabismus classification and, **6:**11
Fixation loss, in perimetry, **5:**93
Fixation target, moving (heterophoria method), for
accommodative convergence/accommodation ratio
measurement, **3:**149
Fixatives, for tissue processing, **4:**35
FKHL7 gene. *See FOXC1 (FKHL7)* gene
Flagella, bacterial, **8:**123
of spirochetes, **8:**128
Flagyl/Flagyl IV. *See* Metronidazole
FLAIR (fluid-attenuated inversion recovery) image,
5:63–64, 66*i*
definition of, **5:**78
parameters of, **5:**64*t*
signal intensity on, **5:**65*t*
Flame hemorrhages
in central retinal vein occlusion, **12:**141, 142*i*
ischemia causing, **4:**131–133, 132*i*
in leukemia, **6:**344
Flap folds, after LASIK, **13:**122–126, 124*t*, 125*i*
Flap tears (horseshoe tears), **12:**253, 254, 255*i*
treatment of, **12:**265, 266, 266*t*, 267*t*
Flaps
advancement, **8:**438
bipedicle (bucket handle), **8:**437–438
for canthal repair, **7:**192–193
conjunctival, **8:**436–438, 437*i*
for corneal edema after cataract surgery, **11:**193
for ICCE, **11:**106
in scleral-tunnel incision for cataract surgery,
11:121–122
for symblepharon, **7:**207
for wound closure after pterygium excision, **8:**429,
430*i*
coronal scalp, for anterior orbitotomy, **7:**110
for eyelid repair, **7:**189–193, 190*i*
Gundersen, **8:**436–437, 437*i*, **11:**193
LASIK
dislocation/subluxation of, **13:**126–127
striae and, **13:**123
femtosecond creation of, **13:**109–110
infected, **13:**128–129, 129*i*
microkeratome creation of, **13:**112–114, 113*i*, 114*i*
complications and, **13:**120–121, 121*i*
penetrating keratoplasty and, **13:**204
replacement of, **13:**115
retinal detachment repair and, **13:**203
retreatment and, **13:**119, 120*i*
striae in, **13:**122–126, 124*t*, 125*i*
partial (bridge), **8:**437
single-pedicle (racquet), **8:**438
for symblepharon, **7:**207
for wound closure after pterygium excision, **8:**429,
430*i*
Flarex. *See* Fluorometholone
Flashing lights. *See* Photopsias
Flat anterior chamber. *See* Anterior chamber, flat or
shallow
"Flatter add plus" rule, **3:**180
Flecainide, ocular effects of, **1:**325*t*
Fleck dystrophy, **8:**310*t*, 323
Fleck retina of Kandori, **12:**200
Fleischer ring/line, in keratoconus, **4:**70, 74, **8:**330,
331*i*, 377*t*, 378

"Flesh-eating disease." *See* Necrotizing fasciitis
Fleurettes, in retinoblastoma, **4:**143–144, 143*i*, **6:**394
Flexible (soft) contact lenses, **3:**184–185
conjunctivitis caused by, **3:**210
as corneal bandages, **3:**202
corneal neovascularization caused by, **3:**208–209
fitting, **3:**189–191, 190*i*, 192*t*, 195
giant papillary conjunctivitis caused by, **3:**210,
8:214–216
hydrogel polymers for, **3:**184–185
keratitis and, **3:**208
for keratoconus, **3:**202
neovascularization associated with, **8:**108
refractive surgery and, **13:**204–205
after PRK, **13:**206
after radial keratotomy, **13:**206
toric, **3:**195–197, 197*i*, 197*t*
Flexible-loop intraocular lenses, **11:**144
Flexner-Wintersteiner rosettes, in retinoblastoma,
4:142–143, 143*i*, 260, **6:**394
Flicker response, 30 Hz, **12:**28*i*, 29
Flicker sensitivity, in glaucoma, **10:**59
Flieringa ring, for scleral support for penetrating
keratoplasty, **8:**455
Floaters
in posterior uveitis, **9:**107
in posterior vitreous detachment, **12:**257
in rhegmatogenous retinal detachment, **12:**268
in spontaneous vitreous hemorrhages, **12:**287
Flocculonodular lobe, **5:**39
"Floor effect," **1:**364
Floppy eyelid syndrome, **7:**160–161, 161*i*, **8:**95–96, 96*i*
Flovent. *See* Fluticasone
Flow cytometry, **4:**38–39, 38*i*
in paroxysmal nocturnal hemoglobinuria screening,
1:159, 162
Flowchart (system of care), **1:**370, 371*i*
Floxacillin, **2:**429
Floxin. *See* Ofloxacin
Flu. *See* Influenza
Fluconazole, **1:**64*t*, 75–76, **2:**438*t*, 439
for endophthalmitis, **9:**218*t*, 219
for yeast keratitis, **8:**186
Flucytosine/5-fluorocytosine, **1:**64*t*, **2:**438*t*, 439
for aspergillosis, **5:**365
for endophthalmitis, **9:**219
Fluid-attenuated inversion recovery (FLAIR) image,
5:63–64, 66*i*
definition of, **5:**78
parameters of, **5:**64*t*
signal intensity on, **5:**65*t*
Fluid (tear) lens, contact lens creation of, **3:**180–181,
181*i*
Fluid-ventilated scleral lenses, **3:**202
Fluidics, in phacoemulsification, **11:**118–121. *See also*
Aspiration; Irrigation
terminology related to, **11:**115
Flumadine. *See* Rimantadine
Flumazenil, for benzodiazepine reversal, **1:**335
FluMist. *See* Influenza virus, vaccination against
Flunisolide, for pulmonary diseases, **1:**157*t*
Flunitrazepam (date rape drug), **1:**269
Fluor-Op. *See* Fluorometholone
Fluorescein, **2:**451, **8:**20–22, 21*i*, **12:**18–19
allergic reactions to, **1:**319

angiography with. *See* Fluorescein angiography
  for applanation tonometry, **8:**20
  in aqueous deficiency diagnosis, **8:**20, 61, 72
  with benoxinate, **2:**446*t*, 448
  in congenital nasolacrimal duct obstruction
    evaluation, **6:**242
  in conjunctival foreign-body identification, **8:**404
  in contact lens fitting, **3:**175, 195, 196*i*
  for dye disappearance test, **7:**268
  for Jones I and Jones II tests, **7:**264–266
  for lacrimal irrigation, **7:**263, 264*i*
  photon (particle) aspects of light and, **3:**7
  punctate staining patterns and, **8:**20, 21*i*
  in tear breakup time testing, **8:**20, 61
Fluorescein angiography, **2:**451, **12:**18–22, 20*i*, 22*i*
  in acute posterior multifocal placoid pigment
    epitheliopathy, **12:**175, 175*i*
  in age-related macular degeneration, **12:**58–59
  anterior segment, **8:**37
  in birdshot retinochoroidopathy, **12:**177–178
  in branch retinal vein occlusion, **12:**137*i*, 138
  in central retinal vein occlusion, **12:**141, 142*i*, 143
  in central serous chorioretinopathy, **12:**22*i*, 52
  in choroidal/ciliary body melanoma, **4:**225–226, 227*i*
  in choroidal hemangioma, **4:**245
  in choroidal neovascularization, **12:**20*i*, 63, 64–67,
    65*i*
  in choroidal perfusion abnormalities, **12:**166, 167*i*,
    168*i*
  in Coat's disease, **12:**156, 157*i*
  in cystoid macular edema, **12:**154, 155*i*
  in diabetic macular edema, **12:**113
  in drusen versus papilledema differentiation,
    5:131–132, 132*i*, 133*i*
  extravasation of dye and, **12:**21
  in hypertensive choroidopathy, **12:**98, 99*i*
  in iris melanoma, **4:**218
  in low vision evaluation, **5:**98, 99*i*
  in lymphoma, **4:**278
  in macular holes, **12:**91
  in metastatic eye disease, **4:**271
  in ocular ischemic syndrome, **9:**222, **12:**151
  before penetrating keratoplasty, **8:**454
  in radiation retinopathy, **12:**305, 306*i*
  in retinal disease, **12:**18–22, 20*i*, 22*i*. *See also specific*
    disease
    capillary hemangioma, **4:**247
    cavernous hemangioma, **4:**247, **12:**163–164, 164*i*
  side effects of, **12:**21
  in Stargardt disease, **12:**216, 216*i*
  in uveitis, **9:**113
  in Vogt-Koyanagi-Harada syndrome, **12:**181
Fluorescence in situ hybridization, **2:**247–249, 248*i*,
  249*i*
Fluorescent treponemal antibody absorption (FTA-
  ABS) test, **1:**17, 17*t*, 302, **9:**189–190
Fluorexon, **8:**20
5-Fluorocytosine. *See* Flucytosine
Fluorometholone, **2:**417*t*
  anti-inflammatory/pressure-elevating potency of,
    2:419*t*
  in combination preparations, **2:**432*t*
  after PRK/LASEK, glaucoma associated with, **13:**105
  for uveitis, **9:**115*t*, 116, 238

Fluorophotometry, aqueous formations measured by,
  10:20
Fluoropolymer, for contact lenses, **3:**184
Fluoroquinolones, **1:**54, 73, **2:**430–433. *See also*
  Quinolones
  for bacterial keratitis, **8:**182, 182*t*, 183
  for endophthalmitis, **9:**217
  for gonococcal conjunctivitis, **8:**172
Fluoroscopy, magnetic resonance, in ischemic heart
  disease, **1:**119
Fluorouracil, **1:**258*t*, **2:**393, 426, 444
  for conjunctival intraepithelial neoplasia, **8:**258
  in trabeculectomy, **10:**190–191
Fluoxetine, ocular effects of, **1:**324*t*
Fluphenazine, **1:**271
Flurbiprofen, **1:**196, 197*t*, **2:**306, 417*t*, 422
Fluress. *See* Fluorescein, with benoxinate
Flutamide, **1:**260*t*
Fluticasone, for pulmonary diseases, **1:**157*t*
Flutrimazole, **1:**76
Flutter
  atrial, **1:**137–138
  ocular, **5:**253
Flutter (F) waves, **1:**137
Fluvastatin, for hypercholesterolemia, **1:**149*t*, 150*t*
Flux
  luminous, **3:**16*t*
  radiant, **3:**16*t*
Fly larvae, ocular infection caused by, **8:**133–134
Flying-spot lasers, for photoablation, **13:**30
FML. *See* Fluorometholone
FMLP. *See* N-Formylmethionylleucylphenylalanine
fMRI. *See* Functional magnetic resonance imaging
FNAB. *See* Fine-needle aspiration biopsy
Focal abnormalities, of optic disc, examination of,
  10:54–55
Focal electroretinogram, **5:**101, **12:**31–32
Focal length, **3:**79
  of mirror, **3:**90
  for operating microscope, **3:**296, 297*i*
Focal planes, **3:**69–71, 70*i*
Focal points, **3:**69–71, 70*i*
Focimeter. *See* Lensmeters
Focus, depth of, **3:**35–36, 35*i*
Fogging
  for astigmatic dial refraction, **3:**134–135, 135*i*
  for binocular balance testing, **3:**141
  for duochrome test, **3:**140
  for functional visual disorder evaluation, **5:**307
  for retinoscopy, **3:**126
  for subjective refraction, **3:**141
Folate/folic acid
  antagonists of, in cancer chemotherapy, **1:**258*t*
  deficiency of, **1:**162
    optic neuropathy caused by, **5:**152
  homocysteine levels and stroke and, **1:**109
  supplementary, for homocystinuria management,
    6:438
Foldable intraocular lens, **11:**145–146
  implantation procedure for, **11:**153
    in children, **6:**298, 301
  instrumentation for, **11:**152
  posterior chamber phakic, **13:**148–149, 149*i*, 150*i*
  in uveitis, **9:**138

Folinic acid, 2:433
  for toxoplasmosis, 12:187, 187*t*
Follicle-stimulating hormone, pituitary adenoma
    producing, 1:229
Follicles
  conjunctival, 8:24*t*, 25*t*, 26, 28*i*
  in external eye defense, 8:114
Follicular carcinoma, of thyroid gland, 1:227
Follicular center lymphoma, of orbit, 4:195
Follicular conjunctivitis, 8:24*t*, 25*t*, 26, 28*i*
  adenoviral, 8:157, 158
  medication toxicity causing, 8:394
Folliculosis, benign lymphoid, 8:26, 28*i*
Follow-up studies (cohort studies), 1:345*i*, 348*i*,
    350–351
Followability, in phacoemulsification, 11:115
Fomivirsen, 1:48
  for cytomegalovirus retinitis, 1:48, 12:193
Food, Drug, and Cosmetic Act, 13:31
Food and Drug Administration, 2:393, 13:31–38
  delays in device approval by, 13:37–38
  lasers approved by, 13:32–34*t*
  medical device classification by, 13:31–35
  medical device pathways to market and, 13:35–36
Foods, headaches caused by, 5:296
Footcandle, 3:16*t*
Foradil. See Formoterol
Foramen (foramina)
  ethmoidal, anterior/posterior, 2:9–10, 5:10, 7:9*i*, 11
  infraorbital, 2:8
  magnum, 5:5
  oculomotor, 7:14
  optic, 2:9, 10*i*, 11*i*
  orbital, 2:9–10, 10*i*, 11*i*
  ovale, 5:13
  spinosum, 5:11
  supraorbital, 2:5, 7*i*, 9
  zygomatic, 2:10
Forced ductions, 6:89
  in blowout fractures, 7:103
    surgery and, 7:103
  in Brown syndrome, 6:144, 145
  in diplopia, 5:217, 218*i*
Forced expiratory volume in 1 second (FEV$_1$), 1:155
Forced vital capacity (FVC), 1:155
Foreheadplasty, 7:239–240
Foreign bodies
  intralenticular, 11:57
  intraocular, 12:296–299, 297*i*
    anesthesia for removal of in children, 6:5
    conjunctival, 4:49, 8:404, 404*i*, 405*i*
    corneal, 4:67, 8:404–406, 406*i*
      in children, 6:445–446
    of iris, 4:219*t*
    posttraumatic endophthalmitis and, 12:300
    retained, 12:298–299
      cataract surgery and, 11:226
      electroretinogram in evaluation of, 12:36, 299
      endophthalmitis caused by, 9:212
      siderosis and, 4:99, 11:58, 59*i*, 12:299, 299*t*
      surgical techniques for removal of, 12:298
      uveitis in children differentiated from, 6:320*t*
    intraorbital, 7:106
      anesthesia for removal of in children, 6:5
  Foreign-body giant cells, 4:13, 15*i*

Foreign-body granuloma, after strabismus surgery,
    6:186, 187*i*
Foreign-body sensation
  in aqueous tear deficiency, 8:72
  in corneal abrasion, 8:406
  fluorescein in investigation of, 8:404
Forkhead genes
  Axenfeld-Rieger syndrome and, 8:292
  glaucoma and, 10:15
Forkhead transcription factor, glaucoma and, 10:15
Formalin, as tissue fixative, 4:35
Forme fruste, 8:332. See also Keratoconus
  refractive surgery contraindicated in, 8:46–47, 47*i*,
    13:9, 186
Formed elements, 1:159. See also Blood cells
Formoterol, 1:157, 157*t*
N-Formylmethionylleucylphenylalanine (FMLP), in
    innate immunity, 9:46
Fornices, 2:29, 32*i*, 36, 4:43, 8:8
  contracture of, anophthalmic socket and, 7:125
  reconstruction of, for cicatricial pemphigoid, 8:223
Fornix incision, for extraocular muscle surgery,
    6:183–184
Fortaz. See Ceftazidime
Fortovase. See Saquinavir
Fosamprenavir, 1:42
Foscarnet, 1:48, 65*t*, 77, 2:440*t*, 443
  for cytomegalovirus retinitis, 1:29, 48, 9:251, 12:193
  for herpetic retinitis (acute retinal necrosis), 12:186
Foscavir. See Foscarnet
Fosinopril, 1:88*t*
Fosphenytoin, 1:283*t*
Fossae
  infratemporal, 7:22
  middle cranial, 7:21
  orbital, 7:21–22
  pterygopalatine, 7:21
Foster Kennedy syndrome, 5:123, 123*i*
4:2:1 rule, 12:102–103
4Δ base-out prism test, 6:61–63, 63*i*
4-mirror contact lens, Zeiss, for fundus biomicroscopy,
    3:288, 288*i*
4-quadrant nucleofractis, 11:131–132, 132*i*
Fourth cranial nerve. See Cranial nerve IV
Fourth nerve (trochlear) palsy, 5:232–234, 234*i*
  bilateral, 5:233
  congenital, 5:233, 234*i*
  Parks-Bielschowsky 3-step test for, 5:232–233
  superior oblique muscle palsy and, 6:132–135, 133*i*
Fovea (fovea centralis), 2:76, 86, 87, 87*i*, 4:119, 5:24,
    12:8, 8*i*, 9*t*, 10
  development of, 2:142–144, 6:47–48
  hypoplasia of, 6:337
    in albinism, 6:345
Fovea externa, 2:87
Fovea lentis (lens pit), formation of, 11:25, 26*i*
Foveal avascular zone, 2:88, 88*i*, 12:8
Foveal burns, photocoagulation causing, 12:319
Foveal cones, 2:80, 87–88
Foveal electroretinogram, 12:31–32
Foveal fibers, 2:98
Foveal pit, 2:144
Foveal pseudocyst, 12:91
Foveal retinoschisis, 6:340
Foveola, 2:86, 87, 87*i*, 4:119, 120*i*, 12:8, 9*t*

Foveomacular retinitis (solar retinopathy/retinitis), 12:307–308

Foveomacular vitelliform dystrophy, adult-onset, 12:219–220, 219*i*

    age-related macular degeneration differentiated from, 12:67, 68*i*

Foville syndrome, 5:227

FOXC1 (FKHL7) gene

    in Axenfeld-Rieger syndrome, 6:253, 271

    in glaucoma, 10:13*t*

    in Peters anomaly, 8:294

FPA. *See* "Flatter add plus" rule

FPG. *See* Fasting plasma glucose test

Fractures. *See specific type or structure affected*

Fragile site/fragility, chromosomal, 2:186

Fragile X syndrome, 2:186

Frames (spectacle), anophthalmic socket camouflage and, 7:127

Frameshift mutation (framing error/frameshift), 2:186

François, central cloudy dystrophy of, 8:310*t*, 323, 324*i*

    in megalocornea, 8:290, 290*i*

François dyscephalic syndrome. *See* Hallermann-Streiff syndrome

FRAS1 gene, 8:286

Fraser syndrome (cryptophthalmos-syndactyly), 6:209, 8:286

    eyelid manifestations of, 4:173*t*, 6:209

Freckle, 4:182

    conjunctival, 4:56*t*, 8:263, 267*t*

    of eyelid, 7:171

    Hutchinson melanotic (lentigo maligna/precancerous melanosis), 7:174

    iris, 4:219*t*, 220*i*, 6:289

    in neurofibromatosis, 6:403

Fredrickson classification, of hyperlipoproteinemias, 8:339, 339*t*

Free radicals (oxygen radicals), 2:365–371

    in Alzheimer disease, 1:287

    cellular sources of, 2:365–366, 367*i*

    as inflammatory mediators, 9:83–85, 84*i*

    in lens, 2:368–370, 369*i*, 11:16–17

    lipid peroxidation and, 2:366–368, 367*i*, 368*i*

    in retina, 2:370–371

Free T_4, 1:222

Freezing, anterior segment injuries caused by, 8:388

Frenzel goggles, in ocular motility assessment, 5:200, 240

Frequency, in phacoemulsification, 11:114

Frequency doubling, 10:58

Frequency-doubling technology (FDT) perimetry, 10:58–59, 71*i*

Frequency-encoding analysis, definition of, 5:79

Frequency of light wave, 3:4

    relationship to wavelength, 3:7

Frequency response, modulation transfer function and, 3:113

Fresnel prisms, 3:89–90, 89*i*

    for esotropia in sixth nerve palsy, 6:107

    for nystagmus, 6:168

    for overcorrection of intermittent exotropia, 6:113

    temporary, 3:89–90, 170

    for thyroid-associated orbitopathy, 5:331

Friedreich's ataxia, retinal degeneration and, 12:232*t*, 235

Frontal artery, 5:15

Frontal bone, 5:9, 10, 7:7, 8*i*, 9*i*

Frontal branch, of cerebral artery, 5:16

Frontal ethmoidal suture, 5:9

Frontal eye fields, 5:202, 208, 211

Frontal nerve, 2:115, 5:52, 53*i*, 7:14

Frontal sinuses, 5:9, 9*i*, 7:9*i*, 20, 20*i*, 21*i*

Frontalis sling, for blepharophimosis syndrome correction, 7:153

Frontalis suspension, for ptosis correction, 7:217, 221*i*, 222

Frontoethmoidal incision, for anterior orbitotomy, 7:112

Frontopolar branch, of cerebral artery, 5:16

Frontozygomatic suture, 5:10

Frozen section, for pathologic examination, 4:41

FTA-ABS (fluorescent treponemal antibody absorption) test, 1:17, 17*t*, 302, 9:189–190

FTC. *See* Emtricitabine

5FU. *See* Fluorouracil

Fuchs adenoma (pseudoadenomatous hyperplasia), 4:146, 241–242

Fuchs coloboma (tilted disc syndrome), 5:139–140, 140*i*, 6:360–361, 361*i*

Fuchs endothelial dystrophy, 2:49, 49*i*, 4:73, 75*i*, 8:310*t*, 324–327, 325*i*, 326*i*

Fuchs heterochromic iridocyclitis/uveitis, 9:107, 144–146, 145*i*

    cataracts in, 11:64, 65*i*

    glaucoma and, 10:107–108, 108*i*

Fuchs superficial marginal keratitis, 8:371

Fucosidosis, 6:436*t*, 8:342

Full-field electroretinography, 5:101, 102

Full-thickness eyelid biopsy, 7:176*i*, 181–182

Fumagillin, for microsporidial keratoconjunctivitis, 8:190

Functional Acuity Contrast Test (FACT), 3:252

Functional disorders, in elderly, 1:239–240

Functional magnetic resonance imaging (fMRI), 5:68, 78

Functional visual loss, 1:266, 5:303–315

    categories of, 5:303

    diagnosis of, 5:304

    examination techniques in, 5:305–315

    identification of patient with, 5:303–304

    management of, 5:315

Fundus

    albipunctatus, 6:336, 12:200, 201*i*

        11-cis retinol dehydrogenase defects causing, 2:351

    in congenital night blindness

        abnormalities of, 12:200–202, 201*i*, 202*i*

        normal, 12:198–200, 199*i*, 200*i*

    evaluation of. *See also* Biomicroscopy, slit-lamp; Fundus photography; Ophthalmoscopy

        before cataract surgery, 11:83–84

        in glaucoma, 10:36

        in low vision evaluation, 5:87–89, 88*i*, 89*i*, 89*t*

        in nystagmus, 6:162, 163*t*

        in penetrating trauma, 6:446

        in premature infants, 6:326–328, 327*i*, 327*t*, 328*i*, 329*i*, 351–356, 354*i*

        before refractive surgery, 13:46

    flavimaculatus (Stargardt disease/juvenile macular degeneration), 6:337–339, 338*i*, 339*i*, 12:216–218, 216*i*, 217*i*, 217*t*

        cone–rod dystrophy and, 6:338, 12:215

retinal pigment epithelium in, 2:363
rod ABC transporter mutations causing, 2:349
illumination of
  in direct ophthalmoscopy, 3:270, 271*i*
  in indirect ophthalmoscopy, 3:272, 275, 275*i*
in Leber hereditary optic neuropathy, 5:134, 135*i*
in multiple sclerosis, 5:321
oculi, 2:76
pulverulentus, 12:222
salt-and-pepper
  in rubella, 6:218, 9:158, 159*i*
  in syphilis, 9:188
    in infants and children, 6:220
sunset-glow, in Vogt-Koyanagi-Harada syndrome,
    9:201*i*, 203, 204*i*
tomato catsup, 4:244, 244*i*
xerophthalmic, 8:92
Fundus biomicroscopy. *See* Biomicroscopy, slit-lamp
Fundus photography
camera for, 3:275–279, 277*i*, 278*i*
  exposure limits for, 2:465
  illumination system of, 3:275–278, 278*i*
  observation system of, 3:278–279, 279*i*
  wide-angle, 3:278
in choroidal/ciliary body melanoma, 4:224–226
Funduscopic lenses, 3:285, 289*i*
Fungi, 1:25–26, 8:128–129, 129*i*, 129*t*, 130*i*. *See also*
  specific organism or type of infection
chorioretinitis caused by, 4:124, 125*i*
disseminated infection caused by, in HIV infection/
  AIDS, 1:50
drugs for infection caused by. *See* Antifungal agents
endocarditis caused by, 1:7
endophthalmitis caused by, 9:208*t*, 210, 212,
  213–214, 214*i*, 219, 223–227
  iris nodule in, 4:219*t*
  vitreous in, 4:107
eyelid infections caused by, 4:170, 8:168–169
isolation techniques for identification of, 8:136
keratitis caused by, 4:66, 66*i*, 8:185–187, 186*i*
as normal ocular flora, 8:115*t*
ocular infection caused by, 8:119*t*, 128–131, 129*t*
  neuro-ophthalmic signs of, 5:364–368
optic nerve infections caused by, 4:205
orbital infections caused by, 4:189, 189*i*
  aspergillosis, 7:46–47
    exenteration in management of, 7:128
  mucormycosis/phycomycosis, 4:189, 6:233, 233*i*,
    7:45–46
    exenteration in management of, 7:45–46, 128
posterior uveitis caused by, 9:160–164
retinal infections caused by, 4:124, 125*i*
scleritis caused by, 8:191
stains and culture media for identification of, 8:137*t*
Fungizone. *See* Amphotericin B
Fungus ball (aspergilloma), 5:365, 366*i*
Furazolidone, 1:75
Furosemide
for diastolic dysfunction, 1:131
for hypertension, 1:88*t*
for idiopathic intracranial hypertension, 5:119
Furoxone. *See* Furazolidone
Furrow degeneration, senile, 8:370
Fusarium, 8:130
infections/inflammation caused by, 8:130

keratitis caused by, 8:186, 186*i*
oxysporum, 8:130
solani, 8:130, 186*i*
Fused bifocals, 3:152, 153*i*
Fusidic acid, for *C difficile* colitis, 1:8
Fusiform gyrus, 5:31
Fusion, 6:43–44
peripheral, in monofixation syndrome, 6:57
strabismus classification and, 6:10
tenacious proximal, in intermittent exotropia, 6:111
Fusion (HIV) inhibitors, 1:42
Fusional amplitudes, 6:43, 43*t*
Fusional convergence, 6:38, 43, 88
Fusional divergence, 6:38, 88
in refractive accommodative esotropia, 6:101
Fusional vergence, 6:43, 88–89
Fuzeon. *See* Enfuvirtide
FVC (forced vital capacity), 1:155

G

G6P. *See* Glucose-6-phosphate
G6PD deficiency. *See* Glucose-6-phosphate
  dehydrogenase deficiency
G protein–coupled receptors, in signal transduction,
  2:311
G proteins
in signal transduction, 2:311, 312*i*
in tear secretion, 2:292, 292*i*, 293, 293*i*
GABA, in cone phototransduction, 2:345
GABA agonists, for nystagmus, 5:255
Gabapentin, 1:283*t*
Gabitril. *See* Tiagabine
GAD. *See* Generalized anxiety disorder
Gadolinium, 5:67, 79
GAGs. *See* Glycosaminoglycans
Gain, ocular movement, definition of, 5:39
Gain of function mutations, 2:214
Galactitol (dulcitol)
in cataract formation, 2:331–332, 11:16, 61
in lens glucose/carbohydrate metabolism, 2:331*i*,
  11:16
Galactokinase deficiency, 2:262*t*
cataract associated with, 2:330–331, 11:62
Galactose
in cataract formation, 11:16, 61
in lens carbohydrate metabolism, 11:16
Galactosemia, 2:262*t*, 6:437*t*
cataracts in, 2:330–332, 11:61–62, 62*i*
  pediatric, 6:288*t*
dietary therapy for, 2:280–281
Galactosialidoses, 6:437*t*
retinal degeneration and, 12:243–244
β-Galactosidase enzymes
deficiency of, in gangliosidoses, 6:350, 437*t*
in sphingolipidoses, 8:340
Galantamine, for Alzheimer disease, 1:288
Galen, vein of, 5:23
Galilean telescope, 3:82–83, 82*i*, 83*i*. *See also* Telescopes
contact lens correction of aphakia and, 3:176*i*, 178
in operating microscope, 3:296, 297*i*
in slit-lamp biomicroscope, 3:280–281, 282*i*
  reverse, 3:280–281
zoom, in operating microscope, 3:296

Gallamine, 2:402*i*, 403
Galtonian inheritance, 2:186
    of mitochondrial DNA diseases, 2:186, 257
Gametes, 2:204, 244
Gamma amino-butyric acid (GABA), in cone
    phototransduction, 2:345
Gamma amino-butyric acid (GABA) agonists, for
    nystagmus, 5:255
Gamma cells, 5:27
Gamma (γ)-crystallins, 2:326*t*, 327, 11:11, 11*i*, 12
Gamma (γ)-interferon, 1:261, 9:82*t*
    in delayed hypersensitivity, 9:65*i*, 66
Gammopathy, benign monoclonal, corneal deposits in,
    8:350
Ganciclovir, 1:47–48, 65*t*, 77, 2:389, 390, 440*t*, 443
    for cytomegalovirus retinitis, 1:29, 47–48, 2:443,
        9:155, 250–252, 12:193
    for herpetic retinitis (acute retinal necrosis), 12:186
Ganciclovir sustained-release intraocular device, 2:390,
    443
Ganglion cells, retinal, 2:80–81*i*, 83, 85, 352–353, 353*i*,
    5:24, 12:11, 11*i*
    development/differentiation of, 2:140–141, 6:46
    K system originating in, 6:46
    M system originating in, 6:44–45
    midget, 6:45
    in optic nerve, 10:44, 46
    P system originating in, 6:45
    parasol, 6:44–45
Ganglioneuromas, in multiple endocrine neoplasia,
    1:230, 230*i*
Ganglionic blocking agents, 2:402*i*
Ganglionic neurons, dilator muscle innervation and,
    2:65
Gangliosidoses, 6:350–351, 437*t*. See also specific type
    under GM
    retinal degeneration and, 12:243–244
Gantrisin. See Sulfisoxazole
Ganzfield stimulus, electroretinogram evoked by, 12:30
Gap junctions, in lens, 2:329
Garamycin. See Gentamicin
Gardner syndrome (familial adenomatous polyposis),
    retinal manifestations of, 2:173, 4:122–123, 230,
        6:390, 12:236–237, 237*i*
Gargoyle cells, in mucopolysaccharidoses, 8:336
Gas permeability constant (Dk), of contact lens
    polymers. See also Gas transmissibility
    for rigid contact lenses, 3:183–184
Gas-permeable contact lenses. See Flexible (soft)
    contact lenses; Rigid gas-permeable contact lenses;
    Scleral contact lenses
Gas retinal tamponade, in retinal detachment, 12:340,
    341
Gas transmissibility, 3:183–185
    of rigid contact lenses, 3:185
Gasserian ganglion (semilunar/trigeminal ganglion),
    2:113*i*, 114, 5:52
Gastric cancer, 1:252, 297
Gastric surgery, for obesity in type 2 diabetes,
    1:208–209
Gastroesophageal reflux disease (GERD), cancer and,
    1:297
Gastrointestinal disease
    cancer screening and, 1:297
    in HIV infection/AIDS, 1:48–49

retinal degeneration associated with, 12:236–237
    in scleroderma, 1:185
Gastrula, 2:133
Gatifloxacin, 1:62*t*, 73, 2:430–433, 431*t*
    for bacterial keratitis, 8:182*i*, 183
Gaucher disease, 6:436*t*
    corneal changes in, 8:341
    racial and ethnic concentration of, 2:259
    retinal degeneration and, 12:243
Gaussian reduction, 3:80
    IOL power selection and, 3:218–219, 218*i*
Gaze
    horizontal, 5:34, 37*i*, 38*i*, 39
    positions of, 6:28
        assessment of, 6:86–87, 88*i*
        cardinal, 5:241*i*, 6:28, 28*i*, 86
            extraocular muscle action and, 6:29–30
            yoke muscles and, 6:28*i*, 36, 86
        diagnostic, 6:87, 88*i*
        extraocular muscle action affected by, 6:23*i*,
            29–30, 31*i*, 32*i*, 33*i*, 35*i*
        midline, 6:86
        primary, 6:13, 28, 86, 88*i*
        secondary, 6:28
        strabismus classification and, 6:10
        tertiary, 6:28
        variation of deviation with, 6:10
    vertical, 5:37*i*, 39, 40*i*
Gaze deviation
    periodic alternating, in comatose patients, 5:256
    seizure activity and, 1:284
Gaze-evoked nystagmus, 5:39, 224, 225*i*, 244, 245*i*
Gaze palsy/preference, 5:208–209, 209*i*, 210*i*, 313
    functional (nonorganic/nonphysiologic), 5:313
    psychic, 5:194
GCA (giant cell arteritis). See Arteritis, giant cell
GCAPs. See Guanylate cyclase assisting proteins
GCL (ganglion cell layer). See Ganglion cells
GDM. See Gestational diabetes mellitus
GDx nerve fiber analysis, 5:69
Gel electrophoresis, denaturing gradient, 2:230
Gel phenomenon, in rheumatoid arthritis, 1:173–174
Gelatinase (MMP-2)
    in recurrent corneal erosion, 8:98
    in Sjögren syndrome, 8:78
    in vitreous, 2:333
Gelatinous droplike dystrophy (primary familial
    amyloidosis), 8:310*t*, 321, 321*i*, 347*t*, 348–349
Gelsolin gene, mutation in, amyloid deposits and,
    8:347*t*
Gemfibrozil, for hypercholesterolemia, 1:149*t*
Gemifloxacin, 1:62*t*, 73
Gender, primary angle closure/angle-closure glaucoma
    and, 10:11, 123
Gene, 2:186, 199–205, 202*i*, 241–242, 8:306. See also
    Genetics
    cancer, 2:215, 216*i*
    candidate, 2:226–227
    expression of. See Gene transcription
    structure of, 2:202–203, 202*i*
Gene dosage, 2:221
Gene duplication. See DNA, replication of
Gene mapping. See Genetic map
Gene replacement therapy, 2:237

Gene therapy, 2:237–238, 238*i*
  evolution of, 10:13
  for glaucoma, 10:176–177
  retinal, 9:42
Gene transcription, 2:197, 205–210, 207*i*, 208*i*
  reverse, 2:195
Gene translation, 2:197, 205, 210–212, 211*i*
  gene product changes/modification after
    (posttranslational modification), 2:193
  of lens proteins, 2:328
General anesthesia. *See* Anesthesia
Generalizability
  of clinical research study, 1:361–362
  of screening/diagnostic test, 1:359
Generalized anxiety disorder (GAD), 1:266–267. *See
  also* Anxiety
Generalized gangliosidosis (GM₁ gangliosidosis type I),
  2:262*t*, 6:350, 437*t*, 8:340–341
  retinal degeneration and, 12:243
Generalized seizures, 1:281, 282, 320
Genetic, definition of, 2:186, 239
Genetic code, 2:200–201, 200*t*, 201*i*, 8:306
  degeneracy of, 2:185
  for mitochondrial DNA translation, 2:215–217
Genetic counseling. *See* Genetic testing/counseling
Genetic/hereditary factors. *See also* Family history/
    familial factors; Genetics, clinical
  in Alzheimer disease, 1:286–287
  in diabetes, 1:205, 205*t*
  in epilepsy, 1:281
  in glaucoma, 6:271, 10:12–15, 13*t*, 147–148
  in human carcinogenesis, 1:252, 254–255, 8:248,
    248*t*
  in Parkinson disease, 1:278
  in pediatric cataract, 6:287, 287*t*
  in retinoblastoma, 4:141, 213, 252–253, 252*i*, 6:394,
    395*i*
Genetic heterogeneity, 2:187, 240–241, 347
Genetic imprinting, 2:188, 210
Genetic map, 2:241
Genetic profiling, of tumors, 1:251
Genetic testing/counseling, 2:276–278
  in albinism, 6:345
  autosomal dominant disorders and, 2:266
  family history/pedigree analysis and, 2:275–276,
    275*i*, 276–277, 8:308
  in glaucoma, 10:15
  polygenic and multifactorial inheritance and,
    2:273–274, 274*t*
  prenatal diagnosis and, 2:278
  in retinitis pigmentosa, 12:212
  in retinoblastoma, 4:252–253, 252*i*, 6:394
  in sickle cell disease, 1:159, 163
  support group referral and, 2:282
Genetic therapy. *See* Gene therapy
Genetics
  clinical, 2:239–282, 8:307. *See also specific disorder
    and* Family history/familial factors; Genetic/
    hereditary factors
    alleles and, 2:242–244
    chromosomal analysis in, 2:246–255, 247*t*, 248*i*,
      249*i*
    congenital anomalies and, 2:159–160
    counseling and. *See* Genetic testing/counseling
    disease management and, 2:280–282

genes and chromosomes and, 2:241–242
    independent assortment and, 2:244–245
    inheritance patterns and, 2:260–269
    linkage and, 2:241, 246
    Lyonization (X chromosome inactivation) and,
      2:242, 269–273
    meiosis and, 2:244, 245*i*
    mitosis and, 2:204, 244
    mutations and, 2:255–259
    pedigree analysis in, 2:275–276, 275*i*, 8:308
    pharmacogenetics and, 2:278–279
    polygenic and multifactorial inheritance and,
      2:273–275, 274*t*
    racial and ethnic concentration of disorders and,
      2:259–260
    segregation and, 2:241, 244
    terminology used in, 2:239–241
  molecular, 2:199–238
    of corneal dystrophies, 8:305–308, 309–310*t*
    correlation of genes with specific diseases and,
      2:220–227, 224*i*, 225*i*
    DNA/genes/chromosomes in, 2:199–204, 200*i*,
      200*t*, 201*i*, 202*i*
    DNA analysis and manipulation and, 2:227–231,
      228*i*, 229*i*, 232*i*, 233*i*
    DNA repair and, 2:212–213
    DNA replication and, 2:212
    gene therapy and, 2:237–238, 238*i*
    mitochondrial genome and, 2:215–220, 219*i*
    mutations and, 2:214–215, 216*i*
    recombinant, 2:227. *See also* Recombinant DNA
    transcription (expression) and, 2:205–210, 207*i*,
      208*i*
    transgenic and knockout animals in study of,
      2:234–237, 236*i*
    translation and, 2:210–212, 211*i*
    value of, 8:305–306
  principles of, 8:306–307
  terms used in, 2:181–198, 239–241
Geniculate body/nucleus/ganglion, 2:118
  lateral, 2:107, 5:16, 17*i*, 27–28, 6:44, 45*i*
    development of, 6:46
      abnormal visual experience affecting, 6:49
Geniculocalcarine pathways (visual radiations), 2:102
Genital ulcers, in Behçet syndrome, 1:193
Gennari line, 5:29
Genocopy, 2:186
Genome, 2:186, 256
  mitochondrial, 2:215–220, 219*i*. *See also*
    Mitochondrial DNA
Genomic clone, 2:186
Genomic DNA library, 2:189, 227, 228*i*
Genoptic. *See* Gentamicin
Genotype, 2:187, 256, 8:307
Gentacidin. *See* Gentamicin
Gentak. *See* Gentamicin
Gentamicin, 1:61*t*, 70, 2:428*t*, 431*t*, 435
  in combination preparations, 2:432*t*
  for endocarditis prophylaxis, 1:11*t*
  for endophthalmitis, 9:217, 218*t*
  ototoxicity of, mitochondrial DNA mutations and,
    2:220
Geographic choroiditis (serpiginous/helicoid
  peripapillary choroidopathy), 9:177*t*, 182–183, 184*i*,
  12:174*t*, 176–177, 177*i*

Geographic epithelial ulcer, in herpes simplex keratitis, 8:143, 144i, 146
Geographic maps, 8:45, 46i
Geometric wavefront, 3:238, 13:14
Geometrical optics, 3:25–104. See also specific aspect
    aberrations and, 3:93–104
    definition of, 3:3
    first-order optics and, 3:55–62. See also First-order optics
    image characteristics and, 3:30–39
    imaging with lenses and, 3:28–30, 29i
    imaging with mirrors and, 3:28–30, 29i, 90–93
    intraocular lenses and, 11:145
        multifocal effects and, 11:146
    light propagation and, 3:39–54
    mirrors and, 3:28–30, 29i, 90–93, 91i
    nonspherical IOLs and, 3:224–225
    pinhole imaging and, 3:25–28, 25i, 28i
    power prediction formulas for IOLs based on, 3:218–219, 218i
    prisms and, 3:84–90
GERD. See Gastroesophageal reflux disease
Geriatrics, 1:233–249. See also Age/aging
    elder abuse and, 1:236–237
    falls and, 1:247, 248t
    medication use and, 1:235–236
    osteoporosis and, 1:240–247, 242t, 243t, 245t
    outpatient visits and, 1:236
    physiologic/pathologic eye changes and, 1:235
    psychology/psychopathology of aging and, 1:238–240
    surgical considerations and, 1:237–238
    systemic disease incidence and, 1:247–249
Germ layer theory, 2:129
German measles. See Rubella
Germinal mosaicism, 2:187
Germinative zone, 2:76, 11:6, 8i
Germinomas, nystagmus caused by, 6:159t
Gerstmann syndrome, 5:166, 194
Gestational age, retinopathy and, 6:326. See also Retinopathy, of prematurity
Gestational diabetes mellitus, 1:203t, 205t, 206
Ghost cell glaucoma, 4:81, 82i, 108, 10:112–113, 112i
Ghost cells, 2:339, 4:108, 109i
Ghost dendrites, in herpes simplex keratitis, 8:143, 145i
Ghost images, after PRK, 13:102
Giant aneurysm, 5:351
Giant cell (temporal) arteritis. See Arteritis, giant cell
Giant cells, 9:15, 52–53
    cytologic identification of, 8:69
    foreign-body, 4:13, 15i
    Langhans, 4:13, 15i
    multinucleated, 4:13
    Touton, 4:13, 15i
        in juvenile xanthogranuloma, 6:389
Giant congenital melanocytic nevi, 4:182
Giant drusen, 4:257–259, 5:132
    in tuberous sclerosis, 6:411
Giant papillary (contact lens–induced) conjunctivitis, 3:210, 4:45, 8:214–216, 215i
Giant retinal tear, 12:253
    vitrectomy for, 12:340, 341
Giant vacuoles, in Schlemm's canal, 2:58, 58i, 59i
Giemsa stain, 8:65t
Gigantism, 1:228
    regional, 6:405

Gillespie syndrome (MIM 206700), aniridia in, 2:254
GIOD. See Ganciclovir sustained-release intraocular device
Glands of Krause, 2:24i, 29t, 34, 290, 4:168t, 7:140i, 145, 253
    aqueous component/tears secreted by, 8:56
Glands of Moll, 2:22, 24i, 29t, 4:168t, 7:166, 8:6, 7i. See also Apocrine glands of eyelid
    hidrocystoma arising in, 7:167–168
Glands of Wolfring, 2:24i, 29t, 34, 290, 4:168t, 7:140i, 145, 253
    aqueous component/tears secreted by, 8:56
Glands of Zeis, 2:22, 24i, 29t, 8:6, 7i
    chalazion caused by obstruction of, 8:87
    sebaceous adenocarcinoma arising in, 7:180
    in tear film-lipids/tear production, 2:289
Glare
    with anterior chamber phakic IOLs, 13:151, 153t
    cataracts and, 11:76, 77t
    intraocular lens design and, 11:194
    with iris-fixated phakic IOLs, 13:153t, 154
    with multifocal IOLs, 13:164, 173
    with posterior chamber phakic IOLs, 13:153t, 154
    after PRK, 13:102
    after radial keratotomy, 13:63
    scattering causing, 3:13
    sunglasses affecting sensitivity to, 3:165
        polarizing lenses and, 3:10–11, 165
Glare testing, 3:317–318, 318i
    in vision rehabilitation, 3:253
Glargine insulin, 1:201, 209t, 210
Glass, refractive index of, 3:40t
Glass–air interface, reflection at, 3:13, 13i
Glass prism, calibration of, 3:86, 86i
Glassblowers
    cataract in, infrared radiation and, 11:56
    exfoliation of lens capsule in, 11:65
Glasses. See Spectacle lenses (spectacles)
Glatiramer acetate, for multiple sclerosis, 5:144, 324
Glaucoma, 5:138, 138i. See also Angle-closure glaucoma; Open-angle glaucoma; Uveitis-glaucoma-hyphema (UGH) syndrome
    angle-recession, 4:82–84, 83i, 10:113–114, 113i
    Axenfeld-Rieger syndrome and, 4:78–79, 6:253, 271, 278, 10:32, 152, 153t
    cataracts and, 11:67–68, 68i
        in children, 11:198
        management of, 11:217–221, 218i, 220i. See also Cataract surgery, in glaucoma patient
    central retinal vein occlusion and, 5:107, 12:143
    characteristics of, 10:6t, 8
    childhood (congenital/infantile/juvenile), 6:271–284, 453, 10:147–156
        aniridia and, 6:277–278
        anomalies associated with, 10:152–156, 153t, 155t
        aphakic, 6:279–280, 280i
            cataract surgery and, 6:279–280, 302–303
        in Axenfeld-Rieger syndrome, 4:78–79, 6:253, 271, 278, 10:32, 152, 153t
        cataract surgery associated with, 6:279–280, 302–303
        characteristics of, 10:6t
        classification of, 10:147
        clinical features of, 6:272–273, 273i, 274t, 10:148–150, 149i

corneal opacities and, **6:**256*t*, 257
corticosteroid-induced, pediatric uveitis treatment
    and, **6:**320
cupping in, **10:**49–50
definitions of, **10:**147
developmental, with associated ocular or systemic
    anomalies, **10:**152–156, 153*t*, 155*t*
diagnosis/differential diagnosis of, **6:**273–277,
    274*t*, **10:**150, 151*t*
epidemiology of, **10:**147–148
follow-up of, **6:**284, **10:**150–151
genetics of, **6:**271, **10:**15, 147–148
juvenile open-angle, **6:**271, 272
in leukemia, **6:**344
in Lowe syndrome, **6:**278–279, 348
medical therapy of, **6:**282–283
natural history of, **6:**277
in neurofibromatosis, **6:**278, 405, 408, **10:**154, 156
pathophysiology of, **6:**272, **10:**148
in Peters anomaly, **10:**152–153, 153*t*
primary, **10:**6*t*
    congenital open-angle, **6:**271, 272–277, 273*i*,
        274*t*, 275*i*, 276*i*, 277*i*
    juvenile, **6:**271, 272, **10:**6*t*
prognosis of, **6:**284, **10:**150–151
pseudophakic, **6:**280
retinopathy of prematurity and, **6:**331–332
secondary, **6:**277–280
    characteristics of, **10:**6*t*
    mechanical, **6:**279
signs and symptoms of, diagnostic considerations
    for, **10:**150, 151*t*
in Sturge-Weber syndrome, **6:**278, 416, **10:**154
surgery for, **6:**281–282, **10:**207–209, 208*i*, 209*i*
    uveitis and, **6:**322
systemic disease and, **6:**278–279
traumatic hyphema in children and, **6:**449
treatment of, **6:**280–283
ciliary block. *See* Aqueous misdirection
classification of, **10:**4–7, 4*t*, 6*t*, 7*i*, 8*i*, 9*t*
    conceptual means of, **10:**4, 4*t*
    mechanisms of outflow obstruction in, **10:**9*t*
clinical evaluation of, **10:**31–81
    anterior chamber, **10:**34–36, 34*i*, 35*i*, 35*t*
    in children, **6:**273–276, 275*i*, 276*i*
    conjunctiva, **10:**33
    cornea, **10:**33–34
    episclera, **10:**33
    external adnexae, **10:**32–33
    fundus, **10:**36
    general examination in, **10:**31–36, 34*i*, 35*i*, 35*t*
    gonioscopy in, **10:**34–44, 34*i*, 35*i*, 35*t*
        peripheral anterior synechiae and, **10:**39
    iris, **10:**36
    lens, **10:**36
    optic nerve, **10:**44, 46–49, 46*i*, 47*i*
    optic neuropathy, **10:**49–57, 50*i*, 52*t*, 53*i*, 54*i*
    patient history in, **10:**31
    pupils, **10:**33
    refraction in, **10:**31–32
    sclera, **10:**33
    tests in, **10:**80, 81*i*
    visual field examination in, **10:**57–81. *See also*
        Visual field, clinical evaluation of, in glaucoma
combined-mechanism, **10:**5, 7

congenital, **6:**271, 272–277, 273*i*, 274*t*, 275*i*, 276*i*,
    277*i*, **8:**299–300, **10:**6*t*. *See also* Glaucoma,
    childhood
contrast sensitivity affected in, **3:**115
cornea plana and, **8:**291
corticosteroid-induced, **2:**419, **10:**116–117
    pediatric uveitis treatment and, **6:**320
defects due to, patterns of, **10:**60, 61–64*i*
definition of, **10:**3
developmental, **10:**147. *See also* Glaucoma,
    childhood
drugs for, **10:**159–174, 160–164*t*, 170*i*. *See also*
    Antiglaucoma agents
dry eye disorders and, **8:**76
environmental factors in, **10:**15
epidemiologic aspects of, **10:**7–12
exfoliative, **4:**80
genetic/hereditary factors in, **6:**271, **10:**12–15, 13*t*,
    147–148
    currently mapped genes and, **10:**12–13, 13*t*
    testing for, **10:**15
ghost cell, **4:**81, 82*i*, 108, **10:**112–113, 112*i*
hemolytic, **4:**82, **10:**112–113
hemorrhage-associated, **4:**81–84, 82*i*, 83*i*
hemosiderin in, **4:**81–82
in herpetic uveitis, **9:**139
hyphema and, in children, **6:**449
infantile, **6:**271, 272–277, 273*i*, 274*t*, 275*i*, 276*i*, 277*i*,
    10:147. *See also* Glaucoma, childhood
intraocular pressure in, **10:**3, 10, 83–84
    congenital/infantile glaucoma and, **6:**274–275
    uveitis and, **9:**237
introduction to, **10:**3–15
juvenile rheumatoid arthritis–associated iridocyclitis
    and, **9:**143–144
after LASIK, **13:**189, 190*i*, 208–209
lens-induced, **4:**81, 82*i*, 96, 101, **9:**52, 136–137,
    10:103–106, 104*i*, 104*t*, 105*i*, **11:**67–68, 68*i*
    angle-closure, **10:**104*t*
    in children, **6:**279
    open-angle, **10:**103–106, 104*i*, 104*t*, 105*i*
lens particle, **10:**104–105, 105*i*, **11:**67–68
low-tension, **10:**92–96, 94*t*. *See also* Glaucoma,
    normal-tension
malignant. *See* Aqueous misdirection
management of
    goal in, **10:**57, 157
    medical, **10:**157–177
        agents used in, **10:**159–174, 160–164*t*, 170*i*. *See
            also specific drug and* Antiglaucoma agents
        compliance in, **10:**176
        future therapy in, **10:**176–177
        general approach to, **10:**174–177
        in nursing mothers, **10:**176
        during pregnancy, **10:**176
    progression of, **10:**158–159
    risk-benefit assessment in, **10:**158
    surgical, **10:**179–209. *See also* Laser trabeculoplasty
        in children, **6:**281–282, **10:**207–209, 208*i*, 209*i*
        nonpenetrating, **10:**206–207
megalocornea and, **8:**290
melanomalytic, **4:**84, 85*i*, 161
microcornea and, **8:**289
nanophthalmos and, **8:**287

neovascular, **10**:132–136, 133*t*, 134*i*, 135*i*
rubeosis iridis and, **4**:155–156
nerve fiber bundle defect in, **10**:60
in neurofibromatosis, **10**:154, 156
in children, **6**:278, 405, 408, **10**:154, 156
normal-tension, **5**:138, **10**:92–96, 94*t*
clinical features of, **10**:92–93
diagnostic evaluation of, **10**:94–95
differential diagnosis of, **10**:93–94, 94*t*
prognosis of, **10**:95
treatment of, **10**:95–96
ocular receptors and, **2**:312–313, 314*t*
ophthalmoscopic signs of, **10**:52, 52*t*
optic nerve changes in, **10**:4, 44, 46–49, 46*i*, 47*i*. *See
also* Optic nerve (cranial nerve II), in glaucoma
optic neuropathy associated with, **10**:49–57, 50*i*, 52*t*,
53*i*, 54*i*
pain caused by, **5**:298
pars planitis and, **9**:151
penetrating keratoplasty and, **8**:460–461, **10**:116,
116*t*
peripapillary atrophy in, **10**:55
persistent fetal vasculature/persistent hyperplastic
primary vitreous and, **6**:324, **12**:282
phacolytic, **4**:81, 82*i*, 96, 101, **9**:52, 136–137, **10**:104,
104*i*, 104*t*, 105*i*, **11**:67
phacomorphic, **10**:122, 128–129, 130*i*, 131*i*, **11**:68,
68*i*
pigment dispersion syndrome and, **4**:84, 85*i*
pigmentary, **10**:101–103, 101–103*i*
primary
congenital, **6**:272–277, 273*i*, 274*t*, 275*i*, 276*i*, 277*i*
definition/description of, **10**:5
juvenile, **6**:271, 272
after PRK/LASEK, **13**:105, 189, 208
pseudophakic, in children, **6**:280
after refractive surgery, **13**:208–209
refractive surgery in patients with, **13**:189–191, 190*i*
retained lens fragments after phacoemulsification
and, **12**:337
retinopathy of prematurity and, **12**:131
in sarcoidosis, **9**:198
scleritis and, **8**:239
secondary
characteristics of, **10**:6*t*
in children, **6**:277–280
mechanical, **6**:279
definition/description of, **10**:5
developmental glaucoma and, **10**:156
with material in trabecular meshwork, **4**:80–84,
161
melanomalytic, **4**:84, 85, 161
rubeosis iridis and, **4**:155–156
in uveal lymphoid infiltration, **4**:279
in Sturge-Weber syndrome, **5**:340, **6**:278, 416, **10**:32,
154
tests for, **1**:355–359, 356*i*, 357*i*, 358*t*, **10**:80, 81*i*
trauma and, **4**:81–84, 82*i*, 83*i*, **10**:113–114, 113*i*
uveitis and, **9**:139, 237–239, 238*t*
visual field changes in, causes of, **10**:4
vitreous injury and, **2**:339
in Vogt-Koyanagi-Harada syndrome, **9**:205
Glaucoma genes, **6**:271, **10**:12–15, 13*t*, 147–148
Glaucoma hemisphere test, **10**:70, 71*i*
Glaucoma Laser Trial (GLT), **10**:158, 180

Glaucoma suspect, **10**:96–98, 97*i*
characteristics of, **10**:6*t*
definition of, **10**:96
Glaucoma tube shunt, **10**:201–204. *See also* Tube-shunt
surgery
Glaucomatocyclitic crisis (Posner-Schlossman
syndrome), **9**:107, 135, **10**:107
Glaucomatous cupping. *See* Cupping of optic disc,
glaucomatous
Glauctabs. *See* Methazolamide
Glaukomflecken, **4**:98, **10**:124, **11**:68
GLC1A gene, **10**:12, 13*t*, 14
testing for, **10**:15
GLC1A TIGR/myocilin (MYOC) gene, in congenital
glaucoma, **6**:271
GLC1B gene, **10**:13*t*, 14
GLC1C gene, **10**:13*t*, 14
GLC1D gene, **10**:13*t*, 14
GLC1E gene, **10**:13*t*, 14
GLC1F gene, **10**:13*t*, 14
GLC1G gene, **10**:14
GLC3A gene, **10**:13*t*, 15
GLC3B gene, **10**:13*t*, 15
Glial cells, retinal, **2**:83–84, 353–354, **5**:24
in neurofibromatosis, **6**:404–407, 405*i*, 406*i*
in retinal ischemia, **4**:129
Glimepiride, **1**:212, 212*t*
Glioblastomas, optic nerve (malignant optic gliomas),
4:209, **5**:151, **7**:72
Gliomas
chiasmal, **5**:149, 150, 163
in neurofibromatosis, **6**:406–407, 406*i*
nystagmus caused by, **6**:159*t*
optic pathway/optic nerve, **4**:208–209, 209*i*,
5:148–151, 149*i*, 150*i*, **7**:72–75, 73*i*
in children, **6**:381, 406–407, 406*i*
malignant (glioblastomas), **4**:209, **5**:151, **7**:72
in neurofibromatosis, **5**:149, **6**:381, 406–407, 406*i*,
7:72–74, 76
orbital involvement in, **6**:381
Gliomatosis, arachnoidal, **6**:406
Gliosis, of retina, **4**:134, 134*i*, 147
of peripapillary nerve fiber layer, **5**:116, 116*i*
Gliotic (sclerotic) lesions, in multiple sclerosis, **5**:318
Glipizide, **1**:212, 212*t*
with metformin, **1**:213
Global Initiative for Chronic Obstructive Lung Disease
(GOLD), **1**:153
Globe
blunt injury to
mydriasis/miosis caused by, **8**:397
rupture caused by, **12**:295
in corneoscleral laceration, repair and, **8**:410–416,
411*i*
developmental anomalies of, **8**:285–288
displacement of
in craniosynostosis, **6**:428
in orbital disorders, **7**:23, 24
embryologic/perinatal realignment of, **2**:158
exposure of for phacoemulsification, **11**:121
gross dissection of, for pathologic examination,
4:33–34, 34*i*
needle penetration/perforation of
during retrobulbar anesthesia, **12**:296
during surgery, **12**:336, 337*i*

orbital tumors originating in, 7:92
orientation of, pathologic examination and, 4:32
ptosis of, in blowout fractures, 7:103
rupture of
  corneoscleral laceration repair and, 8:410–416,
    411i
  after radial keratotomy, 13:64, 65i
stabilization of during phacoemulsification, 11:124
topographic features of, 2:43–44, 43i
Glomerulonephritis, retinal degeneration and, 12:236
Glossopharyngeal neuralgia, 5:300
Glucagon-like peptide, for diabetes, 1:214
Glucocorticoids/glucocorticosteroids, 1:194–196,
  2:416–420, 417t, 419t, 9:96. See also Corticosteroids
Glucophage. See Metformin
Glucose
  in aqueous humor, 2:316t, 318
  in cataract formation, 11:60. See also Diabetes
    mellitus
  for medical emergencies, 1:316t
  metabolism of, 1:202
    in cornea, 2:297–299, 298i
    in lens, 2:330, 11:14–16, 15i
    in retinal pigment epithelium, 2:357–358
  plasma levels of
    in diabetes
      diagnosis/screening and, 1:301
      self-monitoring of, 1:215–216
      surgery and, 1:220, 332–333
      surveillance of (glycemic control), 1:215–216
    normal, 1:203t
  in tear film, 2:290
Glucose control. See Glycemic control
Glucose-6-phosphate, in lens carbohydrate metabolism,
  2:330, 11:14, 15i
Glucose-6-phosphate dehydrogenase deficiency, 1:163
  dapsone use in cicatricial pemphigoid and, 8:222
  pharmacogenetics and, 2:279
  racial and ethnic concentration of, 2:259–260
Glucose tolerance/intolerance
  in gestational diabetes, 1:203t, 206
  impaired, 1:203t, 206
  screening for, 1:301
Glucose tolerance test, 1:206
Glucose toxicity, 1:205–206
Glucose transporter, in rods, 2:344t
α-Glucosidase inhibitors, 1:212t, 213
Glucotrol. See Glipizide
Glucovance. See Glyburide, with metformin
Glulisine insulin, 1:209, 209t
Glutathione
  in aqueous humor, 2:318
  in lens, 2:368–369
  in retina and retinal pigment epithelium, 2:371–372
Glutathione peroxidase
  in lens, 2:368, 369t, 11:17
  in retina and retinal pigment epithelium, 2:371–372
Glutathione-S-transferase, in retina and retinal
  pigment epithelium, 2:371–372
Glyburide, 1:212, 212t
  with metformin, 1:213
Glycemic control (glucose surveillance), 1:215–216
  retinopathy incidence and progression affected by,
    1:215, 215i, 12:105
    Diabetes Control and Complications Trial, 12:105,
      106
  United Kingdom Prospective Diabetes Study,
    12:105, 107
Glycerin, 2:415t, 416
  for dry eye, 2:450
  for glaucoma, 10:164t, 173–174
Glycocalyx, corneal epithelium, 2:299
Glycolysis
  in corneal glucose metabolism, 2:297, 298i
  in lens glucose/carbohydrate metabolism, 2:330,
    11:14, 15i
Glycopeptide antibiotics, 1:60–61t, 71–72
Glycopeptide-intermediate S aureus, 1:5
Glycoprotein IIb/IIIa receptor, 1:123
Glycoprotein IIb/IIIa receptor antagonists, 1:123
  for myocardial infarction, 1:111, 115, 123
Glycoproteins
  corneal glycocalyx, 2:299
  viral envelope, 8:120
  in vitreous, 2:337
Glycosaminoglycans
  corneal haze after PRK and, 13:103
  in macular dystrophy, 8:319
  in mucopolysaccharidoses, 8:335–336
Glycosylated hemoglobin (fast hemoglobin/HbA₁/
  HbA₁c), in glucose control/surveillance, 1:215, 215i,
    216, 219
Glynase. See Glyburide
Glyrol. See Glycerin
Glyset. See Miglitol
GM₁ gangliosidosis type I (generalized), 2:262t, 6:350,
  437t, 8:340–341
  retinal degeneration and, 12:243
GM₁ gangliosidosis type II (Derry disease), 6:350, 437t
GM₁ gangliosidosis type III (adult), 6:437t
GM₁ gangliosidosis type IV (Goldberg-Cotlier
  syndrome), retinal degeneration and, 12:243–244
GM₂ gangliosidosis type I (Tay-Sachs disease), 2:262t,
  6:350, 437t, 8:340
  racial and ethnic concentration of, 2:259
  retinal degeneration and, 12:243–244, 244i
GM₂ gangliosidosis type II (Sandhoff disease), 2:262t,
  6:350, 437t, 438
  retinal degeneration and, 12:243
GM₂ gangliosidosis type III (Bernheimer-Seitelberger
  disease), 6:351, 437t
Goblet cells, 2:29t, 4:168t, 8:8
  cytologic identification of, 8:66, 67i
  mucin tear secretion by, 2:289i, 291, 7:253, 8:56, 58
  deficiency and, 8:58
Goiter. See also Hyperthyroidism
  diffuse toxic, 1:224. See also Graves hyperthyroidism
  nodular toxic, 1:225
GOLD. See Global Initiative for Chronic Obstructive
  Lung Disease
Gold compounds/salts, 1:199
  corneal pigmentation caused by, 8:377t
Gold eyelid weights, 5:286
  for exposure keratopathy, 8:95
  for paralytic ectropion, 7:199
Gold standard, 1:363
Goldberg-Cotlier syndrome (GM₁ gangliosidosis type
  IV), retinal degeneration and, 12:243–244
Goldberg syndrome, 8:342
Goldenhar-Gorlin syndrome, 8:352t

Goldenhar syndrome, **6:**431, 432*i*, **7:**38
colobomas and, **6:**210
dermoids/dermolipomas in, **2:**168, **4:**43–44, **6:**386, 386*i*, 431, **8:**276
Duane syndrome and, **6:**141, 431
Goldmann applanation tonometry, **3:**289–292, 290*i*, 291*i*, 292*i*, **10:**25–28, 26*i*, 27*i*, 28*t*
in children, **6:**274
corneal thickness affecting, **8:**34
after LASIK, **13:**208
after PRK/LASEK, **13:**105, 189, 208
Goldmann equation, **10:**17
Goldmann-Favre disease/syndrome (enhanced S-cone/ blue cone syndrome; vitreoretinal dystrophy), **6:**342, **12:**201, 202*i*, 229
Goldmann lenses, **10:**38
fundus contact lens, **3:**285, 286*i*
3-mirror contact, for fundus biomicroscopy, **3:**285–287, 287*i*
Goldmann perimetry, **5:**91–92, 93*i*
in functional visual disorder evaluation, **5:**310, 312*i*
in hereditary retinal/choroidal degenerations, **12:**205
nodal point concept used in, **3:**105–106
in strabismus/amblyopia evaluation, **6:**89–90, 90*i*
in vision rehabilitation, **3:**252
Goldmann-type lens, **10:**39
Goldmann-Weekers adaptometer, for dark adaptation testing, **12:**41–42, 42*i*
Goldmann-Witmer coefficient, **9:**63
Gomori methenamine–silver nitrate stain, **4:**36
Gonadotroph adenomas, **1:**229
Gonadotropins, pituitary adenoma producing, **1:**229
Goniolens, **10:**38–39
Gonioplasty, laser, for angle-closure glaucoma, **10:**199–200
Gonioscopy, **10:**36–37, 37*i*
in blunt trauma evaluation, **10:**44, 45*i*
before cataract surgery, **11:**82
in central retinal vein occlusion, **12:**143
chamber angle, **2:**59–61
in choroidal/ciliary body melanoma, **4:**224
direct, **10:**37–39, 37*i*
in glaucoma evaluation, **10:**34–36, 34*i*, 35*i*, 35*t*, 36–44
in children, **6:**275
indirect, **10:**37–39, 37*i*
Koeppe-type lenses in, **10:**38
normal angle landmarks in, **10:**39–44, 41–43*i*
in pigment dispersion syndrome, **10:**101, 102*i*
total internal reflection and, **3:**49–50, 50*i*
Goniosynechialysis, for angle-closure glaucoma, **10:**200
Goniotomy, for childhood glaucoma, **6:**281, **10:**207–209, 208*i*, 209*i*
complications of, **10:**209
contraindications to, **10:**207
indications for, **10:**207
preoperative evaluation for, **10:**208
technique for, **10:**208–209, 208*i*, 209*i*
Gonococcus (*Neisseria gonorrhoeae*/gonorrhea), **1:**13–14, **8:**125, 125*i*
conjunctivitis caused by, **8:**119*t*, 171–172, 172*i*
in children, **6:**225
in neonates, **6:**222, 222*i*, **8:**172, 173
invasive capability of, **8:**116
resistant strains of, **1:**13–14

GORE-TEX, for frontalis suspension, **7:**222
Gorlin syndrome (basal cell nevus syndrome), **7:**174
eyelid manifestations of, **4:**176*t*
Gottron sign, in dermatomyositis, **1:**186
Gout, **8:**354–355
gp160 vaccine, **1:**44
GPC. *See* Giant papillary (contact lens–induced) conjunctivitis
Graded-density sunglasses, for glare reduction, **3:**165
Gradenigo syndrome, **5:**234, 358
Gradient method, for accommodative convergence/ accommodation ratio measurement, **3:**149, **6:**87–88
Graft-vs-host disease, **8:**217*t*, 223–224
Grafts
for canthal repair, **7:**193
for cicatricial ectropion, **7:**200–201
for cicatricial entropion, **7:**207
conjunctival, **8:**423*t*, 429–433, 430*i*. *See also* Conjunctiva, transplantation of
indications for, **8:**423*t*
for wound closure after pterygium excision, **8:**429, 430*i*, 431–432
corneal. *See also* Donor cornea; Keratoplasty, penetrating
allografts, **8:**453
autografts, **8:**453, 471–472
disease recurrence in, **8:**461, 462*i*
endothelial failure of
late nonimmune, **8:**464
primary, **8:**461, 461*i*
inflammatory necrosis of, after lamellar keratoplasty, **8:**475
prior LASIK affecting, **13:**204
rejection of, **8:**448, 449, **9:**39, 40*i*, 41. *See also* Rejection (graft)
dermis-fat
for anophthalmos, **7:**37, 121
for exposure and extrusion of orbital implant, **7:**125
for superior sulcus deformity, **7:**124
for eyelid repair, **7:**187, 190*i*, 191*i*
limbal, **8:**423*t*. *See also* Limbal transplantation
for chemical burns, **8:**392, 393
indications for, **8:**423*t*
mucous membrane, **8:**423*t*, 425, 439
indications of, **8:**423*t*, 439
rejection of, **8:**448, 449, 466–470, 468*i*, 469*i*. *See also* Rejection (graft)
transplantation antigens and, **8:**447
retinal/retinal pigment epithelium, **9:**42
for symblepharon, **7:**207
tarsoconjunctival
for cicatricial entropion, **7:**207
for eyelid repair, **7:**187, 190*i*, 191*i*, 192
transplantation antigens and, **9:**93–94
Gram-negative bacteria, **8:**123
as normal ocular flora, **8:**115, 115*t*
ocular infection caused by
cocci, **8:**125, 125*i*
rods, **8:**126–127, 127*i*
Gram-positive bacteria, **8:**123
ocular infection caused by
cocci, **8:**123–124, 124*i*
filaments, **8:**127–128
rods, **8:**125–126, 126*i*

Gram stain, 4:36, 36t, 8:65t, 123
Gramicidin, with polymyxin B and neomycin, 2:431t
Grand mal seizures, 1:282
Granular dystrophy, 4:71, 74i, 8:310t, 316–318, 316t, 317i
Granular-lattice dystrophy, 8:317
Granulations, pacchionian, 5:20
Granulocytic sarcoma (chloroma), 6:375, 7:94–95
Granulomas, 4:13, 14i, 15i. *See also* Granulomatosis
  chalazia, 8:87–88, 87i
  in coccidioidomycosis, 9:163, 226
  conjunctival, 8:24t, 25t, 159, 270t, 271, 271i
    in sarcoidosis, 8:88
  eosinophilic, of orbit, 6:276i, 375, 7:88
  foreign-body, after strabismus surgery, 6:186, 187i
  pyogenic, 8:270t, 271, 271i
    in children, 6:388
  in sarcoidosis, 4:47–49, 5:333, 8:88, 9:196–199, 197i, 198i
  in toxocariasis, 6:317, 318i, 9:170–171, 170i, 171i, 171t, 12:191, 192i
  in tuberculosis, 12:184, 184i
Granulomatosis. *See also* Granulomas
  allergic, and angiitis (Churg-Strauss syndrome), 1:189t, 193
  familial juvenile systemic (Blau syndrome), 6:318
  Wegener, 1:189t, 192, 7:60–61, 61i
    choroidal perfusion abnormalities and, 12:166, 169i
    diagnosis of, 7:36, 60–61
    eyelid manifestations of, 4:173t
    scleritis/retinal vasculitis and, 9:62, 175–176, 176i
Granulomatous disease
  ileocolitis (Crohn disease), 1:177, 9:131–132
  nasolacrimal obstruction caused by, 7:278
  pulmonary, 1:154
  subacute thyroiditis, 1:226–227
Granulomatous hypersensitivity, 9:66
Granulomatous inflammation, 4:12
  choroidal, 4:27–28, 28i
Granulomatous uveitis, 9:104, 108, 197–200
Graphical image analysis, 3:76–78, 77i, 77–78i, 78i
Grating acuity
  contrast sensitivity and, 3:113, 114i
  in strabismic amblyopia, 6:68–69
Graves hyperthyroidism/eye disease, 1:224–225. *See also* Thyroid ophthalmopathy
Gray (Gy), radiation dose measurement, 1:255
Gray line (intermarginal sulcus), 2:22, 287, 7:142i, 146
Grayscale map, 5:92, 94i
Greater (major) arterial circle, 2:40, 64, 67, 5:15
Greater superficial petrosal nerve, 2:119, 5:55
Green lasers, 12:314, 315–316t
Grid pattern photocoagulation, in central retinal vein occlusion, 12:144
Groenouw dystrophy type I, 8:316–317
Grönblad-Strandberg syndrome. *See* Pseudoxanthoma elasticum
Gross dissection, for pathologic examination, 4:33–34, 34i
Group A beta (β)-hemolytic streptococci (*Streptococcus pyogenes*), 1:6, 8:124
  orbital cellulitis caused by, 6:231
  orbital necrotizing fasciitis caused by, 7:44–45
  preseptal cellulitis caused by, in children, 6:230

Grouped pigmentation of retina (bear tracks), 2:173, 4:230, 232i, 6:390, 12:264
Growth factors, 2:126, 129–130, 456–457, 9:80, 82t
  in aqueous humor, 2:320–321
  homeobox gene expression affected by, 2:130, 131
  as inflammatory mediators, 8:198t
  in ocular development, 2:129–130
  in tear film, 2:291
Growth hormone, pituitary adenoma producing, 1:228
Gruber (petroclinoid) ligament, 2:117, 5:43
GSH. *See* Glutathione
Guaiac stool test, in cancer screening, 1:295t, 298
Guanethidine, 2:309
Guanfacine, 1:89t
Guanylate cyclase
  mutations in, 2:349
  in rod phototransduction, 2:343–344, 344t
Guanylate cyclase assisting proteins (GCAPs), 2:343, 344t
Guanylate cyclase gene, photoreceptor-specific (*RETGC1* gene) in Leber congenital amaurosis, 6:335
GUCA1A gene, in cone dystrophies, 12:214
GUCY2D gene
  in cone dystrophies, 12:214
  in cone–rod dystrophies, 12:215
Guerin (maxillary) fracture, 7:98i
Guillain-Barré syndrome
  bulbar variant of, 5:277
  facial diplegia in, 5:285
  immunization and, 1:303
Gullstrand schematic eye, 3:105, 106i, 233
Gummas, syphilitic, 1:16, 9:188, 190
GUN syndrome, in primary central nervous system lymphoma, 9:229
Gundersen flap, 8:436–437, 437i
  for corneal edema after cataract surgery, 11:193
Gustatory nucleus, 2:117
Guyton-Minkowski Potential Acuity Meter (PAM), 3:316–317, 316i
GVHD. *See* Graft-vs-host disease
Gyne-Lotrimin. *See* Clotrimazole
Gyrate atrophy, 2:262t, 12:225–226, 226i
  ornithine amino transferase defects causing, 2:351, 12:225
  retinal pigment epithelium in, 2:363
Gyrus
  cingulate, 5:56
  fusiform, 5:31
  lingual, 5:31
  postcentral, 5:50, 50i, 51i
  precentral, 5:54
  rectus, 2:93, 95i, 5:26
  subangularis, 5:31

H

H&E stain. *See* Hematoxylin and eosin (H&E) stain
H$_1$-receptor blockers. *See also* Antihistamines
  for ocular allergy, 6:236, 236t
H$_2$-receptor blockers, preoperative, 1:331
H zone, basal cell carcinoma in, 7:177
Haab's striae, 4:70, 6:272, 274, 8:300
HAART. *See* Highly active antiretroviral therapy

Haber-Weiss reaction, 12:299
    oxygen radicals produced by, 9:84, 84i
Habit spasm, 5:290
Haemophilus/Haemophilus influenzae, 1:10–12, 8:127
    biotype III (*H aegyptius*), 8:170
    bleb-associated endophthalmitis caused by, 9:208t,
        212–213, 12:331
    conjunctivitis caused by, 8:119t, 170–171
        in children, 6:224–225
    endocarditis caused by, 1:7
    immunization against, 1:12, 291, 304t, 308–309
    as normal ocular flora, 8:115t
    orbital cellulitis caused by, 7:42
    preseptal cellulitis caused by, 6:230, 7:41
    resistant strains of, 1:12
    type b (Hib), 8:127
Haemophilus influenzae type B (Hib) vaccine, 1:12,
        291, 304t, 308–309
    in combination vaccines, 1:309
Hagberg-Santavouri disease, 6:437t
Hageman factor, in kinin-forming system, 9:76
Haidinger brushes, 3:10
Haigis formula, for IOL power determination, 13:202
    clear lens extraction/refractive lens exchange and,
        13:160
Hair follicles, of eyelid (lash follicles), 7:142i
    tumors arising in, 7:168–169, 169i
Halberg trial clips, for overrefraction, 3:142
Halberstaedter-Prowazek inclusion bodies, 8:69, 69i
Halcion. *See* Triazolam
Haldol. *See* Haloperidol
Haller and Zinn, circle of, 2:103, 5:15, 10:48, 49
Hallermann-Streiff syndrome (Hallermann-Streiff-
    François syndrome/François dyscephalic syndrome/
    dyscephalic mandibulo-oculofacial syndrome),
        8:352t
    childhood glaucoma and, 10:155t
Haller's layer, 12:15
Hallucinations, 1:264, 5:189–191
    cortical origin of, 5:190–191
    definition of, 5:187
    nonvisual causes of, 5:188t
    ocular origin of, 5:189–190
    optic nerve origin of, 5:190
    primary visual cortex lesions causing, 5:170
Hallucinatory palinopsia, 5:190–191
Hallucinogenic drugs, abuse of, 1:268t
Haloes
    with anterior chamber phakic IOLs, 13:151, 153t
    with iris-fixated phakic IOLs, 13:153t, 154
    with multifocal IOLs, 13:164, 173
    with posterior chamber phakic IOLs, 13:153t, 154
    after PRK, 13:102
Haloperidol, 1:271
Haltia-Santavuori syndrome, 12:233t, 241
Hamartia, 5:337
Hamartin, 5:338
Hamartomas, 4:12, 45, 5:337, 8:275
    astrocytic (astrocytomas). *See also* Optic nerve (optic
        pathway) glioma
        malignant, 5:151
        nystagmus caused by, 6:159t
        of orbit, 6:381
        pilocytic, 5:148–151, 149i, 150t
            juvenile, 4:208, 209i

retinal, optic disc drusen differentiated from,
    5:132–134, 133i
    retinoblastoma differentiated from, 4:255–258,
        258i, 6:394
    in tuberous sclerosis, 5:339, 6:410, 411i
    combined, of retina and retinal pigment epithelium,
        4:146, 242, 242i, 6:390
    of eyelid and conjunctiva, 8:270t
    in neurofibromatosis, 6:401
    of orbit, 7:63
Hand-Schüller-Christian disease/syndrome, orbital
    involvement in, 7:88
    in children, 6:376
Hand washing, in infection control, 8:50
    HIV transmission prevention and, 1:51
Handheld magnifiers, 3:258
Handicap, visual. *See* Low vision; Visual loss/
    impairment
    reducing. *See* Vision rehabilitation
Hanna limbal fixation trephine system, 8:456
Hansen disease, 8:51t
Hantavirus/hantavirus pulmonary syndrome, 1:35
Haploid/haploid number, 2:187, 244
Haploid insufficiency (haploinsufficiency), 2:187
    in aniridia/*PAX6* gene disorders, 2:255
    gene therapy for disorders caused by, 2:237
Haplotype, 2:187
Hapten, 9:7
    poison ivy toxin as, 9:29–30
    serum sickness caused by, 9:59
Haptic
    of intraocular lens, 3:213
    of scleral contact lens, 3:200–201, 201i
Harada-Ito procedure, 6:135, 174
Harada's disease, 12:181
Hard contact lenses. *See* Rigid corneal contact lenses;
    Rigid gas-permeable contact lenses
Hard (hyaline) drusen, 4:138, 138i, 12:57
Hard exudates, 4:131, 131i
    in diabetic macular edema, 12:113, 114, 114i
Hard palate composite grafts, for eyelid repair, 7:187
"Hard" tubercles, 4:13, 14i
Hardy-Rand-Rittler color plates, 12:43
Harmonin, in Usher syndrome, 12:235
Harmonious anomalous retinal correspondence, 6:60,
    64, 65i
Hartman-Shack wavefront analysis/aberrometry,
    3:240–241, 241i, 320i, 321i, 8:49, 13:14, 14i
Hashimoto thyroiditis, 1:226–227
    in Graves ophthalmopathy, 7:53
    hypothyroidism caused by, 1:225, 226, 227
Hasner, valve of, 6:239, 7:255i, 256
    nasolacrimal duct obstruction and, 7:257, 261
Hassall-Henle bodies/warts (peripheral corneal guttae),
    2:47, 8:362, 375
"Hatchet face," in myotonic dystrophy, 5:335
HATTS (hemagglutination treponemal test for
    syphilis), 1:17, 302
Havrix. *See* Hepatitis A vaccine
Hay fever conjunctivitis, 8:207–209
Haze formation, after keratorefractive surgery
    PRK/LASEK, 13:103–104, 103i
    wound healing and, 13:28, 29
Hb. *See* Hemoglobin
HBA. *See* Hepatitis, type A

HbA₁c. *See* Fast hemoglobin

HbA₁c. *See* Fast hemoglobin
HbA₁/HbA₁c. *See* Fast hemoglobin
HCO₃. *See* Bicarbonate
HCV. *See* Hepatitis, type C
HDE. *See* Humanitarian Device Exemption
HDL cholesterol. *See* High-density-lipoprotein
     cholesterol
Head
     bony anatomy of, 5:5–10
     parasympathetic ganglia of, 5:60*i*
     vascular anatomy of, 5:10–23
          arterial, 5:11–20
          venous, 5:20–23
Head louse. *See* Lice
Head-shaking nystagmus, 5:200
Head shaking test, 5:200
Head thrust maneuver, 5:200
Head-tilt, chin-lift maneuver, for opening airway, 1:314
Head-tilt test, Bielschowsky, 6:92
     in superior oblique muscle palsy, 6:132, 133*i*
Head trauma, seventh nerve palsy in, 5:285
Headache
     analgesic rebound, 5:296
     cluster, 5:297
     elevated intracranial pressure causing, 5:292
     evaluation of, 5:291–298
     giant cell arteritis with, 5:292
     history of, clinical points in, 5:291*t*
     in hypertensive-arteriosclerotic intracerebral
          hemorrhages, 1:105
     idiopathic intracranial hypertension and, 5:119
     idiopathic stabbing, icepick pains and, 5:297
     intracranial hemorrhage causing, 5:292
     migraine. *See* Migraine headache
     with postganglionic Horner syndrome, 5:264–265
     primary, 5:291
     of ruptured aneurysm, 5:351
     secondary, 5:291
     in subarachnoid hemorrhage, 1:105
     tension-type, 5:296
     treatment of, 5:296–297
     with visual loss, 5:84
          transient, 5:172
Healing, ophthalmic wound. *See* Wound healing/repair
Health counseling, in cancer prevention, 1:295*t*
Hearing loss (deafness)
     albinism and, 6:347*t*
     cataract surgery in patients with, 11:201
     mitochondrial DNA mutations and, 2:218, 220
     in peripheral vestibular nystagmus, 5:246
     and retinal degeneration, 12:235. *See also* Usher
          syndrome
Heart block, 1:134–135
Heart disease, 1:111–142
     congestive failure, 1:125–132
     in diabetes, 1:218
     endocarditis prophylaxis recommendations and, 1:7,
          8–11*t*
     hypertension management and, 1:91*t*, 94
     hypertension and risk of, 1:81, 84, 86*t*
     ischemic, 1:111–125
     in Lyme disease, 1:19
     ophthalmic considerations and, 1:141–142
     recent developments in, 1:111
     rhythm disturbances, 1:132–141

in scleroderma, 1:185
screening for, 1:293–294
in systemic lupus erythematosus, 1:179
transient visual loss and, 5:177
Heart failure. *See* Congestive heart failure
Heart rate, reduction of in angina management, 1:120
Heart transplantation, for heart failure, 1:132
Heat, anterior segment injuries caused by, 8:387
Heavy chain disease, corneal deposits in, 8:349–350
Heavy chains, immunoglobulin, 9:54–55, 56*i*
HEDS (Herpetic Eye Disease Study), 8:140, 148, 149*t*,
     150
Heerfordt syndrome, 8:88
Heidelberg retina tomography, 5:69
Heimlich maneuver, 1:316
Heinz bodies, 1:163
Helicases, 2:213
Helicobacter pylori infection, cancer screening and,
     1:297
Helicoid peripapillary choroidopathy (serpiginous
     choroidopathy/geographic choroiditis), 12:174*t*,
     176–177, 177*i*
Heliotrope rash, in dermatomyositis, 1:186, 187, 188*i*
Helix-loop-helix motif, 2:206, 207*i*
Helix-turn-helix motif, 2:206, 207*i*
Helmholtz hypothesis (capsular theory), of
     accommodation, 13:167–168
Helminths, ocular infection/inflammation caused by,
     8:132–133
     panuveitis, 9:195–197
     posterior uveitis, 9:170–173
Helper T cells, 9:22–24, 23*i*. *See also* T cells
     class II MHC molecules as antigen-presenting
          platform for, 9:19–20, 20*i*
     in delayed hypersensitivity (type IV) reactions, 8:201,
          9:63–66, 65*i*, 68*t*
     differentiation of, 9:22–24, 23*i*
     in external eye, 8:114, 196*t*
     in HIV infection/AIDS, 1:37, 9:242–243
     in immune processing, 9:22–24, 23*i*
HEMA. *See* Hydroxyethylmethacrylate
Hemagglutination antibody test, indirect, for Lyme
     disease, 1:20
Hemagglutination treponemal test for syphilis
     (HATTS), 1:17, 302
Hemangioblastomas
     cerebellar, in retinal angiomatosis, 5:340
     retinal, 4:246–247, 246*i*
          with retinal angiomatosis (von Hippel–Lindau
               disease), 5:336*t*, 340, 342*i*, 6:402*t*, 412–413,
               413*i*
          retinoblastoma differentiated from, 6:394
Hemangiomas (hemangiomatosis), 4:12, 45, 243–249.
     See also Angiomas (angiomatosis)
     of choroid, 4:164, 243–246, 243*i*, 244*i*, 12:170, 171*i*
          in children, 6:390
          in Sturge-Weber disease/syndrome, 4:164, 244
     of conjunctiva, 8:270, 270*t*
     diffuse neonatal, 6:277
     of eyelid, 4:180, 7:158, 8:270, 270*t*
     of orbit, 4:12, 196, 197*i*
          capillary, 4:196, 197*i*, 7:26, 64–66, 66*i*
          cavernous, 4:196, 197*i*, 7:67, 68*i*
          in children, 6:376–378, 377*i*, 378*i*
          in pregnancy, 5:345

transient visual loss and, **5**:175
racemose (Wyburn-Mason syndrome), **4**:248, 249*i*,
    12:163
of retina
    capillary (angiomatosis retinae). *See* Retinal
        angiomatosis
    cavernous, **4**:247, 248*i*, **12**:163–164, 164*i*
    systemic disease associated with, **6**:377
Hemangiopericytoma, of orbit, **4**:196, 198*i*, **6**:380, **7**:67
Hematocrit, in anemia, **1**:160
Hematologic disorders, **1**:159–172. *See also specific type*
    in systemic lupus erythematosus, **1**:180, 181*t*
Hematopoietic growth factors
    in cancer therapy, **1**:261
    for HIV infection/AIDS, **1**:44
Hematopoietic stem cells, **1**:160
Hematoxylin and eosin (H&E) stain, **4**:35, 36*i*, 36*t*
Hemeralopia (day blindness), in cone/cone–rod
    dystrophies, **5**:104, **12**:214
Hemianopia
    homonymous, **5**:83
        arteriovenous malformations causing, **5**:355, 356*i*
        cortical injury causing, **5**:29
        hallucinations and, **5**:190
        occipital lobe lesions causing, **5**:168–169, 168*i*,
            169*i*, 170*i*
        parietal lobe lesions causing, **5**:167
        prisms for, **3**:260
        retrochiasmal lesions causing, **5**:164, 165*i*
        in vertebrobasilar disease, **5**:348
    temporal, chiasmal lesions causing, **5**:158, 160*i*
Hemiatrophy, progressive facial, **8**:353*t*
Hemidesmosomes, **2**:45, 46*i*
Hemifacial microsomia, **6**:431, 432*i*, **8**:352*t*
Hemifacial spasm, **5**:287*t*, 288–289, 288*i*, **7**:227–228
Hemispatial neglect, **5**:196
Hemispheric (hemicentral) retinal vein occlusion,
    12:137, 137*i*
Hemizygote/hemizygous alleles, **2**:187, 243–244, **8**:307
Hemoccult slides. *See* Stool guaiac slide test
Hemochromatosis, **8**:356
Hemoglobin, absorption spectrum for, **12**:313, 314*i*
Hemoglobin A$_{1c}$, diabetes control and, **1**:215, 215*i*,
    216, 219
Hemoglobin AS (sickle cell trait), **12**:120, 120*t*
Hemoglobin C, mutant, **12**:119–120, 120*t*
Hemoglobin C trait (hemoglobin AC), **12**:120, 120*t*
Hemoglobin CC, **12**:120*t*
Hemoglobin electrophoresis, in sickling disorders,
    12:120
Hemoglobin S, **1**:163
    mutant, **12**:119–120, 120*t*
Hemoglobin SC disease, **12**:120, 120*t*
Hemoglobin spherules, **4**:108, 109*i*
Hemoglobin SS, **12**:120, 120*t*
Hemoglobinopathies, sickle cell. *See* Sickle cell disease;
    Sickle cell retinopathy
Hemoglobinuria, paroxysmal nocturnal, **1**:162
    hypercoagulability and, **1**:171
    screening test for, **1**:159, 162
Hemolytic anemia, **1**:162–163
    autoimmune, **1**:163
Hemolytic glaucoma, **4**:82, **10**:112–113
Hemophilia A (classic hemophilia/factor VIII
    deficiency), **1**:168

Hemophthalmos, **12**:286
Hemorrhages. *See also* Hyphema
    cataract surgery and, **11**:164*t*, 168–171
        at-risk patients and, **11**:215–217
        flat anterior chamber and, **11**:163
        patient receiving anticoagulation therapy and,
            11:168–169, 201–202
    choroidal, expulsive, **4**:25, 26*i*
    coagulation disorders and, **1**:166
    conjunctival, **8**:396
        in hereditary hemorrhagic telangiectasia, **8**:91
    flame
        in central retinal vein occlusion, **12**:141, 142*i*
        ischemia causing, **4**:131–133, 132*i*
        in leukemia, **6**:344
    glaucoma associated with, **4**:81–84, 82*i*, 83*i*,
        10:53–54, 54*i*
    in hemophilia, **1**:168
    hemostatic derangement and, **1**:166
    intracranial, **1**:105–106
        headache caused by, **5**:292
        hypertensive-arteriosclerotic, **1**:105, 106
        ruptured aneurysm causing, **1**:105, 106, **5**:351
        in shaking injury, **6**:433
        Terson syndrome caused by, **12**:95
    intraparenchymal, MRI/CT appearance of, **5**:77*t*
    iron deficiency anemia and, **1**:161
    MR imaging of, **5**:63*t*
    ocular, with subarachnoid hemorrhage, **5**:351
    orbital, **7**:72, 106
        after blepharoplasty, visual loss and, **7**:232–233
        from orbital lymphangioma, **7**:67–68
    platelet disorders and, **1**:166, 166–168
    retinal
        in arterial macroaneurysms, **12**:158, 159
        in branch retinal vein occlusion, **12**:136
        in central retinal vein occlusion, **12**:141, 142*i*
        dot-and-blot, **5**:183, 184*i*
        in HIV infection/AIDS, **9**:248
        ischemia causing, **4**:131, 132*i*
        in leukemia, **4**:281, **6**:344
        in nonproliferative diabetic retinopathy, **12**:103,
            104*i*
        in ocular ischemic syndrome, **12**:151, 151*i*
        in shaking injury, **6**:433, 433*i*, 444, **12**:301, 302*i*
    retrobulbar
        after blepharoplasty, visual loss and, **7**:232–233
        cataract surgery and, **11**:169
    salmon patch
        in sickle cell disease, **12**:121, 122*i*
        syphilitic keratitis and, **6**:260, **8**:227, 299
    splinter, in glaucoma, **10**:53–54, 54*i*
    subarachnoid, **1**:105, 106, **5**:353
        with ocular hemorrhage, **5**:351
    subconjunctival, **8**:90, 91*t*, 396
    submacular, **12**:326–327, 328*i*
    suprachoroidal, **12**:332–334, 333*i*
        cataract surgery and, **11**:164*t*, 169–170
            delayed, **11**:171
            expulsive, **11**:170–171
            patients at risk for, **11**:215–217
            flat anterior chamber and, **11**:163, 166
    vascular disorders and, **1**:166
    vitreous, **4**:108, 109*i*
        blunt trauma causing, **12**:291, 292*i*

in branch retinal vein occlusion, 12:138
  photocoagulation for, 12:140
in diabetic retinopathy, 12:111–112, 116–117
in pars planitis, 12:182
in posterior vitreous detachment, 12:257–258
retinal cavernous hemangioma causing, 12:164
in shaking injury, 6:443
spontaneous, 12:287
vitrectomy for, in diabetic patients, 12:111–112,
  116–117
Hemorrhagic conjunctivitis, acute, 8:163
Hemorrhagic disease of newborn, 1:169
Hemorrhagic fever, Ebola, 1:35
Hemorrhagic telangiectasia, hereditary (Osler-Weber-
  Rendu disease), 1:166, 8:91
Hemosiderin, in glaucoma, 4:81–82
Hemostasis, 1:164–165, 164i
  disorders of, 1:163–172
    cataract surgery in patients with, 11:201–202
    clinical manifestations of, 1:166
    coagulation disorders and, 1:168–172
    hemorrhage and, 1:166
    hypercoagulable states and, 1:170–172
    platelet disorders and, 1:166–168
    vascular disorders and, 1:166
  laboratory evaluation of, 1:165
Henderson-Patterson bodies, 8:121
Henle fiber layer, 2:84, 85, 4:119
Henle pseudoglands, 4:45
Henley's layer, 5:24
Henoch-Schönlein purpura, 1:189t
HEP. See Hepatoerythropoietic porphyria
Hepacare. See Hepatitis B vaccine
Heparan sulfate
  in microbial adherence, 8:116
  in mucopolysaccharidoses, 8:335–336
  retinal dystrophy and, 12:243
Heparin, as inflammatory mediator, 8:200t
Heparin surface modification, intraocular lens, 9:138
Heparin therapy, 1:171
  for antiphospholipid antibody syndrome, 1:184
  cataract surgery and, 11:202
  for deep venous thrombosis prophylaxis in stroke
    patients, 1:101, 104
  for non-ST-segment elevation acute coronary
    syndrome, 1:123
  in perioperative setting, 1:332
Hepatic disease. See Hepatitis; Liver disease
Hepatitis, 1:31–32
  delta, 1:31–32
  HIV coinfection and, 1:50
  transfusion-transmitted virus causing, 1:32
  type A, 1:31
    immunization against, 1:31, 291, 305
      travel and, 1:309–310
  type B, 1:303–305
    cancer and, 1:254
    immunization against, 1:291, 303–305, 304t
      travel and, 1:309
  type C, 1:31–32
  type E, 1:32
Hepatitis A vaccine, 1:31, 291, 305
  travel and, 1:309–310
Hepatitis B immune globulin, 1:305

Hepatitis B vaccine, 1:291, 303–305, 304t
  in combination vaccines, 1:305, 309
  travel and, 1:309
Hepatitis D virus, 1:31–32
Hepatitis E virus, 1:32
Hepatitis G virus, 1:32
Hepatocellular carcinoma, 1:297
  viral carcinogenesis and, 1:254
Hepatoerythropoietic porphyria (HEP), 8:355
Hepatolenticular degeneration (Wilson disease), 6:260,
  8:355–356, 356i, 11:62
  cataracts associated with, 6:288t
  penicillamine for, 2:281, 8:356
HepB. See Hepatitis B vaccine
Herbert's pits, 8:175, 176i
Hereditary, definition of, 2:187, 239. See also Genetics
Hereditary dystrophies, 12:203–229. See also specific
  type
  choroidal, 12:224–227
  diagnostic/prognostic testing in, 12:204–205, 206t
  diffuse photoreceptor, 12:205–215
  endothelial, congenital, 6:256t, 257
  inner retinal, 12:228–229
  macular, 12:215–224
    in children, 6:337–340
  stromal, congenital, 6:256t, 257
  vitreoretinal, 6:340–342, 12:228–229
Hereditary factors. See Genetic/hereditary factors
Hereditary hemorrhagic telangiectasia (Osler-Weber-
  Rendu disease), 1:166, 8:91
Hereditary hyaloideoretinopathies with optically empty
  vitreous, 12:283–284, 284i
Hereditary optic neuropathy, Leber, 5:134–136, 135i,
  6:364–365
  mitochondrial DNA mutations and, 2:218–220, 219i,
    5:134–135, 6:365
Hereditary progressive arthro-ophthalmopathy. See
  Stickler syndrome
Hereditary sensory and autonomic neuropathy, type 3.
  See Familial dysautonomia
Hereditary spherocytosis, 1:162
Hering's law of motor correspondence, 6:36–37, 37i
  eyelid retraction and, 7:224
Heritable, definition of, 2:187
Hermansky-Pudlak syndrome, 4:120, 6:346t, 348,
  12:240
  racial and ethnic concentration of, 2:260
Heroin abuse, 1:269
Herpes simplex virus, 1:27–28, 8:139–151, 152t
  acute retinal necrosis caused by, 4:123, 124i, 9:140,
    154–156, 155i, 156i, 12:185–186, 185i
  acyclovir for infection caused by, 1:28, 76, 2:441
  antiviral agents for, 2:440–444, 8:141, 142t
  blepharoconjunctivitis caused by, 8:140–141, 141i,
    143
  cancer association and, 1:254
  congenital infection caused by, 6:219–220, 223
  conjunctivitis caused by
    in children, 6:226, 227i
    in neonates, 6:219–220, 223
  disciform keratitis caused by, 8:147, 147i
  famciclovir for infection caused by, 1:28, 77
  in HIV infection/AIDS, 5:359–360, 361i, 9:260
  iridocyclitis caused by, 8:150

keratitis caused by, **4:**65–66, 66*i*, **8:**51*t*, 143–150
  Acanthamoeba keratitis differentiated from,
    8:188–189
  epithelial, **8:**143–146, 143*i*, 144*i*, 145*i*
  interstitial, **8:**146–147, 146*i*
  neurotrophic keratopathy/ulcers and, **8:**103, 103*i*,
    151
  in newborn, **6:**219
  stromal, **8:**146–150, 146*i*, 147*i*, 148*i*, 149*t*
    penetrating keratoplasty for, **8:**151
  topical antiviral agents for, **2:**439, 440*t*
necrotizing keratitis caused by, **8:**147–148, 148*i*, 150
ocular infection/inflammation caused by, **8:**139–151,
    152*t*
  adenovirus infection differentiated from, **8:**140,
    158–159
  complications of, **8:**151
  evasion and, **8:**116
  in infants and children, **6:**219–220, 223
  iridocorneal endothelial syndrome and, **8:**300–301
  pathogenesis of, **8:**139–140, 142, 146
  primary infection, **8:**140–141, 141*i*
  recurrent infection, **8:**142–150
  treatment of, **8:**141, 142*t*, 145–146, 148–150, 149*t*
  varicella-zoster virus infection differentiated from,
    8:152, 152*t*
perinatal infection caused by, **1:**28, **6:**219–220
retinitis caused by (acute retinal necrosis), **4:**123,
    124*i*, **9:**140, 154–156, 155*i*, 156*i*, **12:**185–186,
    185*i*
skin infection after laser resurfacing caused by, **7:**238
type 1, **1:**27, **6:**219, 226, **8:**139
type 2, **1:**27, **6:**219, 226, **8:**139
uveitis caused by, **9:**138–140
valacyclovir for infection caused by, **1:**28, 77
Herpes zoster, **1:**28–29, **8:**151, 153–156. *See also*
  Varicella-zoster virus
acute retinal necrosis caused by, **4:**123, 124*i*, **9:**140,
    154–156, 155*i*, 156*i*, **12:**185–186, 185*i*
acyclovir for, **1:**28, 76–77
conjunctivitis and, **6:**226–227, 228*i*
cranial nerve VII involvement and, **5:**284
in elderly, **1:**248–249
famciclovir for, **1:**28, 77, **2:**442
in HIV infection/AIDS, **5:**359–360, 361*i*, **9:**260
ophthalmic manifestations in, **5:**300–301, 300*i*,
    8:153–156, 153*i*, 154*i*, 155*i*
retinitis caused by (acute retinal necrosis), **4:**123,
    124*i*, **9:**140, 154–156, 155*i*, 156*i*, **12:**185–186,
    185*i*
uveitis and, **9:**138–140, 139*i*
valacyclovir for, **1:**28, 77, **2:**442
without vesicles (zoster sine herpete), **5:**300
Herpes zoster ophthalmicus, **5:**300–301, 300*i*,
  8:153–156, 153*i*, 154*i*, 155*i*
acyclovir for, **1:**76
in elderly, **1:**248–249
neurotrophic keratopathy in, **8:**102–103, 153, 154
Herpesviruses, **1:**27–30, **8:**120. *See also specific type*
cancer association and, **1:**254
ocular infection caused by, **8:**120, 139–157
  glaucoma and, **9:**139
  refractive surgery in patient with, **13:**185–186
  uveitis, **9:**138–140, 139*i*

Herpetic Eye Disease Study (HEDS), **8:**140, 148, 149*t*,
  150
Herpex. *See* Idoxuridine
Hertel exophthalmometer, **7:**25
Hess screen test, **6:**86
Heterochromatin, **2:**204
Heterochromia iridis, **6:**267, 267*i*, 267*t*
  in leukemia, **6:**344
  in siderosis bulbi, **11:**59*i*
Heterocyclic antidepressants, **1:**275*t*
Heterogeneity, **2:**190
  allelic, **2:**182, 241, 347
  clinical, **2:**184, 241
  genetic, **2:**187, 240–241, 347
  locus, **2:**190, 240–241
Heteronuclear (heterogeneous nuclear) RNA (hnRNA),
  2:187, 209
Heteronymous diplopia, **6:**59*i*, 60
Heterophoria method, for accommodative
  convergence/accommodation ratio measurement,
  3:149, **6:**88
Heterophorias/phorias, **6:**9, 10
  cover tests in assessment of, **6:**80–82, 81*i*
  prismatic effects of bifocal lenses and, **3:**157, 157*i*,
    158*i*
    decentration and, **3:**164
  prisms for, **3:**169–170
Heteroplasmy, **2:**187
Heterotropia, **6:**9
  alternating, **6:**81
  simultaneous prism-cover test in assessment of, **6:**82
Heterozygosity, loss of, **2:**215
Heterozygote/heterozygous alleles, **2:**187, 242, **8:**307.
  See also Carrier (genetic)
  compound, **2:**184, 261
  double, **2:**243
Hexagonal cells, specular photomicroscopy in
  evaluation of percentage of, **8:**37
Hexagonal keratotomy, **13:**66
Hexokinase, in lens carbohydrate metabolism, **2:**330,
  11:14, 15*i*
Hexosaminidase, deficiency of, in gangliosidoses,
  6:350–351, 437*t*
Hexose monophosphate shunt
  in corneal glucose metabolism, **2:**297–299, 298*i*
  in lens glucose/carbohydrate metabolism, **2:**330,
    11:14, 15*i*
Hib. *See Haemophilus/Haemophilus influenzae,* type b
Hib (*Haemophilus influenzae* type B) vaccine, **1:**12,
  291, 304*t*, 308–309
  in combination vaccines, **1:**309
Hib-DTaP vaccine, **1:**309
Hidradenoma, clear cell (eccrine acrospiroma), **7:**167
Hidrocystoma
  apocrine, **7:**167–168, 169*i*
  eccrine, **7:**167
High accommodative convergence/accommodative
  esotropia, **6:**98*t*, 102–104
High-density-lipoprotein cholesterol, **1:**144, 144*t*. *See
  also* Cholesterol
  beta-blockers affecting, **1:**150
  low levels of, **1:**144*t*, 150
  risk assessment and, **1:**144, 144*t*
  screening, **1:**293

High hyperopia
  cataract surgery in patients with, **11**:222
    clear lens extraction and, **11**:138, 222
  correction of, intraocular lenses for, **11**:147–148
High-index glass lenses, **3**:168
High (pathologic/degenerative) myopia, **3**:121,
  12:71–72*t*, 84–86, 85*i*
  ametropia and, **6**:70
  cataract surgery in patients with, **11**:222
    clear lens extraction and, **11**:138, 222
  correction of
    bioptics for, **13**:143, 155–156, 157*t*
    clear lens extraction/refractive lens exchange for,
      13:158, 159
    intraocular lenses for, **11**:147–148
    LASIK for, **13**:117
    phakic IOLs for, **13**:144–146
    retinal detachment and, **13**:191–192, 203
  esotropia and, **6**:155
  in infants, **3**:146
High-output failure, causes of, **1**:128
High-pass resolution perimetry, **10**:58
High-plus-power lenses, for slit-lamp delivery of
  photocoagulation, **12**:317
High-positioning contact lenses, **3**:194–195
High-speed rotary devices, for coronary
  revascularization, **1**:122
Higher-order aberrations, **3**:93, 101–102, 103*i*,
  238–241, **13**:15–17, 17*i*, 18*i*, 19*i*. *See also specific*
  type and Irregular astigmatism
Highly active antiretroviral therapy (HAART), **1**:43–44,
  9:246
  CMV retinitis and, **1**:3, 48, **9**:253, **12**:193
  immune reconstitution syndromes and, **1**:51
Hirschberg test, **6**:82, 84*i*
His bundle, **1**:133, 134
Histamine, **8**:198*t*, 199*i*, 200*t*, **9**:77
Histiocytes, **4**:13
  cytologic identification of, **8**:68
  epithelioid, **4**:13, 14*i*
Histiocytic (large) cell lymphoma. *See* Lymphomas,
  intraocular
Histiocytic disorders, of orbit, **7**:88
Histiocytoma, fibrous (fibroxanthoma), **8**:271
  orbital, **4**:199, 199*i*, **7**:81
  scleral, **4**:92
Histiocytosis, Langerhans cell (histiocytosis X/diffuse
  soft tissue histiocytosis), orbital involvement in,
  7:88
  in children, **6**:375–376, 376*i*
Histo spots, **9**:160, 160*i*, 161, **12**:79
Histocompatibility antigens, **8**:447. *See also* Human
  leukocyte (HLA) antigens
Histocryl. *See* Cyanoacrylate adhesives
Histogram, **1**:368, 369*i*
Histones, **2**:204
Histoplasma capsulatum (histoplasmosis), ocular,
  9:160–163, 160*i*, 161*i*, 162*i*, 177*t*, **12**:79–82, 80*i*
  histo spots in, **9**:160, 160*i*, 161
  HLA association in, **9**:94*t*, 160
  management of, **12**:72*t*, 80–82
Historical/calculation method, for IOL power
  calculation after refractive surgery, **11**:151–152,
  13:200–201, 201*t*

History
  in amblyopia, **6**:77–78
  in cataract, **11**:75–77, 77*t*
    evaluation for surgery and, **11**:79–80
  in child abuse, **6**:442
  family. *See also* Genetic/hereditary factors; Genetics,
    clinical
    congenital anomalies and, **8**:282–283
    in genetic counseling, **2**:276–277
    in human carcinogenesis, **1**:254–255
    in nystagmus, **6**:160–161, 161*t*
    pedigree analysis and, **2**:275–276, 275*i*, **8**:308
    in primary angle closure, **10**:123–124
    in primary open-angle glaucoma, **10**:10, 87
    in uveitis, **9**:122
  in infant with decreased vision, **6**:452
  keratorefractive surgery and, **13**:40–41
  in nystagmus, **6**:160–161, 161*t*
  in pediatric cataract, **6**:294
  in penetrating/perforating injury, **8**:407–408, 408*t*
  preoperative assessment and, **1**:327, 328*t*
  in strabismus, **6**:77–78
  in uveitis, **9**:122–126
HIV (human immunodeficiency virus), **1**:36–37, **8**:122,
  9:241–242. *See also* HIV infection/AIDS
  drug resistance and, **1**:41, 43, 44
  superinfection and, **1**:40
  testing for antibody to, **1**:39, **9**:245–246
  vaccine development and, **1**:44–45
  viability of after excimer laser ablation, **13**:196–197
HIV-1, **1**:36–37, **9**:242. *See also* HIV infection/AIDS
  superinfection and, **1**:40
HIV-1 delta 4 vaccine, **1**:44
HIV-2, **1**:37, **9**:242. *See also* HIV infection/AIDS
HIV infection/AIDS, **1**:36–53, **5**:360–361, **8**:122,
  9:241–262
  atypical mycobacterial infections and, **1**:23, 49–50
  CDC definition of, **1**:37, 40*t*, **9**:243, 244–245*t*
  choroiditis in
    Cryptococcus neoformans, **9**:257
    multifocal, **9**:257–258
    Pneumocystis carinii (Pneumocystis jiroveci),
      9:256–257, 256*i*, 257*i*
  classification of, **1**:40*t*, **9**:243–245, 244–245*t*
  clinical syndrome of, **1**:37–39, 40*t*
  cytomegalovirus infection in, **1**:29, 47–48, **5**:359,
    360*i*
    retinitis, **4**:123, 124*i*, **9**:71, 156, 249, 251*i*,
      12:192–193, 192*i*
    in children, **6**:219
  diagnosis of, **1**:39, **9**:245–246
    ophthalmologist's role in, **9**:261
  encephalopathy in, **1**:37, **5**:361
  etiology of, **1**:36–37
  herpes zoster ophthalmicus in, **8**:154
  herpesvirus infection in, **5**:359–360, 361*i*, **9**:260,
    260*i*, **12**:185, 186
  immunization against, development of vaccine for,
    1:44–45
  incidence of, **1**:36, **9**:241
  influenza vaccine in patients with, **1**:305
  intraocular tuberculosis in, **12**:184
  Kaposi sarcoma in, **7**:183, 183*i*, **8**:272, 272*i*,
    9:258–259, 258*i*, 259*i*
  lymphoma in, **1**:50–51, **5**:359

malignancies associated with, 1:50–51
management of, 1:40–45, 2:244, 9:246–248, 247t
 chemoprophylaxis and, 1:45, 46–47t
 drug resistance and, 1:41, 43, 44
 HAART in, 1:43–44, 9:246
  CMV retinitis and, 9:253, 12:193
  immune reconstitution syndromes and, 1:51
 ophthalmologist's role in, 9:261
 recent developments in, 1:3, 42, 44
microsporidiosis in, 1:48, 49, 8:190, 9:260, 260i
molluscum contagiosum in, 8:161, 161i, 9:259
natural history of, 9:243–245, 244–245t
nephropathy associated with, 1:37–38
neuro-ophthalmic signs of, 5:359–362
occupational exposure to, 1:39
 precautions in health care setting and, 1:51–52,
  9:261–262
 prophylaxis for, 1:45, 46–47t
ocular infection/manifestations and, 1:51–52, 8:122,
 9:241–262
 external eye manifestations, 9:258–260
 ophthalmic complications, 9:248–249
opportunistic infections associated with, 1:45–51,
 9:248, 260, 260i
pathogenesis of, 1:36–37, 9:242–243
Pneumocystis carinii (Pneumocystis jiroveci) infections
 and, 1:45–47, 9:256–257, 256i, 257i
primary (retroviral syndrome), 1:38
prognosis of, 1:40–45
progressive multifocal leukoencephalopathy in,
 5:362, 363i
progressive outer retinal necrosis in, 9:155, 253–254,
 254i
refractive surgery in patients with, 13:196–197
retinitis in, 9:71, 140, 154–156, 155i, 156i, 248–253,
 251i, 260, 12:185, 186
retinopathy associated with, 9:248, 249i
seroepidemiology of, 1:39
seventh nerve palsy in, 5:284
spore-forming intestinal protozoa and, 1:48–49
superinfection and, 1:40
syphilis/syphilitic chorioretinitis in, 1:18, 5:361–362,
 9:189, 255–256
systemic conditions associated with, 9:246
Toxoplasma retinochoroiditis/toxoplasmosis in,
 5:362, 9:165–166, 165i, 166i, 254–255, 255i,
 12:187
transmission of, 1:39–40, 9:245
transplacental transmission of, chemoprophylaxis
 for, 1:45
tuberculosis and, 1:24, 49–50, 301, 302, 5:361, 9:193
virology of, 9:242
HIV p24 antigen testing, 1:39
HIV RNA
 as predictor of response to therapy, 1:40, 43
 testing for, 1:39
HIV vaccine, development of, 1:44–45
Hivid. See Zalcitabine
HLA. See Human leukocyte (HLA) antigens
HLH. See Helix-loop-helix motif
HMB-45, in immunohistochemistry, 4:37
HMG-CoA (3-hydroxy-3-methyl glutaryl coenzyme-A)
 reductase inhibitors. See also Statins
 cataracts and, 1:151, 11:54
 for hypercholesterolemia, 1:149t

HMP shunt. See Hexose monophosphate shunt
HMR 3467. See Telithromycin
HMS (hydroxymethyl progesterone). See Medrysone
hnRNA. See Heteronuclear (heterogeneous nuclear)
 RNA
Hodgkin disease
 in HIV infection/AIDS, 1:50–51
 in orbit, 4:194
Hoffer Q formula, for IOL power selection, 13:202
 clear lens extraction/refractive lens exchange and,
  13:160
Holandric inheritance/trait, 2:188, 266
Holes
 macular, 4:112–114, 12:253
  idiopathic, 12:89–93, 92i, 325–326, 327i
   vitrectomy for, 12:93, 325–326, 327i
  impending, 12:89
  posttraumatic, 12:292, 294i
  treatment of, 12:93, 266, 325–326, 327i
  vitreous in formation of, 2:339
 optic (optic pits), 2:127, 136, 175, 4:204, 5:140
  in children, 6:363, 363i
 retinal
  atrophic, 12:253
   treatment of, 12:265, 266, 266t, 267t
  operculated, 12:253, 254, 255i
   treatment of, 12:265, 265–266, 266t, 267t
Holladay II formula, for IOL power determination,
 11:149, 13:202
 clear lens extraction/refractive lens exchange and,
  13:160
Hollenhorst plaques (cholesterol emboli)
 in branch retinal artery occlusion, 4:133, 12:146,
  147i
 in central retinal artery occlusion, 12:149
 transient visual loss and, 5:173, 173i
Holmium:YAG (Ho:YAG) laser, for thermokeratoplasty,
 13:27, 29, 50t, 138
 risks/benefits of, 13:50t, 138
Holmium-YLF solid-state laser, 3:22. See also Lasers
Holoprosencephaly, 2:126
Homatropine, 2:310, 401t
 for amblyopia, 6:73
 for cycloplegia/cycloplegic refraction, 3:142t, 6:94,
  94t
Home environment, manipulating, in reducing visual
 handicap, 3:263i
Homeobox, 2:126, 130. See also Homeobox genes
Homeobox genes/homeotic selector genes, 2:130–131,
 181, 188
 congenital anomalies associated with mutations in,
  2:159
  microphthalmos, 8:287
 growth factors affecting expression of, 2:130, 131
 in ocular development, 2:130–131
 in retinal dystrophies, 12:204
Homeodomain, 2:130–131
Homeotic genes/homeotic selector genes. See
 Homeobox genes
Homer-Wright rosettes, in retinoblastoma, 4:143, 143i,
 6:394
Homing, 9:27–28
 MALT and, 9:36
Homocysteine
 carotid artery disease and, 1:109

hypercoagulability and, 1:171
Homocystinuria, 2:262*t*, 6:307, 307*i*, 437*t*, 11:41–42
ectopia lentis in, 4:94, 95*t*
retinal degeneration and, 12:232*t*
treatment of, 6:438
vitamin B₆ replacement therapy for, 2:281
Homogentisic acid/homogentisic acid oxidase,
alkaptonuria and, 2:261–263, 8:345
Homologous antigens, 8:447. *See also* Human
leukocyte (HLA) antigens
Homologous chromosomes, 2:188
Homonymous diplopia, 6:58–60, 59*i*
Homonymous hemianopia, 5:83
arteriovenous malformations causing, 5:355, 356*i*
cortical injury causing, 5:29
hallucinations and, 5:190
occipital lobe lesions causing, 5:168–169, 168*i*, 169*i*,
170*i*
parietal lobe lesions causing, 5:167
partial prism for, 3:260
retrochiasmal lesions causing, 5:164, 165*i*
in vertebrobasilar disease, 5:348
Homonymous nerve fiber layer, 5:164
Homoplasmy, 2:188
Homoplastic corneal inlays, for keratophakia, 13:71–72
Homozygote/homozygous alleles, 2:188, 242, 261,
8:307
Honan balloon, 11:217
Hordeolum, 8:168
external (stye), 4:170, 7:160, 8:168
internal, 7:158–159, 160, 8:168. *See also* Chalazion
Horizontal cells, 2:80, 83*i*, 352, 352*i*, 5:24
in cone phototransduction, 2:345
Horizontal deviations
A-pattern and V-pattern, 6:119–125. *See also* A-
pattern deviations; V-pattern deviations
in craniosynostosis, 6:429
dissociated, 6:116, 116*i*, 131
in internuclear ophthalmoplegia, 6:155
strabismus surgery planning and, 6:177
Horizontal eyelid shortening/tightening
for cicatricial ectropion, 7:200–201
for involutional ectropion, 7:198
for involutional entropion, 7:204
Horizontal gaze, 5:34, 37*i*, 38*i*, 39
Horizontal gaze palsy, 5:208, 209*i*
congenital, 5:208
Horizontal heterophoria/phoria
prismatic effects of bifocal lenses and, 3:157, 157*i*,
158*i*
prisms for, 3:169
Horizontal incomitance, strabismus surgery planning
and, 6:177
Horizontal rectus muscles, 6:13–14, 13*i*, 17*t*, 18*i*
A-pattern deviations associated with dysfunction of,
6:119
action of, 6:13–14, 17*t*, 28, 30, 31*i*
anatomy of, 6:13–14, 14*i*, 17*t*, 18*i*
surgery of
for A- and V-pattern deviations, 6:123–124, 123*i*,
182
for nystagmus, 6:168–171, 170*i*, 170*t*
V-pattern deviations associated with dysfunction of,
6:119
Horizontal strabismus. *See* Horizontal deviations

Hormonal action, of cytokines, 9:80
Hormone replacement therapy. *See also* Estrogen/
estrogen replacement therapy
breast cancer risk and, 1:295
Hormones
in cancer chemotherapy, 1:260*t*
for metastatic eye disease, 4:273–275
headaches caused by, 5:296
ocular effects of, 1:325*t*
osteoporosis and, 1:241, 245*t*, 246
pituitary adenoma producing, 1:228–229
Horner syndrome, 5:262–265, 263*i*, 264*i*, 300
congenital, 5:264, 7:217
eyelid fissure changes in, 2:23*i*
internal carotid artery dissection causing, 5:263–264,
264*i*
localization of lesions causing, 5:263, 263*i*
Müller's muscle actuation and, 2:26
in neuroblastoma, 6:374, 374*i*, 7:94, 94*i*
neuronal lesions causing, 5:263–264, 263*i*, 264*i*
pharmacologic testing for, 5:262–263, 7:212–213,
212*i*
postganglionic, 5:264–265
isolated, 5:264
preganglionic, 5:263
underlying disorders causing, 5:265
Horner-Trantas dots, 4:46, 8:209–210
in vernal keratoconjunctivitis, 6:235
Horner's muscle, 2:24, 7:255, 256*i*
Horner's tensor tarsi, 7:140
Horopter, empirical, 6:42, 42*i*, 43
Horror autotoxicus, 9:87
Horror fusionis (central fusional disruption), 6:53, 115
Horseshoe tears (flap tears), 12:253, 254, 255*i*
treatment of, 12:265, 266, 266*t*, 267*t*
Hospital-acquired infections, treatment of, 1:77–78
Host cell, 2:188
Host defenses
impaired, 8:117–118. *See also* Immunocompromised
host
of outer eye, 8:113–114
Host susceptibility, in carcinogenesis, 1:254
HOTV test, in children, 6:78*t*, 79
Hounsfield unit, definition of, 5:79
Houseplants, ocular injuries caused by, 8:395–396
HOX genes, 2:130, 131, 181, 188
HOX7.1 gene, 2:131
HOX8.1 gene, 2:131
HOX10 gene, in microphthalmos, 8:287
HPMC. *See* Hydroxypropyl methylcellulose
HPMPC. *See* Cidofovir
HPV. *See* Human papillomaviruses
Hruby lens, 3:285, 286*i*, 12:17–18
HSV. *See* Herpes simplex virus
HTH. *See* Helix-turn-helix motif
HTLV-I. *See* Human T-cell lymphotropic retrovirus
type I
HTLV-II. *See* Human T-cell lymphotropic retrovirus
type II
HTLV-III. *See* Human T-cell lymphotropic virus type
III
Hudson-Stähli line, 4:74, 8:377*t*, 378
Hughes procedure/modified Hughes procedure, in
eyelid repair, 7:191*i*, 192
Humalog. *See* Lispro insulin

Human artificial chromosomes (HACs), for glaucoma, **10**:177
Human bites, eyelid injuries caused by, **7**:187
Human gene mapping. *See* Genetic map
Human Genome Project, **2**:226, **8**:306
Human granulocytic ehrlichiosis, **1**:19
Human herpes virus 8, Kaposi sarcoma caused by, **8**:162, 272
Human immunodeficiency virus (HIV), **1**:36–37, **8**:122, **9**:241–242. *See also* HIV infection/AIDS
  drug resistance and, **1**:41, 43, 44
  superinfection and, **1**:40
  testing for antibody to, **1**:39, **9**:245–246
  vaccine development and, **1**:44–45
  viability of after excimer laser ablation, **13**:196–197
Human leukocyte (HLA) antigens, **8**:447, 449, **9**:90–95, 92*t*. *See also* Major histocompatibility complex
  allelic variations and, **9**:91
  in ankylosing spondylitis, **1**:175, 176, **9**:93, 129
  in anterior uveitis, **1**:175, 176, 178, **6**:314, **9**:93, 94*t*, 129–132
  in Behçet syndrome, **1**:193, **9**:94*t*, 134, **12**:181
  in birdshot retinochoroidopathy, **9**:94*t*, 180–181, **12**:178
  detection and classification of, **9**:91
  in diabetes mellitus, **1**:203–205
  disease associations of, **9**:94–95, 94*t*
  in enteropathic arthritis, **1**:177
  in glaucomatocyclitic crisis (Posner-Schlossman syndrome), **9**:135
  in inflammatory bowel disease, **9**:131–132
  in intermediate uveitis/pars planitis, **9**:94*t*, 147
  in juvenile idiopathic (chronic/rheumatoid) arthritis, **6**:314, **9**:94*t*, 141
  in multiple sclerosis, **5**:317, **9**:94*t*
  normal function of, **9**:90–91
  in ocular histoplasmosis syndrome, **9**:94*t*, 160–161
  in psoriatic arthritis, **1**:178
  in reactive arthritis/Reiter syndrome, **1**:176, **9**:94*t*, 130–131
  in retinal vasculitis, **9**:94*t*
  in rheumatoid arthritis, **1**:174
  in sarcoidosis, **9**:94*t*
  in Sjögren syndrome, **8**:78
  in spondyloarthropathies, **1**:175, 178
  in sympathetic ophthalmia, **9**:94*t*
  in systemic lupus erythematosus, **1**:179
  transplantation and, **9**:93–94
  in Vogt-Koyanagi-Harada syndrome, **4**:153–154, **9**:94*t*, 205, **12**:181
Human papillomaviruses, **1**:33, **4**:51
  cancer association of, **1**:33, 254, 291, 294
  conjunctival intraepithelial neoplasia caused by, **8**:257
  eyelid infections caused by, **4**:170–171
  ocular infection/papillomas caused by, **8**:121, 162, 255
Human T-cell lymphotropic retrovirus type I (HTLV-I), **1**:37
Human T-cell lymphotropic retrovirus type II (HTLV-II), **1**:37
Human T-cell lymphotropic virus type III (HTLV-III), **1**:37. *See also* Human immunodeficiency virus
Humanitarian Device Exemption, **13**:35–36
Humira. *See* Adalimumab

Humoral immunity, **1**:4. *See also* Antibody-mediated immune effector responses
Humorsol. *See* Demecarium
Humphrey Field Analyzer (HFA), **10**:65
Humphrey Field Analyzer (HFA) II (700 series), **10**:70, 71*i*
Humphrey STATPAC 2 program, **10**:69, 69*i*
Hunter syndrome, **2**:262*t*, 281, **6**:436*t*, **8**:335–336, 337*t*, **12**:233*t*, 243
Hurler-Scheie syndrome, **8**:335–336
Hurler syndrome, **2**:262*t*, 281, **6**:436*t*, **8**:309*t*, 335–336, 337*t*, **12**:232*t*, 243
  congenital/infantile corneal opacities and, **6**:255, 256*i*, 436*t*, **8**:298
Hurricane (vortex) keratopathy, **8**:394
Hutchinson melanotic freckle (lentigo maligna/precancerous melanosis), **7**:174
Hutchinson sign, **9**:138
Hutchinson triad, **6**:220
Hyaline bodies. *See* Optic disc (optic nerve head), drusen of
Hyaline deposits, corneal, in Avellino dystrophy, **4**:72–73
Hyaline (hard) drusen, **4**:138, 138*i*
Hyalocytes, **2**:89, 147, **4**:106
Hyaloid artery/system
  development of, **2**:138, 142*i*, 155–156
  persistence/remnants of, **2**:147, 156, 156*i*, 175, 176*i*, 177*i*, **4**:107, **6**:361, **12**:280, 281. *See also* Persistent fetal vasculature
  tunica vasculosa lentis development and, **11**:29
Hyaloid corpuscle (Mittendorf dot), **2**:91, 92*i*, 175, 177*i*, **4**:107, **6**:361, **11**:29–30, 31, **12**:280
Hyaloid face, of vitreous, **4**:105
Hyaloideocapsular ligament, **4**:105
Hyaloideoretinopathies, hereditary, with optically empty vitreous, **12**:283–284, 284*i*
Hyalosis, asteroid, **4**:110, 110*i*, **12**:285–286, 286*i*
Hyaluronan/hyaluronic acid, in vitreous, **2**:147, 335–336, 336*i*, **12**:279
Hyaluronate/sodium hyaluronate, **2**:452
  as viscoelastic, **11**:144–145, 159, 160, 161*t*
Hyaluronidase
  in aqueous humor, **2**:319
  in ocular infections, **8**:124
  streptococcal production of, **8**:124
  in vitreous, **2**:333
Hybridization, **2**:188
  fluorescence in situ, **2**:247–249, 248*i*, 249*i*
Hybridomas, **1**:261
  monoclonal antibody and, **9**:56
Hydatid cyst, orbital infection caused by rupture of, **7**:47
Hydralazine
  for heart failure, **1**:130
  for hypertension, **1**:89*t*, 94
Hydraulic support (catenary) theory, of accommodation, **13**:171
Hydrocephalus, otitic, **5**:358
Hydrochlorothiazide, **1**:88*t*, 90*t*
Hydrocortisone
  for anaphylaxis, **1**:319
  anti-inflammatory/pressure-elevating potency of, **2**:419*t*
  in combination preparations, **2**:432*t*

for medical emergencies, 1:316*t*
perioperative, 1:334
Hydrocortisone sodium succinate
for medical emergencies, 1:316*t*
for uveitis, 9:115*t*
Hydrodelineation, in phacoemulsification, 11:127
Hydrodissection
in clear lens extraction/refractive lens exchange, 13:159
in phacoemulsification, 11:127
Hydrodiuril. *See* Hydrochlorothiazide
Hydrogel polymers
for contact lenses, 3:183–185, 183*t*, 184*t*
for keratoconus, 3:202
after keratorefractive surgery, 3:202
for foldable intraocular lenses, 3:213
Hydrogen peroxide, 2:365–366. *See also* Free radicals
as inflammatory mediator, 8:198*t*
Hydroperoxides, 2:365, 366
Hydropres. *See* Reserpine
Hydrops, in keratoconus, 4:70, 8:330
management of, 8:332
Hydroton. *See* Chlorthalidone
3-Hydroxy-3-methyl glutaryl coenzyme-A (HMG-CoA)
reductase inhibitors. *See also* Statins
cataracts and, 1:151, 11:54
for hypercholesterolemia, 1:149*t*
Hydroxyamphetamine, 2:309, 401*t*
in Horner syndrome diagnosis, 5:263
for pupillary testing, 2:406–407
Hydroxyapatite, 1:241
deposition of (calcific band keratopathy), 8:356, 373–374, 374*i*
in sarcoidosis, 8:88
Hydroxyapatite orbital implants, 7:122
exposure and extrusion of, 7:125*i*
Hydroxychloroquine, 1:174, 198
ocular effects of, 1:324*t*
retinal toxicity of, 1:198, 12:247–248, 248*i*
Hydroxyethylmethacrylate (HEMA), contact lenses
made from, 3:184
Hydroxyl radicals, 2:366, 9:83, 85. *See also* Free radicals
Hydroxymethyl progesterone. *See* Medrysone
Hydroxypropyl methylcellulose (HPMC)
for dry eye, 2:450
as viscoelastic, 2:452, 11:159, 160, 161*t*
Hyfrecator, for punctal occlusion, 8:77
Hyper- (prefix), definition of, 6:9
Hyperacuity (Vernier acuity), 3:111
Hyperaldosteronism, hypertension in, 1:83, 84*t*
Hyperbaric oxygen therapy, for nonarteritic anterior
ischemic optic neuropathy, 5:124
Hypercalcemia, corneal changes in, 8:356. *See also*
Band keratopathy
Hypercholesterolemia, 1:143–152. *See also*
Hyperlipoproteinemias
classification of, 1:144, 144*t*
management of, 1:145–147, 146*i*, 147*t*, 148*t*, 149*t*,
150*t*, 151*t*. *See also* Lipid-lowering therapy
metabolic syndrome and, 1:146, 148, 152*t*
ophthalmologic considerations and, 1:150–151
recent developments in, 1:143
risk assessment and, 1:144, 144*t*, 145, 145*t*, 146*i*
in Schnyder crystalline dystrophy, 8:322
screening for, 1:293

specific dyslipidemias and, 1:150
Hypercoagulable states (hypercoagulability), 1:170–172.
See also Thrombophilia; Thrombosis
fetal loss/preeclampsia and, 1:159
primary, 1:170–171
secondary, 1:171–172
transient visual loss and, 5:185
Hyperemia, conjunctival, 8:24*t*, 90
Hyperfluorescence, angiographic, 12:20–21, 20*i*, 22*i*
in age-related macular degeneration, 12:58–59
in angioid streaks, 12:83
in central serous chorioretinopathy, 12:22*i*, 52
in choroidal neovascularization, 12:20*i*
in cystoid macular edema, 12:154, 155*i*
Hyperglycemia. *See also* Diabetes mellitus; Glycemic
control
diabetic retinopathy incidence and progression and,
1:215, 215*i*, 12:101, 105
Diabetes Control and Complications Trial, 12:105,
106
United Kingdom Prospective Diabetes Study,
12:105, 107
obesity and, 1:202
rebound, 1:210
Hyperglycinemia, 2:262*t*
Hyperhomocysteinemia, 1:171
carotid artery disease and, 1:109
Hyperkeratosis
definition of, 4:168, 8:247*t*
exuberant (cutaneous horn), 7:164
Hyperlipidemia, in Schnyder crystalline dystrophy,
8:322
Hyperlipoproteinemias, 8:338–339, 339*t*
Schnyder crystalline dystrophy and, 8:322, 338
xanthelasma associated with, 4:171, 173*t*
Hyperlysinemia, 6:308, 11:42
Hypermature cataract, 11:48, 51*i*
phacolytic glaucoma and, 4:96, 11:67
Hypermetabolism, in hyperthyroidism, 1:223
Hypermetric saccades, 5:206, 207
Hyperopia, 3:116, 117*i*
amblyopia and, 6:69, 70
contact lens-corrected aphakia and, 3:179
converging lens for correction of, 3:143
cornea plana and, 8:291
high
cataract surgery in patients with, 11:222
clear lens extraction and, 11:138, 222
correction of, intraocular lenses for, 11:147–148
high accommodative convergence/accommodative
esotropia and, 6:102, 103
in infants and children, 3:119–120, 146–147, 6:199
intermittent exotropia and, 6:112
microcornea and, 8:289
nanophthalmos and, 8:287
primary angle closure/angle-closure glaucoma and,
10:12, 124
refractive accommodative esotropia and, 6:101, 103
retinal reflex in, 3:126–127
surgical correction of
clear lens extraction/refractive lens exchange for,
13:158, 159
conductive keratoplasty for, 13:139, 140
incisional corneal surgery for, 13:66
keratophakia for, 13:71–73, 73*i*

LASIK for, **13**:26, 27*i*, 118
light-adjustable IOLs for, **13**:165–166
monovision for, **13**:172
multifocal IOLs for, **13**:163–164, 163*i*
phakic IOLs for, **13**:144–146
PRK for, **13**:26, 99
wavefront aberration produced by (negative defocus), **13**:15
Hyperopic astigmatism
conductive keratoplasty for, **13**:140
LASIK for, **13**:118
PRK for, **13**:99
Hyperopic shift, after radial keratotomy, **13**:60, 63, 64
Hyperosmolar agents, **2**:451
Hyperosmolarity, tear film, dry eye and, **8**:71
Hyperosmotic agents, **2**:415–416, 415*t*, **10**:164*t*, 173–174
Hyperparathyroidism, in multiple endocrine neoplasia, **1**:230
Hyperpigmentation
congenital, **2**:175–176
after laser skin resurfacing, **7**:238
Hyperplasia
definition of, **6**:205, **8**:247*t*
epithelial
ciliary pigmented, **4**:241–242
of eyelid, **7**:163–164, 164*i*, 165*i*
lymphoid, of orbit, **7**:81–89. *See also* Lymphomas, orbital
pseudoadenomatous (Fuchs adenoma), **4**:146, 241–242
pseudoepitheliomatous, **7**:164
reactive/reactive lymphoid. *See* Lymphoid hyperplasia
sebaceous, of eyelid, **7**:166–167
Hypersensitivity reactions, **8**:198–201, 199*i*, 199*t*, **9**:54, 54*t*. *See also* Allergic reactions
anaphylactic or atopic (type I), **8**:198–200, 199, 199*t*, **9**:27, 54*t*, 72–73, 73*i*
fluorescein angiography and, **12**:21
topical medication and, **8**:205, 206*i*
contact, **9**:66
response to poison ivy as, **9**:29, 30
cutaneous basophil, **9**:66
to cycloplegics, **6**:95
cytotoxic (type II), **8**:199*i*, 199*t*, 200, **9**:54*t*
delayed (type IV), **8**:199, 199*t*, 201, **9**:54*t*
in chronic mast cell degranulation, **9**:73
contact dermatoblepharitis as, **8**:205–207, 206*i*
contact lenses and, **8**:107, 107*i*
in graft rejection, **8**:448
response to poison ivy as, **9**:29, 30
topical medication and, **8**:205–207, 206*i*
tuberculin form of, **9**:31, 65
granulomatous, **9**:66
immediate (type I/anaphylactic/atopic). *See* Hypersensitivity reactions, anaphylactic or atopic
immune-complex (type III), **8**:199*i*, 199*t*, 201, **9**:54*t*. *See also* Immune (antigen–antibody) complexes
stimulatory (type V), **9**:54, 54*t*
Hyperstat. *See* Diazoxide
Hypertelorism (telorbitism), **2**:126, **6**:207, 424, **7**:25
clefting syndromes and, **7**:38
Hypertension, **1**:81–99
cardiovascular risk and, **1**:81, 84, 86*t*

in children and adolescents, **1**:81, 97
choroidal perfusion abnormalities and, **12**:166, 168*i*
definition of, **12**:97
in diabetes, **1**:218
diabetic retinopathy affected by, **12**:105
United Kingdom Prospective Diabetes Study, **12**:105, 107
diagnosis/definition of, **1**:82, 82*t*, 292
etiology and pathogenesis of, **1**:82–84, 83*i*, 84*t*
evaluation of, **1**:84
incidence and prevalence of, **1**:81–82
intracranial hemorrhage and, **1**:105, 106
left ventricular hypertrophy and, **1**:95
MAO inhibitor interactions and, **1**:97, 276
metabolic syndrome and, **1**:95
minority populations and, **1**:97
obesity and, **1**:85, 95
ocular, **10**:96. *See also* Elevated intraocular pressure
refractive surgery in patients with, **13**:189–191, 190*i*
in older patients, **1**:96
ophthalmic considerations and, **1**:98–99, 98*t*
orthostatic, **1**:96
peripheral arterial disease and, **1**:96
phenylephrine causing, **2**:405
during pregnancy, **1**:96–97
primary (essential), **1**:82–83, 83*i*
rebound, **1**:97–98
resistant, **1**:83, 85*t*
retinal arterial macroaneurysms and, **12**:159
retinal disease associated with, **1**:98–99, 98*t*, **12**:97–99, 98*i*, 99*i*, 100*i*
screening for, **1**:292–293
secondary, **1**:83, 84*t*
sleep disorders and, **1**:95
treatment of, **1**:84–94, 91*i*
cerebrovascular disease and, **1**:95
chronic renal disease and, **1**:91*t*, 95
diabetes and, **1**:91*t*, 95
heart failure and, **1**:91*t*, 95, 130
ischemic heart disease and, **1**:91*t*, 94
lifestyle modifications and, **1**:85–86, 87*t*
pharmacologic, **1**:86, 87–94, 88–89*t*, 90*t*, 91*i*, 91*t*. *See also* Antihypertensive drugs
white coat, **1**:82
withdrawal syndromes and, **1**:97–98
in women, **1**:96–97
Hypertensive-arteriosclerotic intracerebral hemorrhages, **1**:105, 106
Hypertensive choroidopathy, **12**:98, 98*i*, 99*i*
Hypertensive crisis, **1**:98
MAO inhibitor interactions and, **1**:276
parenteral antihypertensive agents for, **1**:94
Hypertensive optic neuropathy, **12**:98–99, 100*i*
Hypertensive retinopathy, **1**:98–99, 98*t*, **12**:97–98
in renal disease in children, **6**:349
Hyperthermia
diode laser
for melanoma, **4**:238
for retinoblastoma, **4**:262
malignant, **1**:336–337, 337*t*, **6**:191–192, 193*t*
preoperative assessment of risk for, **1**:329–330
Hyperthyroidism, **1**:223–225
in elderly, **1**:249
Graves, **1**:224–225

ophthalmopathy and. *See* Thyroid ophthalmopathy
   toxic nodular goiter, **1**:225
Hypertonic medications, for recurrent corneal erosions,
   8:99
Hypertriglyceridemia, screening for, **1**:293
Hypertrophy, definition of, **8**:247*t*
Hypertropia, **6**:127
   vertical rectus muscle surgery for, **6**:181–182
Hyperuricemia, **8**:354–355
Hyperviscosity
   retinopathy and, central retinal vein occlusion
      differentiated from, **12**:143
   transient visual loss and, **5**:185
Hyphae, **8**:128–129, 129*i*
Hyphema. *See also* Uveitis-glaucoma-hyphema (UGH)
   syndrome
   after cataract surgery, **11**:171
   in children, **6**:447–449, 448*i*
      abuse and, **6**:442
   glaucoma and, **4**:82, **10**:110–112, 111*i*
   intraoperative, iris-fixated phakic IOL insertion and,
      13:154
   microscopic, **8**:398
   recurrent, transient visual loss and, **5**:174
   sickle cell disease and, **6**:447, 448*i*, **8**:402–403, **12**:123
   spontaneous, **8**:398
   traumatic, **8**:398–403, 399*i*, 400*i*
      in children, **6**:447–449, 448*i*
      medical management of, **8**:401–402
      rebleeding after, **8**:399–401, 400*i*, 401*i*
      sickle cell disease and, **6**:447, 448*i*, **8**:402–403,
         12:123
      surgery for, **8**:402, 403*t*
Hypnotic drugs, **1**:273–277, 274*t*
   abuse of, **1**:269
Hypo- (prefix), definition of, **6**:9
Hypoblast, **2**:134, 134*i*, 136
Hypocalcemia, cataracts associated with, **11**:62
Hypochondriasis, **1**:266
   in elderly, **1**:240
Hypoesthesia, in infraorbital nerve distribution, in
   blowout fractures, **7**:21, 104
Hypofluorescence, angiographic, **12**:19–20
   in age-related macular degeneration, **12**:59
Hypoglycemia
   childhood cataracts associated with, **6**:288*t*
   insulin therapy causing, **1**:211
   sulfonylurea-induced, **1**:212
Hypoglycemia unawareness, **1**:211
Hypoglycemic agents. *See* Insulin therapy; Oral
   hypoglycemic agents
Hypolipoproteinemias, corneal changes in, **8**:339–340
Hypomania, **1**:265
Hypometabolism, in hypothyroidism, **1**:226
Hypometric saccades, **5**:206, 207
Hypoparathyroidism, childhood cataracts associated
   with, **6**:288*t*
Hypoperfusion, **5**:170. *See also* Ischemia
   scotoma caused by, **5**:170
   transient visual loss caused by, **5**:174*t*, 183–184, 184*i*
Hypophosphatasia, **8**:352*t*
Hypophyseal artery, inferior, of tentorium, **5**:13
Hypopigmentation
   congenital, **2**:176–178, 177*i*
   oculocerebral (Cross syndrome), **6**:346*t*

Hypopigmented macule (ash-leaf spot), in tuberous
   sclerosis, **5**:339, **6**:409–410, 410*i*
Hypoplasia. *See also specific structure affected*
   definition of, **2**:126, **6**:205
Hypopyon
   in Behçet syndrome, **1**:193, 194, **9**:107, 132, 133,
      134*i*, **12**:181
   in endophthalmitis, **9**:211, 212, 223–224
   in uveitis, **9**:107, 127, 127*i*
Hypotelorism, **6**:207
Hypotension, ocular. *See* Hypotony
Hypotensive lipids, for glaucoma, **10**:163–164*t*,
   171–172
Hypothalamic-pituitary axis, disorders of, **1**:227–230,
   229*t*
Hypothalamus, **1**:227, **5**:56, 58*i*
Hypothyroidism, **1**:225–226
   ophthalmopathy and, **7**:53. *See also* Thyroid
      ophthalmopathy
Hypotony
   cataract surgery in patients with, **11**:223
   during/after surgery
      flat anterior chamber and, **11**:165, 166
      suprachoroidal hemorrhage and, **12**:333
   in uveitis, **9**:239
Hypotropia, **6**:127
   in Graves eye disease, **6**:149, 149*i*
   vertical rectus muscle surgery for, **6**:181–182
Hypovitaminosis A, **8**:92–94, 93*i*
Hypovolemic shock, **1**:317. *See also* Shock
Hypoxia, corneal, in flexible contact lens wearers,
   3:209–210
Hysteria, **5**:303
"Hysterical blindness." *See* Functional visual loss
Hytrin. *See* Terazosin
Hyzaar. *See* Losartan
HZO. *See* Herpes zoster ophthalmicus

I

I-cell (inclusion-cell) disease, **6**:436*t*, **8**:342
I-S number, **13**:12
Ibuprofen, **1**:197*t*, **2**:421*t*
   ocular effects of, **1**:324*t*
   for scleritis, **8**:240
Ibutilide, for atrial flutter, **1**:137–138
ICAM-1, **8**:198*t*
   in neutrophil rolling, **9**:48
   in Sjögren syndrome, **8**:78
ICAM-2, in neutrophil rolling, **9**:48
ICCE. *See* Intracapsular cataract extraction
ICDs. *See* Implantable cardioverter-defibrillators
Ice-pack test, for myasthenia gravis, **5**:326, 327, 327*i*,
   7:213
ICE syndrome. *See* Iridocorneal endothelial (ICE)
   syndrome
Icepick pain, idiopathic stabbing headache and, **5**:297
ICG angiography. *See* Indocyanine green angiography
Ichthyosis, **8**:89, 309*t*
   retinal degeneration and, **12**:237
   vulgaris, **8**:89
ICL. *See* Implantable Contact Lens
ICL/ICR. *See* Intracorneal lens/ring
Iclaprim, **1**:75

IDDM. *See* Diabetes mellitus, type 1
Idiopathic choroidal neovascularization, **12**:82–83
Idiopathic enlargement of blind spot syndrome
    (IEBSS), **5**:107, **12**:176
Idiopathic intracranial hypertension (pseudotumor
    cerebri), **5**:118–120, 118*t*, **6**:366–367
Idiopathic iridocyclitis, **9**:146
Idiopathic macular hole, **12**:89–93, 92*i*, 325–326, 327*i*
    vitrectomy for, **12**:93, 325–326, 327*i*
Idiopathic multiple cranial neuropathy syndrome,
    5:235
Idiopathic orbital inflammation. *See* Orbital
    inflammatory syndrome
Idiopathic retinal telangiectasia with exudation, **6**:332.
    See also Coats disease
Idiopathic retinal vasculitis/aneurysms/neuroretinitis
    (IRVAN), **12**:153
Idiopathic sclerosing inflammation of orbit, **7**:57, 58.
    See also Orbital inflammatory syndrome
Idiopathic thrombocytopenic purpura, **1**:167
Idiotopes, **9**:56
Idiotypes, **9**:56
Idioventricular escape rhythm, **1**:134
Idoxuridine, **2**:439
α-L-Iduronidase, in mucopolysaccharidoses, **8**:335–336
Ifex. *See* Ifosfamide
IFG. *See* Impaired fasting glucose
IFNs. *See* Interferons
Ifosfamide, **1**:258*t*
Ig. *See under* Immunoglobulin
IGF–1. *See* Insulin-like growth factor 1
IGFBPs. *See* Insulin-like growth factor binding proteins
IGT. *See* Impaired glucose tolerance
IHD. *See* Ischemic heart disease
IK (interstitial keratitis). *See* Keratitis, interstitial
IL. *See under* Interleukin
Ileocolitis, granulomatous (Crohn disease), **1**:177,
    9:131–132
Illegitimate transcripts, **2**:188
Illiterate E chart (E-game), for visual acuity testing in
    children, **6**:78*t*, 79
Illuminance, **2**:462, **3**:14–15, 16*t*
    retinal, **3**:16*t*
Illumination, **3**:14–17, 15*i*, 16*t*, 17*t*
    for direct ophthalmoscope, **3**:270, 271*i*
    for fundus camera, **3**:275
    improving, for low-vision patients, **3**:264
    for indirect ophthalmoscope, **3**:272, 275*i*, 279*i*
    for operating microscope, **3**:297
    recommended levels of, **3**:15–17, 17*t*
    for retinoscopy, **3**:125, 125*i*, 126*i*
    for slit-lamp biomicroscope, **3**:284, 284*i*
        direct, **8**:16–18, 17*i*, 18*i*
        indirect, **8**:18–19
Illumination test, for pediatric cataract, **6**:292
Illusions, **5**:187–189
    cortical origin of, **5**:189
    definition of, **5**:187
    nonvisual causes of, **5**:188*t*
    ocular origin of, **5**:187–189
    optic nerve origin of, **5**:189
ILM. *See* Internal limiting membrane
Ilotycin. *See* Erythromycin
Image jump, with bifocal lenses, **3**:158–159, 158*i*
    progressive addition lenses and, **3**:152

Image size
    calculation of, **3**:106–108, 108*i*
    contact lenses affecting, **3**:177–179
Image space, reversal of by mirrors, **3**:90
Images
    characteristics of, **3**:30–39. *See also specific type*
        brightness and irradiance, **3**:39
        depth of focus, **3**:35–36, 35*i*
        graphical analysis of, **3**:76–78, 77*i*, 77–78*i*, 78*i*
        location, **3**:34–35
        quality, **3**:36–38, 37*i*, 38*i*
        transverse magnification, **3**:30–31, 30*i*, 32*i*
    displacement of by prisms, **3**:86–87, 86*i*
    at infinity, **3**:74–75
    magnification of, **3**:30–34. *See also* Magnification
        with intraocular lenses, **3**:216
    virtual, **3**:67–69
        displacement of by prisms, **3**:87, 87*i*
Imaging
    with lenses, **3**:28–30, 29*i*
        image quality and, **3**:38, 38*i*
    with mirrors, **3**:28–30, 29*i*, 90–93
        image quality and, **3**:38, 38*i*
    pinhole, **3**:25–27, 25*i*, 28*i*, 33, 34, 34*i*
        image quality and, **3**:36–38, 37*i*, 38*i*
        visual acuity and, **3**:109–110
    radiographic. *See specific modality and* Neuroimaging
    stigmatic, **3**:38, 38*i*, 62, 62*i*, 116–117
    with single refractive surface, **3**:53–54, 54*i*
Imbibition pressure, **8**:11
Imidazoles, **1**:64*t*, 75–76, **2**:437–439, 438*t*
    for *Acanthamoeba* keratitis, **8**:189
Imipenem-cilastin, **1**:59*t*, 69, **2**:428*t*
Imipramine, ocular effects of, **1**:324*t*
Immediate hypersensitivity (type I) reaction,
    8:198–200, 199, 199*t*, **9**:27, 54*t*, 72–73, 73*i*. *See also*
    Allergic reactions
    fluorescein angiography and, **12**:21
    topical medication and, **8**:205, 206*i*
Immune-complex hypersensitivity (type III) reaction,
    8:199*i*, 199*t*, 201, **9**:54*t*. *See also* Immune
    (antigen–antibody) complexes
Immune (antigen–antibody) complexes
    circulating, **9**:58–59, 58*i*
        anterior uveitis and, **9**:59
    tissue-bound, **9**:59–62, 60*i*
        Arthus reaction and, **9**:60, 60*i*
    in type III hypersensitivity reaction, **8**:199*i*, 201
Immune cytolysis, **9**:59, 60*i*
Immune hypersensitivity reactions. *See* Hypersensitivity
    reactions
Immune-mediated diabetes. *See* Diabetes mellitus,
    type 1
Immune privilege
    in anterior uvea, **9**:37–39
    corneal, **8**:195–196, 447–448, **9**:39
    in retina/retinal pigment epithelium/choroid, **9**:41
    therapeutic potential of, **9**:39
    tolerance to lens crystallins and, **9**:90
Immune processing, **9**:22–24, 23*i*
    response to poison ivy and, **9**:29, 30
    response to tuberculosis and, **9**:30–31
Immune reconstitution syndromes (IRS), **1**:51

Immune response (immunity). *See also* Immune response arc
  adaptive, 9:9–10. *See also* Adaptive immune response
  cellular, 1:4, 8:199*i*, 199*t*, 201
  definition of, 9:9
  disorders of, neuro-ophthalmic signs of, 5:317–332
  glucocorticoids affecting, 2:418
  humoral, 1:4
  immunoregulation of, 9:34*t*, 87–89
  inflammation differentiated from, 9:12
  innate, 9:9, 10. *See also* Innate immune response
  mediator systems in, 9:7, 74–86, 75*t*
  ocular, 8:195–203, 9:33–42
    of anterior chamber/anterior uvea/vitreous, 9:34*t*, 36–39
    of conjunctiva, 8:195, 196*t*, 201, 9:33–36, 34*t*
    of cornea/sclera, 8:195–196, 196*t*, 201–202, 9:34*t*, 39, 40*i*
    disorders of. *See also specific type*
      clinical approach to, 8:205–241
      diagnostic approach to, 8:202–203, 202*t*, 203*t*
      patterns of, 8:201–202
      hypersensitivity reactions and, 8:198–201, 199*i*, 199*t*
    of retina/retinal pigment epithelium/choroid, 9:34*t*, 40–41
    soluble mediators of inflammation and, 8:197, 198*t*, 200*t*
  primary
    immune response arc and, 9:27–28
    secondary response differentiated from, 9:27
  regional, 9:28
  secondary
    immune response arc and, 9:27–28
    primary response differentiated from, 9:27
  tumor immunology and, 8:248–249
Immune response arc, 9:17–32. *See also* Immune response
  clinical examples of, 9:29
  immunologic microenvironments and, 9:28
  overview of, 9:17, 18*i*
  phases of, 9:17, 18*i*, 19–25
    afferent, 9:17, 18*i*, 19–22, 20*i*, 21*i*
      response to poison ivy and, 9:29, 30
      response to tuberculosis and, 9:30–31
    effector, 9:17–19, 18*i*, 25, 26*i*, 43–86. *See also* Effector phase of immune response arc
      response to poison ivy and, 9:29, 30
      response to tuberculosis and, 9:30–31
    processing, 9:22–24, 23*i*
      response to poison ivy and, 9:29, 30
      response to tuberculosis and, 9:30–31
  primary or secondary immune responses and, 9:27–28
  regional immunity and, 9:28
Immune system. *See also* Immune response; Immune response arc
  components of, 9:13–16
Immunization, 1:302–311. *See also specific disease*
  active, 1:303
  adaptive immunity and, 9:17–31. *See also* Immune response arc
  childhood, recommendations for, 1:303, 304*t*
  in immunocompromised host/HIV infection/AIDS, 1:41, 303, 305

new developments in, 1:291, 310
  passive, 1:303
  for travel, 1:309–310
Immunocompromised host. *See also* HIV infection/ AIDS
  immunization in, 1:303, 305
  ocular infection in, 8:118
    candidiasis, 9:163–164, 223–224
    cryptococcosis, 9:163, 257
    cytomegalovirus retinitis, 1:29, 4:123, 124*i*, 6:219, 9:71, 156–157, 249–250
Immunodot assay, for Lyme disease, 1:20
Immunofluorescence assay
  in HIV infection/AIDS, 1:39
  in Lyme disease, 1:20
Immunogen, 9:19
Immunoglobulin A (IgA)
  secretory, in tear film, 2:290, 8:56, 198
    in external eye defense, 8:113
  structural and functional properties of, 9:57*t*
  in tear film, 2:290, 8:56, 198, 9:33
  in viral conjunctivitis, 9:35
Immunoglobulin A (IgA) protease, as microbial virulence factor, 1:4
Immunoglobulin D (IgD)
  structural and functional properties of, 9:57*t*
  in tear film, 2:290
Immunoglobulin E (IgE)
  mast cell degranulation mediated by, 9:13–14, 72–73, 73*i*
  structural and functional properties of, 9:57*t*
  in tear film, 2:290
  in type I hypersensitivity/anaphylactic reactions, 1:319, 8:198, 199*i*, 9:27, 72–73, 73*i*
Immunoglobulin G (IgG)
  structural and functional properties of, 9:57*t*
  in tear film, 2:290
Immunoglobulin M (IgM)
  structural and functional properties of, 9:57*t*
  in tear film, 2:290
Immunoglobulin superfamily molecules, in neutrophil rolling, 9:48, 49*i*
Immunoglobulins, 9:25. *See also specific type*
  classes of, 9:54–55
  in conjunctiva, 8:195
  disorders of synthesis of, 8:349–350
  intravenous, for cicatricial pemphigoid, 8:223
  isotypes of, 9:7, 55
    in immunologic tolerance, 9:89
  structural and functional properties of, 9:54–55, 56*i*, 57*t*
  in tear film, 8:198
    in external eye defense, 8:113
Immunohistochemistry, 4:37–38, 37*i*
Immunologic competence, ocular infection and, 8:118
Immunologic memory, 9:11, 27–28
Immunologic microenvironments, 9:28
  of anterior chamber/anterior uvea/vitreous, 9:34*t*, 36–37
  of conjunctiva, 9:33, 34*t*
  of cornea/sclera, 9:34*t*, 39, 40*i*
  of retina/retinal pigment epithelium/choroid, 9:34*t*, 40–41
Immunologic tolerance, 9:87–89
  to lens crystallins, 9:90

Immunology, **9**:7–97. *See also* Immune response;
    Immune response arc
  basic concepts in, **9**:9–16
  definitions/abbreviations of terms and, **9**:7–8, 9–12
Immunoregulation/immunoregulatory systems, **9**:34*t*,
    87–89
  for anterior uvea, **9**:34*t*, 37–39
  for conjunctiva, **9**:34*t*, 36
  for cornea, **9**:34*t*, 39
  for retina/retinal pigment epithelium/choroid, **9**:34*t*,
    42
  T- and B-cell antigen receptor repertoire and, **9**:87
  tolerance and, **9**:87–89
Immunotherapy/immunosuppression, **1**:199–200,
    9:95–97
  for allergic conjunctivitis, **8**:208
  for atopic keratoconjunctivitis, **8**:213
  for Behçet syndrome, **1**:193–194
  for cancer, **1**:251, 257–262, 260*t*
  for cicatricial pemphigoid, **8**:222–223
  for corneal graft rejection, **8**:469
  diabetes affected by, **1**:203
  for HIV infection/AIDS, **1**:44
  for melanoma, **4**:238
  for multifocal choroiditis and panuveitis syndrome,
    12:178
  for multiple sclerosis, **5**:144
  for pars planitis, **9**:151
  for peripheral ulcerative keratitis, **8**:231
  for primary central nervous system lymphoma,
    9:228
  for pulmonary diseases, **1**:158
  for rheumatic disorders, **1**:199–200
  for rheumatoid arthritis, **1**:174–175
  for scleritis, **8**:241
  for serpiginous choroidopathy, **12**:177
  for uveitis, **9**:118–121, 119*t*
    in children, **6**:321
  for vernal keratoconjunctivitis, **8**:211
  for Vogt-Koyanagi-Harada syndrome, **9**:205
Impact-resistant spectacle lenses, **3**:168
Impaired fasting glucose, **1**:203*t*, 206
Impaired glucose tolerance, **1**:203*t*, 206
Impairment, visual. *See* Low vision; Visual loss/
    impairment
Impending macular holes, **12**:89
Implant surgery, for childhood glaucoma, **6**:281
Implantable cardioverter-defibrillators (ICDs), **1**:111,
    139–140
  for heart failure, **1**:131
  laser surgery in patient with, **13**:41
  for tachyarrhythmias, **1**:139–140
Implantable Contact Lens (ICL), **13**:148–149, 149*i*,
    150*i*, 154–155. *See also* Phakic intraocular lenses,
    posterior chamber
Implantation membrane, of iris, **4**:219*t*
Implants, orbital, **7**:121–122
  in children, **7**:121
  exposure and extrusion of, **7**:125, 125*i*
  for superior sulcus deformity, **7**:124
Implicit time (τ), in electroretinogram, **12**:28*i*, 29
Impression cytology, **8**:64, 70*i*
  in Sjögren syndrome diagnosis, **8**:73
  in stem cell deficiency, **8**:109
Imprinting (genetic), **2**:188, 210

Imuran. *See* Azathioprine
In situ hybridization, **2**:247–249, 248*i*, 249*i*
Inborn errors of metabolism, **6**:435–439, 436–437*t*,
    457*t*
  dietary therapy in, **2**:280–281
  enzyme defect in, **2**:262*t*, 263, **6**:435, 436–437*t*
  inheritance of, **6**:435, 436–437*t*
  ocular findings in, **2**:262*t*, **6**:435, 436–437*t*
  treatment of, **6**:438
INC. *See* Interstitial nucleus of Cajal
Incisional biopsy, **7**:176, 176*i*, **8**:251, 252*i*
Incisional surgery
  for angle-closure glaucoma, **10**:200
  corneal, **13**:59–70. *See also* Keratotomy
    for astigmatism correction, **13**:66–69, 67*i*, 69*t*
    biomechanics affected by, **8**:13, 14*i*
    for hyperopia, **13**:66
    for myopia, **13**:59–66. *See also* Radial keratotomy
  for open-angle glaucoma, **10**:183–194, 187–191*i*,
    193*i*, 193*t*
    antifibrotic agents in, **10**:188, 190–192
    complications of, **10**:192–194, 193*i*, 193*t*
    contraindications to, **10**:185
    flap management in, **10**:192
    indications for, **10**:184
    postoperative considerations in, **10**:192
    preoperative evaluation for, **10**:185–186
    trabeculectomy technique, **10**:186–188, 187–191*i*
Incisions
  for cataract surgery, **11**:106, 110, 121–126. *See also*
      type of incision and type of surgery
    clear corneal, **11**:100–101, 123–125, 125*i*, 126*i*
      minimizing bleeding risk and, **11**:202
    for ECCE with nucleus expression, **11**:110
    for ICCE, **11**:106
    minimizing bleeding and, **11**:202
    modification of preexisting astigmatism and,
        11:102–103
    for phacoemulsification, **11**:121–126
    scleral tunnel, **11**:99–100, 100*i*, 121–123, 123*i*,
        124*i*
      modification of preexisting astigmatism and,
          11:102
    self-sealing
      beveled/biplanar, clear corneal incisions and,
          11:124–125, 126*i*
      scleral tunnel incisions and, **11**:99
    single-plane, **11**:99
    wound closure and, **11**:99–100, 100*i*
  corneal biomechanics affected by, **8**:13, 14*i*
  for extraocular muscle surgery, **6**:183–184
  for keratorefractive surgery, corneal biomechanics
      affected by, **8**:13, 14*i*, **13**:19–23, 23*i*, 24*i*
  for orbital surgery, **7**:109, 111*i*
  for radial keratotomy, **13**:61, 62*i*
    depth affecting outcome and, **13**:61
  for rhytidectomy, **7**:244
Inclusion-cell (I-cell) disease, **6**:436*t*, **8**:342
Inclusion conjunctivitis, trachoma (TRIC), **6**:222
Inclusion criteria, **1**:364
Inclusion cysts
  epidermal, of eyelid, **7**:164–166, 165*i*
  epithelial, **4**:45, 46*i*, **8**:254, 254*i*
    conjunctival, **4**:45, 46*i*, **6**:386
      after strabismus surgery, **6**:187, 188*i*

nevi and, **4:**55–56, 56*i*
orbital, **4:**188
Inclusions
cytoplasmic
in chlamydial infection, **8:**69, 69*i*
cytologic identification of, **8:**65*t*, 69, 69*i*
nuclear, cytologic identification of, **8:**69
Incomitant (noncomitant) deviations, **5:**213, 217, 218*i*,
6:10
esodeviations, **6:**98*t*, 107–108
strabismus surgery planning and, **6:**176–177
vertical, **6:**127
strabismus surgery planning and, **6:**177
Incomplete penetrance (skipped generation), **2:**266
Incontinentia pigmenti (Bloch-Sulzberger syndrome),
2:269, **6:**402*t*, 418–419, 418*i*, 419*i*, **12:**233*t*, 237
Incorrect corrective lens, in visual field testing, **10:**70
Increased intraocular pressure. *See* Elevated intraocular
pressure
Incretins, for diabetes, **1:**214
Incyclo- (prefix), definition of, **6:**10
Incycloduction. *See* Intorsion
Incyclovergence, **6:**38
Indapamide, **1:**88*t*
Indentation (Schiøtz) tonometry, **10:**29
HIV prevention precautions and, **9:**262
Independent assortment, **2:**244–245
Inderal/Inderal LA. *See* Propranolol
Inderide. *See* Propranolol
Index case (proband), **2:**193, 275
Index features, in diagnosis, **4:**17–18
Index of refraction. *See* Refractive index
Indinavir, **1:**42
for postexposure HIV prophylaxis, **1:**46–47*t*
Indirect hemagglutination antibody test, for Lyme
disease, **1:**20
Indirect ophthalmoscopy. *See* Ophthalmoscopy
Indirect traumatic optic neuropathy, **2:**102
Individual versus average effect, **1:**361–362
Indocin. *See* Indomethacin
Indocyanine green, **2:**451–452
Indocyanine green angiography, **2:**452, **12:**22–23
in central serous chorioretinopathy, **12:**53
of choriocapillaris, **12:**15
in choroidal neovascularization, **12:**63
in choroidal perfusion abnormalities, **12:**166, 167*i*,
168*i*, 169*i*
in low vision evaluation, **5:**98
Indoles, **2:**421. *See also* Nonsteroidal anti-inflammatory
drugs
Indomethacin, **1:**197*t*, **2:**421*t*, 422
cornea verticillata caused by, **8:**375
for cystoid macular edema prophylaxis, **12:**155
prostaglandin synthesis affected by, **2:**306
Induced tropia test, **6:**79
Inducer region, **2:**202
Induction
definition of, **2:**126
in ocular development, **2:**129
Infantile cataract, **4:**95, **11:**33–39, 35*t*. *See also* specific
type and Cataract, congenital and infantile
definition of, **11:**33
Infantile (congenital) esotropia, **6:**97–101, 98*t*, 99*i*
essential (classic), **6:**97–100, 98*t*, 99*i*

Infantile glaucoma, **6:**271, 272–277, 273*i*, 274*t*, 275*i*,
276*i*, 277*i*, **10:**147. *See also* Glaucoma, childhood
Infantile nystagmus, **6:**334, 334*t*. *See also* Nystagmus,
childhood
Infantile phytanic acid storage disease (Refsum
disease), **2:**262*t*, **6:**437*t*, **12:**242
gene defects causing, **2:**351
Leber congenital amaurosis and, **6:**335
Infants. *See also* Children
corneal transplantation in, **8:**470–471
decreased/low vision in, **3:**266, **6:**451–459
electroretinogram in, **12:**31
intraocular lens use in, **6:**301–302
retinal degeneration onset in, **12:**233–234
peroxisomal disorders/Refsum disease and, **12:**242,
242*i*
shaking injury and, **6:**442–445, 443*i*, 444*i*,
12:301–302, 302*i*
visually evoked cortical potentials in, **6:**78*t*, 202, 451
Infection (ocular), **8:**139–192. *See also* specific type,
structure affected, or causative agent and Infectious
disease; Inflammation
basic concepts of, **8:**113–137
defense mechanisms and, **8:**113–114, 117–118
diagnostic laboratory techniques in, **8:**134–136, 135*t*,
136*i*, 137*t*
globally important, **8:**51, 51*t*
in infants and children, **6:**215–233, 457*t*
conjunctivitis, **6:**224–229, 224*t*, 227*i*, 228*i*, 229*i*,
230*i*
intrauterine and perinatal, **6:**215–221
corneal anomalies and, **8:**298–299
ophthalmia neonatorum, **6:**221–224, 222*i*
orbital and adnexal, **6:**230–233, 232*i*, 233*i*
microbiology of, **8:**118–134, 119*t*
normal flora and, **8:**114–115, 115*t*
pathogenesis of, **8:**115–118
prevention of, **8:**50–51
in Stevens-Johnson syndrome, **8:**217
after strabismus surgery, **6:**185–186, 186*i*
virulence factors in, **8:**116–117
Infection control, **8:**50–51
in clinical tonometry, **8:**50, **10:**29
Infectious crystalline keratopathy, **8:**180, 181*i*
after penetrating keratoplasty, **8:**464, 464*i*
Infectious disease, **1:**3–79. *See also* specific organism and
specific disorder and Infection (ocular)
antimicrobial treatment for, **1:**53–78, 55–65*t*
chorioretinopathy and, **12:**183–193
diabetes mellitus and, **1:**204*t*
endophthalmitis and, **9:**207–214, 208*t*
differential diagnosis of, **9:**215
microbiologic principles and, **1:**3–4
neuro-ophthalmic signs of, **5:**358–368
panuveitis and, **9:**187–197
posterior uveitis and, **9:**154–173
recent developments in, **1:**3
screening for, **1:**301–302
Infectious mononucleosis
Epstein-Barr virus causing, **1:**30
ocular involvement in, **8:**156–157, 156*i*
conjunctivitis, **6:**228
Inferior hypophyseal artery of tentorium, **5:**13
Inferior meatus, **2:**6, **5:**10
Inferior muscular artery, **5:**15

Inferior oblique muscles, 2:8, 15*i*, 17*i*, 18*t*, 5:41, 42,
42*i*, 6:14*i*, 15–16, 17*t*, 18*i*, 7:13, 141*i*
action of, 6:15–16, 17*t*, 30*t*, 31, 35*i*
anatomy of, 6:14*i*, 15–16, 17*t*, 18*i*
surgery and, 6:23, 24*i*
field of action/activation of, 6:29
insertion relationships of, 2:16, 17*i*, 18*t*
overaction of, 6:127–129, 128*i*
V-pattern deviations associated with, 6:119, 120*i*
vertical deviations caused by, 6:127–129, 128*i*
palsy of, 6:135–136, 136*i*, 137*t*
surgery of, 6:180
for dissociated vertical deviation, 6:131, 181–182
for superior oblique paralysis, 6:134, 180
for V-pattern deviations, 6:122, 124
for vertical deviations, 6:128–129
Inferior oblique subnucleus, 5:45
Inferior ophthalmic vein, 5:20, 22*i*
Inferior orbital fissure, 2:12, 5:8*i*, 10, 7:10*i*, 11, 22
Inferior orbital vein, 6:16
Inferior petrosal sinus, 5:23
Inferior punctum, 2:22, 34
Inferior rectus muscles, 2:15*i*, 17*i*, 18*t*, 19*i*, 5:42, 42*i*,
6:14, 17*t*, 18*i*, 7:13
A-pattern deviations associated with dysfunction of,
6:119
action of, 6:14, 17*t*, 30, 30*t*, 32*i*
anatomy of, 6:14, 17*t*, 18*i*
surgery and, 6:23
paresis of, in orbital floor fractures, 6:139, 139*i*, 140
restriction of, in monocular elevation deficiency
(double elevator palsy), 6:136, 137, 137–138
surgery of
for dissociated vertical deviation, 6:181
eyelid position changes after, 6:189–190, 190*i*
for superior oblique paralysis, 6:134, 135
Inferior rectus subnucleus, 5:45
Inferior tarsal muscle, 7:145
Inferior turbinate, 5:10
infracture of, for congenital tearing/nasolacrimal
duct obstruction, 6:245–246, 7:263, 265*i*
Inferior vestibular nerve, 5:32, 54
Inferolateral displacement of globe, in orbital disorders,
7:23
Inferolateral trunk, 5:13
Inferomedial displacement of globe, in orbital
disorders, 7:23
Inferonasal crescent, in congenital tilted disc syndrome,
5:139, 140*i*
Infiltrative dermopathy, in hyperthyroidism, 1:224
Infiltrative lesions, orbital, 5:129, 130*i*
Infiltrative optic neuropathy, 5:156
Infinity
focal planes and focal points at, 3:70*i*, 75
objects and images at, 3:74–75
Inflamase Forte/Inflamase Mild. *See* Prednisolone
Inflammation (ocular), 4:12–16, 14*i*, 15*i*, 16*i*. *See also*
specific type or structure affected and
Endophthalmitis; Uveitis
acute, 4:12, 19
age-related macular degeneration differentiated
from, 12:69
cataract surgery and, 11:164*t*, 178
in glaucoma patient, 11:218
trauma and, 11:225

choroidal disorders and, 12:173–193. *See also*
Chorioretinitis; Chorioretinopathy;
Choroidopathy
pain and, 5:298
chronic, 4:12
clinical evaluation of, 8:22–31, 24–25*t*, 32*t*
conjunctival, 4:45–49
corneal, 4:65–67
eyelid, 4:170*i*, 171, 172*i*
granulomatous, 4:12
choroidal, 4:27–28, 28*i*
lens-related, 4:96–97, 96*i*, 97*i*, 98*i*
nonsteroidal anti-inflammatory agents for,
1:196–198
optic nerve, 4:205, 205*i*, 206*i*
orbital, 4:188–190, 189*i*, 190*i*, 191*i*
pupil irregularity caused by, 5:259
retinal, 4:123–126, 125*i*
pain caused by, 5:298
in retinoblastoma, 4:253, 253*t*, 254*i*
scleral, 4:89–91, 90*i*
secondary angle-closure glaucoma caused by,
10:138–140, 139*i*
secondary open-angle glaucoma and, 10:106–108,
108*i*
soluble mediators of. *See* Mediators
treatment of. *See* Anti-inflammatory agents
uveal tract, 4:152–156
vitreal, 4:107–108, 108*i*
Inflammatory bowel disease, 1:177, 9:131–132
Inflammatory (stimulated) macrophages, 9:50, 51*i*,
52–53
Inflammatory mediators. *See* Mediators
Inflammatory pseudoguttae, 8:29
Inflammatory pseudotumor. *See* Orbital inflammatory
syndrome
Inflammatory response. *See also* Inflammation
immune response triggering, 9:11
immunity differentiated from, 9:12
local antibody production and, 9:63
Infliximab, 1:173, 199
for Behçet syndrome, 1:194
for uveitis, 9:120
in children, 6:322
Influenza virus
antiviral agents for infection caused by, 1:77, 291
conjunctivitis in children caused by, 6:228
vaccination against, 1:291, 305–306
Informed consent
for cataract surgery, 11:88
for refractive surgery, 13:49–50
clear lens extraction/refractive lens exchange and,
13:158
model forms for, 13:51–56
phakic intraocular lens insertion and, 13:146
Infraciliary blepharoplasty incision, for anterior
orbitotomy, 7:110–111
Infracture of turbinates, for congenital tearing/
nasolacrimal duct obstruction, 6:245–246, 7:263,
265*i*
Infraduction. *See* Depression of eye
Infranuclear pathways, in ocular motility, 5:197
Infraorbital artery, 5:13, 15–16
extraocular muscles supplied by, 2:16–18, 6:16
orbit supplied by, 2:39*i*

Infraorbital canal, 2:10
Infraorbital foramen, 2:8
Infraorbital groove, 2:8, 9*i*
Infraorbital nerve, 2:116, 5:52, 56
  hypoesthesia in distribution of, in blowout fractures, 7:21, 104
Infrared lasers, 12:314, 315–316*t*
Infrared radiation. *See also* Radiation
  lens affected by, 2:463–464, 11:56
Infratemporal fossa, 7:22
Infratrochlear artery, 5:13
Inhaled insulin, 1:214
Inhaled steroids, for pulmonary diseases, 1:158
Inhalers, metered-dose, β₂-adrenergics for pulmonary disease and, 1:157
Inheritance. *See also specific disorder and* Genetics
  codominant, 2:184, 260
  digenic, 2:185
  dominant, 2:185, 260–261
    autosomal, 2:265–266, 267*t*
    disorders associated with, 2:185
      gene therapy for, 2:237–238, 238*i*
      X-linked, 2:268–269
    X-linked, 2:268, 268*t*
  galtonian, 2:186
    of mitochondrial DNA diseases, 2:186, 257
  holandric, 2:188, 266
  maternal, 2:217, 257, 269
  multifactorial, 2:191, 273–275
  patterns of, 2:260–269, 8:306–307
  polygenic, 2:192, 273–275, 274*t*
  recessive, 2:194, 260
    autosomal, 2:261–265, 265*t*
    disorders associated with, 2:194, 261–265
      gene therapy for, 2:237
      X-linked, 2:267–268, 268*t*
  sex linked, 2:195
    X-linked, 2:198, 220, 266–269, 268*t*
    disorders associated with, 2:268–269
      gene therapy for, 2:237
    Y-linked, 2:198, 266
Inhibitor region, 2:202
Inhibitors, 2:392
Initiator codon, 2:189
INL. *See* Inner nuclear layer
Inlays, corneal, 13:71–85
  alloplastic, 13:72–73, 73*i*, 175
  homoplastic, 13:71–72
  for keratophakia, 13:71–72, 72–73, 73*i*
  for presbyopia, 13:175–176
Innate immune response, 9:9, 10
  acute phase reactants in, 9:47
  bacteria-derived molecules in, 9:43–46, 44*t*
  complement in, 9:46–47, 75
  effector reactivities of, 9:43–54
  macrophage recruitment and activation and, 9:48–54, 51*i*
  mediator systems affecting, 9:74–86, 75*t*
  neutrophil recruitment and activation and, 9:48–50, 49*t*
  triggers of, 9:11, 43–54, 44*t*
Inner ischemic retinal atrophy, 4:128, 129*i*
  in branch retinal artery occlusion, 4:133
Inner marginal zone, 2:140
Inner neuroblastic layer, 2:140

Inner nuclear layer, 2:80–81*i*, 84, 351–354, 352*i*, 353*i*, 354*i*
Inner plexiform layer, 2:80–81*i*, 85
Inner segments. *See* Cone inner segments; Photoreceptor inner segments; Rod inner segments
Innominate artery, 5:17, 178*i*
INO. *See* Internuclear ophthalmoplegia
Inoculum size, 8:117
Inositol-1,4,5-triphosphate (IP₃), in signal transduction
  in iris–ciliary body, 2:311–312, 312*i*, 313*i*
  in tear secretion, 2:292, 292*i*
Inotropic agents, for heart failure, 1:130–131
INR. *See* International normalized ratio
Insect hairs/stings, ocular injury/infection caused by, 8:395
Inspection, in orbital disorders, 7:24–26
Inspra. *See* Eplerenone
Instantaneous radius of curvature (tangential power), 8:43, 43*i*, 44*i*, 13:7, 7*i*
Instrument (proximal) convergence, 6:38
Instrument myopia, in automated refraction, 3:312
Instrumentation. *See* Ophthalmic instrumentation; Surgical instruments
Insulin. *See also* Insulin therapy
  in glucose metabolism/diabetes, 1:202
    genetic defects and, 1:204*t*
Insulin-dependent diabetes mellitus (IDDM). *See* Diabetes mellitus, type 1
Insulin-like growth factor 1, 2:456
  in aqueous humor, 2:320, 321
  in ocular development, 2:130
Insulin-like growth factor binding proteins, in aqueous humor, 2:321
Insulin-neutralizing antibodies, 1:211
Insulin pump, 1:210–211
Insulin resistance
  immunologic, insulin therapy and, 1:211
  metabolic syndrome and, 1:148, 206
Insulin therapy, 1:208–211, 209*t*
  complications of, 1:211
  inhaled, 1:214
  intensive (tight control), 1:214–215
  recent developments in, 1:201
  surgery in diabetic patient and, 1:220–221, 333
  types of insulin for, 1:209–210, 209*t*
Intacs. *See* Intrastromal corneal ring segments
Intal. *See* Cromolyn
Integrase inhibitors, for HIV infection/AIDS, 1:42
Integrilin. *See* Eptifibatide
Integrins, 8:116
  in neutrophil rolling, 9:48, 49*t*
Intensity. *See also* Brightness
  of laser light, 3:18–19
  luminous (candle power), 3:16*t*
  radiant, 3:16*t*
    for medical lasers, 3:18*t*
  of retinal reflex, in axis determination, 3:131
Intention-to-treat analysis, 1:352
Intercellular adhesion molecules, in neutrophil rolling, 9:48, 49*t*
Intercrines. *See* Chemokines
Interface debris, after LASIK, 13:131, 131*i*
Interface keratitis
  diffuse (diffuse lamellar keratitis/sands of the Sahara), 13:127, 128*i*, 129*t*

infectious, **13**:128–129, 129*i*
Interfaces, optical, **3**:41–42
  light propagation at, **3**:41–42, 42*i*, 43*i*
  reflection at, **3**:13–14, 13*i*
Interference, **3**:7–9, 8*i*, 9*i*
  applications of, **3**:8–9, 9*i*
  constructive, **3**:7, 8*i*
  destructive, **3**:7, 8*i*
Interference filters, **3**:8–9, 9*i*
Interferometry, laser, **3**:8, 315–316, 322
  for potential acuity estimation, before cataract
    surgery, **11**:85
Interferons (IFNs), **1**:261, **2**:455, **9**:80, 82*t*
  α, **1**:261
    for Behçet syndrome, **1**:193
    in cancer therapy, **1**:260*t*, 261
    for capillary hemangioma, **7**:66
    for hepatitis B, **1**:305
    for hepatitis C, **1**:31
    for orbital hemangiomas in children, **6**:378
  β, **1**:261
    for conjunctival intraepithelial neoplasia, **8**:258
  γ, **1**:261
    in delayed hypersensitivity, **9**:65*i*, 66
  for multiple sclerosis, **5**:144, 324
  ocular effects of, **1**:324*t*
  in tear film, **2**:290–291
Interlenticular membranes, piggyback IOLs and, **13**:160
Interleukin-1, **8**:197, 198*t*
  in external eye defense, **8**:114
Interleukin-1α, **9**:81*t*
  in Sjögren syndrome, **8**:78
Interleukin-1β, in Sjögren syndrome, **8**:78
Interleukin-2, **9**:81*t*
  in cancer therapy, **1**:261
Interleukin-4, **9**:81*t*
  atopy and, **8**:200
  in delayed hypersensitivity, **9**:65*i*, 66
Interleukin-5, **9**:81*t*
  in delayed hypersensitivity, **9**:65*i*, 66
Interleukin-6, **9**:81*t*
  in Sjögren syndrome, **8**:78
Interleukin-8, **9**:81*t*
  in Sjögren syndrome, **8**:78
Interleukins, **9**:80–83, 81*t*
  in cancer therapy, **1**:261
  in external eye defense, **8**:114
  for HIV infection/AIDS, **1**:44
  in Sjögren syndrome, **8**:78
Intermarginal sulcus (gray line), **2**:22, 287, **7**:142*i*, 146
Intermediate uveitis (pars planitis/chronic cyclitis),
  9:107, 147–152, 148*i*, **12**:182
  causes of, **9**:112*t*
  in children, **6**:311, 312*t*, 316–317, 317*i*
    differential diagnosis of, **6**:312*t*
    laboratory tests for, **6**:321*t*
  clinical characteristics of, **9**:147–148, 148*i*
  complications of, **9**:151–152
  cystoid macular edema and, **12**:154
  differential diagnosis of, **6**:312*t*, **9**:110*t*, 148–149
  HLA association in, **9**:94*t*, 147
  in Lyme disease, **9**:192
  multiple sclerosis and, **9**:152
  prognosis of, **9**:149
  signs of, **9**:105–106

treatment of, **9**:149–150
Intermediate zone, **2**:74–76
Intermittent ataxia, **2**:262*t*
Intermittent tropias, **6**:10
  esotropia, **6**:97
  exotropia, **6**:109–114, 110*i*
Intermuscular septum, **2**:20, **6**:21, **7**:12
  surgery and, **6**:23
Internal auditory meatus, **2**:118
Internal carotid artery, **5**:11, 11–12*i*, 13, 14*i*, 178*i*
  aneurysm of, **5**:350–351
    chiasmal syndromes caused by, **5**:162
    third nerve palsy and, **5**:228–229, 229*i*
  dissection of, **5**:354–355
    Horner syndrome caused by, **5**:263–264, 264*i*
  eyelids supplied by, **8**:7
  supraclinoid, **5**:16
Internal hordeolum, **8**:168
Internal jugular veins, venous sinuses draining into,
  2:119, 120*i*
Internal limiting membrane, **2**:80–81*i*, 83, 85, **12**:9
  optic disc, **2**:98, 100*i*
  in Valsalva retinopathy, **12**:93
  vitreous detachment and, **2**:338
Internal maxillary artery, **5**:9
Internal reflection, total (TIR), **3**:14, 47–49, 48*i*, 50*i*
  gonioscopy and, **3**:49–50, 50*i*
Internal scleral sulcus, **2**:54
Internal ulcer of von Hippel. *See* Keratoconus,
  posterior
International normalized ratio (INR), **1**:165
Internuclear ophthalmoplegia, **5**:39, 210, 224–225,
  225*i*, 226*i*, **6**:155
  myasthenia gravis and, **5**:224
  nystagmus in, **5**:224, 225*i*, **6**:155
  unilateral, **5**:225, 226*i*
  wall-eyed bilateral, **5**:224, 225*i*
Interocular distance, abnormal, **6**:207–209, 208*i*, 209*i*
Interpalpebral fissure, vertical, height of, in ptosis,
  7:209, 210*i*
Interphotoreceptor matrix (IPM/subretinal space), **2**:78
  development of, **2**:137*i*
  retinal pigment epithelium in maintenance of,
    2:361–362
Interphotoreceptor retinoid-binding protein, **2**:359,
  361*t*, **4**:140–142
Interplexiform cells, **5**:24
Interpulse time (TI), definition of, **5**:81
Interpupillary distance, bifocal segment decentration
  and, **3**:163
Interrater reliability, **1**:363
Interrupted sutures, for penetrating keratoplasty, **8**:457,
  457*i*
Intersex, **2**:252
Interstitial growth, in development of lamellae, **2**:151
Interstitial keratitis. *See* Keratitis, interstitial
Interstitial nucleus of Cajal, **5**:34, 202
  skew deviation and, **5**:223
Intervening sequence. *See* Intron
Intervention, in clinical research, **1**:342
Interventional (experimental) studies (clinical trials),
  1:345, 351–352, 351*i*. *See also* Clinical research
  for new drug, **2**:393
  systematic reviews/meta-analyses of, **1**:352

Intorsion (incycloduction), 6:28, 34
  extraocular muscles in
    superior oblique, 6:15, 30t, 31, 34i
    superior rectus, 6:14, 28, 30, 30t, 32i
Intorsional strabismus, 6:10
Intracameral injections, 2:386–387
  lidocaine, for cataract surgery, 11:94, 95–96
Intracanalicular portion of optic nerve, 2:93, 97t, 102
  blood supply of, 2:103
  compressive lesions of, 5:145–151
Intracapsular cataract extraction (ICCE), 11:103–108,
    107i. See also Cataract surgery
  advantages of, 11:104
  contraindications to, 11:105
  cystoid macular edema and, 12:154
  disadvantages of, 11:104–105
  early techniques for, 11:90–91, 92i, 93i
  indications for, 11:105
  instrumentation for, 11:105
  patient preparation for, 11:105–106
  postoperative course for, 11:108
  postoperative flat or shallow anterior chamber and,
    11:165
  procedure for, 11:106–108, 107i
  retinal detachment and, 11:175
  vitreous changes associated with, posterior vitreous
    detachment, 12:257
Intraconal fat/surgical space (central surgical space),
    7:12, 109, 110i
Intracorneal implants, alloplastic
  corneal biomechanics affected by, 13:23–24, 25i
  for epikeratoplasty (epikeratophakia), 13:77
  for keratophakia, 13:72–73, 73i
  for presbyopia, 13:175–176
Intracorneal lens/ring, 13:20t. See also Intrastromal
    corneal ring segments
Intracranial hemorrhage, 1:105–106
  headache caused by, 5:292
  hypertensive-arteriosclerotic, 1:105, 106
  ruptured aneurysm causing, 1:105, 106, 5:351
  in shaking injury, 6:433
  Terson syndrome caused by, 12:95
Intracranial hypertension (increased intracranial
    pressure). See also Papilledema
  in children, 6:366
  in craniosynostosis, optic nerve abnormalities and,
    6:429
  headache caused by, 5:292
  idiopathic (pseudotumor cerebri), 5:118–120, 118t,
    6:366–367
  symptoms associated with, 5:112–113
Intracranial portion of optic nerve, 2:93, 97t, 102, 103i
  blood supply of, 2:103
Intracranial tumors, nystagmus caused by, 6:159t, 167
Intradermal nevus, 4:183, 184i, 7:170
Intraepithelial dyskeratosis, benign hereditary, 8:255t,
    309t
Intraepithelial neoplasia
  conjunctival, 4:51–52, 52i, 8:255t, 257–259, 257i,
    258i
  corneal, 4:76, 8:255t, 259, 259i
Intralenticular foreign bodies, 11:57
Intramuscular agents, in ocular pharmacology, 2:389
Intramuscular circle of the iris, 2:38–40
Intramuscular plexus, ciliary body, 2:67

Intranasal influenza vaccine, 1:305
Intranuclear inclusions, cytologic identification of, 8:69
Intraocular culture, in postoperative endophthalmitis,
    9:216
Intraocular foreign bodies. See Foreign bodies
Intraocular inflammation. See Inflammation (ocular)
Intraocular injections, 2:386–387
Intraocular lenses (IOLs), 3:213–229, 4:103, 104i. See
    also Cataract surgery
  accommodating, 3:229, 13:165, 178–180, 179i
  in adults, 11:139–156
  anterior chamber, 3:214–215, 215i, 10:132,
    11:107–108
    history of development of, 11:143
    implantation procedure for, 11:107–108, 154–155
    phakic, 11:148, 13:147–148, 148i. See also Phakic
      intraocular lenses
    preoperative gonioscopy and, 11:82
    UGH syndrome and, 3:215, 11:143, 192
  bifocal, 3:226, 11:146–147
  biometric assumptions in selection of, 3:217–221
  in children, 6:297–300, 299i, 301–302, 11:156–157,
    199–200
    visual outcomes and, 6:303
  complications of, 11:191–194
    after ICCE, 11:105
  contraindications to
    in adults, 11:155
    in children, 11:156
  corneal abnormalities and, 11:214–215, 216i
  corneal endothelial changes caused by, 8:419–420
  cystoid macular edema and, 11:173–174
  decentration of, 11:164t, 191–192, 192i
  design considerations for, 3:214, 11:143–144
    glare and, 11:194
    innovations in, 13:180
  developmentally abnormal eye and, 11:213–214
  dislocation of, 11:164t, 191–192, 192i
  flexible-loop, 11:144
  foldable, 3:213, 11:145–146
    implantation procedure for, 11:153
      in children, 6:298, 301
    instrumentation for, 11:152
    in uveitis, 9:138
  history of, 11:139–142, 140–142i
  image magnification and, 3:216
  implantation of, 11:139–156
    anterior chamber, 11:107–108, 154–155
    complications of, 11:191–194
    after ECCE, 11:111–112
    after ICCE, 11:105, 107–108
    instrumentation for, 11:152–153
    posterior chamber, 11:111–112, 153–154, 154i
    procedure for
      in adults, 11:153–155, 154i
      in children, 6:297–300, 299i, 301–302, 11:157
    secondary, 11:155
      in children, 11:200
  in infants, 6:301–302
  iritis and, 9:137
  juvenile rheumatoid arthritis–associated iridocyclitis
    and, 9:143
  in keratoconus patient, 11:214
  laser capsulotomy and, 11:190
  light-adjustable, 13:165–166, 165i, 180

multifocal, 3:225–229, 11:146–147, 13:163–164, 163*i*
  bifocal, 3:226, 11:146–147
  clinical results of, 3:228–229
  diffractive, 3:227, 228*i*
  multiple-zone, 3:226–227, 227*i*
  for presbyopia, 13:163–164, 173
multiple-zone, 3:226–227, 227*i*
nonspherical optics and, 3:224–225
optical considerations and, 3:215–221
with penetrating keratoplasty and cataract surgery
  (triple procedure), 11:208–209
phakic, 11:147–148, 13:50*t*, 143–155, 145*t*. *See also*
  Phakic intraocular lenses
  in children, 11:199–200
  penetrating keratoplasty and, 13:204
  retinal detachment and, 13:151, 192
  risks/benefits of, 13:50*t*
piggyback, 3:214, 221, 11:153
  in children, 11:200
posterior chamber, 3:215, 215*i*, 11:144–146
  for diabetic patients, 11:205
  dislocated, 12:339–340
  history of development of, 11:139–143
  implantation procedure for, 11:111–112, 153–154,
    154*i*
  phakic, 11:148, 13:148–149, 149*i*, 150*i*. *See also*
    Phakic intraocular lenses
power of
  determination of, 3:216–221, 218*i*, 220*i*
    in adults, 11:148–152
    biometric assumptions and, 3:217–218
    in children, 6:301, 11:157
    clear lens extraction/refractive lens exchange
      and, 13:160
    refractive surgery and, 3:221–222, 11:82,
      150–152, 13:65, 160, 199–203, 201*t*
    triple procedure and, 11:209
  incorrect, 11:193–194
  pupil evaluation and, 11:81
  after radial keratotomy, 13:65, 202
  in retinitis pigmentosa patient, 12:212
  for sclerocornea patient, 11:214, 216*i*
  standards for, 3:225
  toric, 11:147, 13:161–163
  traumatic cataract and, 11:228
  types of, 3:213–215, 215*i*
  in uveitis, 9:235, 236, 11:223
    postoperative inflammation and, 9:137–138, 137*i*
    uveitis-glaucoma-hyphema (UGH) syndrome and,
      9:47, 137–138, 11:143, 192
  visual disturbances related to, 3:222–224, 223*i*, 224*i*
Intraocular portion of optic nerve, 2:93, 95–101, 95*t*,
  98*i*, 99*i*, 100*i*
Intraocular pressure
  aqueous humor dynamics and, 2:305, 315, 10:23–30
  calculation of, 10:18*t*
  in central retinal vein occlusion, 12:143
  corneal thickness and, 8:11, 34
  corticosteroids affecting, 2:419–420, 419*t*
    in children, 6:320
  cycloplegics affecting, 2:401
  decreased, after cataract surgery, flat anterior
    chamber and, 11:165
  digital pressure in estimation of, 10:29
  distribution in population, 10:23–24, 23*i*

diurnal variation in, 10:25
elevated/increased. *See* Elevated intraocular pressure
factors influencing, 10:3–4, 3*i*, 24–25, 24*t*
in glaucoma, 10:3, 10, 83–84
  congenital/infantile, 6:274–275
  uveitis and, 9:237
in hyphema, 8:400, 401–402
  surgery and, 8:402, 403*t*
lowering of, in glaucoma management, 10:157. *See
  also* Antiglaucoma agents
measurement of, 10:25–29, 26*i*, 27*i*, 28*t*
  before refractive surgery, 13:44
  after refractive surgery, 13:208–209
    PRK/LASEK, 13:105, 189, 208
  as screening tool, 1:355, 356*i*
normal range for, 10:3
  in infants and children, 6:202
in ocular ischemic syndrome, 12:150
in rhegmatogenous retinal detachment, 12:268
traumatic hyphema in children and, 6:447
in uveitis, 9:103*t*, 104, 136, 237
  corticosteroids affecting, 9:238
Intraocular specimens, for endophthalmitis diagnosis,
  9:215–216, 12:328–329
Intraocular surgery. *See* Ocular (intraocular) surgery
Intraocular tumors, 1:262, 4:211. *See also specific type of
  tumor and structure affected*
  angiomatous, 4:243–249, 249*i*
  in children, 6:388–399
    choroidal and retinal pigment epithelial lesions,
      6:390, 391*i*, 392*i*
    iris and ciliary body lesions, 6:388–389, 389*i*
    leukemia and. *See* Leukemia
    retinoblastoma, 6:390–399, 393*i*,
  direct extension from extraocular tumors and, 4:275
  enucleation for, 7:119–122
  exenteration for, 7:128–129, 128*i*
  leukemia and. *See* Leukemia
  lymphoma (reticulum cell sarcoma/histiocytic [large]
    cell lymphoma/non–Hodgkin lymphoma of
    CNS), 4:277–279, 277*i*, 279*i*, 9:228–231, 228*i*,
    230*i*, 12:182–183, 182*i*
    vitreous involvement and, 4:114–115, 115*i*
  melanocytic, 4:215–242
  metastatic, 4:163–164, 163*i*, 267–275. *See also*
    Metastatic eye disease
  open-angle glaucoma caused by, 10:106
  rare, 4:283
  retinoblastoma, 4:140–144, 146*i*, 251–265, 265*t*,
    6:390–399, 393*i*, 9:232
  secondary, 4:267–275. *See also* Metastatic eye disease
  staging of, 4:285–293*t*
Intraorbital foreign bodies, 7:106
Intraorbital portion of optic nerve, 2:93, 97, 97*t*,
  101–102, 101*i*, 5:26, 7:12
  blood supply of, 2:103, 104*i*
  compressive lesions of, 5:145–151
  length of, 7:7*t*, 12
Intraorbital pressure
  in central retinal vein occlusion, 12:143
  in traumatic optic neuropathy, 7:107
Intraparenchymal hemorrhage, MRI/CT appearance of,
  5:77*t*
Intrarater reliability, 1:363

Intraretinal microvascular abnormalities (IRMAs), 4:131, 132*i*
  in nonproliferative diabetic retinopathy, 12:103, 104*i*
Intrastromal corneal ring segments, 13:23–24, 26*i*, 77–84, 78*i*, 79*t*
  complications of, 13:82–83, 83*i*
  corneal transplantation after, 13:204
  expulsion of, 13:82, 83*i*
  instrumentation for, 13:79–80, 80*t*
  and keratoconus, 13:81–82, 186
  outcomes of, 13:80–81
  patient selection for, 13:78–79
  penetrating keratoplasty after, 13:204
  risks/benefits of, 13:50*t*
  technique for, 13:80, 80*i*
Intrastromal photodisruption, 13:21*t*, 29
Intrauterine ocular infection, 6:215–221. *See also specific type*
  corneal anomalies and, 8:298–299
    keratectasia, 8:296
Intravascular ultrasound, in ischemic heart disease, 1:119
Intravenous immunoglobulin (IVIg), for cicatricial pemphigoid, 8:223
Intravenous injections, in ocular pharmacology, 2:388–389
Intraventricular block (cardiology), 1:134
Intravitreal medications, 2:387
  for branch retinal vein occlusion, 12:141
  for central retinal vein occlusion, 12:144
  corticosteroids
    for pars planitis, 9:151
    for uveitis, 9:117–118
  for cytomegalovirus retinitis, 1:29, 48, 9:252
  for postoperative endophthalmitis, 12:329, 331
Intrinsic sympathomimetic activity, beta-blocker, 1:92
Intron, 2:189, 202, 202*i*, 203
  excision of, 2:209. *See also* Splicing
Intron-A. *See* Interferons (IFNs), α
Intropin. *See* Dopamine
Intrusions, saccadic, 5:199, 204, 252–254
  with normal intersaccadic intervals, 5:252–253, 252*i*
  without normal intersaccadic intervals, 5:253
Intubation, silicone
  for acquired nasolacrimal obstruction, 7:278
  for canalicular constriction, 7:275
  for canalicular trauma, 7:277
  for congenital lacrimal duct obstruction/tearing, 6:246–247, 7:263–264, 266*i*
Intumescent cortical cataract, 11:28
  phacomorphic glaucoma and, 11:68, 68*i*
Invagination
  definition of, 2:126
  in optic development, 2:137
Invasion, as microbial virulence factor, 8:116
Inversion recovery (IR), definition of, 5:79
Inverted follicular keratosis, 4:174, 175*i*, 7:163
Inverting prism
  in operating microscope, 3:296, 297*i*
  in slit-lamp biomicroscope, 3:280, 281*i*
Invirase. *See* Saquinavir
Involutional ectropion, 7:195–198, 196*i*, 197*i*
Involutional entropion, 7:202–205, 203*i*
Involutional stenosis, nasolacrimal obstruction caused by, 7:278

IO. *See* Inferior oblique muscles
Iodine, radioactive
  for thyroid (Graves) disease, 1:225, 7:54
  for thyroid scanning, 1:223
  thyroid uptake of, 1:223
Iodine-123, 1:223
Iodine-131, 1:225
IOL. *See* Intraocular lenses
IOLMaster, 11:150
Ionic charge, of ocular medication, absorption affected by, 2:384–385
Ionizing radiation. *See also* Radiation
  anterior segment injury caused by, 8:388–389
  cataracts caused by, 11:55–56
  in free radical generation, 2:366
  tissue damage from, 2:459–465, 460*t*
Ionizing radiation. *See* Radiation
Iontophoresis, for drug delivery, 2:391
IOP. *See* Intraocular pressure
Iopidine. *See* Apraclonidine
IP. *See* Incontinentia pigmenti
IP₃. *See* Inositol-1,4,5-triphosphate
IPL. *See* Inner plexiform layer
IPM. *See* Interphotoreceptor matrix
Ipratropium, 1:157–158, 157*t*
  in combination agents, 1:157*t*
IPV (Salk vaccine), 1:304*t*, 307
  in combination vaccines, 1:309
IR. *See* Inferior rectus muscles
Irbesartan, 1:88*t*, 90*t*
IRBP. *See* Interphotoreceptor retinoid-binding protein
IRID1 gene, 10:13*t*
Iridectomy
  for bacterial keratitis, 8:184
  laser. *See also* Laser iridectomy
    for angle-closure glaucoma, 10:197–199, 198*i*
  peripheral
    for angle-closure glaucoma, 10:200
    for ICCE, 11:106–107
Irides. *See* Iris
Iridocorneal endothelial (ICE) syndrome, 4:79–80, 8:300–301, 301*i*
  glaucoma in, 10:136–138, 136*i*, 137*i*
  variants of, 10:136
Iridocyclitis, 9:106. *See also* Anterior uveitis; Iritis
  acute, 9:127–141, 127*i*, 128*i*
  in ankylosing spondylitis, 1:176
  in Behçet syndrome, 1:194, 9:133
  chronic, 9:141–146
  in coccidioidomycosis, 9:163, 226–227
  drug-induced, 9:141
  Fuchs heterochromic, 9:107, 144–146, 145*i*
    cataracts in, 11:64, 65*i*
    glaucoma and, 10:107–108, 108*i*
  herpetic, 8:150, 9:138–140
  HLA-associated diseases and, 1:177, 9:128–132
  idiopathic, 9:146
  in inflammatory bowel disease, 9:131–132
  iris nodules in, 4:219*t*
  in juvenile rheumatoid arthritis, 9:141–144, 142*i*, 144*t*
  lens-associated, 9:135–136, 135*i*, 136*i*
  in Lyme disease, 9:192, 12:191
  muscarinic antagonists for, 2:401
  in sarcoidosis, 9:198, 199*i*, 200*i*

in tuberculosis, **9:**194–195, 194*i*
in varicella, **9:**138
viral, **9:**140
Iridodialysis, **2:**62, 64*i*, **4:**25, 26*i*, 83, 83*i*, **5:**259, **8:**398
 cataract surgery and, **11:**181
 repair of, **8:**416, 418*i*
Iridodonesis
 cataract surgery and, **11:**226–227, 227*i*, 228*i*
 in dislocated lens in children, **6:**304
Iridogoniodysgenesis anomaly and syndrome. *See*
 Axenfeld-Rieger syndrome
Iridogoniodysplasia, familial glaucoma. *See* Axenfeld-
 Rieger syndrome
Iridoplasty, peripheral, for angle-closure glaucoma,
 10:199–200
Iridoplegia, familial, **6:**268
Iridotomy
 for iris bombé in uveitis, **9:**237–238
 for phakic IOL insertion, **13:**147
Iris
 abnormalities of, in infants and children, **6:**261–270
 absence of (aniridia), **4:**151, **6:**261–262, 262*i*,
  277–278, **11:**33, 34*i*
  cataract and, **6:**293*i*
  nystagmus and, **6:**162, 262
  pediatric glaucoma and, **6:**277–278
  Wilms tumor and, **6:**262, 277–278
 anatomy of, **2:**55*i*, 62–66, 62*i*, 63*i*
 anterior pigmented layer of, **2:**64, 65*i*
 atrophy of, **4:**79
  in Fuchs heterochromic iridocyclitis/uveitis,
   9:144–145, 145*i*
  in herpetic inflammation, **9:**139*i*, 140
 in Axenfeld-Rieger syndrome, **6:**253, 253*i*
 biochemistry and metabolism of, **2:**303–314
 coccidioidal granuloma of, **9:**226, 227*i*
 collarette of, **2:**64
 coloboma of, **2:**171, 171*i*, **6:**262–264, 263*i*
  cataract surgery in patients with, **11:**212, 213*i*
 color of, in infants, **6:**200
 congenital anomalies of, **2:**169–170
 cysts of, **4:**219*t*
  muscarinic therapy and, **2:**398, 400
  primary, **6:**265–266, 266*i*
  secondary, **6:**266
 development of, **2:**154–155
 dyscoria and, **6:**261
 ectropion of, congenital, **6:**269–270, 270*i*
  glaucoma in neurofibromatosis and, **6:**408
 epithelial invasion of, **4:**219*t*
 evaluation of, **5:**258–259
  before cataract surgery, **11:**82
  in glaucoma, **10:**36
   in children, **6:**275–276
  gonioscopic, **2:**59
 immunologic microenvironment of, **9:**37
 incarceration of, after penetrating keratoplasty, **8:**460
 innervation of, **2:**64
  altered, pupillary irregularity caused by, **5:**259–260
 intramuscular circle of, **2:**38–40
 juvenile xanthogranuloma affecting, **6:**264, 389, 389*i*
  leukemic involvement differentiated from, **6:**345
 in leukemia, **4:**219*t*, 221*i*, **6:**344–345, 388
 malformation of, **5:**259
 melanoma of, **4:**157, 158*i*, 217–222, 218*i*, 220*t*

metastatic disease of, **4:**220*t*, 265*i*, 269–271, 270*i*
neoplastic disorders of, **4:**156–157, 158*i*, 215–216
 in children, **6:**388–389, 389*i*
neovascularization of (rubeosis iridis), **2:**40, 61,
 4:155–156, 155*t*
 in branch retinal vein occlusion, **12:**139
 in central retinal artery occlusion, **12:**150
 in central retinal vein occlusion, **5:**107, **12:**142,
  144–145
 in diabetic patients, **12:**111
 disorders predisposing to, **10:**132, 133*t*, 134*i*, 135*i*
 in ocular ischemic syndrome, **12:**150, 151
nodules of. *See* Iris nodules
pigment epithelium of. *See* Iris pigment epithelium
pigmentation of, **2:**62, 63*i*
 development of, **2:**154–155, **6:**200
 latanoprost affecting, **2:**414
plateau, **10:**128, 129*i*, 130*i*
posterior pigmented layer of, **2:**62*i*, 64, 65*i*
 development of, **2:**154–155
prolapse of, cataract surgery and, **11:**164*t*
signal transduction in, **2:**308–310, 310–312, 312*i*,
 313*i*
stroma of, **2:**62
 cysts of, **6:**265–266
topography of, **4:**149, 150*i*
transillumination of, **6:**270
 in albinism, **6:**270, 345
traumatic damage to
 anisocoria and, **5:**265–266
 cataract surgery and, **11:**226
 iris-fixated phakic IOL insertion and, **13:**154
 repair of, **4:**22, **8:**416, 417*i*, 418*i*
in uveitis, **9:**103*t*, 104
vessels of, **2:**64
 development of, **2:**155
wound healing and, **4:**22, **8:**416, 417*i*, 418*i*
Iris bombé
 aphakic glaucoma in children and, **6:**280
 uveitis and, **9:**237–238
Iris clip intraocular lenses, **11:**140*i*, 143
 phakic, **11:**148
Iris diaphragm/iris diaphragm pattern, **2:**62
Iris dilator. *See* Dilator muscle
Iris-fixated phakic intraocular lenses, **13:**148, 149*i*
 complications of, **13:**153*t*, 154
 patient selection for, **13:**146
 results of, **13:**152*t*
Iris freckle, **4:**219*t*, 220*i*, **6:**389
Iris hypoplasia. *See* Axenfeld-Rieger syndrome
Iris mamillations/folliculi (diffuse iris nodular nevi),
 6:264–265, 265*i*
 central (pupillary) cyst rupture and, **6:**265
Iris nevus, **4:**156–157, 215–216, 215*i*, 219*t*
 in children, **6:**389
 diffuse nodular (iris mamillations), **6:**264–265, 265*i*
  central (pupillary) cyst rupture and, **6:**265
Iris nevus syndrome (Cogan-Reese syndrome), **4:**79,
 219*t*, **8:**301
Iris nodosa, in syphilis, **9:**188
Iris nodules, **4:**219–220*t*, 220–221*i*. *See also* Lisch
 nodules
 in children, **6:**264–265, 264*i*, 265*i*
  with posteior synechiae, **6:**270
 differential diagnosis of, **4:**219–220*t*

in leukemia, **4:**219*t*, 221*i*
in metastatic disease, **4:**269–271, 269*i*, 270*i*
in neurofibromatosis, **5:**337, 338*i*, **6:**264, 264*i*, 265,
   403–404, 404*i*, 408
in retinoblastoma, **4:**220*t*, 221*i*
in sarcoidosis, **4:**155, **9:**105*i*, 198, 199*i*
in syphilis, **9:**188
in uveitis, **9:**105, 105*i*
Iris papulosa, in syphilis, **9:**188
Iris pigment epithelium, **2:**62*i*, 64, 65*i*, **4:**149, 150*i*
cysts of, **4:**219*t*, 221*i*, **6:**265, 266*i*
development of, **2:**154–155
proliferation of, **4:**219*t*
Iris plane, phacoemulsification at, **11:**128
whole nucleus emulsification and, **11:**129, 129*i*, 130*i*
Iris plane lenses, **3:**214
Iris processes, **2:**53*i*, 59
Iris retractor, for cataract surgery in glaucoma patient,
   11:219, 220*i*
Iris root, gonioscopic visualization of, **2:**59
Iris roseola, in syphilis, **9:**188
Iris sphincter. *See* Sphincter muscle
Iritis, **5:**299, 333, **9:**106. *See also* Iridocyclitis
acute, **9:**127–141, 127*i*, 128*i*
in ankylosing spondylitis, **9:**129
after anterior chamber phakic IOL insertion, **13:**151
in Behçet syndrome, **9:**132, 133, 133*i*, **12:**181
chronic, lens epithelium affected in, **4:**98–99, 99*i*
drug-induced, **9:**141
in glaucomatocyclitic crisis (Posner-Schlossman
   syndrome), **9:**135
in herpetic disease, **9:**138–140
HLA-associated diseases and, **9:**128–132
in inflammatory bowel disease, **9:**131–132
intraocular lenses and, **9:**137
after iris-fixated phakic IOL insertion, **13:**154
lens-associated, **9:**135–136, 136*i*
muscarinic antagonists for, **2:**401
in psoriatic arthritis, **9:**132
in reactive arthritis/Reiter syndrome, **8:**228, **9:**131
in syphilis, **9:**187, 188
traumatic, **8:**397–398
in tuberculosis, **9:**194–195, 194*i*
in varicella, **9:**138
viral, **9:**140
treatment of, **9:**140
Iritis. *See* Anterior uveitis; Iridocyclitis
IRMAs. *See* Intraretinal microvascular abnormalities
Iron
in aqueous humor, **2:**317
corneal deposits of, **8:**377*t*, 378
in keratoconus, **8:**330
foreign body of, **8:**377*t*, 378, 406, 406*i*
siderosis caused by, **4:**99, **11:**58, 59*i*, **12:**299, 299*t*
Iron deficiency anemia, **1:**161
anemia of chronic disease differentiated from, **1:**159
treatment of, **1:**159, 161
Iron dextran, **1:**159, 161
Iron lines, **4:**74, **8:**377*t*, 378
in pterygium, **8:**366, 366*i*
Irradiance, **2:**460, 460*t*, **3:**14, 16*t*
effective, **2:**462
as image characteristic, **3:**39
for medical lasers, **3:**18*t*, 19

Irregular astigmatism, **3:**118, 170–171, 236–242, 242*i*.
   See also Wavefront aberrations
chalazia causing, **3:**170
corneal topography in detection/management of,
   8:46, 48, **13:**9, 10–11
keratorefractive surgery and, **3:**241–242, **13:**10–11,
   47, 48*i*
after penetrating keratoplasty, refractive surgery for,
   13:187–189
retinoscopy in detection of, **3:**133, **8:**49
wavefront analysis and, **3:**237–240, 237*i*, 238*i*, 239*i*,
   240*i*, 241*i*, 318–320, 319*i*, 321*i*, 322*i*, **8:**49,
   13:13–17. *See also* Wavefront analysis
Irrigation. *See also* Ophthalmic irrigants
for chemical injuries, **8:**391
for conjunctival foreign body, **8:**404
in ECCE, **11:**109
of lacrimal drainage system
for acquired tearing evaluation, **7:**270–271, 270*t*
for canalicular obstruction, **7:**270–271, 270*t*, 271*i*,
   275
for congenital tearing management, **7:**262–263,
   264*i*
in phacoemulsification, **11:**118, 137
with toxic solutions, corneal edema caused by,
   11:168
for plant materials, **8:**396
solutions for, **2:**451
endothelial changes caused by, **8:**420
IRS. *See* Immune reconstitution syndromes
IRVAN. *See* Idiopathic retinal vasculitis/aneurysms/
   neuroretinitis
Irvine-Gass syndrome, **11:**172, **12:**154, 288
ISA. *See* Intrinsic sympathomimetic activity
Ischemia
cardiac. *See* Ischemic heart disease
carotid territory, **5:**177
evaluation of, **5:**179–180
cataracts caused by, **11:**69
cerebral, **1:**101–105. *See also* Stroke
choroidal, **12:**166–167, 167*i*, 168*i*, 169*i*
macular, in diabetes, **12:**116
occipital, transient visual loss caused by, **5:**185–186
ocular (ocular ischemic syndrome), **5:**183–184, 184*i*,
   9:221–222, **12:**150–152, 151*i*
carotid artery disease and, **1:**107
retinal neovascularization in diabetes and,
   12:102–112
Ischemic heart disease, **1:**111–125. *See also* Acute
   coronary syndrome; Angina pectoris
asymptomatic patients with, **1:**116
clinical syndromes in, **1:**113–116
in diabetes, **1:**218
diagnosis of
invasive procedures for, **1:**119–120
noninvasive procedures for, **1:**116–119
heart failure and, **1:**127, 128
hypercholesterolemia and, **1:**143, 143–144
hypertension management in, **1:**91*t*, 94
management of, **1:**120–125
pathophysiology of, **1:**112
risk factors for, **1:**112–113
screening for, **1:**293–294

Ischemic optic neuropathy
    anterior, 5:120–124, 121*t*, 347
        arteritic, 5:120–122, 121*i*, 121*t*
        nonarteritic, 5:121*t*, 122–124, 123*i*, 124*t*
        in giant cell arteritis, 1:190, 5:120–122
        posterior, 5:155
Ischemic theory, of glaucomatous optic nerve damage,
    10:51
Iseikonic spectacles, 3:145
Ishihara color plates, 12:43
Island of vision, in low vision evaluation, 5:91
Islet cells, injection of, for diabetes, 1:214
Ismelin. *See* Guanethidine
Ismotic. *See* Isosorbide
Isoantibody production, posttransfusion, 1:167
Isochromosomes, 2:189
Isoflurophate, 2:396*i*
Isoforms, 2:209
Isolated stromal rejection, 8:468. *See also* Rejection
    (graft)
Isolation techniques, in ocular microbiology, 8:136
Isoniazid, 1:24, 49
    pharmacogenetics of, 2:279
Isopter, 5:91, **10**:60
Isoptin. *See* Verapamil
Isopto Atropine. *See* Atropine
Isopto Carbachol. *See* Carbachol
Isopto Carpine. *See* Pilocarpine
Isopto Cetamide. *See* Sulfacetamide
Isopto Eserine. *See* Physostigmine
Isopto Homatropine. *See* Homatropine
Isopto Hyoscine. *See* Scopolamine
Isosorbide, 2:416
Isospora belli (isosporiasis), in HIV infection/AIDS,
    1:48, 49
Isotretinoin
    ocular effects of, 1:324*t*
    retinopathy caused by, 12:250
Isotypes, 9:7, 54–55
    in immunologic tolerance, 9:89
Isradipine, 1:89*i*
ITP. *See* Idiopathic thrombocytopenic purpura
Itraconazole, 1:25, 64*t*, 75–76, 2:438*t*, 439
    for aspergillosis, 5:365
    for endophthalmitis, 9:218*t*
    for fungal keratitis, 8:186–187
Ivermectin
    for loiasis, 8:191
    for onchocerciasis, 9:196–197
IVIg. *See* Intravenous immunoglobulin
Ixodes ticks, Lyme disease transmitted by, 1:18–19,
    9:191

J

J-loop intraocular lenses, **11**:142*i*
Jabs and jolts syndrome, 5:297
Jackson cross cylinder, for refraction, 3:136–139, 138*i*
Jaeger numbers, 3:251
Janetta procedure, for hemifacial spasm, 5:289
Jansen disease, 12:283
Jansky-Bielschowsky disease/syndrome, 6:437*t*, 12:233*t*,
    241
Japanese encephalitis vaccine, 1:309

Jarisch-Herxheimer reaction, in Lyme disease
    treatment, 1:21
Javal-Schiøtz keratometers, 3:300, 300*i*, 301*i*
Jaw thrust, modified, for opening airway, 1:314
Jaw-winking ptosis/syndrome, Marcus Gunn, 5:276,
    277*i*, 279, 281, 6:214, 7:217, 218*i*
    synkinesis in, 6:214, 7:211, 217, 218*i*
JC virus, in progressive multifocal
    leukoencephalopathy, 5:362
Jerk nystagmus, 5:239, 6:159, 160, 165, 166*i*. *See also*
    Nystagmus
JIA. *See* Juvenile idiopathic (chronic/rheumatoid)
    arthritis
Jones I and Jones II tests, 7:268–270, 269*t*
Josamycin, 1:60*t*, 71
Joule, laser energy reading in, 3:18*t*, 19
JRA. *See* Juvenile idiopathic (chronic/rheumatoid)
    arthritis
Jugular bulb, 5:22
Jugular veins
    external, 5:23
    eyelids drained by, 8:7
    venous sinuses draining into, 2:119, 120*i*
Junction (contact lens), 3:174*i*
Junctional complexes
    in corneal endothelium, 2:48–49
    in retinal pigment epithelium, 2:78
Junctional complexes (cardiac arrhythmia), premature
    (PJCs), 1:135
Junctional nevus, 7:170–171
    of conjunctiva, in children, 6:387
Junctional rhythm, atrioventricular, 1:133
Junctional tachycardia, 1:137
Junk DNA, 2:203
Juvenile ankylosing spondylitis, 1:178
Juvenile epithelial dystrophy (Meesmann dystrophy),
    8:310*t*, 313, 314*i*
Juvenile fibroma/fibromatosis, of orbit, 4:200, 6:380
Juvenile glaucoma. *See* Glaucoma, childhood
Juvenile idiopathic (chronic/rheumatoid) arthritis,
    1:178–179, 6:312–315, 9:141–144, 142*i*, 144*t*
    cataract and, 9:142, 142*i*, 143
    criteria for, 6:313, 313*t*
    eye examination schedule for children with, 6:315,
        316*t*
    HLA association in, 9:94*t*, 141
    iridocyclitis in, 9:141–144, 142*i*, 144*t*
    management of, 9:143–144
    nomenclature for, 6:312–313, 313*t*
    pauciarticular, 9:141, 144*t*
    polyarticular, 9:141, 144*t*
    systemic onset (Still disease), 1:178–179, 9:141, 144*t*
    uveitis in, 6:311, 313–315, 313*t*, 314*i*, 9:107,
        141–144, 142*i*, 144*t*
Juvenile macular degeneration (Stargardt disease/
    fundus flavimaculatus), 6:337–339, 338*i*, 339*i*,
    12:216–218, 216*i*, 217*i*, 217*t*
    cone–rod dystrophy and, 6:338, 12:215
    retinal pigment epithelium in, 2:363
    rod ABC transporter mutations causing, 2:349
Juvenile nephronophthisis, retinal degeneration and,
    12:236
Juvenile-onset diabetes mellitus. *See* Diabetes mellitus,
    type 1
Juvenile-onset (developmental) myopia, 3:120–122, 146

Juvenile open-angle glaucoma. *See* Glaucoma, childhood
Juvenile pilocytic astrocytoma, of optic nerve, **4:**208, 209*i*
Juvenile retinoschisis. *See* Retinoschisis, X-linked
Juvenile rheumatoid arthritis, **6:**312. *See also* Juvenile idiopathic (chronic/rheumatoid) arthritis
Juvenile spondyloarthropathy, **1:**178
Juvenile systemic granulomatosis (Blau syndrome), **6:**318
Juvenile xanthogranuloma (nevoxanthoendothelioma), **6:**389, 389*i*, **8:**271, **9:**233
  glaucoma associated with, **10:**32
  of iris, **4:**219*t*, **6:**264, 389, 389*i*
    leukemic involvement differentiated from, **6:**345
  of orbit, **7:**88–89
  uveitis in children differentiated from, **6:**320*t*
Juxtacanalicular tissue, **2:**56, 57*i*
Juxtafoveal/parafoveal retinal telangiectasis, **4:**121–122, **12:**157–158, 158*i*, 159*i*
JXG. *See* Juvenile xanthogranuloma

K

K. *See* Potassium
K readings, **3:**175, 232, 234
K system (koniocellular system), **6:**45, 46
  development of, **6:**46
Kaletra. *See* Lopinavir/ritonavir
Kallikrein, **9:**76
Kalt forceps, **11:**91, 92*i*
Kanamycin, **1:**70, **2:**428*t*, 435
  ototoxicity of, mitochondrial DNA mutations and, **2:**220
Kandori, fleck retina of, **12:**200
Kaposi sarcoma, **8:**162, 270*t*, 272, 272*i*
  of eyelid, **7:**183, 183*i*
  human herpes virus 8 causing, **8:**162, 272
  ocular adnexal, **9:**258–259, 259*i*
  treatment of, **1:**50
  viral carcinogenesis and, **1:**254, **8:**162, 272
Kaposi sarcoma–associated herpesvirus/human herpes virus 8, **8:**162, 272
Kappa (κ) statistic, **1:**364
Karyotype, **2:**189, 247, 248*i*
Kasabach-Merritt syndrome, **6:**377, **7:**66
Kawasaki syndrome (mucocutaneous lymph node syndrome/infantile periarteritis nodosa), **1:**189*t*, **6:**238
Kayser-Fleischer ring, **4:**74, **6:**260, **8:**356, 356*i*, 377*t*, **11:**62
kb. *See* Kilobase
KC. *See* Keratoconus
KCS (keratoconjunctivitis sicca). *See* Dry eye syndrome
Kearns-Sayre syndrome, **5:**334, 335*i*, **6:**150, **12:**245, 246*t*, 247*i*
  mitochondrial DNA deletions and, **2:**218
Keflex. *See* Cephalexin
Kefurox. *See* Cefuroxime
Kefzol. *See* Cefazolin
Kelman intraocular lens, **11:**141*i*, 143
Keloids, corneal, **8:**373
  congenital, **8:**299
Kenalog. *See* Triamcinolone

Keplerian telescope, **3:**82–84, 83*i*
Keppra. *See* Levetiracetam
KERA gene, in cornea plana, **8:**291
Keratan sulfate
  in cornea, **2:**300, **8:**10
  macular dystrophy and, **8:**320
  mucopolysaccharidoses and, **8:**335–336
  mutation in gene for, in cornea plana, **8:**291
Keratectasia, **8:**296
  after LASIK, **13:**131–132
Keratectomy, **8:**440–441, **13:**21–22*t*
  hexagonal, **13:**66
  laser, **13:**21*t*. *See also* Photorefractive keratectomy
  mechanical, **8:**440
  multizone, **13:**25–26, 26*i*
  photorefractive (PRK). *See* Photorefractive keratectomy
  phototherapeutic (PTK), **8:**440
    for calcific band keratopathy, **8:**374
    for corneal epithelial basement membrane dystrophy, **8:**313
    lasers approved for, **13:**32*t*, 33*t*
    for recurrent corneal erosions, **8:**100
  superficial, **8:**440–441
Keratic precipitates, **8:**29, **9:**104, 105*i*
  in sarcoidosis, **9:**105*i*, 198, 199*i*
  stellate
    in Fuchs heterochromic iridocyclitis/uveitis, **9:**145, 145*i*
    in herpetic ocular infection, **9:**139
  in uveitis, **9:**104, 105*i*, 127
Keratinization (keratinized/degenerated epithelial cells), **8:**23
  cytologic identification of, **8:**64, 65*i*, 67*i*
    in immune-mediated keratoconjunctivitis, **8:**203*t*
  in meibomian gland dysfunction, **8:**80
  in vitamin A deficiency, **8:**93
Keratinocytes, **8:**245
  stromal, corneal haze after PRK and, **13:**104
Keratinoid degeneration, **8:**368–369. *See also* Spheroidal degeneration
Keratitis, **5:**299, **8:**24–25*t*, 26–29, 30*i*, 31*i*, 32*i*, 32*t*
  Acanthamoeba, **4:**66, 67*i*, **8:**119*t*, 131, 187–189, 188*i*. *See also* Acanthamoeba
    contact lens wear and, **3:**207, **4:**66, 67*i*, **8:**187
    herpes simplex keratitis differentiated from, **8:**188–189
    stains and culture media for identification of, **8:**137*t*
    treatment of, **2:**444–445, **8:**188–189
  autosomal dominant, **8:**309*t*
  bacterial, **4:**65–66, **8:**51*t*, 179–185. *See also* Keratitis, infectious/microbial
    clinical presentation of, **8:**179–180, 180*i*, 181*i*
    contact lens wear and, **8:**179
      after radial keratotomy, **13:**206
    after intrastromal corneal ring segment placement, **13:**81, 82*i*
    intrauterine, **8:**298–299
    laboratory evaluation/causes of, **8:**180–181, 181*t*
    management of, **8:**181–184, 182*t*
    pathogenesis of, **8:**179
    after radial keratotomy, **13:**64
    stains and culture media for identification of, **8:**137*t*

Candida causing, **8**:119*t*
in Cogan syndrome, **8**:228, 229
dendritic
    contact lens wear and, **3**:208
    herpes simplex virus causing, **8**:143, 143*i*, 144*i*,
        145*i*, 146
    herpes zoster causing, **8**:154
diffuse lamellar/interface (DLK), after LASIK,
    13:127, 128*i*, 129*t*
disciform, herpes simplex virus causing, **8**:147, 147*i*
epithelial
    adenoviral, **8**:158, 160*i*
    herpes simplex virus causing, **8**:143–146, 143*i*,
        144*i*, 145*i*
    measles virus causing, **8**:162
    varicella-zoster virus causing, **8**:154
Epstein-Barr virus causing, **8**:156–157, 156*i*
exposure, **8**:94–95
    in craniosynostosis-induced proptosis, **6**:427–428
Fuchs superficial marginal, **8**:371
fungal, **4**:66, 66*i*, **8**:185–187, 186*i*
gonococcal conjunctivitis and, **8**:171
herpes simplex, **4**:65–66, 66*i*, **8**:51*t*, 119*t*
    Acanthamoeba keratitis differentiated from,
        8:188–189
    complications of, **8**:151
    in HIV infection/AIDS, **9**:260, 260*i*
    in infants and children, **6**:219, 227, 227*i*
    after LASIK, **13**:185–186
    neurotrophic keratopathy/ulcers caused by, **8**:103,
        103*i*, 151
    after PRK, **13**:185
    refractive surgery in patient with, **13**:185–186
    topical antiviral agents for, **2**:439, 440*t*
herpes zoster, **8**:154, 154*i*, 155*i*
in HIV infection/AIDS, **8**:190, **9**:260, 260*i*
infectious/microbial, **8**:119*t*. *See also specific infectious
    agent*
    after LASIK, **13**:128–129, 129*i*, 185–186
    after penetrating keratoplasty, **8**:463–464
    stains and culture in identification of, **8**:137*t*
interstitial
    herpetic, **8**:146–147, 146*i*
    in infectious disease, **8**:226–227, 227*i*
    syphilitic, **6**:220, 260, 260*i*, **8**:226–227, 227*i*, 299,
        9:187–188, 188*i*
intrauterine, **8**:298–299
    keratectasia caused by, **8**:296
measles virus causing, **8**:162
Microsporida causing, **8**:190, **9**:260, 260*i*
necrotizing, herpes simplex causing, **8**:147–148, 148*i*,
    150
NSAID use and, **1**:197–198
in onchocerciasis, **8**:132
peripheral, **8**:32*t*
    differential diagnosis of, **8**:230*t*
    Mooren ulcer and, **8**:231, 232–234, 233*i*, 234*i*
    scleritis and, **8**:239
    in systemic immune-mediated diseases, **8**:203,
        229–232, 230*t*, 232*i*
    in Wegener granulomatosis, **1**:192
punctate, **8**:24*t*, 29, 30*i*, 32*t*
    contact lens wear and, **3**:208
in reactive arthritis/Reiter syndrome, **8**:228, **9**:131
in rosacea, **8**:84–85, 84*i*, 85*i*, 86

sicca. *See* Dry eye syndrome
staphylococcal, **8**:165–168, 166*i*, 167*i*, 179
stromal
    in Cogan syndrome, **8**:228, 229
    Epstein-Barr virus causing, **8**:156–157, 156*i*
    herpes simplex virus causing, **8**:146–150, 146*i*,
        147*i*, 148*i*, 149*t*
        penetrating keratoplasty for, **8**:151
    in herpes zoster ophthalmicus, **8**:154, 154*i*, 155*i*
    microsporidial, **8**:190
    necrotizing, **8**:147–148, 148*i*, 150
    nonnecrotizing, **8**:146–147, 146*i*, 147*i*
    nonsuppurative, **8**:25*t*, 29, 31*i*, 32*t*
        systemic infections and, **8**:189–190
    scleritis and, **8**:239
    suppurative, **8**:25*t*, 29, 31*i*, 32*t*
    syphilitic, **8**:227
syphilitic, **4**:67, **6**:220, 260, 260*i*, **8**:226–227, 227*i*,
    299, **9**:187–188, 188*i*
Thygeson superficial punctate, **8**:224–225, 225*i*
toxic, **8**:394. *See also* Toxic conjunctivitis/
    keratoconjunctivitis
ulcerative, **8**:362
    differential diagnosis of, **8**:230*t*
    Mooren ulcer and, **8**:231, 232–234, 233*i*, 234*i*
    in rosacea, **8**:86
    in systemic immune-mediated diseases, **8**:203,
        229–232, 230*t*, 232*i*
varicella-zoster virus causing, **8**:151–156, 154*i*, 155*i*
yeasts causing, **8**:185, 186
Keratoacanthoma, **4**:175–176, 176*i*, **7**:173, 173*i*
    conjunctival, **8**:256
Keratoconjunctivitis
    adenoviral, **8**:158, 158*i*, 159, 159*i*, 160*i*
    atopic, **6**:235, **8**:211–213, 212*i*, 213*i*, **9**:74
    chlamydial, **8**:174
    contact lens superior limbic (CLSLK), **3**:208
    epidemic, **8**:158, 158*i*, 159, 159*i*, 160*i*
        in children, **6**:225–226
            preseptal cellulitis caused by, **6**:230
    immune-mediated, ocular surface cytology in, **8**:203,
        203*t*
    microsporidial, **8**:190
    phlyctenular, in children, **6**:388
    sicca. *See* Aqueous tear deficiency; Dry eye syndrome
    superior limbic, **8**:96–98, 97*i*
    toxic
        contact lens solutions causing, **8**:107
        medications causing, **8**:393–395
    vernal, **8**:209–211, 209*i*, 210*i*, **9**:13
        in children, **6**:234–235, 235*i*
Keratoconus, **4**:70, 71*i*, **6**:250, **8**:329–332, 329*i*, 330*i*,
    331*i*, 334*i*, 334*t*
    corneal abnormalities and, **3**:199–200, 200*i*
    corneal contact lenses for, **3**:202
    Descemet's membrane rupture and, **4**:27*i*, 70, 71*i*
    epikeratoplasty (epikeratophakia) for, **13**:75–76, 186
    Fleischer ring in, **8**:330, 331*i*, 377*t*, 378
    in floppy eyelid syndrome, **8**:95–96
    inherited, **8**:310*t*, 329
    intraocular lens implantation and, **11**:214
    intrastromal corneal ring segments and, **13**:81–82,
        186
    keratotomy for, **13**:59
    Marfan syndrome and, **8**:354

posterior (internal ulcer of von Hippel), **2:**168, 169, **4:**64, 64*i*
central (posterior corneal depression), **6:**254
circumscribed, **8:**294, 294*i*, 295*i*
intrauterine keratitis and, **8:**298–299
refractive surgery contraindicated in, **8:**46–47, 47*i*, **13:**44, 186–187
corneal topography in detection of, **13:**9, 12, 47
scleral lenses for, **3:**202
thermokeratoplasty for, **13:**137
in vernal keratoconjunctivitis, **8:**210
Keratocytes, **2:**47, 151, 152*i*, 300, **8:**10, 10*i*, 11*i*
in wound healing/repair, **8:**384
Keratoepithelin, gene responsible for formation of. *See BIGH3* (keratoepithelin) gene
Keratoglobus, **6:**250, **8:**334–335, 334*i*, 334*t*
Keratoiritis, in herpetic disease, **9:**138–140
Keratolimbal allograft, **8:**423*t*, 433. *See also* Limbal transplantation
Keratolysis (corneal melting)
cataract surgery and, **11:**180–181
in patients with dry eye, **11:**180, 206–207
peripheral ulcerative keratitis and, **8:**231
Keratomalacia, in vitamin A deficiency, **8:**93
Keratome, scleral tunnel incision and, **11:**123
Keratometry, **3:**298–302, 298*i*, 299*i*, 300*i*, 301*i*, **8:**40–41, **13:**5. *See also* K readings
before cataract surgery, **11:**82, 207
IOL power determination and, **11:**149
errors in, **11:**193–194
refractive surgery and, **11:**150–151
in IOL selection, **3:**218
for refractive surgery, IOL power calculation and, **13:**200
values for in infants and children, **6:**199, 201*i*
Keratomileusis, **13:**20*t*, 23, 106. *See also* Laser in situ keratomileusis (LASIK); Laser subepithelial keratomileusis (LASEK)
in situ, **13:**20*t*, 106. *See also* Automated lamellar keratoplasty/automated lamellar therapeutic keratoplasty; Laser in situ keratomileusis (LASIK)
Keratopathy
actinic (Labrador keratopathy/spheroidal degeneration), **4:**68, 69*i*, **8:**368–369
annular, traumatic, **8:**396
band, **4:**67–68, 68*i*
calcific (calcium hydroxyapatite deposition), **8:**356, 373–374, 374*i*
in sarcoidosis, **8:**88
in juvenile idiopathic (chronic/rheumatoid) arthritis, **6:**314, 314*i*, **9:**142, 142*i*, 143
surgery for, **6:**322
bullous, **4:**68–69, 70*i*
after cataract surgery, **11:**164*t*, 192–193, 193*i*
disciform keratitis and, **8:**151
flexible contact lenses for, **3:**202
climatic droplet, **8:**368–369. *See also* Spheroidal degeneration
drug-related, **4:**70
exposure, **8:**94–95
filamentary, **8:**72*i*, 73*i*, 75–76
infectious crystalline, **8:**180, 181*i*
after penetrating keratoplasty, **8:**464, 464*i*
Labrador, **4:**68, 69*i*, **8:**368–369

lipid, **8:**373
in herpes zoster ophthalmicus, **8:**154, 155*i*
measles, **8:**162
medications causing, **8:**393–395
neurotrophic, **8:**102–104, 103*i*
diabetic neuropathy and, **8:**102
esthesiometry in evaluation of, **8:**35
herpetic eye disease and, **8:**102–103, 103*i*, 151, 153, 154
punctate epithelial, **8:**24*t*, 29, 30*i*, 32*t*
exposure causing, **8:**95
microsporidial, **8:**190
staphylococcal blepharoconjunctivitis and, **8:**165, 166*i*, 168
topical anesthetic abuse causing, **8:**105
striate, intraocular surgery causing, **8:**419
toxic ulcerative, **8:**101–102, 375–376
vortex (hurricane), **8:**394
Keratophakia, **13:**23, 71–73, 73*i*
Keratoplasty
conductive, **13:**27–28, 28*i*, 50*t*, 139–142, 140*i*, 141*i*, 141*t*, 142*i*
penetrating keratoplasty after, **13:**204
for presbyopia, **13:**173
risks/benefits of, **13:**50*t*
Descemet membrane stripping (DSEK), **8:**476
for infantile corneal opacities, **6:**257–258
lamellar, **8:**472–476, 473*i*
advantages of, **8:**474
automated (automated therapeutic), **8:**472, **13:**107
deep anterior (DALK), **8:**472, 475
deep endothelial (DLEK), **8:**472, 475
disadvantages of, **8:**474
endothelial (ELK), **8:**475
indications for, **8:**472–473, 473*i*
posterior, **8:**475–476
postoperative care and complications and, **8:**474–475
rejection and, **8:**475
surgical technique for, **8:**474
wound healing/repair and, **13:**28, 29
penetrating, **8:**453–470, 453*t*, 465*t*, **13:**22*t*
for *Acanthamoeba* keratitis, **8:**189
astigmatism after
arcuate keratotomy for, **13:**66, 67*i*, 68, 187
control of, **8:**464–466, 465*t*, 467*i*
corneal topography in management of, **13:**12
refractive surgery for, **13:**187–189
for bacterial keratitis, **8:**184
cataract surgery following, **11:**209–211
cataract surgery and IOL implantation combined with (triple procedure), **11:**208–209
in children, **8:**470–471, 470*t*
for cicatricial pemphigoid, **8:**223
complications of
in children, **8:**470–471
intraoperative, **8:**460
postoperative, **8:**460–464
conjunctival flap removal and, **8:**438
for corneal changes in mucopolysaccharidoses, **8:**336
corneal topography after, **13:**12
donor cornea preparation in, **8:**455
endophthalmitis after, **9:**207
glaucoma after, **8:**460–461, **10:**116, 116*t*

graft placement and, **8**:456
graft rejection and, **8**:466–470, 468*i*, 469*i*, **9**:41
for herpetic keratitis complications, **8**:151
indications for, **8**:453–454, 453*t*
for keratoconus, **8**:332
for keratoglobus, **8**:335
for neurotrophic keratopathy, **8**:104, 151
for pellucid marginal degeneration, **8**:333
for peripheral ulcerative keratitis, **8**:232
postoperative care and, **8**:460–464
preoperative evaluation and preparation and,
    8:454
procedures combined with, **8**:459
after radial keratotomy, **13**:65, 203
recipient eye preparation and, **8**:455–456
recurrence of primary disease after, **8**:461, 462*i*
refractive aspects of, **8**:465*t*
refractive error after, control of, **8**:464–466, 465*t*
after refractive surgery, **13**:203–204
refractive surgery after, **13**:187–189, 187*i*
in rosacea patients, **8**:86
for Stevens-Johnson syndrome, **8**:218–219
surgical technique for, **8**:455–459, 457*i*, 458*i*, 459*i*
suturing techniques for, **8**:455–459, 457*i*, 458*i*,
    459*i*
    postoperative problems and, **8**:462–463, 462*i*,
        463*i*
tectonic
    for herpetic keratitis complications, **8**:151
    for keratoglobus, **8**:335
    for peripheral ulcerative keratitis, **8**:232
radial thermal, **13**:137–138
Keratoprosthesis
for chemical burns, **8**:393
for cicatricial pemphigoid, **8**:223
Cobo irrigating, **8**:471
with penetrating keratoplasty, **8**:459
for Stevens-Johnson syndrome, **8**:219
Keratorefractive surgery (KRS). *See also specific
    procedure*
basic science of, **13**:5–30
cataract/cataract surgery and, **11**:211, **13**:173
    intraocular lens power calculation and, **11**:82,
        150–152
classification of, **13**:19, 20–22*t*
contact lens use after, **13**:204–208
    fitting and, **3**:202, 203*i*, **13**:205–208
corneal biomechanics affected by, **8**:13, 14*i*, **13**:19–28
corneal shape and, **13**:5–6
corneal topography and, **8**:46–48, 47*i*, 48*i*, **13**:6–12,
    47, 48*i*
    indications for, **13**:9–10, 9*i*
corneal transplant after, **13**:203–204
corneal wound healing and, **13**:28–29
glaucoma after, **13**:208–209
in glaucoma patient, **13**:189–191, 190*i*
for induced anisophoria, **3**:162
intraocular lens power calculations after, **3**:221–222,
    13:65, 160, 199–203, 201*t*
iron lines associated with, **8**:378
irregular astigmatism and, **3**:102
    corneal topography in detection/management of,
        8:46, 48
laser biophysics and, **13**:29–30
laser–tissue interactions and, **13**:29

in ocular hypertension patient, **13**:189–191, 190*i*
in ocular and systemic disease, **13**:183–198. *See also
    specific disorder*
optical considerations in, **3**:231–242, **13**:5–30
patient expectations and, **13**:39–40
after penetrating keratoplasty, **13**:187–189, 187*i*
penetrating keratoplasty after, **13**:203–204
postoperative considerations and, **13**:199–209
preoperative evaluation for, **13**:39–56, 40*t*
retinal detachment after, **13**:203
risks/benefits of, discussion of with patient,
    13:49–50, 50*t*. *See also* Informed consent
wavefront aberrations after, **13**:13–17
Keratoscopy, **8**:41, 41*i*
computerized, **8**:41–46, 42*i*, 43*i*, 44*i*, 45*i*, 46*i*, **13**:6
photographic, **3**:302–303, **8**:41
Keratosis, **8**:24*t*
actinic (solar), **4**:176–177, 177*i*, **7**:172–173, 172*i*
inverted follicular, **4**:174, 175*i*, **7**:163
seborrheic, **4**:174–175, 175*i*, **7**:163, 165*i*
Keratosteepening, contact lens assisted,
    pharmacologically induced (CLAPIKS), **13**:207–208
Keratotomy, **13**:21*t*
arcuate, **13**:21*t*, 66, 68–69
    after penetrating keratoplasty, **13**:66, 67*i*, 68, 187
astigmatic, **13**:21*t*, 66–69, 67*i*, 69*t*
    for astigmatism/refractive errors after penetrating
        keratoplasty, **8**:465*t*, 466
    cataract surgery and, **11**:102–103
    wound healing/repair and, **13**:28
hexagonal, **13**:66
radial. *See* Radial keratotomy
transverse, **13**:21*t*, 66–67, 67*i*
Keratouveitis, **9**:107
in congenital syphilis, **9**:187, 188*i*
Kerlone. *See* Betaxolol
Kestenbaum-Anderson procedure, **5**:255, **6**:168–170,
    170*i*
Ketek. *See* Telithromycin
Ketoacidosis, diabetic, **1**:216
Ketoconazole, **1**:64*t*, **2**:438*t*, 439
for endophthalmitis, **9**:218*t*
for keratitis, **8**:186
Ketolides, **1**:60*t*, 71, 75
Ketoprofen, **1**:197*t*, **2**:421*t*
Ketorolac tromethamine, **1**:196–197, **2**:307, 417*t*,
    422–423, 424*t*
for cystoid macular edema, **11**:174, **12**:155
for ocular allergy, **6**:236
perioperative, **1**:332*t*, 338
for postoperative pain, **1**:197, 338
for recurrent corneal erosions, **8**:99
Ketotifen, **2**:424*t*, 425
Keyhole pupil (iris coloboma), **2**:171, 171*i*, **6**:262–264,
    263*i*
Khodadoust line, **8**:468, 469*i*, **9**:39, 40*i*
KID syndrome, **8**:89
Kidneys, scleroderma (scleroderma renal crisis), **1**:185
Killer cells, **8**:200
in antibody-dependent cellular cytotoxicity, **9**:72
lymphokine-activated, **9**:66–70
natural, **9**:70
    in viral conjunctivitis, **9**:35
Kilobase, **2**:189
Kineret. *See* Anakinra

Kinetic perimetry, **3**:252, **5**:90–91, **10**:57, 58*i*
  in glaucoma, **10**:57, 58*i*
  in vision rehabilitation, **3**:252
Kinetic testing, definition of, **10**:59
Kininogens, **9**:76
Kinins, **8**:198*t*, **9**:76
"Kissing" nevi, **4**:182, 182*i*
Klebsiella, **8**:126
Klippel-Trénaunay-Weber syndrome, **5**:335, 340, **6**:415
  glaucoma associated with, **10**:32
KM. *See* Keratomileusis
KM-1, **1**:42
K_m (Michaelis/affinity constant), "sugar" cataract
  development and, **11**:14–16
Knapp procedure
  inverse, for inferior rectus muscle paresis in orbital
    floor fracture, **6**:140
  for monocular elevation deficiency (double elevator
    palsy), **6**:138
Knapp's law, **3**:80–81, 81*i*
Knockout mutation, **2**:234–237, 236*i*
Koeppe lens/Koeppe-type lenses, for gonioscopy, **10**:38
  in congenital/infantile glaucoma, **6**:275
Koeppe nodules
  in iridocyclitis, **4**:219*t*
  in sarcoidosis, **4**:155, **9**:105*i*, 198, 199*i*
    in children, posterior synechiae and, **6**:270
  in uveitis, **9**:105, 105*i*
Koganei, clump cells of, **4**:149
Koniocellular (K) system, **6**:45, 46
  development of, **6**:46
KP. *See* Keratic precipitates
Krabbe disease/leukodystrophy, **2**:262*t*, **6**:436*t*
Krause, glands of, **2**:24*i*, 29*t*, 34, 290, **4**:168*t*, **7**:140*i*,
  145, 253
  aqueous component/tears secreted by, **8**:56
Krill disease (acute retinal pigment epitheliitis/ARPE),
  9:177*t*, 178, 179*i*
Krimsky test, **6**:82–83, 84*i*
  for dissociated vertical deviation, **6**:131
KRS. *See* Keratorefractive surgery
Krukenberg spindles, **4**:73, 76*i*, 84, 85*i*, **8**:375, 377*t*,
  10:101, 101*i*
Krumeich, guided trephine system of, **8**:456
Krypton fluoride excimer laser, **3**:23. *See also* Lasers
Krypton laser, **3**:22–23. *See also* Lasers
KSHV. *See* Kaposi sarcoma–associated herpesvirus
Kufs disease, **6**:437*t*
Kyphosis
  cataract surgery in patients with, **11**:203
  in osteoporosis, **1**:242

L

L-cone opsin genes, **2**:346, 346*i*, 347
  mutations in, **2**:346, 346*i*, 350
L cones, **2**:345–346
  bipolar cells for, **2**:352, 353*i*
  horizontal cells for, **2**:352
  retinal ganglion cells for, **2**:353, 354*i*
L-Dopa, for Parkinson disease, **1**:279
L1 repeat element/sequence, **2**:189, 203
L-selectin, in neutrophil rolling, **9**:48

L-type calcium channels, **2**:310
  mutations in, **2**:349
Labbé vein, **5**:22
Labetalol, **1**:89*t*
  for hypertensive emergency, **1**:94
Labrador (actinic) keratopathy, **4**:68, 69*i*, **8**:368–369
Labyrinthine bone, **5**:54
Labyrinthine reflex system, **6**:39
Lacerations
  canalicular, **7**:277
  conjunctival, **8**:403
  corneoscleral. *See also* Anterior segment, trauma to;
    Perforating injuries
    repair of, **8**:410–416, 411*i*
      anesthesia for, **8**:411
      in children, **6**:447
      postoperative management and, **8**:416–417
      secondary repair measures and, **8**:415–416,
        417*i*, 418*i*
      steps in, **8**:411–414, 412*t*, 413*i*, 414*i*, 415*i*
      Seidel test in identification of, **8**:22, 22*i*
  eyelid
    lid margin involved in, **7**:185, 185*i*
    lid margin not involved in, **7**:184–185
    ptosis caused by, **7**:219
    repair of, **7**:184–187, 185*i*
      secondary, **7**:186–187
  iris, repair of, **8**:416, 417*i*, 418*i*
  posterior segment, **12**:295–296
Lacquer cracks, in pathologic myopia, **12**:84, 85*i*
Lacrimal artery, **2**:39*i*, 41*i*, **5**:15
  extraocular muscles supplied by, **2**:16–18, **6**:16
Lacrimal bone, **5**:6*i*, 10, **7**:7, 8*i*, 9*i*
Lacrimal canaliculi. *See* Canaliculi, lacrimal
Lacrimal crests, anterior and posterior, **2**:5, 7*i*
Lacrimal–cutaneous fistula, congenital, **6**:240, **7**:258,
  258*i*, 266–267
Lacrimal drainage system, **2**:30*i*, 34–36, 35*i*, **6**:239–247,
  7:253–256, 255*i*, 256*i*. *See also* Nasolacrimal duct
  in children, **6**:239–247
  developmental abnormalities of, **6**:239–240,
    7:257–258
  diagnostic tests for evaluation of, **7**:268–274
  irrigation of
    for acquired tearing evaluation, **7**:270–271, 270*t*,
      271*i*
    for canalicular obstruction, **7**:270–271, 271*i*, 275
    for congenital tearing management, **7**:262–263,
      264*i*
  obstruction of. *See also* Tearing
    acquired, **7**:268–284
    congenital, **7**:258, 261–265
Lacrimal ducts, **2**:30*i*, 31–33, **7**:253. *See also* Lacrimal
  drainage system
Lacrimal fossa, **6**:239
Lacrimal glands, **2**:29*t*, 31–34, 33*i*, 34*i*, 35*i*, 289–290,
  289*i*, **4**:168*t*, 187–188, **7**:16, 253, 254*i*. *See also*
  Lacrimal system
  accessory, **2**:29*t*, 34, 289–290, 289*i*, **4**:168*t*, **7**:140*i*,
    145, 253
  aqueous component/tears produced by, **8**:56, 57
  biopsy of, **8**:73
  development of, **2**:157–158
  dysfunction of
    non–Sjögren syndrome, **8**:80

in sarcoidosis, 8:88
in Sjögren syndrome, 8:78–80
tests of, 8:62–63, 62i, 62t
ectopic, 6:382, 8:277
Epstein-Barr virus infection and, 8:156
in external eye defense, 8:113
orbital, 2:31, 33i, 289
palpebral, 2:31, 33i, 34i, 289
parasympathetic innervation of, 5:59–60, 60i
sarcoidosis involving, 7:59, 8:88
in tear secretion, 2:289–290, 289i
tumors of, 4:192–194, 193i, 194i, 7:89–92, 90i
epithelial, 7:89–91, 90i
exenteration for, 7:90, 128
nonepithelial, 7:91–92
staging of, 4:292t
Lacrimal nerve, 2:115, 5:52, 53i, 7:14
Lacrimal papillae, 2:34
Lacrimal probing
for acquired nasolacrimal duct/canalicular
obstruction, 7:271, 275
for congenital dacryocele, 6:241
for congenital nasolacrimal duct obstruction, 6:243,
243–245, 244i, 245i, 7:261, 262–265, 263i
Lacrimal pump, 7:256, 257i
ocular medication absorption affected by, 2:382
Lacrimal puncta. See Puncta
Lacrimal sac (tear sac), 2:33i, 35, 35i, 6:239, 7:255, 255i
cast formation in (dacryoliths), 7:283
distension of, in dacryocystitis, 7:278, 279i
trauma to, 7:284
tumors of, 7:283–284
Lacrimal sac massage
for congenital dacryocele, 6:241
for congenital nasolacrimal duct obstruction, 6:242
Lacrimal scintigraphy, for acquired tearing evaluation,
7:272, 273i
Lacrimal system. See also specific structure
anatomy of, 7:253–256
disorders of. See also Tearing
acquired, 7:267–284
congenital, 7:259–267
developmental abnormalities, 7:257–258, 258i
lower system abnormalities, 7:278–284
upper system abnormalities, 7:274–278
excretory apparatus of, 2:30i, 34–36, 35i, 7:253–256,
255i, 256i. See also Lacrimal drainage system
physiology of, 7:256–257, 257i
secretory apparatus/function of, 2:291–294, 292i,
293i, 7:253, 254i. See also Lacrimal glands
silicone intubation of
for acquired nasolacrimal obstruction, 7:278
for canalicular constriction, 7:275
for canalicular trauma, 7:277
for congenital lacrimal duct obstruction/tearing,
6:246–247, 7:263–264, 266i
tumors of, 7:277–278, 283–284
wound healing/repair and, 4:24
Lacrimopalato-nasal nucleus, 5:59
Lactate
in aqueous humor, 2:316t, 317
in tear film, 2:290
Lactate dehydrogenase analysis, in myocardial
infarction, 1:118

Lactation
fluorescein dye transmission to breast milk and,
12:21
glaucoma medications and, 10:176
refractive surgery contraindicated during, 13:41
Lactoferrin, in tear film, 2:290, 8:56
decreased, 8:63
in external eye defense, 8:113
Lactotroph adenomas (prolactinomas), 1:228
LADA. See Latent autoimmune diabetes in adults
Lagophthalmos
after blepharoplasty, 7:233
causes of, 8:94–95
exposure keratopathy and, 8:94–95
in paralytic ectropion, 7:199
gold weight loading for, 7:199
after ptosis repair, 7:217, 223
LAK cells. See Lymphokine-activated killer cells
Lake-Cavanagh disease, 12:233t, 241
LAL. See Light-adjustable intraocular lenses
Lambdoid suture, 5:9
Lamellae
corneal, 2:300
development of, 2:151
eyelid, 2:27i
zonular, 11:6
Lamellar bodies, in sarcoidosis, 9:198
Lamellar (zonular) cataracts, 11:37–38, 39i
in children, 6:289, 290i, 292t
hereditary factors in, 6:287t
Lamellar deficiency, surgery for eyelid retraction and,
7:225
Lamellar surgery, 13:20t, 106. See also specific type
corneal biomechanics affected by, 13:23, 24i, 25i
corneal wound healing and, 13:28, 29
keratectomy, 8:440
keratoplasty. See Keratoplasty
Lamictal. See Lamotrigine
Lamina cribrosa, 2:99, 4:87, 5:26, 10:48
blood supply of, 2:103
Lamina densa, 2:151
Lamina fusca, 2:50–51, 4:88, 151
Lamina granularis interna, 5:29
Lamina lucida, 2:151
Lamina papyracea (ethmoidal bone), 2:6, 5:10, 7:7, 8i,
9, 9i, 11
Laminar portion of optic nerve, 2:99, 10:48, 49
Lamisil. See Terbinafine
Lamivudine (3TC)
for hepatitis B, 1:305
for HIV infection/AIDS, 1:41
for postexposure HIV prophylaxis, 1:45, 46–47t
with zidovudine, 1:41, 45
Lamotrigine, 1:283t
Lamour frequency, definition of, 5:80
Lancaster red-green test, 6:85–86
Lancefield groups, 8:124
Lang stereopsis tests, 6:93–94
Langerhans cell histiocytosis (histiocytosis X), orbital
involvement in, 7:88
in children, 6:375–376, 376i
Langerhans cells, 2:45, 8:114, 195, 196i, 245, 9:15
Langhans giant cells, 4:13, 15i
Lanoconazole, 1:76

Lanthony desaturated 15-hue test, in low vision evaluation, 5:96
Lanthony tritan plates, in low vision evaluation, 5:96
Lantibiotics, staphylococci producing, 8:124
Lantus. *See* Glargine insulin
Large (histiocytic) cell lymphoma. *See* Lymphomas, intraocular
Large-print materials, 3:260
Larva migrans. *See also Toxocara* (toxocariasis)
 ocular, 8:133
 visceral, 6:317, 8:133
LASEK. *See* Laser subepithelial keratomileusis
Laser burns, corneal endothelial damage caused by, 8:420
Laser capsulotomy (Nd:YAG), 11:187–191, 189*i*
 in children, 11:197
 complications of, 11:190–191
 contraindications to, 11:188
 indications for, 11:188
 lens-particle glaucoma and, 11:67–68
 procedure for, 11:188–190, 189*i*
 retinal detachment and, 11:175, 190, 12:334
Laser dacryocystorhinostomy, 7:281–282, 282*i*
Laser gonioplasty, for angle-closure glaucoma, 10:199–200
Laser in situ keratomileusis (LASIK), 13:20*t*, 23, 25*i*, 26, 27*i*, 50*t*, 87–90, 89*i*, 106–133
 ablation techniques for, 13:114, 115*i*
 for amblyopia, 13:194
 for anisometropic amblyopia, 13:194
 for astigmatism/refractive errors after penetrating keratoplasty, 8:465*t*, 466
 Bowman's layer and, 2:300
 cataract surgery after, 11:211
 intraocular lens power calculation and, 11:151, 152
 in children, 13:195
 CLAPIKS after, 13:207–208
 complications of, 13:120–132. *See also specific type*
 corneal biomechanics affected by, 13:23, 25*i*, 26, 27*i*
 in diabetic patients, 13:197
 diffuse lamellar keratitis (DLK) after, 13:127, 128*i*, 128*t*
 dry eye and, 8:80, 13:127
 ectasia after, 13:131–132
 intrastromal corneal ring segment placement and, 13:83–84
 elevated intraocular pressure after, 13:189, 190*i*
 epithelial erosions and, 13:122
 in diabetic patients, 13:197
 epithelial ingrowth after, 13:129–131, 130*i*
 filtering surgery and, 13:191
 flap creation for
 femtosecond laser, 13:109–110
 microkeratome, 13:112–114, 113*i*, 114*i*
 complications of, 13:120–121, 121*i*
 flap dislocation and, 13:126–127
 flap replacement in, 13:115
 glaucoma after, 13:189, 190*i*, 208–209
 in glaucoma patient, 13:189–191, 190*i*
 herpetic keratitis after, 13:185–186
 history of, 13:106–107
 for hyperopia, 13:26, 27*i*, 118
 for hyperopic astigmatism, 13:118

infectious keratitis after, 13:128–129, 129*i*
 atypical mycobacteria causing, 8:185
 informed consent forms for, 13:51–56
 instrumentation for, 13:107–110
 interface debris after, 13:131, 131*i*
 interface inflammation and, 13:127
 intraocular pressure measurements after, 13:191, 208
 intrastromal corneal ring segment placement and, 13:83
 for keratoconus, 8:332
 lasers approved for, 13:32*t*, 33*t*, 34*t*
 microkeratome for, 13:107–109, 108–109*i*
 flap creation by, 13:112–114, 113*i*, 114*i*
 complications of, 13:120–121, 121*i*
 for mixed astigmatism, 13:118
 for myopia
 with astigmatism, 13:117–118
 high myopia, 13:117
 low myopia, 13:116
 moderate myopia, 13:116–117
 in ocular hypertension patient, 13:189–191, 190*i*
 outcomes of, 13:116–119
 patient selection for, 13:110–112
 after penetrating keratoplasty, 8:465*t*, 13:187–189, 187*i*
 penetrating keratoplasty after, 13:204
 with phakic IOL insertion (bioptics), 13:143, 155–156, 157*t*
 preoperative laser inspection and, 13:110
 preoperative laser programming for, 13:112
 preoperative patient preparation and, 13:112
 PRK for enhancement of, 13:119
 after radial keratotomy, 13:64–65
 residual stromal bed thickness after, 13:49
 retinal detachment and, 13:192, 203
 retreatment and, 13:119, 120*i*
 risks/benefits of, 13:50*t*
 spherical aberration after, 3:102
 striae and, 13:122–126, 124*t*, 125*i*
 surgical techniques for, 13:112–115, 113*i*, 114*i*, 115*i*
 wavefront-guided, 13:112, 133–135
Laser interferometry, 3:8, 315–316, 322
 for potential acuity estimation, before cataract surgery, 11:85
Laser iridectomy, for angle-closure glaucoma, 10:197–198, 198*i*
 complications of, 10:199
 contraindications to, 10:198
 indications for, 10:197
 postoperative care and, 10:199
 preoperative consideration in, 10:198
 technique for, 10:198–199
Laser keratectomy, 13:21*t*. *See also* Photorefractive keratectomy
Laser ophthalmoscopy, 3:279
 in retinal examination, 12:24–25
Laser phacolysis, 11:138
Laser photoablation. *See* Photoablation
Laser pointers, retinal injury caused by, 12:309
Laser pupilloplasty, for cataracts, 11:77
"Laser ridges," in intraocular lenses, 11:145
Laser skin resurfacing, 7:237–238
Laser speckle, 3:18

Laser subepithelial keratomileusis (LASEK), **13**:50*t*, 90–106. *See also* Photorefractive keratectomy
Bowman's layer and, **2**:300
epithelial preservation techniques for, **13**:94–95, 94*i*
patient selection for, **13**:90–91
penetrating keratoplasty after, **13**:203–204
risks/benefits of, **13**:50*t*
Laser therapy (laser surgery). *See also specific procedure and* Photocoagulation; Photodynamic therapy
for capillary hemangioma, **7**:66
for childhood glaucoma, **6**:281, 282
for coronary revascularization, **1**:122
for diabetic retinopathy, **4**:136, 136*i*
for iris bombé in uveitis, **9**:237–238
for keratoconus, **8**:332
ocular damage after (laser burns), **8**:420
for ocular histoplasmosis, **9**:161
for orbital hemangiomas in children, **6**:378
for orbital lymphangiomas, **7**:69
for pars planitis, **9**:150
for posterior segment disease, **12**:313–322
for punctal occlusion, **7**:274
for retinal angioma, **6**:413
for retinoblastoma, **4**:262
for retinopathy of prematurity, **6**:330
for skin resurfacing, **7**:237–238
for trichiasis, **7**:208
for xanthelasmas, **7**:166
Laser thermokeratoplasty, **13**:27–28, 138–139
penetrating keratoplasty after, **13**:204
risks/benefits of, **13**:50*t*, 138
Laser trabeculoplasty, for open-angle glaucoma, **10**:180–183, 181*i*
complications of, **10**:182–183
contraindications to, **10**:181
indications for, **10**:180
long-term follow-up after, **10**:183
mechanism for, **10**:180
preoperative evaluation for, **10**:181
results of, **10**:183
selective, **10**:182
technique of, **10**:181–182, 181*i*
Lasers, **3**:17–24. *See also specific type and* Laser therapy
absorption in, **3**:19, 21*i*
active medium of, **3**:17, 19, 22*i*
biophysics of, **13**:29–30
corneal biomechanics affected by, **13**:24–26, 26*i*, 27*i*
elements of, **3**:19–22, 22*i*
emission by, **3**:19–20, 22*i*
interference and coherence and, **3**:8, 18
occupational light injury and, **12**:309
optical feedback in, **3**:19, 22, 22*i*
photic damage in therapeutic mechanism of, **12**:307
population inversion and, **3**:21–22, 22*i*
power readings on, **3**:18–19, 18*t*
principles of, **3**:17–24, 24*i*
properties of light from, **3**:17–19, 20*i*
pumping in, **3**:19, 21–22, 22*i*
for refractive surgery, FDA-approved, **13**:32–34*t*
sources for, **3**:22–24
tissue interactions and, **3**:23–24, 24*i*, **13**:29, 87
visual pigment absorption spectra and, **12**:313, 314*i*
wavefront-guided, **13**:134
wavelengths used in, **3**:24*i*
for photocoagulation, **12**:313–317, 315–316*t*

Lashes. *See* Eyelashes
LASIK. *See* Laser in situ keratomileusis
Lasix. *See* Furosemide
Latanoprost, **2**:389, 413–414, 414*t*, **10**:162*t*, 171–172
for childhood glaucoma, **6**:283
Late-onset Alzheimer disease, **1**:286
Latency
perimetry effects of, **10**:65
in saccades testing, **5**:202
Latency (viral), herpesvirus infection and, **1**:27, 28, **8**:142
Latent autoimmune diabetes in adults (LADA), **1**:206
Latent/manifest latent nystagmus, **5**:242–243, **6**:165, 166*i*
Lateral canthal defects, repair of, **7**:192
Lateral canthal tendon, **7**:146
Lateral choroidal artery, **5**:18
Lateral (spatial) coherence, **3**:7–8, 8*i*
Lateral geniculate body/nucleus, **6**:44, 45*i*
anatomy of, **2**:107
development of, **6**:46
abnormal visual experience affecting, **6**:49
Lateral incomitance, strabismus surgery planning and, **6**:177
Lateral muscular branch, of ophthalmic artery, extraocular muscles supplied by, **6**:16
Lateral orbitotomy, **7**:114–115
Lateral pontine cistern, **2**:118
Lateral rectus muscles, **2**:17*i*, 18*t*, 19*i*, **5**:42, 42*i*, **6**:13–14, 13*i*, 17*t*, 18*i*, **7**:13
A-pattern deviations associated with dysfunction of, **6**:119
action of, **6**:13–14, 17*t*, 30*t*, 31*i*
anatomy of, **6**:13–14, 14*i*, 17*t*, 18*i*
field of action/activation of, **6**:29
paralysis of, treatment of, **6**:182–183
surgery of
for A- and V-pattern deviations, **6**:123–124, 123*i*, 124, 182
for constant exotropia, **6**:114
for Duane syndrome, **6**:143–144
for incomitant esodeviation, **6**:107–108
for intermittent exotropia, **6**:113–114
V-pattern deviations associated with dysfunction of, **6**:119
Lateral (transverse) sinus thrombosis, **5**:358
Lateral subnucleus, of cranial nerve VII, **5**:54
Lateral tarsal strip operation
for cicatricial ectropion, **7**:200–201
for involutional ectropion, **7**:197–198, 197*i*
for involutional entropion, **7**:205
Lateropulsion
ocular, **5**:205
in Wallenberg syndrome, **5**:205
Latex allergy, in ocular surgery candidate, **1**:330
Lattice degeneration, **4**:127–128, 127*i*, **12**:258–259, 259*i*, 260*i*
radial perivascular, **4**:127–128
in Stickler syndrome, **12**:284*i*
treatment of, **12**:265, 266–267, 266*t*, 267*t*
Lattice dystrophy, **4**:71–72, 75*i*, **8**:310*t*, 316*t*, 318–319, 349
Lattice lines, **8**:318, 318*i*
LAV. *See* Lymphadenopathy-associated virus
Lavage, bronchial, **1**:155

Law of motor correspondence, Hering's, **6**:36–37, 37*i*
eyelid retraction and, **7**:224
Law of reciprocal innervation, Sherrington's, **6**:35
Law of rectilinear propagation, **3**:41, 42*i*
Law of reflection, **3**:42–44, 44*i*
Law of refraction (Snell's law), **3**:44–46, 46*i*, 47, 47*i*, **8**:39–40
contact lens power and, **3**:174
Fermat's principle and, **3**:51–52
small-angle approximation and, **3**:59–60
LBBB. *See* Left bundle branch block
LBD. *See* Lewy body dementia
LC. *See* Langerhans cells
LCA. *See* Leber congenital amaurosis
LCAT deficiency. *See* Lecithin–cholesterol acyltransferase (LCAT) deficiency
LDL cholesterol. *See* Low-density-lipoprotein cholesterol
Le Fort fractures, **7**:97, 98*i*
LEA Low-Contrast Test, **3**:252
Lea symbols, for visual acuity testing in children, **6**:79
Leakage, fluorescein, **12**:20, 20*i*. *See also* Hyperfluorescence
in central serous chorioretinopathy, **12**:22*i*, 52
in choroidal neovascularization, **12**:20*i*, 65*i*, 66
in cystoid macular edema, **12**:154
in hypertensive choroidopathy, **12**:98, 99*i*
Leão, spreading depression of, **5**:191
Learning effect, in automated perimetry, **10**:74, 75*i*
Leash phenomenon, **6**:141
Leber (epithelioid) cells, **8**:68, **9**:15, 52–53. *See also* Macrophages
Leber congenital amaurosis (Leber amaurosis congenita/congenital retinitis pigmentosa), **6**:334–335, 335*i*, 452, 454–455, **12**:211–212, 233–234
guanylate cyclase mutations causing, **2**:349
RPE65 gene defects causing, **2**:350, **6**:335
Leber hereditary optic neuropathy, **5**:134–136, 135*i*, **6**:364–365
mitochondrial DNA mutations and, **2**:218–220, 219*i*, **5**:134–135, **6**:365
Leber idiopathic stellate neuroretinitis, **6**:366, 366*i*
Leber miliary aneurysm, **4**:121–122
Lecithin–cholesterol acyltransferase (LCAT) deficiency, **8**:339–340
Leflunomide, **1**:199–200
for uveitis in children, **6**:321
Left anterior hemiblock, **1**:134
Left bundle branch block, **1**:134–135
Left gaze (levoversion), **6**:36
Left posterior hemiblock, **1**:134
Left ventricular hypertrophy, hypertension and, **1**:95
Legal blindness, **3**:245
Leigh syndrome (Leigh necrotizing encephalopathy), **2**:262*t*
mitochondrial DNA mutations and, **2**:219*i*, 220
Leiomyoma, **4**:283
of ciliary body, **4**:165
of iris, **4**:219*t*
of orbit, **4**:198
Leiomyosarcoma
conjunctival, **8**:269
of orbit, **4**:198
Leishmania infection, **8**:132

Leiske intraocular lens, **11**:144
Lens (crystalline)
absence of, **6**:304, **11**:30. *See also* Aphakia
aging changes in, **11**:5, 45–49, 46*i*
presbyopia and, **3**:147
anatomy of, **2**:73–76, 74*i*, 75*i*, 77*i*, 323–325, 324*i*, **11**:5–9, 6*i*, 7*i*, 8*i*
antioxidants in, **2**:368–369, 369*i*
biochemistry and metabolism of, **2**:323–332, **11**:11–17
sugar cataracts and, **2**:330–332, 331*i*
capsule of. *See* Lens capsule
carbohydrate metabolism in, **2**:330, **11**:14–16, 15*i*
changing shape of. *See* Accommodation
chemical composition of, **2**:325–328
chemical injuries affecting, **11**:57
in children, **6**:199, 201*i*
disorders of, **6**:285–309, 285*t*. *See also specific type*
colobomas of, **2**:171–172, **6**:304, 304*i*, **11**:31, 31*i*
coloration change in, **11**:45, 46*i*
congenital anomalies and abnormalities of, **2**:172–173, **4**:94–95, 95*i*, 95*t*, **6**:285*t*, 304, 304*i*, **11**:30–39
cortex of, **2**:75*i*, 76, 324–325, 324*i*, **4**:94, **11**:9
degenerations of, **4**:100–101, 101*i*, 102*i*
degenerations of, **4**:97–103, 102*i*. *See also* Cataract
degenerative ocular disorders and, **11**:69
development/embryology of, **2**:145–146, **6**:199, 201*i*, **11**:5, 25–43
cataract development and. *See* Cataract, congenital and infantile
congenital anomalies and abnormalities and, **2**:172–173, **4**:94–95, 95*i*, 95*t*, **6**:285*t*, 304, 304*i*, **11**:30–39
developmental defects and, **11**:40–43
normal, **11**:25–30, 26–27*i*, 28*i*, 29*i*
diabetes mellitus affecting, **11**:60–61. *See also* Cataract, diabetic
dislocated, **4**:94, 95*i*, 95*t*, **11**:40. *See also* Ectopia lentis
cataract surgery and, **11**:226–227, 227*i*, 228*i*
in children, **6**:304–309, 305*t*
abuse and, **6**:442
disorders of, **4**:93–104, **11**:45–69. *See also specific disorder and* Cataract
in children, **6**:285–309, 285*t*
illusions caused by, **5**:188
systemic disorders and, **4**:103
drug-induced changes in, **11**:50–54
electrical injury of, **11**:59, 60*i*
energy production in, **2**:330
epithelium of, **2**:74–76, 74*i*, 324, 324*i*, **4**:93–94, **11**:6–9, 8*i*
abnormalities of, **4**:98–100, 99*i*, 100*i*
active transport and, **11**:19–20
development of, **11**:27*i*, 28
opacification of (capsular cataract), **11**:37
evaluation of
before cataract surgery, **11**:82–83
in glaucoma, **10**:36
before refractive surgery, **13**:44–45
exfoliation syndromes and, **11**:65–66, 66*i*
foreign body in, **11**:57
free radicals affecting, **2**:368–370, 369*i*, **11**:16–17

glaucoma and, **4:**81, 82*i*, 96, 100–101, **11:**67–68, 68*i*
  in children, **6:**279
in homocystinuria, **6:**307, 307*i*, **11:**42
in hyperlysinemia, **6:**308, **11:**42
infection/inflammation of, **4:**96–97, 96*i*, 97*i*, 98*i*
ionic current flow around/through, **2:**329–330, 329*i*
ischemic damage to, **11:**69
luxed/luxated, **4:**94, 95*i*, **6:**304, 305*t*, 309, **11:**40. *See
    also* Ectopia lentis
  cataract surgery and, **11:**226–227, 227*i*, 228*i*
in Marfan syndrome, **6:**306–307, 306*i*, **11:**41, 41*i*
membranes of, **2:**325, 328
metabolic diseases affecting, **11:**60–63
molecular biology of, **11:**11–13, 11*i*
normal, **11:**5–9, 6*i*, 7*i*, 8*i*
nucleus of, **2:**76, 324–325, 324*i*, **4:**94, **11:**9
  congenital cataract of, **11:**37, 38*i*
  degenerations of, **4:**101–103, 101*i*
  embryonic, **2:**146, **11:**9, 26–27, 27*i*
    opacification of (congenital nuclear cataract),
      11:37, 38*i*
  emulsification of. *See* Phacoemulsification
  expression/removal of. *See* Cataract surgery;
      Lensectomy
  fetal, **11:**9, 27*i*, 28
    opacification of (congenital nuclear cataract),
      11:37, 38*i*
nutritional diseases affecting, **11:**63–64
opacification of. *See* Cataract
oxidative damage to, **2:**368, **11:**16–17
perforating and penetrating injury of, **11:**55, 57*i*, 58*i*
physiology of, **2:**328–330, 329*i*, **11:**19–23
placode/plate, formation of, **2:**136–137, 145–146,
    11:25, 26*i*
radiation affecting, **1:**255–256, **11:**55–57
removal of. *See* Cataract surgery; Lensectomy
retained, cataract surgery and, **11:**182–183,
    12:337–339, 338*t*, 339*i*
in schematic eye, **3:**106*i*
skin diseases and, **11:**66
spherophakic, **6:**304, 304*i*
subluxed/subluxated, **4:**94, **6:**304, 305*t*, 309, **11:**40.
    See also Ectopia lentis
  cataract surgery and, **11:**226–227, 227*i*, 228*i*
in sulfite oxidase deficiency, **6:**308, **11:**42
sutures of, **2:**75*i*, 76, **11:**9
  development of, **2:**146, **11:**27*i*, 28–29, 28*i*
  opacification of (sutural/stellate cataract),
    11:35–36, 37*i*
topography of, **4:**93–94, 93*i*, 94*i*
transport functions in, **11:**19–21, 21*i*
traumatic damage to, **11:**54–60
uveitis and, **4:**96, 96*i*, 97*i*, **9:**64, 135–136, 135*i*, 136*i*,
    11:64, 65*i*, 67. *See also* Phacoantigenic
    endophthalmitis
vesicle, formation of, **2:**137, 145–146, 147*i*, **11:**25,
    26*i*
water and cation balance in, maintenance of,
    11:19–21, 21*i*
in Weill-Marchesani syndrome, **6:**308
wound healing/repair and, **4:**23
zonular fibers/zonules of, **2:**75*i*, 76, 323, **4:**94, 94*i*,
    11:5, 6, 7*i*
  in accommodation, **13:**167–171, 168*i*, 169*i*, 170*i*
  development of, **2:**146, **11:**30

Lens capsule, **4:**93, **11:**5–6, 8*i*. *See also* Capsulorrhexis;
    Capsulotomy
  anatomy of, **2:**74, 74*i*, 75*i*, 323, 324*i*
  development of, **2:**146, 147*i*, **11:**25, 26–27*i*, 28
  disorders of, **4:**97–98
  exfoliation of, **11:**65
  rupture of, cataract formation and, **4:**25–26
Lens crystallins. *See* Crystallins
Lens-fiber plasma membranes, **2:**325, 328
Lens fibers, **2:**75*i*, 76, 77*i*, 324–325, 324*i*, **4:**94
  accommodation and, **11:**22, 23
  degenerations of, **4:**100–101, 101*i*, 102*i*
  development of, **2:**146, **11:**8–9, 8*i*
    primary fibers, **11:**26–27, 27*i*
    secondary fibers, **11:**27*i*, 28
      microspherophakia and, **11:**32
  zonular (zonules of Zinn), **2:**75*i*, 76, 323, **4:**94, 94*i*,
    11:5, 6, 7*i*
    in accommodation, **13:**167–171, 168*i*, 169*i*, 170*i*
    development of, **2:**146, **11:**30
Lens glides, for IOL implantation, **11:**152
Lens hooks, for IOL implantation, **11:**152
Lens-induced angle closure, **10:**128–132, 129–131*i*, 131*t*
Lens-induced glaucoma, **4:**81, 82*i*, 96, 101, **9:**52, 136,
    10:103–106, 104*i*, 104*t*, 105*i*, **11:**67–68, 68*i*
  angle-closure, **10:**104*t*, 122, 128–132, 129*i*, 131*i*, 131*t*
  in children, **6:**279
  open-angle, **10:**103–106, 104*i*, 104*t*, 105*i*
Lens-induced granulomatous endophthalmitis, **4:**96,
    97*i*
Lens-induced uveitis, **11:**64, 67
Lens maker's equation (LME), **3:**60–62, 61*i*
  thin-lens approximation and, **3:**66–67
  transverse magnification and, **3:**65–66, 66*i*
  vergence and reduced vergence and, **3:**62–65, 63*i*,
    64*i*
Lens Opacities Classification System III (LOCS III),
    11:73
Lens-particle glaucoma, **10:**104–105, 105*i*, **11:**67–68
Lens pit (fovea lentis), formation of, **11:**25, 26*i*
Lens proteins, **2:**325–328, 326*t*, **11:**11, 11*i*. *See also
    specific type*
  aging affecting, **11:**13
  concentration of
    age affecting, **11:**13
    cataracts and, **11:**13
  crystallins, **2:**76, 323, 325–327, 326*t*, **11:**11–12, 11*i*.
    See also Crystallins
  cytoskeletal and membrane, **2:**327–328
  in phacolytic glaucoma, **4:**96, 101, **9:**52, 136, **11:**67
  posttranslational modification of, **2:**328
  tolerance to, **9:**87
  urea-insoluble (membrane structural), **11:**11*i*, 12
  urea-soluble (cytoskeletal), **11:**11*i*, 12
  in uveitis, **9:**64, 135, 135*i*, 136*i*
  water-insoluble, **11:**11, 11*i*
    age affecting, **11:**12–13
  water-soluble, **11:**11, 11*i*. *See also* Crystallins
    conversion of to water-insoluble, **11:**12–13
Lens rim, in visual field testing, **10:**70, 72*i*
Lensectomy. *See also* Cataract surgery
  in children, **6:**295–296, 298*i*, **11:**197
    without intraocular lens, **6:**295–296, 298*i*
    with intraocular lens, **6:**297–300, 299*i*
    for rubella, **6:**218

for subluxed lenses, **6**:309
clear lens, **11**:138, 222
  refractive (refractive lens exchange), **13**:156–161
    advantages of, **13**:161
    complications of, **13**:160–161
    disadvantages of, **13**:161
    indications for, **13**:156
    informed consent for, **13**:158
    IOL calculations for, **13**:160
    patient selection for, **13**:156–158
    retinal detachment and, **13**:158, 160, 161, 192
    surgical planning/techniques for, **13**:158–160
  in Marfan syndrome, **11**:41
  pars plana, **11**:138–139
    juvenile rheumatoid arthritis–associated uveitis
      and, **9**:235
Lenses. *See also* Bifocal lenses; Contact lenses;
  Ophthalmic lenses
  aphakic. *See* Aphakic spectacles
  combinations of
    analysis of, **3**:67
    spherocylindrical lenses, **3**:99–100
      at oblique axes, **3**:99–100, 101*i*
  correcting, in retinoscopy, **3**:128–129, 129*i*
  cylindrical, **3**:94–95, 97*i*. *See also* Cylinders
  for fundus biomicroscopy, **3**:285–289, 285*i*, 286*i*,
    287*i*, 288*i*, 289*i*
  imaging with, **3**:28–30, 29*i*
    image quality and, **3**:38, 38*i*
  index of refraction and, **3**:6
  intraocular. *See* Intraocular lenses
  negative (minus), **3**:72–74, 73*i*
  prismatic effect of (Prentice's rule), **3**:87–88, 88*i*,
    155, 157*i*
    bifocal design and, **3**:155–162
  special materials used for, **3**:168–169
  spectacle. *See* Spectacle lenses
  spherocylindrical, **3**:95–98. *See also* Spherocylindrical
    lenses
  standard (field), in manual lensmeter, **3**:305, 306*i*
  of telescope, **3**:82–83, 82*i*, 83*i*
  thick, power approximation for, **3**:78–79, 78*i*
  thin, **3**:66–67
    negative, **3**:72–74, 73*i*
Lensmeters
  automatic, **3**:306*i*, 307–308
  manual, **3**:304–307, 305*i*
    Badal principle and, **3**:80–81, 305
    bifocal add measured with, **3**:305*i*, 306–307
Lensometer. *See* Lensmeters
Lente insulin, **1**:209*t*
Lenticonus, **2**:172, **4**:97, 98*i*, **11**:30, 30*i*
  posterior/lentiglobus, **4**:97, 98*i*, **11**:30, 31
    in children, **6**:289–290, 291*i*, 292*t*
Lenticular astigmatism, contact lenses and, **3**:182
Lenticular contact lens, **3**:175
Lenticular irregularities, decreased vision with, **5**:103
Lenticular myopia, **11**:45
Lenticule
  for epikeratoplasty, **13**:74, 75*i*
  for keratophakia, **13**:71
Lentiglobus, **4**:97, 98*i*, **11**:30, 31
  in children, **6**:289–290, 291*i*, 292*t*

Lentigo (lentigines)
  maligna (Hutchinson's melanotic freckle/
    precancerous melanosis), **7**:174
  senile (liver spots), **7**:171
  simplex (simple lentigines), **7**:171
  solar, **7**:171
Lentigo maligna melanoma, **4**:185, **7**:182
Leptospirosis, panuveitis in, **9**:193
Lescol. *See* Fluvastatin
Leser-Trélat sign, **4**:175
Lesionectomy, for seizures, **1**:283
Lesser arterial circle, **5**:15
Letter chart visual acuity. *See* Visual acuity
Letterer-Siwe disease/syndrome. *See also* Histiocytosis
  orbital involvement in, **7**:88
    in children, **6**:376
Leucine zipper motif, **2**:206, 207*i*
Leukemia, **4**:17*i*, 17*t*, **6**:343–345, 344*i*
  neoplastic masquerade syndromes secondary to,
    9:231
  ocular involvement in, **1**:262, **4**:281–282, 281*i*,
    6:343–345, 344*i*, 390
    choroid, **4**:281–282, **6**:343
    iris, **4**:219*t*, 221*i*, **6**:344–345, 388
    optic disc/optic nerve, **6**:344, 344*i*
    orbit, **4**:194–196, **6**:345, 375, **7**:94–95
    retina, **4**:281–282, **6**:343–344
    uveitis differentiated from, **6**:320
    vitreous, **4**:281, 281*i*, 282*i*
Leukeran. *See* Chlorambucil
Leukocoria, **5**:259, **6**:323–333. *See also specific cause*
  in Coats disease, **4**:121–122, 122*i*, **12**:156
  differential diagnosis of, **6**:323, 394, 396*t*
  in persistent fetal vasculature/persistent hyperplastic
    primary vitreous, **6**:324–325, **12**:281–282
  in retinoblastoma, **4**:253, 253*t*, 254*i*, **6**:390–391, 393*i*
    differential diagnosis and, **4**:256*t*
  in retinopathy of prematurity, **6**:325–332
  in toxocariasis, **9**:170, 170*i*, 171*i*
Leukocyte common antigen, in immunohistochemistry,
  4:37
Leukocyte function–associated antigen 1 (LFA-1), in
  neutrophil rolling, **9**:48
Leukocyte oxidants, as inflammatory mediators, **8**:198*t*
Leukocytes, **1**:159, **9**:13–16. *See also specific type*
Leukodystrophy
  Krabbe, **2**:262*t*, **6**:436*t*
  metachromatic, **2**:262*t*, **6**:436*t*
Leukoencephalopathy, progressive multifocal, in HIV
  infection/AIDS, **5**:362, 363*i*
Leukomalacia, periventricular, **6**:363
Leukomas, **2**:126, 168
  in Peters anomaly, **11**:32
Leukotriene modifiers, for pulmonary diseases, **1**:157*t*,
  158
Leukotrienes, **2**:305, 306*i*, 307, **8**:198*t*, 200*t*, **9**:7, 80
Leuprolide, ocular effects of, **1**:325*t*
Levaquin. *See* Levofloxacin
Levatol. *See* Penbutolol
Levator aponeurosis, **2**:22, 26, 26*i*, 27*i*, 289, **6**:16, **7**:140,
  140*i*, 142–143, 144, 144*i*
  lacrimal gland development and, **7**:253
  ptosis and, **5**:278, **7**:215, 216*i*, 217*t*, 219
  repair of, for ptosis correction, **7**:222
Levator complex, **5**:45

Levator muscle (levator palpebrae superioris), **2**:16,
  16*i*, 19*i*, 21, 26, 26*i*, 27*i*, **4**:168, **6**:16, 17*t*, 18*i*
  anatomy of, **6**:16, 17*t*, 18*i*, **7**:140*i*, 142
  disinsertion of, eyelid fissure changes and, **2**:23*i*
  external (transcutaneous) advancement of, for ptosis
    correction, **7**:221
  function of, in ptosis, **7**:210–211, 210*i*
  innervation of, **7**:12
  internal (conjunctival) resection of, for ptosis
    correction, **7**:221
  in myogenic ptosis, **7**:214–215
  in traumatic ptosis, **7**:219
Levetiracetam, **1**:283*t*
Levobunolol, **2**:410, 410*t*, **10**:160*t*, 165
  for childhood glaucoma, **6**:282
Levocabastine, **2**:423, 424*t*
Levocycloversion, **6**:36
Levodopa (L-dopa), for Parkinson disease, **1**:279
Levodopa/carbidopa, for Parkinson disease, **1**:279
Levofloxacin, **1**:62*t*, 73, **2**:430–433, 431*t*
  for bacterial keratitis, **8**:183
Levothyroxine, for hypothyroidism, **1**:226
Levoversion (left gaze), **6**:36
Lewy bodies, in Parkinson disease, **1**:278, 285
Lewy body dementia (LBD), **1**:285
Lexan lenses. *See* Polycarbonate spectacle lenses
Lexiva. *See* Fosamprenavir
Lexxel. *See* Felodipine
LFA-1. *See* Leukocyte function–associated antigen 1
LGB. *See* Lateral geniculate body
LHON. *See* Leber hereditary optic neuropathy
Liability, in inheritance, **2**:189
Library, DNA, **2**:189, 227, 228*i*
  cDNA, **2**:189, 227
  genomic, **2**:189, 227, 228*i*
Lice, ocular infection caused by, **8**:133, 169
  cholinesterase inhibitors for, **2**:400
Lid, Lids. *See* Eyelids
Lid margin. *See* Eyelids, margin of
Lid twitch, Cogan's, **5**:275, 325, **6**:151
Lidocaine, **2**:445*t*, 446*t*, 447, 448
  for blepharoplasty, **7**:231
  intracameral, for cataract surgery, **11**:94, 95–96
  intraocular, **2**:448–449
  maximum safe dose of, **1**:322*t*
  for medical emergencies, **1**:316*t*
  toxic reaction to, **1**:323, 336
Lieberman cam-guided corneal cutter, **8**:456
Lifestyle modification
  in hypercholesterolemia management, **1**:143,
    145–146, 148*t*
  in hypertension management, **1**:85–86, 87*t*, 91*i*
Ligaments. *See specific ligament*
Ligand-gated channels, in signal transduction, **2**:311
Light. *See also specific aspect and* Light waves
  absorption of, **3**:14
  anisocoria affected by brightness of, **5**:260, 262–269,
    263*i*
  corneal reflex to, in ocular alignment testing,
    6:82–84, 84*i*
  corpuscular theory of, **3**:3
  eye injury caused by exposure to, **2**:459–465, 460*t*,
    3:167. *See also* Light toxicity
  laser, properties of, **3**:17–19, 20*t*
  measurement of, types of, **3**:15, 16*t*
  opsin changes caused by, **2**:345
  photon (particle) aspects of, **3**:3, 6*i*, 7
  photo-oxidative processes triggered by, **2**:366–367
    in retina, **2**:370–371
  point source of, in geometric optics, **3**:26
  polarization of, **3**:10–11
  propagation of, **3**:39–54
  pupillary response to. *See* Pupillary light reflex
  reflection of, **3**:13–14, 13*i*. *See also* Reflection
  retinal cell changes caused by, **2**:354–355, 355*i*
  retinal pigment epithelial transport systems affected
    by, **2**:361
  rhodopsin changes caused by, **2**:342–344, 343*i*
  scattering of, **3**:12–13
  speed of, **3**:4–6
  tissue damage caused by, **2**:459–465, 460*t*. *See also*
    Light toxicity
  transmission of, **3**:14
  as visible portion of electromagnetic spectrum, **3**:4,
    6*i*
  wave theory of, **3**:3–7, 4*i*, 5*i*
Light adaptation, **2**:345
Light-adapted electroretinogram, **12**:28*i*, 29, 205, 206*t*
  in hereditary retinal/choroidal degenerations, **12**:205,
    206*t*
Light-adjustable intraocular lenses, **13**:165–166, 165*i*,
  180
Light amplification by stimulated emission of
  radiation, **3**:17. *See also* Lasers
Light chains, immunoglobulin, **9**:54, 56*i*
Light–dark ratio, electrooculogram, **12**:36–37, 38*i*
  in Best disease, **12**:37–38, 219
Light-gathering power, **3**:31. *See also* Transverse
  magnification
Light–near dissociation, **2**:111, **5**:269–270, 269*t*
Light response, of standing potential, **12**:36–37, 38*i*
Light-ROP study, **12**:132
Light toxicity, **2**:459–465, 460*t*, **3**:167
  age-related macular degeneration and, **12**:61
  ambient exposure to ultraviolet or visible light and,
    12:309
  cataract surgery and, **11**:171–172
  free radical damage and, **2**:370–371, 459
  occupational, **12**:309
  ophthalmic instrumentation causing, **2**:459–465,
    460*t*, **12**:308–309
  retinal damage caused by, **2**:459, **12**:307–309
    in retinitis pigmentosa, **12**:210, 213
  retinopathy of prematurity and, **6**:326, **12**:132
Light waves. *See also* Light
  characteristics of, **3**:3–4, 4*i*
  coherence of, **3**:7–8, 8*i*, 9*i*
  diffraction of, **3**:11–12, 12*i*
  interference and, **3**:7–9, 8*i*, 9*i*
  theory of, **3**:3–7, 4*i*, 5*i*
Lighthouse Letter Contrast Sensitivity Test, **3**:252
Lightning streaks of Moore, **5**:189
Ligneous conjunctivitis, **8**:213–214
  in children, **6**:388
Lignocaine. *See* Lidocaine
Likelihood ratio, **1**:358–359
  combining screening tests and, **1**:359
  log of (LOD score), **2**:190
Limbal dermoids, **4**:43–44, **6**:257, 258*i*, 386, 386*i*
  Goldenhar syndrome and, **6**:257, 431

Limbal incision, for extraocular muscle surgery, **6**:184
Limbal papillae, **4**:45–46
Limbal relaxing incisions, **13**:21*t*, 66, 67*i*, 68–69, 69*t*
  cataract surgery and, **11**:103
Limbal stem cells, **8**:9–10, 58
  in corneal and conjunctival wound healing/repair,
    8:58, 384, 424
  in corneal epithelium maintenance, **2**:45, **8**:9–10
  deficiency of, **8**:58, 108–109, 109*i*, 433. *See also*
    Limbal transplantation
    toxic insults causing, **8**:102, 394
    in toxic keratoconjunctivitis from medications,
      8:394
  transplantation of. *See* Limbal transplantation
Limbal transplantation (limbal autograft/allograft/stem
  cell transplantation), **8**:109, 423*t*, 425, 433,
  434–435*i*
  for chemical burns, **8**:392, 393
  indications for, **8**:423*t*
Limbal vernal conjunctivitis/keratoconjunctivitis,
  6:234–235, **8**:209–210, 210*i*
Limbic system (cingulate gyrus), **5**:56
Limbitis, in onchocerciasis, **9**:195–197
Limbus, **2**:51–52, 52*i*, **8**:8, 39, 39*i*, 58. *See also under*
  Limbal
  conjunctival vessels near, **8**:59
  marginal corneal infiltrates in blepharoconjunctivitis
    and, **8**:229
  mechanical functions of, **8**:59–60
  physiology of, **8**:58
  squamous cell carcinoma of, **8**:260, 260*i*
  wound healing/repair and, **4**:22, 23*i*
Limiting membrane
  external, **2**:80–81*i*, 83, 84
    development of, **2**:141
  internal, **2**:80–81*i*, 83, 85
    optic disc, **2**:98, 100*i*
Line of Gennari, **5**:29
Line of sight (visual axis), **6**:29
Linear staining, **8**:72
Linearly polarized light, **3**:10
LINEs. *See* Long interspersed elements
Linezolid, **1**:63*t*, 74–75
Lingual gyrus, **5**:31
Link protein, in vitreous, **2**:333
Linkage disequilibrium (allelic association), **2**:189
Linkage (gene), **2**:189, 222–224, 224*i*, 225*i*, 241, 246
  corneal conditions and, **8**:308, 309–310*t*
Linoleate
  auto-oxidation of, **2**:366, 367*i*
  photo-oxidation of, **2**:367, 368*i*
Lipid keratopathy, **8**:373
  in herpes zoster ophthalmicus, **8**:154, 155*i*
Lipid layer of tear film, **2**:287–289, 288*i*, 289*i*, **8**:56, 56*i*
  deficiency of, **8**:56
  secretion of, **8**:57
Lipid-lowering therapy, **1**:145–147, 146*i*, 147*t*, 148*t*,
  149*t*, 150*t*, 151*t*. *See also specific agent*
Lipid peroxidation, **2**:366–368, 367*i*, 368*i*
  in lens opacification, **11**:16
Lipid strip, **2**:289
Lipidoses. *See* Lipids, disorders of metabolism and
  storage of

Lipids
  disorders of metabolism and storage of (lipidoses),
    6:436*t*, **8**:338–343, 339*t*
    corneal changes in, **8**:338–343, 339*t*
      in Schnyder crystalline dystrophy, **8**:321, 322,
        338
  hypotensive, for glaucoma, **10**:163–164*t*, 171–172
  as inflammatory mediators, **9**:77–79, 78*i*
  meibomian gland secretion of, **8**:56, 57
  in retinal pigment epithelium, **2**:358
  solubility of, ocular medication absorption affected
    by, **2**:384, 385*i*
  in tear film. *See* Lipid layer of tear film
  in vitreous, **2**:337
Lipitor. *See* Atorvastatin
Lipoatrophy, at insulin injection site, **1**:211
Lipocalins, in tear film, **2**:290, **8**:56
Lipodermoids (dermolipomas), **2**:168, **4**:43–44, 44*i*,
  8:277, 277*i*
  in children, **6**:386–387, 386*i*
  Goldenhar syndrome and, **4**:43–44, **6**:386, 386*i*, 431
  of orbit, **7**:64, 65*i*
Lipofuscin granules (wear-and-tear pigment), **2**:79, 86
Lipofuscinosis, neuronal ceroid, **6**:437*t*, 438, **12**:233*t*,
  234, 236, 241, 241*i*
Lipohypertrophy, at insulin injection site, **1**:211
Lipomas, of orbit, **4**:201
Lipopeptide antibiotics, **1**:63–64*t*, 75
Lipopolysaccharide, bacterial, **8**:123
  in innate immune response, **9**:43–44, 45
  uveitis caused by, **9**:45
Lipoprotein analysis, **1**:144, 144*t*
Liposarcomas, of orbit, **4**:201, **7**:81
Liposomes
  for drug delivery, **2**:391
  for gene therapy, **2**:237
Liposuction, neck, **7**:245–246, 246*i*
Lipoxygenase
  in eicosanoid synthesis, **9**:78–79
  in free radical generation, **2**:366
  in leukotriene synthesis, **2**:306*i*, 307
Lipschütz bodies, **8**:69
Liraglutide, for diabetes, **1**:214
Lisch corneal dystrophy, **8**:310*t*, 313–315, 314*i*
Lisch nodules, **4**:219*t*, 221*i*
  in children, **6**:264, 264*i*
  in neurofibromatosis, **5**:337, 338*i*, **6**:264, 264*i*,
    403–404, 405*i*, 408
Lisinopril
  for heart failure, **1**:130
  for hypertension, **1**:88*t*, 90*t*
  for non-ST-segment elevation acute coronary
    syndrome, **1**:123
Lispro insulin, **1**:209, 209*t*
Lissamine green, **2**:451, **8**:22
  in ocular surface evaluation, **8**:22
  in tear-film evaluation, **8**:22, 72
Listing's plane, **6**:27, 27*i*, 28
Lithiasis, conjunctival, **8**:367
Lithium, **1**:277
Lithonate. *See* Lithium
Liver disease
  cancer, viral carcinogenesis and, **1**:254
  hemostatic abnormalities and, **1**:169
  hepatitis C and, **1**:31

Liver spots, 7:171
Living will, surgery in elderly patients and, 1:238
Livostin. *See* Levocabastine
LK. *See* Keratoplasty, lamellar
LME. *See* Lens maker's equation
LMWHs. *See* Low-molecular-weight heparins
LMX1B gene, in glaucoma, 10:13*t*
LN. *See* Latent/manifest latent nystagmus
Loa loa (loiasis), 8:132–133, 191
Load, in phacoemulsification, 11:114
Lobectomy, for seizures, 1:283
Local anesthesia. *See* Anesthesia (anesthetics), local
Lockwood, suspensory ligament of (Lockwood's
    ligament), 2:37–38, 38*i*, 6:21, 7:145
LOCS III (Lens Opacities Classification System III),
    11:73
Locus (gene), 2:189, 241. *See also* Gene
Locus heterogeneity, 2:190, 240–241
LOD score, 2:190
Lodine. *See* Etodolac
Lodosyn. *See* Carbidopa
Lodoxamide, 2:424, 424*t*
    for allergic conjunctivitis, 8:208
Lofgren syndrome, 8:88
Log of the likelihood ratio (LOD score), 2:190
logMAR, 3:112, 112*t*
Lomefloxacin, 1:62*t*, 73
Lomustine, 1:260*t*
Long (q) arm, 2:194, 205
Long arm 13 deletion syndrome (13q14 syndrome),
    2:253–254, 253*t*
Long interspersed elements, 2:189, 203
Longitudinal (temporal) coherence, 3:8, 8*i*
Longitudinal fasciculus, 2:108
    medial, 5:34, 6:155
        rostral interstitial nucleus of, 5:34, 37*i*
Longitudinal (axial) magnification, 3:30, 34
Longitudinal/spin-lattice relaxation time (T1), 5:81,
    7:30–31
Longitudinal Study of Cataract, 11:73
Loniten. *See* Minoxidil
Loop diuretics
    for diastolic dysfunction, 1:131
    for hypertension, 1:87, 88*t*, 89–92
Loop of Meyer, 2:108, 5:29, 166
Lopinavir/ritonavir, 1:42
    for postexposure HIV prophylaxis, 1:46–47*t*
Lopressor. *See* Metoprolol
Lorabid. *See* Loracarbef
Loracarbef, 1:59*t*, 69
Losartan, 1:88*t*, 90*t*
Loss of heterozygosity, 2:215
Lost muscle, surgery and, 6:190
Lotemax. *See* Loteprednol
Lotensin. *See* Benazepril
Loteprednol, 2:417*t*, 419*t*, 424*t*, 425
    for uveitis, 9:116
Lotrel. *See* Amlodipine
Lotrimin. *See* Clotrimazole
Louis-Bar syndrome (ataxia-telangiectasia), 5:336*t*, 340,
    342, 342*i*, 8:91–92, 270
    ATM mutation in, 2:213, 6:417–418
    in children, 6:402*t*, 416–418, 417*i*
Louse. *See* Lice

Lovastatin
    cataracts and, 1:151
    for hypercholesterolemia, 1:149*t*, 150*t*
Lovenox. *See* Enoxaparin
Low birth weight, retinopathy and, 6:325, 326. *See also*
    Retinopathy, of prematurity
Low-density-lipoprotein cholesterol, 1:144, 144*t*. *See
    also* Cholesterol
    beta-blockers affecting, 1:150
    goals for, hypercholesterolemia management and,
        1:145, 146, 147*t*
    reducing levels of, 1:143, 145–147, 146*i*, 147*t*, 148*t*,
        149*t*, 150*t*, 151*t*
    risk assessment and, 1:144, 144*t*, 145*t*, 146*i*, 147*t*
    screening, 1:293
    very high levels of, 1:144*t*, 150
Low-molecular-weight heparins
    for acute coronary syndrome, 1:111, 123
    in perioperative setting, 1:332
Low-tension glaucoma, 10:92–96, 94*t*. *See also*
    Glaucoma, normal-tension
Low vision. *See also* Blindness; Visual loss/impairment
    assessment of, 3:247*i*, 5:83–102
        adjunctive testing in, 5:96–102
        best-corrected visual acuity in, 5:84
        color vision testing in, 5:96
        electrophysiologic testing in, 5:99–102
        electroretinography in, 5:101–102, 102*i*
        fluorescein angiography in, 5:98, 99*i*
        fundus examination in, 5:87–89, 88*i*, 89*i*, 89*t*
        history in, 5:83–84
        objective visual deficit and, 3:245*t*
        photostress recovery test in, 5:97
        potential acuity meter testing in, 5:97–98
        pupillary testing in, 5:84–87, 86*i*
        spatial contrast sensitivity testing in, 5:97
        visual evoked potential testing for, 5:100–101
        visual field testing in, 5:89–96
    binocular, 5:308–309
    classification of, 3:245, 251–252, 5:103–170. *See also
        specific causative factor*
    definitions in, 3:244–246, 244*i*
    in infants and children, 3:266–267, 6:451–459
        achromatopsia and, 6:336, 455
        acquired, 6:456–459, 457*t*
        albinism and, 6:345
        anterior segment anomalies and, 6:453
        approach to infant with, 6:452–456
        cataracts and, 6:294, 453
        congenital infection/TORCH syndrome and,
            6:455–456
        cortical visual impairment and, 6:456
        craniosynostosis syndromes and, 6:429
        delayed visual maturation and, 6:456
        in glaucoma, 6:284, 453
        Leber congenital amaurosis and, 6:334, 452,
            454–455
        optic atrophy and, 6:454
        optic nerve hypoplasia and, 6:362, 453–454
        sources of information on, 6:458*t*
    management of, 3:245*t*, 254–260, 5:103–170. *See also*
        Low vision aids; Vision rehabilitation
        goals of, 3:243
        handicap reduction and, 3:263*i*
        nonvisual assistance in, 3:260–263

optical devices in, 3:254–260
    professionals providing, 3:264–265
  moderate, 3:245, 251
    magnifiers for reading and, 3:258–260
    spectacles for reading and, 3:257
  profound, 3:245, 252
    spectacles for reading and, 3:257
  severe, 3:245, 251–252
    distance visual acuity testing in, 3:251
    magnifiers for reading and, 3:258–260
    spectacles for reading and, 3:257
  sources of information on, 6:458t
Low vision aids, 3:82, 254–260, 11:78. *See also* Vision
    rehabilitation
  in functional visual disorder evaluation, 5:309
  reducing handicap and, 3:263i
Low-zone tolerance, in anterior chamber–associated
    immune deviation, 9:38
Lowe syndrome (oculocerebrorenal syndrome), 2:172,
    6:348–349
  childhood glaucoma and, 6:278–279, 348, 10:155t
  congenital corneal keloids in, 8:299
  ocular findings in carriers of, 2:270t
  pediatric cataract and, 6:288t, 348
Lower eyelids. *See* Eyelids, lower
Lozol. *See* Indapamide
LPS. *See* Levator muscle; Lipopolysaccharide
LR. *See* Lateral rectus muscles
LRI. *See* Limbal relaxing incisions
LSC (Longitudinal Study of Cataract), 11:73
LTK. *See* Laser thermokeratoplasty
Lubricants. *See also* Artificial tears
  for chemical burns, 8:382
  for craniosynostosis-induced corneal exposure,
    6:427–428
  for dry eye, 8:74, 75t
  eye ointment as, 5:286
  for peripheral ulcerative keratitis, 8:231
  for persistent corneal epithelial defects, 8:102
  for recurrent corneal erosions, 8:99
  for Stevens-Johnson syndrome, 6:237, 8:218
Luliconazole, 1:76
Lumbar puncture
  in cerebral ischemia/stroke, 1:103
  in subarachnoid hemorrhage, 1:106
  in syphilis, 1:17–18
Lumboperitoneal shunting, for idiopathic intracranial
    hypertension, 5:119–120
Lumens, 3:14–15, 16t
Lumican, 8:10
Lumigan. *See* Bimatoprost
Luminance, 2:462, 3:15, 16t
  background, perimetry affected by, 10:63
  stimulus, perimetry affected by, 10:63
Luminous flux, 2:462, 3:16t
Luminous intensity (candle power), 3:16t
Lung cancer, 1:252, 296–297
  eye involvement and, 1:262, 4:267–268, 268t,
    273–275, 274i
  screening for, 1:296–297
Lung diseases. *See* Pulmonary diseases
Lupron. *See* Leuprolide
Lupus anticoagulant, in antiphospholipid antibody
    syndrome, 1:183–184

Lupus erythematosus, systemic, 1:179–182, 180i, 181t,
    9:61, 173–175, 174i
  eyelid manifestations of, 4:173t
Lupus nephritis, 1:179
Lutein, 2:86
  cataract risk affected by, 11:63
  in macula, 12:7
  structure of, 2:373i
Luteinizing hormone, pituitary adenoma producing,
    1:229
Lux, 3:16t
Luxed/luxated globe, in craniosynostosis, 6:428
Luxed/luxated lens, 4:94, 95i, 6:304, 305t, 309, 11:40.
    See also Ectopia lentis
  cataract surgery and, 11:226–227, 227i, 228i
Lyme disease/Lyme borreliosis, 1:18–21, 8:128,
    9:191–193, 191i, 192i, 12:191
  cranial nerve VII involvement in, 5:284
  ocular manifestations of, 5:362–364
  stages of, 5:363
Lymecycline, 1:72
Lymph nodes, 9:16
  eyelids drained by, 8:7
Lymphadenopathy-associated virus (LAV), 1:36. *See
    also* Human immunodeficiency virus
Lymphadenopathy syndrome (ARC), 1:38–39
Lymphangiectasia, 8:91–92, 273
Lymphangiomas, 8:273. *See also* Vascular
    malformations
  orbital, 4:196, 197i, 6:379, 379i, 7:67–69
Lymphatic/lymphocytic tumors. *See also specific type
    and* Lymphoproliferative lesions
  conjunctival, 8:273–275, 273i, 274i
Lymphatics, 9:7, 19
  eyelid, 2:29, 33i, 7:147, 8:7
Lymphocyte-mediated immune effector responses,
    9:55t, 63–70
  cytotoxic lymphocytes and, 9:66–70, 69i
  delayed hypersensitivity T lymphocytes and, 9:63–66,
    65i, 68t
Lymphocytes, 9:15. *See also* B cells; T cells
  activation of, 9:22–24, 23i, 25
  cytologic identification of, 8:65t, 67, 68i
    in immune-mediated keratoconjunctivitis, 8:203t
  effector, 9:11, 15, 25, 26i
  in inflammation, 4:15, 16i
Lymphocytic thyroiditis, subacute ("painless"), 1:226
Lymphohistiocytosis, EBV-associated hemophagocytic
    (EBV-HLH), 1:30
Lymphoid folliculosis, benign, 8:26, 28i
Lymphoid hyperplasia (lymphoid infiltration/reactive
    lymphoid hyperplasia/benign lymphoid
    pseudotumor/pseudolymphoma)
  of conjunctiva, 4:54, 54i, 55i, 8:273–274, 273i
  of orbit, 7:81–89. *See also* Lymphomas, orbital
  of uveal tract, 4:165, 279–280
Lymphoid proliferation, uveal tract involvement and,
    4:165
  masquerade syndromes secondary to, 9:231–232
Lymphoid stem cells, 1:160
Lymphoid tissues, 9:16
  mucosa-associated (MALT), 8:59, 201
    of conjunctiva (conjunctiva-associated/CALT),
      2:36, 8:5, 8, 59, 201, 9:34t, 36
    lymphoma of, 4:194–195, 195i, 7:85–87, 86t

Lymphokine-activated killer cells, 9:66–70
Lymphokines, 9:70, 80
Lympholysis, radiotherapy for Graves ophthalmopathy and, 7:54
Lymphomas, 4:17i, 17t, 277–279
  Burkitt
    Epstein-Barr virus associated with, 1:30
    of orbit, 4:195, 6:375
  conjunctival, 4:53–55, 54i, 55i, 8:274–275, 274i
  in HIV infection/AIDS, 1:50–51, 5:359
  intraocular (reticulum cell sarcoma/histiocytic
    [large] cell lymphoma/non–Hodgkin lymphoma
    of CNS), 4:277–279, 277i, 279i, 9:228–231, 228i,
    230i, 12:182–183, 182i
    uveitis in children differentiated from, 6:320t
    vitreous involvement and, 4:114–115, 115i
  numb chin associated with, 5:301
  ocular involvement in, 1:262
  orbital, 4:194–196, 195i, 6:375, 7:81–89, 83i, 86t
    clonality of, 7:84
    identification and classification of, 7:82–85, 83i
    lacrimal gland origin and, 7:89, 92
    MALT-type (marginal zone), 7:85–87, 86t
    management of, 7:87
    orbital inflammatory syndrome differentiated
    from, 4:195–196
  systemic, neoplastic masquerade syndromes
    secondary to, 9:231
  of uveal tract, 4:165, 165i
  vitreous, 4:277, 277i, 278
Lymphomatous tumors, 4:277–280. See also
  Lymphoproliferative lesions
Lymphoproliferative lesions, 4:277–280. See also specific
  type and Lymphoid hyperplasia; Lymphomas
  of lacrimal glands, 7:89, 91
  of orbit, 4:194–196, 195i, 7:81–89, 83i, 86t
    histiocytic disorders, 7:88
    juvenile xanthogranuloma, 7:88–89
    lymphoid hyperplasia/lymphomas, 7:82–87
    plasma cell tumors, 7:88
Lynch incision, for anterior orbitotomy, 7:112
Lynell intraocular lens, 11:141i
Lyonization (X chromosome inactivation), 2:190, 210,
  242, 269–273
Lysis, cell
  complement-mediated, 9:59, 60i
  by cytotoxic lymphocytes, 9:68, 69i
Lysosomal fusion, blocking, as microbial virulence
  factor, 1:4
Lysosomal storage disorders, 8:335–336, 337t. See also
  Mucopolysaccharidoses
  retinal degeneration and, 12:243–244, 244i
Lysozyme
  in aqueous humor, 2:320
  in tear film, 2:290, 8:56
    decreased, 8:63
  in external eye defense, 8:113
Lysyl hydroxylase, defects in gene for, in Ehlers Danlos
  syndrome, 8:288, 350

M

M1S1 gene, in amyloidosis, 8:347t
M cells (magnocellular neurons/system), 5:24, 6:44–45,
  47i, 10:44, 46

  development of, 6:46
    abnormal visual experience affecting, 6:49
M-cone opsin genes, 2:346, 346i, 347
  mutations in, 2:346, 346i, 350
M cones, 2:345–346
  bipolar cells for, 2:352, 353i
  horizontal cells for, 2:352
  retinal ganglion cells for, 2:353, 354i
M proteins
  overproduction of, corneal deposits and, 8:349–350
  streptococcal, 8:123, 124
  in subacute sclerosing panencephalitis, 9:159
M unit, 3:251
MAC. See Membrane attack complex
Mac-1, in neutrophil rolling, 9:48
MAC (Mycobacterium avium complex) infections, in
  HIV infection/AIDS, 1:49
Macroadenoma, pituitary, 1:228
  in pregnancy, 5:344
Macroaneurysms, retinal arterial, 12:158–160, 160i
  age-related macular degeneration differentiated
    from, 12:67, 68i
Macroglia, retinal, 2:353
α_2-Macroglobulin
  in aqueous humor, 2:319
  in innate immune response, 9:47
Macroglobulinemia, Waldenström, corneal deposits in,
  8:350
Macrolides, 1:60t, 71, 2:436. See also specific agent
  polyene, 2:437
Macrophage-activating factor, 9:66
Macrophage chemotactic protein-1, 9:81t
Macrophages, 4:13, 9:14–15
  cytologic identification of, 8:67–68
  innate mechanisms for recruitment and activation
    of, 9:48–54, 51i
Macropsia, 5:188, 189
Macrosaccadic oscillations, 5:204, 252–253, 252i
Macrosquare-wave jerks, 5:252, 252i
Macrostomia
  in oculoauriculovertebral (OAV) spectrum, 6:431
  in Treacher Collins syndrome, 6:432
Macrostriae/macrofolds, in LASIK flaps, 13:123–125,
  124t, 125i
Macugen. See Pegaptanib
Macula, 4:119, 120i, 12:7–8, 8i, 9t. See also under
  Macular
  anatomy of, 2:76, 86–88, 86i, 87i, 12:7–8, 8i, 9t
  choroidal neovascularization in. See Age-related
    macular degeneration
  coloboma of, 2:173
  detachment of, visual acuity after reattachment
    surgery and, 12:273
  development of, 6:200
  diseases of, 12:51–95. See also specific type
    electroretinogram in evaluation of, 12:33–34, 34i
    nystagmus and, 6:162
    transient visual loss and, 5:174
    vitrectomy for, 12:323–327
  evaluation of function of, 3:315–317
    before cataract surgery, 11:85–86
  lutea, 2:86, 12:7, 8i
  vitreous interface with, 12:7
    abnormalities of, 12:87–93. See also specific type
Macular atrophy, in cone dystrophies, 12:214, 215i

Macular degeneration
  age-related. *See* Age-related macular degeneration
  cataract surgery in patients with, 11:83, 224
  juvenile (Stargardt disease/fundus flavimaculatus),
    6:337–339, 338*i*, 339*i*, 12:216–218, 216*i*, 217*i*,
    217*t*
    cone–rod dystrophy and, 6:338, 12:215
    retinal pigment epithelium in, 2:363
    rod ABC transporter mutations causing, 2:349
  vitelliform
    adult-onset, 12:219–220, 219*i*, 220*i*
      age-related macular degeneration differentiated
        from, 12:67, 68*i*
      Best disease/vitelliruptive macular degeneration,
        6:339–340, 339*i*, 12:218–219, 218*i*
      bestrophin defect causing, 2:350, 6:340, 12:218
      electrooculogram in, 6:340, 12:37–38, 219
      retinal pigment epithelium in, 2:363
Macular detachment, vitelliform exudative, 12:220,
  220*i*
Macular dystrophy, 4:71, 73*i*, 8:310*t*, 316*t*, 319–320,
  320*i*, 12:215–224. *See also specific type*
  hereditary, 12:215–224
    in children, 6:337–340
  North Carolina, 12:226–227, 227*i*
  Sorsby, 12:223–224, 223*i*
    retinal pigment epithelium in, 2:363
    TIMP3 defects causing, 2:227, 350
  vitelliform. *See* Macular degeneration, vitelliform
Macular edema
  in branch retinal vein occlusion, 12:136
    photocoagulation for, 12:138–140, 139*i*
      wavelength selection and, 12:315*t*
  in central retinal vein occlusion, 12:141
    grid pattern photocoagulation for, 12:144
  clinically significant, 12:114, 114*i*, 115*i*
    photocoagulation and, 12:117–118
  cystoid, 5:104–105, 12:154–156, 155*i*
    angiographic, 12:154
    cataract surgery and, 11:104, 164*t*, 172–174, 173*i*
      in glaucoma patient, 11:218–219
      Nd:YAG capsulotomy and, 11:190–191
    in pars planitis, 9:147, 151, 12:154
    postoperative, 12:332, 333*i*
    prostaglandins and, 9:79
    in retinitis pigmentosa, 12:154, 212, 213*i*
    in sarcoidosis, 8:88
    in uveitis, 9:239
  diabetic, 12:112–113, 113*i*
    laser treatment of, 12:113–116, 114*i*, 115*i*, 116*t*
      wavelength selection and, 12:315*t*
    surgical treatment of, 12:116
Macular electroretinography, 5:101
Macular epiretinal membrane. *See* Epiretinal
  membrane
Macular fibers/projections, 2:98, 104
Macular fibrosis, preretinal, 12:87
Macular holes, 4:112–114, 5:105, 12:253
  idiopathic, 12:89–93, 92*i*, 325–326, 327*i*
    vitrectomy for, 12:93, 325–326, 327*i*
  impending, 12:89
  posttraumatic, 12:292, 294*i*
  treatment of, 12:93, 266, 325–326, 327*i*
  vitreous in formation of, 2:339
Macular infarction, after cataract surgery, 11:178

Macular ischemia, diabetic, 12:116
Macular neuroretinopathy, acute, 9:182
Macular Photocoagulation Study (MPS), 12:70, 80, 82
Macular pucker, 5:105, 12:87
Macular translocation procedures
  for age-related macular degeneration, 12:76
  strabismus and, 6:157
Macule
  of eyelid, 8:24*t*
  hypopigmented (ash-leaf spot), in tuberous sclerosis,
    5:339, 6:409–410, 410*i*
Maculopathies, 5:104–105. *See also specific type*
  age-related. *See* Age-related macular degeneration/
    maculopathy
  bull's-eye
    differential diagnosis of, 12:217, 217*t*
    hydroxychloroquine causing, 1:198
  cellophane, 5:105, 12:87
  crystalline, drug toxicity causing, 12:249, 250*i*
  in ocular histoplasmosis, 9:160–161
  in subacute sclerosing panencephalitis, 9:159
Madarosis, in staphylocooccal blepharitis, 8:164
Maddox rod, 3:94, 97*i*
Maddox rod testing, 5:214, 214*i*, 215*i*, 6:84–85
  before cataract surgery, 11:86
  double, 6:85
    in superior oblique muscle palsy, 6:132
Maffucci syndrome, 6:377
Magainins, 2:457
MAGE. *See* Melanoma antigen genes
Maggots (fly larvae), ocular infection caused by,
  8:133–134
Magnesium, in aqueous humor, 2:317
Magnetic field, of light wave, 3:4, 5*i*
Magnetic resonance angiography (MRA)
  in carotid stenosis, 5:179
  in cerebral ischemia/stroke, 1:103–104
  definition of, 5:80
  limitations of, 5:77*t*
  in orbital evaluation, 7:34
Magnetic resonance fluoroscopy, in ischemic heart
  disease, 1:119
Magnetic resonance imaging (MRI), 5:62–65
  basic principles of, 5:62
  in cerebral ischemia/stroke, 1:103–104
  in choroidal/ciliary body melanoma, 4:227
  diffusion-weighted image in, 5:64, 67*i*
  functional, 5:68, 78
  in intraparenchymal hemorrhage, 5:77*t*
  in ischemic heart disease, 1:119
  limitations of, 5:77*t*
  in orbital evaluation, 7:30–31, 30*i*
    CT scanning compared with, 7:31–33, 32*i*, 33*t*
  parameters in, 5:64*t*
  in retrobulbar optic neuritis, 5:143
  signal intensity in, 5:65*t*
  T1- and T2-weighted images in, 5:62–63, 63*i*, 64*i*,
    65*i*, 66*i*, 7:30–31
  in trilateral retinoblastoma, 4:259–260
Magnetic resonance spectroscopy (MRS), 5:68
  definition of, 5:80
Magnetic source imaging (MSI), in epilepsy diagnosis,
  1:282
Magnetoencephalography (MEG), in epilepsy
  diagnosis, 1:282

Magnification
  axial (longitudinal), **3:**30, 34
  definition of, **3:**31
  with intraocular lenses, **3:**216
  in low vision, for reading, **3:**255–259
  meridional (meridional aniseikonia). *See also*
    Distortion
    astigmatic spectacle lenses causing, **3:**145
      avoidance of with contact lenses, **3:**181
    distortion caused by, **3:**145
      contact lenses in reduction of, **3:**181
  of operating microscope, **3:**296
  transverse, **3:**30–34, 30*i*, 65–66, 66*i*
    in afocal system, **3:**81–82
    calculation of, **3:**65–66, 66*i*
  unit, planes of, **3:**75
Magnifiers, **3:**258–260. *See also* Vision rehabilitation
  handheld, **3:**258
  stand, **3:**259
Magnocellular neurons (M cells/system), **5:**24, **6:**44–45,
    47*i*, **10:**44, 46
  development of, **6:**46
    abnormal visual experience affecting, **6:**49
Magnocellular nevus. *See* Melanocytoma
Main sensory nucleus, of cranial nerve V (trigeminal),
    2:113, 113*i*, **5:**50, 50*i*, 51*i*
Major amblyoscope testing, **6:**64–65, 65*i*, 84, 86
Major (greater) arterial circle, **2:**40, 64, 67, **5:**15
  development of, **2:**155
Major basic protein, **8:**200*t*
Major depression, **1:**265. *See also* Depression
  drugs for (antidepressants), **1:**274–276, 275*t*
    ocular effects of, **1:**324*t*
  in elderly, **1:**239
Major histocompatibility complex (MHC), **8:**447,
    9:90–91, 92*t*. *See also* Human leukocyte (HLA)
    antigens
  class I molecules of, **9:**19–22, 21*i*, 90, 92*t*
  class II molecules of, **9:**19, 20*i*, 90, 92*t*
    primed macrophages as, **9:**51*i*, 52
  class III molecules of, **9:**91
  transplantation and, **9:**93–94
Major intrinsic protein (MIP), **2:**324, 328, **11:**11*i*, 12
  in lens transport, **2:**329
Major tranquilizers. *See* Antipsychotic drugs
Malar rash, in systemic lupus erythematosus, **1:**179,
    181*t*
Malassezia furfur
  as normal ocular flora, **8:**115, 115*t*, 168
  ocular infection caused by, **8:**168
Malattia leventinese, **12:**220. *See also* Drusen
  EFEMP1 defects causing, **2:**351, **12:**220–221
  retinal pigment epithelium in, **2:**363
Malformation, definition of, **6:**205. *See also* Congenital
  anomalies
Malignancy. *See* Cancer
Malignant glaucoma. *See* Aqueous misdirection
Malignant hyperthermia, **1:**336–337, 337*t*, **6:**191–192,
    193*t*
  preoperative assessment of risk for, **1:**329–330
Malignant lymphomas. *See* Lymphomas
Malignant melanomas. *See* Melanomas
Malignant myopia. *See* High (pathologic/degenerative)
  myopia
Malingering, **1:**266, **5:**303

Malondialdehyde (MDA), oxidative lens damage and,
    11:16
MALT. *See* Mucosa-associated lymphoid tissue
MALT lymphoma/MALT-type tumors. *See* Mucosa-
    associated lymphoid tissue (MALT) lymphoma
Mamillations, iris (iris folliculi/diffuse iris nodular
    nevi), **6:**264–265, 265*i*
  central (pupillary) cyst rupture and, **6:**265
Mammography, for cancer screening, **1:**295*t*, 296
Mandibular nerve. *See* Cranial nerve V (trigeminal
    nerve), V₃
Mandibular primordia, **2:**132
Mandibulofacial dysostosis (Treacher Collins/Treacher
    Collins–Franceschetti syndrome), **6:**432, 433*i*, **7:**38,
    38*i*, **8:**353*t*
  eyelid manifestations of, **4:**173*t*
Mandibulo-oculofacial syndrome, dyscephalic. *See*
    Hallermann-Streiff syndrome
Mandol. *See* Cefamandole
Mania, **1:**265
Manic depression. *See* Bipolar disorder
Manifest latent nystagmus, **5:**243, **6:**165, 166*i*
Manifest (noncycloplegic) refraction, **3:**141–142
  before refractive surgery, **13:**42–43
    PRK/LASEK, **13:**91, 92
Manifest strabismus, **6:**9
  cover tests in assessment of, **6:**80–82, 81*i*
Mannitol, **2:**415–416, 415*t*, **10:**164*t*, 173–174
Mannosidosis, **2:**262*t*, **6:**437*t*, **8:**342
  pediatric cataracts in, **6:**288*t*
  retinal degeneration and, **12:**232*t*
Manual lensmeters, **3:**304–307, 305*i*, 306*i*
  Badal principle and, **3:**80–81, 305
  bifocal add measured with, **3:**306–307, 307*i*
Manual objective refractors, **3:**313
Manual perimetry, **10:**78–79, 79*i*, 80*i*
MAO inhibitors. *See* Monoamine oxidase inhibitors
Map-dot-fingerprint dystrophy (epithelial basement
    membrane/anterior membrane dystrophy), **4:**70,
    72*i*, **8:**310*t*, 311–313, 312*i*
  cataract surgery in patients with, **11:**208, 209*i*
  refractive surgery in patients with, **13:**44, 46*i*
Maple syrup urine disease, **2:**262*t*
MAR. *See* Melanomas, retinopathy associated with
MAR (minimum angle of resolution/recognition),
    3:112, 112*t*
  logarithm of, **3:**112, 112*t*
Marax. *See* Theophylline
Marcaine. *See* Bupivacaine
Marcus Gunn jaw-winking ptosis/syndrome, **5:**276,
    277*i*, 279, 281, **6:**214, **7:**217, 218*i*
  synkinesis in, **6:**214, **7:**211, 217, 218*i*
Marcus Gunn pupil (relative afferent pupillary defect)
  cataract surgery and, **11:**81
  in central retinal artery occlusion, **5:**106
  in central retinal vein occlusion, **5:**107, **12:**143
  in multiple evanescent white dot syndrome, **5:**107
  retrochiasmal lesions causing, **5:**165
  testing for, **5:**84–87, 86*i*
    in functional visual disorder evaluation, **5:**307
    practical tips in, **5:**85–86
Marfan syndrome, **1:**166, **6:**306–307, **8:**352*t*, 354,
    11:40–41, 41*i*
  lens defects and, **2:**172
    ectopia lentis, **4:**94, 95*t*, **6:**306–307, 306*i*

subluxation, 10:122
  megalocornea and, 8:290, 354
  pleiotropism in, 2:259
Margin
  ciliary, 7:146
  lid. *See* Eyelids, margin of
Margin–reflex distance, in ptosis, 7:209–210, 210*i*
Marginal arterial arcade, 2:24*i*, 29, 32*i*, 36
Marginal corneal infiltrates
  blepharoconjunctivitis and, 8:229
  staphylococcal blepharitis and, 8:165, 166*i*, 168, 229
Marginal degeneration
  pellucid, 8:332–333, 333*i*, 334*i*, 334*t*, 13:11–12, 47,
    48*i*
    refractive surgery contraindicated in, 8:46–47, 47*i*
  Terrien, 8:370–371, 371*i*
Marginal keratitis, Fuchs superficial, 8:371
Marginal myotomy, 6:175*t*
Marginal rotation, for cicatricial entropion, 7:206, 206*i*
Marginal tear strip (tear meniscus), 2:287
  inspection of, 8:61
  in pseudoepiphora evaluation, 7:273
Marginal zone B-cell lymphoma, 7:85
Marijuana use/abuse, 1:268*t*, 271
MARINA Study, 12:77*t*
Marker site, 2:223
Markers (gene). *See also specific type*
  microsatellites/minisatellites/satellites, 2:190, 203,
    223, 225*i*
  restriction fragment length polymorphisms, 2:195,
    222–223
Maroteaux-Lamy syndrome, 6:436*t*, 8:337*t*
Marshall syndrome, vitreous collapse in, 2:339
Masked bilateral superior oblique muscle palsy, 6:132
Masquerade syndromes, 9:108, 221–233
  eyelid tumors and, 7:184
  lymphoma and, 4:277, 277*i*
  neoplastic, 9:108, 228–233
  nonneoplastic, 9:221–227
  orbital tumors and, 7:69–70, 71*i*, 72*i*
  retinal vasculitis and, 12:153
  uveitis in children and, 6:319, 320*t*
Masson trichrome stain, 4:36, 36*t*
Mast cell stabilizers, 2:423–425, 424*t*. *See also specific
    agent*
  for giant papillary conjunctivitis, 8:216
  for ocular allergy, 6:236, 236*t*, 8:208
  for pulmonary diseases, 1:157*t*, 158
  for vernal keratoconjunctivitis, 8:211
Mast cells, 2:423, 4:13, 9:13–14
  cytologic identification of, 8:65*t*, 66
  in immune-mediated keratoconjunctivitis, 8:203*t*
  degranulation of
    acute IgE-mediated, 9:14, 72–73, 73*i*
    chronic, plus Th2 delayed hypersensitivity, 9:73
  mediators released by, 8:200*t*
  in external eye, 8:196*t*
Mastoid bone, 5:54
Maternal age, Down syndrome incidence and, 2:250
Maternal drug/alcohol use
  childhood glaucoma and, 10:155*t*
  malformations associated with, 1:270, 2:160–161,
    161*i*, 162*i*
    craniofacial malformations and, 6:433–434, 434*i*
Maternal inheritance, 2:217, 257, 269

Mating, assortative, 2:183
Matrix metalloproteinases. *See also specific type under
    MMP*
  in cornea, 2:301
  in ocular infection, 8:117
  in Sjögren syndrome, 8:78
  in Sorsby dystrophy, 12:223
  in vitreous, 2:333
Mature cataract, 11:48, 50*i*
  capsulorrhexis and, 11:210–211
  phacolytic glaucoma and, 11:67
Mavik. *See* Trandolapril
Maxair. *See* Pirbuterol
Maxaquin. *See* Lomefloxacin
Maxide. *See* Triamterene
Maxidex. *See* Dexamethasone
Maxilla/maxillary bone, 5:5, 6*i*, 10, 7:7, 8*i*
  fracture of, 7:97, 98*i*
Maxillary artery, 5:11
  internal, 5:9
Maxillary nerve. *See* Cranial nerve V (trigeminal
    nerve), V₂
Maxillary osteomyelitis, 6:233
Maxillary primordia, 2:132
Maxillary sinuses, 5:9, 7:20–21, 20*i*, 21*i*
Maximal combined response, in electroretinogram,
    12:27, 28*i*, 29
Maxipime. *See* Cefepime
Maxzide. *See* Triamterene
Maze procedure, 1:138
Mazzocco foldable intraocular lens, 11:142*i*, 146
Mazzotti reaction, 9:196
MB isoenzyme, in myocardial infarction, 1:117
McCannel suture/technique
  for intraocular lens decentration, 11:191, 192*i*
  for iridodialysis repair, 8:416, 418*i*
  for iris laceration repair, 8:416, 417*i*
McCarey-Kaufman tissue transport medium, for donor
    corneas, 8:449
McDonald diagnostic criteria, for multiple sclerosis,
    5:323*t*, 324
McNeill-Goldmann blepharostat, for penetrating
    keratoplasty, 8:455
MCP. *See* Multifocal choroiditis, and panuveitis
    syndrome
MCP-1. *See* Macrophage chemotactic protein-1
MCTD. *See* Mixed connective tissue disease
MDA. *See* Malondialdehyde
MDMA (3,4-methylenedioxymethamphetamine/
    ecstasy), 1:270
MDRTB. *See* Multidrug resistant infections,
    tuberculosis
Mean curvature/mean curvature map, 8:43, 45*i*, 13:7
Mean of the ten largest melanoma cell nuclei (MLN),
    4:161
Measles-mumps-rubella (MMR) vaccine, 1:304*t*, 306
Measles (rubeola) virus, 9:159
  immunization against, 1:304*t*, 306
  ocular infection caused by, 8:162–163
    conjunctivitis, 6:228
    posterior uveitis, 9:159
Measurement bias, outcome measures in clinical
    research and, 1:343
Measurement system, designing, 1:363–364
Mecamylamine, 2:402*i*

Mechanical blepharoptosis/ptosis, 7:219, 8:23
Mechanical ectropion, 7:196*i*, 201
Mechanical theory, of glaucomatous optic nerve
    damage, 10:50–51
Mechlorethamine (nitrogen mustard), 1:258*t*
Meckel's cave, 2:114
Meclofenamate, 1:197*t*
Meclomen. *See* Meclofenamate
Medial canthal tendon, 7:146, 255, 256*i*
    trauma involving, 7:186
Medial canthal tumors, 7:277–278
Medial complex, 5:45
Medial longitudinal fasciculus, 5:34, 6:155
    disruption of, 5:224
    rostral interstitial nucleus of, 5:34, 37*i*, 202
Medial muscular branch, of ophthalmic artery,
    extraocular muscles supplied by, 6:16
Medial orbital fractures, 7:101–102, 101*i*
Medial rectus muscles, 2:15*i*, 17*i*, 18*t*, 19*i*, 5:42, 42*i*,
    6:13–14, 13*i*, 17*t*, 18*i*, 7:12
    A-pattern deviations associated with dysfunction of,
        6:119
    action of, 6:13, 17*t*, 30*t*, 31*i*
    anatomy of, 6:13–14, 15*i*, 17*t*, 18*i*
    field of action/activation of, 6:29
    laceration of during sinus surgery, 6:157
    restriction of, incomitant esodeviation and, 6:98*t*,
        108
    surgery of
        for A- and V-pattern deviations, 6:123–124, 123*i*,
            124, 182
        for classic congenital (essential infantile)
            esotropia, 6:100
        for constant exotropia, 6:114
        for Duane syndrome, 6:143
        for esotropia, 6:178–179, 179*i*
        for overcorrection of intermittent exotropia, 6:114
        for sixth nerve paralysis, 6:107–108
        for undercorrection of intermittent exotropia,
            6:114
    V-pattern deviations associated with dysfunction of,
        6:119
Medial spindle procedure, 7:197, 197*i*
Medial superior temporal area, 5:34
Median perforators, of basilar artery, 5:18
Median plane, 6:27–28
Median thalamostriate branch, of posterior cerebral
    artery, 5:18
Mediators, 8:197–198, 198*t*, 200*t*, 9:8, 74–86, 75*t*. *See
    also specific type*
    cytokines, 8:197, 198*t*, 9:80–83, 81–82*t*
    lipid, 9:77–79, 78*i*
    macrophage synthesis of, 9:52–54
    neutrophil-derived granule products, 9:86
    plasma-derived enzyme systems, 9:75–77, 76*i*
    reactive nitrogen products, 9:85–86
    reactive oxygen intermediates, 9:83–85, 84*i*
    in Sjögren syndrome, 8:78
    in uveitis, 9:102
    vasoactive amines, 9:77
Medical Device Amendments, 13:31
Medical devices
    delays in FDA approval of, 13:37–38
    FDA classification of, 13:31–35
    labeling, 13:37

pathways to market for, 13:35–36
Medical history. *See* History
Medications. *See* Drugs
Medium, optical
    opaque. *See* Cataract; Opacities
    refractive index of, 3:39–41, 40*t*. *See also* Refractive
        index
    definition of, 3:6
Medium Choroidal Melanoma Trial, 4:240–241
Medroxyprogesterone, for chemical burns, 8:392
Medrysone, 2:417*t*
    anti-inflammatory/pressure-elevating potency of,
        2:419*t*
Medullary carcinoma of thyroid gland, 1:227
    in multiple endocrine neoplasia, 1:230
Medullary velum, superior, 2:111
Medullated (myelinated) nerve fibers, 4:121, 121*i*,
    6:360, 360*i*
Medulloblastoma
    eyelid manifestations of, 4:176*t*
    nystagmus caused by, 6:159*t*
Medulloepithelioma (diktyoma), 4:144–146, 147*i*, 283,
    6:369
    teratoid, 4:146
Meesmann dystrophy (juvenile epithelial dystrophy),
    8:310*t*, 313, 314*i*
Mefenamic acid, 1:197*t*
Mefoxin. *See* Cefoxitin
MEG. *See* Magnetoencephalography
Megaloblastic anemia, 1:161
Megalocornea, 2:167–168, 167*i*, 6:250, 8:289–290, 289*i*,
    290*i*, 309*t*
    Marfan syndrome and, 8:290, 354
    simple, 6:250
Megaloglobus (buphthalmos)
    in glaucoma, 6:277, 10:147
    in neurofibromatosis, 6:408
Megalopapilla, 6:361
Megalophthalmos
    anterior, 6:250
    intraocular lens implantation and, 11:213–214, 215*i*
Meglitinides, 1:213
Meibomian glands, 2:22, 24*i*, 27–28, 29*t*, 30*i*, 31*i*,
    4:168*t*, 7:142*i*, 147, 166, 8:6, 7*i*, 8
    chalazion caused by obstruction of, 6:388, 7:158,
        8:87
    dysfunction of, 2:294, 8:56, 80–84, 82*i*
        blepharitis in, 8:83, 164*t*
        refractive surgery and, 13:44
    in external eye defense, 8:113
    sebaceous adenocarcinoma arising in, 7:180
    in tear film-lipids/tear production, 2:287–289, 289*i*,
        7:253, 8:56, 57
Meibomianitis, cataract surgery in patients with,
    11:206
Meige syndrome, 5:286, 287*i*
Meiosis, 2:190, 204, 244, 245*i*
    nondisjunction during, 2:245*i*, 249. *See also*
        Nondisjunction
Melanin
    absorption spectrum for, 12:313, 314*i*
    corneal pigmentation caused by, 8:375, 377*t*
    defective synthesis of, in albinism, 2:176, 263, 362,
        12:239
    in eyelid skin, 8:245

photoprotective function of, 2:362, 370
in retinal pigment epithelium, 2:357, 362, 370
hypertrophy and, 12:264
Melanin pigment granules, cytologic identification of,
8:69–70, 69i
α-Melanocyte-stimulating hormone, 8:198t
in tear secretion, 2:293
Melanocytes
choroidal, 2:149, 12:15
dendritic, 8:245
in iris stroma, 2:62
tumors arising from, 8:263, 263t
Melanocytic nevus, 4:182–185
of anterior chamber/trabecular meshwork, 4:84
congenital, 4:182, 182i
Melanocytic proliferation, bilateral diffuse uveal, 9:233,
12:165–166, 165i
Melanocytic tumors, 4:215–242
of anterior chamber/trabecular meshwork, 4:84, 85i
of conjunctiva, 4:55–59, 56i, 56t, 57i, 58i
of eyelid, 4:182–185, 182i, 183i
benign, 7:169–170
premalignant, 7:174
in neurofibromatosis, 6:403–404, 404i
Melanocytoma
in children, 6:390, 392i
of ciliary body or choroid, 4:158, 209i, 217
of optic disc/optic nerve, 4:208, 209i
melanoma differentiated from, 4:230, 232i
of uveal tract, 4:158
Melanocytosis
dermal, 7:171–172
ocular (melanosis oculi), 8:264–265, 265i, 267t
in children, 6:387–388, 388i
oculodermal (nevus of Ota/congenital
oculomelanocytosis), 2:175, 4:56t, 7:171,
171–172, 172i, 8:264, 267t
in children, 6:387–388
glaucoma associated with, 10:32
of iris, 4:220t
Melanogenesis, 2:144, 150
latanoprost and, 2:414
Melanokeratosis, striate, 8:264
Melanoma antigen genes, 9:72
Melanomalytic glaucoma, 4:84, 85i, 161
Melanomas, 1:299, 12:15
acral-lentiginous, 4:185
of anterior chamber/trabecular meshwork, 4:84, 85i
choroidal, 4:159–163, 222–241, 223i. See also
Choroidal/ciliary body melanoma
age-related macular degeneration differentiated
from, 12:70
nevus differentiated from, 4:216–217
open-angle glaucoma caused by, 10:106
spindle cell, 4:160, 160i
spread of, 4:161–163, 161i
staging of, 4:289–290t
ciliary body, 4:159–163, 222–241, 223i. See also
Choroidal/ciliary body melanoma
staging of, 4:289–290t
conjunctival, 4:58–59, 58i, 8:268–269, 268i
in children, 6:387
intraocular extension of, 4:275
primary acquired melanosis and, 4:58–59, 58i
staging of, 4:286t

enucleation for, 7:119–120
exenteration for, 7:128
of eyelid, 4:185, 7:182–183
incidence of, 1:299
of iris, 4:157, 158i, 217–222, 218i, 220t
lentigo maligna, 4:185, 7:182
metastatic, 9:233
nodular, 7:182–183
ocular melanocytosis and, 8:264–265
retinoblastoma associated with, 4:265t
retinopathy associated with, 5:101, 109, 12:237–239
ring, 4:157, 159, 161, 162i, 222
screening for, 1:299
superficial spreading, 4:185
tapioca, 4:220t
unsuspected, 4:228–229
uveal, 4:159–163, 222–241, 9:72, 232. See also
Choroidal/ciliary body melanoma
staging of, 4:289–290t
uveitis in children differentiated from, 6:320t
Melanosis, 8:263
benign, 4:56t, 8:264, 264i, 267t
congenital, 8:263
oculi (ocular melanocytosis), 6:387–388, 388i,
8:264–265, 265i, 267t
precancerous (lentigo maligna/Hutchinson's
melanotic freckle), 7:174
primary acquired, 4:56–58, 56t, 57i, 58i, 8:266–268,
267i, 267t
Melanosomes
in choroid, 2:149
in retinal pigment epithelium, 2:78–79, 144, 12:13
MELAS (mitochondrial myopathy with
encephalopathy/lactic acidosis/stroke-like episodes)
syndrome, 5:297, 12:245
mitochondrial DNA mutation and, 2:211, 218, 219i
Melasma, of eyelids, 7:170
Melkersson-Rosenthal syndrome, 5:285
Mellaril. See Thioridazine
Melphalan, 1:258t
MEM. See Minimum essential medium
Memantine, for Alzheimer disease, 1:288
Membrane attack complex, 9:59
Membrane sacs, in rods, 2:341, 344
Membrane structural (urea-insoluble) lens proteins,
2:328, 11:11i, 12
Membrane-type frizzled protein (MFRP), mutation in
gene for, in nanophthalmos, 8:287
Membranes
conjunctival, 8:24t, 25t
in epidemic keratoconjunctivitis, 8:159
Descemet. See Descemet's membrane
implantation, of iris, 4:219t
retrocorneal fibrous (posterior collagenous layer),
2:301–302, 8:33–34
Membranous cataract, 11:38, 40i
Memory, immunologic, 9:11, 27–28
MEN. See Multiple endocrine neoplasia
Mendelian disorder (single-gene disorder), 2:190, 257
Ménière disease, 5:246
Meningeal artery
dorsal, 5:13
middle, 5:11, 13
Meningeal nerve, middle, 5:52
Meninges, optic nerve, 2:101–102, 101i

Meningiomas, **7**:77–79, 77–78*i*
  cerebellopontine angle, **5**:284
  MR imaging of, **5**:76*i*
  optic nerve, **4**:209–210, 210*i*
    optic glioma differentiated from, **6**:406
  optic nerve sheath, **5**:130*i*, 145–148, 147*i*, 148*t*, **7**:77
    in children, **5**:148
  orbital, **7**:77–79, 77–78*i*, 93
    in children, **6**:381
    transient visual loss and, **5**:175
  parasellar, chiasmal syndromes caused by, **5**:162
Meningitis
  cranial nerve VII involvement in, **5**:284
  cryptococcal, **5**:368
  Haemophilus influenzae causing, **1**:11, 12, 309
  headache and, **5**:291
  meningococcal, **1**:13
    immunization against, **1**:13, 309
Meningoceles, **7**:38
  orbital, **6**:384
Meningococcemia, **1**:13
Meningococcus (*Neisseria meningitidis*), **1**:12–13, **8**:125
  conjunctivitis in children caused by, **6**:225
  immunization against, **1**:13, 309
  invasive capability of, **8**:116
Meningoencephaloceles, **7**:38, 38*i*
Mental acuity disturbances, in multiple sclerosis, **5**:320
Mental disorders due to general medical condition
    (organic mental syndromes), **1**:264. *See also*
    Alzheimer disease; Behavioral/psychiatric disorders
  in elderly, **1**:240
Mental nerve neuropathy, **5**:301
Mentax. *See* Butenafine
Meperidine, for postoperative pain, **1**:338
Mepivacaine, **2**:445*t*, 447
  maximum safe dose of, **1**:322*t*
Mepron. *See* Atovaquone
6-Mercaptopurine, **1**:258*t*
Meretoja syndrome, **8**:319
Meridians, **11**:5
  alignment of, combination of spherocylindrical
      lenses and, **3**:99–100
  of astigmatic surface or lens, **3**:94–98, 96*i*
  locating axes of, in retinoscopy, **3**:130–132, 131*i*,
      132*i*
Meridional amblyopia, **6**:70
Meridional complex, **12**:9, 263*i*
Meridional folds, **12**:9, 262, 263*i*
Meridional magnification (meridional aniseikonia). *See
    also* Distortion
  astigmatic spectacle lenses causing, **3**:145
    avoidance of with contact lenses, **3**:181
  distortion caused by, **3**:145
    contact lenses for reduction of, **3**:181
Meropenem, **1**:60*t*, 69
Merrem. *See* Meropenem
MERRF. *See* Myoclonic epilepsy with ragged red fibers
Mesectodermal dysgenesis. *See* Anterior segment,
    dysgenesis of
Mesectodermal leiomyoma, **4**:185
Mesencephalic nucleus, of cranial nerve V (trigeminal),
    2:112, 113*i*, **5**:50, 50*i*
Mesencephalon, cranial nerve III arising from, **2**:108
Mesenchymal cells, in ocular development, **8**:6

Mesenchymal dysgenesis. *See* Anterior segment,
    dysgenesis of
Mesenchymal tumors
  eyelid and conjunctiva, **8**:269–272, 270*i*
  orbital, **7**:79–81, 79*i*, 82*i*
Mesenchyme, **2**:126
Mesoderm, **2**:126, 134, 134*i*, 135*i*, 137*i*
  ocular structures derived from, **2**:133*t*
Mesodermal dysgenesis. *See* Anterior segment,
    dysgenesis of; Axenfeld-Rieger syndrome;
    Leukomas
Messenger RNA (mRNA), **2**:126, **8**:306
  in antibiotic mechanism of action, **1**:54
  processing of, **2**:209
Meta-analyses, of clinical trials, **1**:352
Metabolic disorders. *See also specific type and* Inborn
    errors of metabolism
  cataracts and, **11**:60–63
  corneal changes and, **8**:309–310*t*, 335–357, 337*t*,
      339*t*, 346*t*, 347*t*, 351–353*t*, 358*t*
  diagnostic approach to, **8**:308
  enzyme defects/ocular signs in, **2**:262*t*
  molecular genetics of, **8**:305–308, 309–310*t*
  retinal manifestations of, **12**:239–245
  screening for, **1**:300–301
Metabolic syndrome, **1**:95, 146, 148, 152*t*, 206
Metachromatic leukodystrophy, **2**:262*t*, **6**:436*t*
Metaglip. *See* Glipizide, with metformin
Metaherpetic ulcer, **8**:151
Metallic reflection, **3**:13
Metalloproteinases, matrix. *See also specific type under
    MMP*
  in cornea, **2**:301
  in ocular infection, **8**:117
  in Sjögren syndrome, **8**:78
  in Sorsby dystrophy, **12**:223
  in vitreous, **2**:333
Metallosis, lens damage/cataracts caused by, **11**:58–59,
    59*i*
Metamorphopsia, **5**:90
  in age-related macular degeneration, **12**:63
  in epiretinal membrane, **12**:88
  illusions and, **5**:188–189
Metaplasia, definition of, **8**:247*t*
Metarhodopsin II, **2**:342
Metastatic eye disease, **4**:267–275, 279–288, **9**:233. *See
    also specific type and structure affected*
  carcinoma, **4**:267–275
    ancillary tests in evaluation of, **4**:271–273, 274*i*
    clinical features of, **4**:269–271, 269*i*, 270*i*, 271*i*,
        272*i*, 274*i*
    diagnostic factors in, **4**:273–275
    mechanisms of spread and, **4**:268–271
    primary sites and, **4**:267–268, 268*t*
    prognosis for, **4**:274–275
    treatment of, **4**:273–275
  of choroid, **4**:163–164, 163*i*, 269–271, 270*i*, 271*i*,
      272*i*
  of conjunctiva, **8**:275
  of iris, **4**:220*t*
  of optic nerve, **4**:273
  of orbit, **4**:202, **7**:94–96
    in adults, **7**:95–96, 95*i*
    in children, **6**:374–376, **7**:94, 94*i*
    management of, **7**:96

of retina, 4:273, 274*i*
of uvea, 4:163–164, 163*i*
Metered-dose inhalers, β₂-adrenergics for pulmonary
disease and, 1:157
Metformin, 1:212*t*, 213
Methadone maintenance, for heroin dependence, 1:269
Methamphetamine, abuse of, 1:270
Methanol toxicity, optic neuropathy caused by, 5:152
Methazolamide, 2:411*t*, 412, 10:163*t*, 168
for childhood glaucoma, 6:283
Methenamine–silver nitrate stain, 4:36
Methicillin, 1:67, 2:428*t*, 429
for *Staphylococcus aureus* preseptal cellulitis, 7:42
Methicillin-resistant *S aureus*, 1:5, 67, 71, 72
Methimazole, for Graves disease, 1:225, 7:54
Methionine, in homocystinuria, 11:41, 42
dietary restriction in management of, 6:438
Methohexital, perioperative, 1:332*t*, 335
Methotrexate, 1:198, 258*t*
in cancer chemotherapy, 1:258*t*
for cicatricial pemphigoid, 8:223
intraocular injection of, 2:387
for intraocular lymphoma, 4:278
for juvenile rheumatoid arthritis, 9:143
for peripheral ulcerative keratitis, 8:231
for primary central nervous system lymphoma,
9:230
for rheumatoid arthritis, 1:174
for scleritis, 8:241
for uveitis, 9:119, 119*t*
in children, 6:321
for Wegener granulomatosis, 1:192
Methoxyflurane, crystalline maculopathy caused by,
12:249, 250*t*
Methylation, DNA, 2:210
Methylcellulose, hydroxypropyl (HPMC)
for dry eye, 2:450
as viscoelastic, 2:452
Methyldopa, 1:89*t*, 90*t*
3,4-Methylenedioxymethamphetamine (MDMA/
ecstasy), 1:270
Methylprednisolone
for corneal graft rejection, 8:469
for giant cell arteritis, 5:122
for optic neuritis, 5:143
for pars planitis, 9:149
for traumatic optic neuropathy, 5:154
for traumatic visual loss, 7:108
for uveitis, 9:115*t*
Metipranolol, 2:410*t*, 10:160*t*, 165
for childhood glaucoma, 6:282
Metoclopramide, perioperative, 1:331, 332*t*, 338
Metolazone, 1:88*t*
Metoprolol
for heart failure, 1:131
for hypertension, 1:88*t*, 90*t*
Metric units, for visual acuity notations, 3:112
Metrogel. *See* Metronidazole
Metronidazole, 1:62*t*, 74
for *C difficile* colitis, 1:8
for rosacea, 8:86
Mevacor. *See* Lovastatin
MEWDS. *See* Multiple evanescent white dot syndrome
Meyer, loop of, 2:108, 5:29, 166
Mezlin. *See* Mezlocillin

Mezlocillin, 1:56*t*, 67, 2:429
MFRP. *See* Membrane-type frizzled protein
MG. *See* Myasthenia gravis
MGD. *See* Meibomian glands, dysfunction of
MH. *See* Malignant hyperthermia
MHA-TP (microhemagglutination assay for *T
pallidum*), 1:17, 302, 9:189
MHC. *See* Major histocompatibility complex
MI. *See* Myocardial infarction
Miacalcin. *See* Calcitonin/calcitonin nasal spray
MIC. *See* Minimal inhibitory concentration
Micafungin, 1:76
Micardis. *See* Telmisartan
Micatin. *See* Miconazole
Michaelis constant (K_m), "sugar" cataract development
and, 11:14–15
Michaelis-Menton equation, "sugar" cataract
development and, 11:14–15
Michelson interferometer, 3:322
Miconazole, 1:64*t*, 2:438*t*, 439
Microadenoma, pituitary, 1:228
Microaneurysms, retinal
in HIV infection/AIDS, 9:248
ischemia causing, 4:131, 132*i*
in nonproliferative diabetic retinopathy, 12:103, 104*i*
in children, 6:343
Microbial keratitis. *See* Keratitis, infectious/microbial
Microbiology, 8:118–134, 119*t*. *See also* specific
organism
bacteriology, 8:119*t*, 122–128
cytologic identification of organisms and, 8:70, 70*i*
mycology, 8:119*t*, 128–131, 129*t*
parasitology, 8:119*t*, 131–134
principles of, 1:3–4
prions, 8:134
virology, 8:118–122, 119*t*
virulence factors and, 8:116–117
Microcirculatory failure, in shock, 1:317
Micrococcus, as normal ocular flora, 8:115*t*
Microcoria (congenital miosis), 6:268
Microcornea, 2:167, 167*i*, 6:250–251, 251*i*, 8:288–289
cornea plana and, 8:291
Microcystic dystrophy, Cogan, 8:311, 312
Microcystic epitheliopathy, 8:107
Microcytic anemia, 1:161
Microenvironments, immunologic. *See* Immunologic
microenvironments
Microfilariae
loa loa, 8:191
onchocercal, 8:132
in anterior chamber, 9:196
Microfolds/microstriae, in LASIK flaps, 13:123, 124*t*,
125–126, 125*i*
Microglial cells, 2:83, 84, 353, 4:203
degeneration of in retinal ischemia, 4:129–130
Micrographic surgery, Mohs'
for canthal tumors, 7:193
for neoplastic disorders of eyelid, 8:250
basal cell carcinoma, 4:180, 7:178–179
sebaceous adenocarcinoma, 7:182
squamous cell carcinoma, 7:178–179
Microhemagglutination assay for *T pallidum* (MHA-
TP), 1:17, 302, 9:189
Microkeratomes
for lamellar keratoplasty, 8:474

for LASIK, **13**:89, 106, 107–109, 108–109*i*
  flap creation by, **13**:112–114, 113*i*, 114*i*
  complications of, **13**:120–121, 121*i*
Micronase. *See* Glyburide
Micronutrients. *See also specific type*
  in age-related macular degeneration management,
    12:60–61
Micropannus. *See* Pannus
Microperoxisomes, in retinal pigment epithelium,
    2:357
Microphakia, in fetal alcohol syndrome, **2**:161
Microphthalmos, **2**:126, 160*i*, 162–163, 164*i*, **7**:37–38,
    8:286–287, 286*i*, 289
  anterior, **8**:289
  in congenital cytomegalovirus infection, **6**:218
  in congenital rubella, **6**:218
  with cyst (colobomatous cyst), **6**:383, 383*i*, **7**:37–38
  in fetal alcohol syndrome, **2**:161
  intraocular lens implantation and, **11**:213
  with linear skin defects, **6**:254–255
  microcornea with, **2**:167, 167*i*
  persistent hyperplastic primary vitreous associated
    with, **12**:281, 282
Micropsia, **5**:188, 189
  in epiretinal membrane, **12**:88
Micropuncture, anterior stromal, for recurrent corneal
    erosions, **8**:99–100, 100*i*
Microsaccadic refixation movements, **5**:199
Microsatellites, **2**:190, 203, 223
Microscope
  confocal, **8**:37–38
  operating, **3**:296–297, 296*i*, 297*i*
    phototoxicity and, **2**:459, **11**:171–172, **12**:308
  specular, **3**:294–295, 295*i*, **8**:18, 36–37, 36*i*
    examination with before cataract surgery, **11**:87
    examination with before phakic intraocular lens
      insertion, **13**:146
    in optical focusing technique for pachymetry,
      3:293
Microscopic polyangiitis (microscopic polyarteritis),
    1:189*t*, 192
Microsomal triglyceride transfer protein (MTP),
    mutations in, **2**:351
Microsomia, hemifacial, **6**:431, 432, **8**:352*t*
Microspherophakia, **2**:172, **11**:32–33, 33*i*
  pupillary block and angle-closure glaucoma caused
    by, **10**:130, 131*i*, **11**:33
  in Weill-Marchesani syndrome, **6**:308
Microsporida (microsporidiosis), **8**:131–132, 190
  in HIV infection/AIDS, **1**:48, 49, **8**:190, **9**:260, 260*i*
  keratitis/keratoconjunctivitis caused by, **4**:47, **8**:190,
    9:260, 260*i*
Microstriae/microfolds, in LASIK flaps, **13**:123, 124*t*,
    125–126, 125*i*
Microtropias, in monofixation syndrome, **6**:57
Microvascular cranial nerve palsy, pain associated with,
    5:299
Microvascular disease, diabetic. *See* Diabetic
    retinopathy
Microwave radiation, biological effects of on lens,
    11:57
Microzide. *See* Hydrochlorothiazide
Mid chiasmal syndrome, **5**:158, 160*i*
Midamor. *See* Amiloride

Midazolam, **1**:273
  perioperative, **1**:332*t*, 335
Midbrain lesions
  corectopia caused by, **5**:260
  pupillary reactivity affected by, **5**:270
Middle cerebral artery, **5**:16, 17, 20*i*
Middle cranial fossa, **7**:21
Middle limiting membrane, **12**:12
Midface lift, **7**:241–242
Midfacial fractures, **7**:97, 98*i*
Midget bipolar cell, **12**:10
Midget ganglion cells, **6**:45
Midline positions of gaze, **6**:86
Miglitol, **1**:212*t*, 213
Migraine equivalent (acephalgic migraine), **5**:294–295.
    See also Migraine headache
Migraine headache, **5**:292–295
  acephalgic, **5**:294–295
  with aura (classic migraine), **5**:185, 293–294, 293*i*
  without aura (common migraine), **5**:294
  basilar-type (complicated migraine), **5**:293–294
  branch retinal artery occlusion and, **12**:147
  evaluation of, **5**:295, 295*i*
  inherited encephalopathies resembling, **5**:297–298
  ophthalmoplegic, **5**:231
  pathophysiology of, **5**:294
  retinal, **5**:184, 294–295
  transient visual loss caused by, **5**:185
  treatment of
    acute, **5**:296
    prophylactic, **5**:296–297
Mikulicz syndrome, **7**:91, **8**:88
Milia, **7**:164–166
Millard-Gubler syndrome, **5**:227
Miller Fisher syndrome, **5**:277, 285
Miller-Nadler Glare Tester, **3**:253
Milrinone, for heart failure, **1**:130–131
Mimetic muscles, **7**:135–137, 138*i*
  facial nerve supplying, **7**:137–138
Mimicry, molecular, **9**:89
  autoimmune uveitis and, **9**:91
  HLA disease associations and, **9**:95
  retinal vasculitis in systemic lupus erythematosus
    and, **9**:61
Minerals
  antioxidant, oral supplements containing, **2**:373–375,
    374*t*, 454
  disorders of metabolism of, corneal changes in,
    8:355–356
Minimal inhibitory concentration (MIC), **1**:66–67
Minimal lethal concentration (MLC), **1**:67
Minimal pigment albinism, **6**:347*t*
Minimum angle of resolution/recognition (MAR),
    3:112, 112*t*
  logarithm of, **3**:112, 112*t*
Minimum essential medium, **2**:454
Minimum legible threshold, **3**:111
Minimum separable threshold, **3**:111
Minimum visible threshold, **3**:111
Minipress. *See* Prazosin
Minisatellites, **2**:190, 203, 223
Minizide. *See* Prazosin
Minocin. *See* Minocycline
Minocycline, **1**:61*t*, **2**:433
  for meibomian gland dysfunction, **8**:83

ocular effects of, 1:324*t*
for rosacea, 8:86
Minoxidil, for hypertension, 1:89*t*
Minus cylinder form, for contact lenses, 3:181
Minus cylinder refraction, 3:135*i*, 136
Minus (concave) lenses, anophthalmic socket
    camouflage and, 7:127
Miochol. *See* Acetylcholine
Miosis/miotic agents, 2:309, 398*t*
    adrenergic antagonists, 2:408
    cataracts caused by, 11:53–54
    cholinergic agonists, 2:309, 394–398, 398*t*
    cholinesterase inhibitors, 2:309, 398–400, 398*t*, 399*i*
    congenital (microcoria), 6:268
    for glaucoma, 10:166–167
        cataract symptoms and, 11:217
        in children, 6:283
    modes of action of, 2:314*t*
    muscarinic agents and, 2:397–398, 398*t*
    for overcorrection of intermittent exotropia, 6:113
    for refractive accommodative esotropia, 6:102
    traumatic injury and, 8:397
Miostat. *See* Carbachol
MIP. *See* Major intrinsic protein
Mirapex. *See* Pramipexole
Mirror test, in functional visual disorder evaluation,
    5:305, 306*i*
Mirrors, 3:28–30, 29*i*, 90–93
    central ray for, 3:91, 91*i*
    cold, 3:9
    in direct ophthalmoscope, 3:270, 271*i*
    imaging with, 3:28–30, 29*i*, 90–93
        image quality and, 3:38, 38*i*
    in lasers, 3:22, 22*i*
    reflecting power of, 3:90
    in retinoscope, 3:125, 125*i*, 126*i*
    reversal of image space by, 3:90
    vergence calculations for, 3:92–93, 92*i*
Mismatch repair, 2:213
Missense mutation, 2:191
Mitochondrial DNA, 2:215–220, 219*i*
    diseases associated with deletions/mutations of,
        2:217–220
        galtonian inheritance of, 2:186, 257
        Leber hereditary optic neuropathy, 2:218–220,
            219*i*, 5:134–135, 6:365
        maternal inheritance/transmission and, 2:217, 257,
            269
        retinal degeneration and, 12:233*t*, 245
    genetic code for translation of, 2:215–217
    genomic structure of, 2:217
    in replicative segregation, 2:195
Mitochondrial myopathy, 12:245
    with encephalopathy/lactic acidosis/strokelike
        episodes (MELAS), 5:297, 12:245
        mitochondrial DNA mutation and, 2:211, 218,
            219*i*
Mitomycin/mitomycin C, 1:257, 259*t*, 2:393, 426
    for conjunctival intraepithelial neoplasia, 8:258
    for dacryocystitis, 7:283
    in phototherapeutic keratectomy, 8:440
    for PRK, 13:95
        enhancement of LASIK flaps and, 13:119
        undercorrection and, 13:101
    in pterygium surgery, 8:432

toxic keratoconjunctivitis caused by, 8:394
    in trabeculectomy, 10:191–192
        in children, 6:281
Mitosis, 2:191, 204
    nondisjunction during, 2:252. *See also*
        Nondisjunction
Mitoxantrone, for multiple sclerosis, 5:324
Mitten deformity, 6:427*i*
Mittendorf dot, 2:91, 92*i*, 175, 177*i*, 4:107, 6:361,
    11:29–30, 31, 12:280
Mixed astigmatism
    LASIK for, 13:118
    PRK for, 13:99
Mixed connective tissue disease, 1:185
Mixed dementia, 1:285
Mixed lymphocyte reaction, 9:94
Mixed tumor
    benign (pleomorphic adenoma)
        of eyelid, 7:167
        of lacrimal gland, 4:192–193, 193*i*, 7:89–90
    malignant, of lacrimal gland, 7:90
Mizuo-Nakamura phenomenon, 12:201
MLC. *See* Minimal lethal concentration
MLF. *See* Medial longitudinal fasciculus
MLN. *See* Manifest latent nystagmus; Mean of the ten
    largest melanoma cell nuclei
MLS. *See* Microphthalmos, with linear skin defects;
    Mucolipidoses
MLS I. *See* Dysmorphic sialidosis
MLS II. *See* Inclusion-cell (I-cell) disease
MLS III. *See* Pseudo-Hurler polydystrophy
MLS IV, 8:342
MM isoenzyme, in myocardial infarction, 1:117
MMC. *See* Mitomycin/mitomycin C
MMP. *See* Matrix metalloproteinases
MMP-2 (gelatinase)
    in recurrent corneal erosion, 8:98
    in Sjögren syndrome, 8:78
    in vitreous, 2:333
MMP-2 proenzyme, in cornea, 2:301
MMP-3, in Sjögren syndrome, 8:78
MMP-9
    in recurrent corneal erosion, 8:98
    in Sjögren syndrome, 8:78
MMP-13, in Sjögren syndrome, 8:78
MMR vaccine, 1:304*t*, 306
Mn SOD, 2:372
MOABs. *See* Monoclonal antibodies
Mobile lens syndrome, 10:122
Mobitz type II atrioventricular block, 1:134
Möbius syndrome, 5:283, 6:154–155, 154*i*
    esotropia in, 6:98*t*, 154, 154*i*
Modulation transfer function, 3:113, 317
Moduretic. *See* Amiloride
Moexipril, 1:88*t*, 90*t*
Mohs' micrographic surgery
    for canthal tumors, 7:193
    for neoplastic disorders of eyelid, 8:250
        basal cell carcinoma, 4:180, 7:178–179
        sebaceous adenocarcinoma, 7:182
        squamous cell carcinoma, 7:178–179
Molds, 5:365, 8:128–129, 129*i*, 129*t*
    endogenous ophthalmitis caused by, 12:188–189,
        189*i*

Molecular biologic techniques/molecular genetics. *See* Genetics, molecular
Molecular mimicry, **9**:89
  autoimmune uveitis and, **9**:91
  HLA disease associations and, **9**:95
  retinal vasculitis in systemic lupus erythematosus and, **9**:61
Molecular pathology techniques, **4**:39–40, 39*i*
Moll, glands of, **2**:22, 24*i*, 29*t*, **4**:168*t*, **7**:166, **8**:6, 7*i*. *See also* Apocrine glands of eyelid
  hidrocystoma arising in, **7**:167–168
Molluscum contagiosum, **8**:121, 160–161, 161*i*
  conjunctivitis in children in, **6**:228–229, 229*i*
  of eyelid, **4**:171, 172*i*, **7**:166
  in HIV infection/AIDS, **9**:259
Molteno implant, for childhood glaucoma, **6**:281
Monistat. *See* Miconazole
Monitoring system, **1**:364–366
Monoamine oxidase inhibitors, **1**:275*t*, 276
  discontinuing before surgery, **1**:334
  drug interactions and, **1**:276
    apraclonidine/brimonidine interactions, **2**:408
    hypertension and, **1**:97, 276
Monobactams, **1**:59*t*, 70
Monochromaticity, of laser light, **3**:17, 20*i*
Monochromatism
  blue-cone, **6**:336, **12**:198
    ocular findings in carriers of, **2**:270*t*
    electroretinogram patterns in, **12**:30*i*
  rod, **12**:196
    in children, **6**:335–336
Monocid. *See* Cefonicid
Monoclonal antibodies, **9**:54
  in cancer therapy, **1**:261
Monoclonal gammopathy, benign, corneal deposits in, **8**:350
Monocular aphakia, aniseikonia and, with contact lenses, **3**:178
Monocular blindness, evaluation of, as functional disorder, **5**:306–307, 308*i*
Monocular cover-uncover test, **6**:80–81, 81*i*
Monocular diplopia, **3**:170–171, **5**:216
  in cataracts, **11**:45, 47, 77
  in epiretinal membrane, **12**:88
  multifocal IOLs and, **3**:228–229
Monocular distortion, **3**:325–326. *See also* Distortion
  adaptation to, **3**:336–337
  minimizing, **3**:332–336
  sources of, **3**:326–327
Monocular elevation deficiency (double elevator palsy), **6**:137–138, 138*i*, **7**:214
Monocular eye movements (ductions), **6**:34–35. *See also specific type*
Monocular fixation, **6**:11
Monocular nystagmus, **5**:243, **6**:167
Monocular recess-resect procedures
  for esodeviation, **6**:179, 179*t*
  for exodeviation, **6**:179, 181*t*
Monocular suppression, **6**:54–55
Monocular telescopes, **3**:260
Monocular transient visual loss, **5**:173–184. *See also* Transient visual loss
  binocular visual loss compared with, **5**:171
  carotid artery disease and, **1**:107

  embolic causes of, **5**:174*t*, 175–183, 176*i*, 178*i*
    clinical aspects of, **5**:177*t*
    clinical and laboratory evaluation of, **5**:179–180
    prognosis for, **5**:180–181, 180*t*
    treatment of, **5**:181–182, 182*t*
  hypoperfusion causing, **5**:174*t*, 183–184, 184*i*
  ocular causes of, **5**:173–175, 174*t*
  orbital causes of, **5**:174*t*, 175
  systemic causes of, **5**:174*t*, 175–184
  vasculitis causing, **5**:174*t*, 183
Monocular vision, reduced, **5**:308, 309*t*
Monocytes, **9**:14–15. *See also* Macrophages
  cytologic identification of, **8**:65*t*, 67–68, 68*i*
    in immune-mediated keratoconjunctivitis, **8**:203*t*
  in inflammation, **4**:13, 14*i*
Monofixation syndrome, **6**:57–58
  Bagolini striated glasses in evaluation of, **6**:61
  4Δ base-out prism test in evaluation of, **6**:61–63, 63*i*
  simultaneous prism and cover test in evaluation of, **6**:82
  Worth 4-dot test in evaluation of, **6**:60, 61*i*
Monogenic (mendelian) disorder, **2**:190
Monokines, **9**:80
Mononucleosis, infectious
  Epstein-Barr virus causing, **1**:30
  ocular involvement in, **8**:156–157, 156*i*
    conjunctivitis, **6**:228
Monopril. *See* Fosinopril
Monosomy, **2**:249
Monovision, **3**:183, 225
  refractive surgery and (modified monovision), **13**:42, 171–172
Montelukast, **1**:157*t*
Mood disorders (affective disorders), **1**:265–266
  drugs for treatment of, **1**:277
Moore, lightning streaks of, **5**:189
Mooren ulcer, **8**:231, 232–234, 233*i*, 234*i*
Moraxella
  bleb-associated endophthalmitis caused by, **9**:213
  blepharoconjunctivitis caused by, **8**:165
  conjunctivitis in children caused by, **6**:224
  lacunata, **8**:165
  as normal ocular flora, **8**:115*t*
Morgagnian cataract, **4**:101, 102*i*, **11**:48, 52*i*
Morgagnian globules, **4**:101, 101*i*, **11**:48
Morning glory disc, **5**:140–141, **6**:359, 359*i*
Morpheaform (fibrosing) basal cell carcinoma, **7**:175, 175*i*
Morphine
  for diastolic dysfunction, **1**:131
  for non-ST-segment elevation acute coronary syndrome, **1**:122
  for postoperative pain, **1**:338
Morquio syndrome, **6**:436*t*, **8**:337*t*
Morula, **2**:133, 134*i*
Mosaic degeneration (anterior crocodile shagreen), **8**:370
Mosaicism (mosaic), **2**:191, 251–252
  germinal, **2**:187
  sex chromosome, **2**:252
  trisomy 21, **2**:252
Motility disorders. *See* Ocular motility, disorders of
Motility examination. *See* Ocular motility, assessment of
Motor apraxia, ocular. *See* Ocular motor apraxia

Motor correspondence, Hering's law of, **6:**36–37, 37*i*
  eyelid retraction and, **7:**224
Motor fusion, **6:**43, 43*t*
Motor nerves, facial, anatomy of, **5:**49–56
Motor nucleus
  of cranial nerve V (trigeminal), **2:**113*i*, 114
  of cranial nerve VII (facial), **2:**117
Motor nystagmus, congenital, **6:**160, 161, 162–164,
  163*i*, 164*t*, 452
Motor physiology, **6:**27–39
  basic principles and terms related to, **6:**27–33
  eye movements and, **6:**33–38
  strabismus and, **6:**27–39
  supranuclear control systems and, **6:**39
Motor root
  of cranial nerve III (oculomotor), **2:**14, 14*i*
  of cranial nerve V (trigeminal), **2:**114
  of cranial nerve VII (facial), **2:**117
Motor system disorders. *See* Movement disorders;
  Parkinson disease
Motor units, **6:**32
Motrin. *See* Ibuprofen
MOTSA. *See* Multiple overlapping thin slab acquisition
Mouth-to-mouth resuscitation, **1:**314
Mouth-to-nose resuscitation, **1:**314
Movement disorders. *See also* Parkinson disease
  bradykinetic, **1:**278
  in multiple sclerosis, **5:**320
  in schizophrenia, **1:**264–265
Moxifloxacin, **1:**62*t*, 73, **2:**430–433, 431*t*
  for bacterial keratitis, **8:**182*t*, 183
6-MP. *See* 6-Mercaptopurine
MPS. *See* Mucopolysaccharidoses
MPS I H. *See* Hurler syndrome
MPS I H/S. *See* Hurler-Scheie syndrome
MPS I S. *See* Scheie syndrome
MPS II. *See* Hunter syndrome
MPS III. *See* Sanfilippo syndrome
MPS IV. *See* Morquio syndrome
MPS V. *See* Scheie syndrome
MPS VI. *See* Maroteaux-Lamy syndrome
MPS VII. *See* Sly syndrome
MPS (Macular Photocoagulation Study), **12:**70, 80, 82
MR. *See* Medial rectus muscles
MRA. *See* Magnetic resonance angiography
MRD. *See* Margin–reflex distance
MRI. *See* Magnetic resonance imaging
mRNA. *See* Messenger RNA
MRS. *See* Magnetic resonance spectroscopy
MRSA. *See* Methicillin-resistant *S aureus*
MS. *See* Multiple sclerosis
α-MSH (alpha-melanocyte-stimulating hormone),
  8:198*t*
  in tear secretion, **2:**293
MSI. *See* Magnetic source imaging
MST. *See* Medial superior temporal area
mtDNA. *See* Mitochondrial DNA
MTF. *See* Modulation transfer function
MTP (microsomal triglyceride transfer protein),
  mutations in, **2:**351
MTX. *See* Methotrexate
MUC1, **8:**57
MUC4, **8:**57
MUC5AC, **8:**56

Mucins/mucin gel, tear film, **2:**44, 288*i*, 291, **8:**56–57,
  56*i*
  deficiency of, **2:**291, 294, **8:**58
  in external eye defense, **8:**113
  secretion of, **2:**289*i*, 291, **8:**58
Mucoceles
  congenital, **7:**260
    lacrimal, **6:**240–241, 240*i*
    nasal, **6:**241
  in dacryocystitis, **7:**278
  orbital invasion by, **6:**384, **7:**92–93, 93*i*
Mucocutaneous lymph node syndrome (Kawasaki
  syndrome/infantile periarteritis nodosa), **1:**189*t*,
  6:238
Mucoepidermoid carcinoma, **4:**53, **8:**255*t*, 261
Mucolipidoses, **6:**436*t*, **8:**341–342
  corneal changes in, **8:**341–342
    congenital/infantile opacities and, **6:**255, 256*t*,
    8:298
  retinal degeneration and, **12:**243, 244
Mucopolysaccharidoses, **6:**436*t*, 438, **8:**309*t*, 335–336,
  337*t*
  corneal changes in, **8:**309*t*, 335–336, 337*t*
    congenital/infantile opacities and, **6:**255, 256*i*,
    256*t*, 436*t*, **8:**298
  retinal degeneration and, **12:**232*t*, 233*t*, 242–243
Mucopyoceles, orbital invasion by, **7:**92–93, 93*i*
Mucor (mucormycosis), **8:**130–131
  neuro-ophthalmic signs of, **5:**366–367, 367*i*
  optic nerve involved in, **4:**205
  orbit involved in, **4:**189, **6:**233, 233*i*, **7:**45–46
    exenteration in management of, **7:**45–46, 128
Mucosa-associated lymphoid tissue (MALT), **8:**59, 201
  of conjunctiva (conjunctiva-associated/CALT), **2:**36,
    8:5, 8, 59, 201, **9:**34*t*, 36
Mucosa-associated lymphoid tissue (MALT)
  lymphoma, **4:**194–195, 195*i*
  of orbit, **7:**85–87, 86*t*
Mucosal mast cells, **9:**13
Mucous membrane grafting (transplantation), **8:**423*t*,
  425, 439
  indications for, **8:**423*t*, 439
Mucus excess, conjunctival, **8:**24*t*
Mucus-fishing syndrome, **8:**105
Muir-Torre syndrome, eyelid manifestations of, **4:**176*t*,
  7:167
Mulberry lesions, **5:**132
Müller cells/fibers, retinal, **2:**83, 353, **5:**24, **12:**10, 12
Müllerectomy, tarsoconjunctival (Fasanella-Servat
  procedure), for ptosis correction, **7:**222
Müller's muscle (superior tarsal muscle), **2:**26, 27*i*,
  4:168, **5:**57, 58*i*, **7:**140*i*, 144
  in congenital Horner syndrome, **7:**217
  internal (conjunctival) resection of, for ptosis
    correction, **7:**222
  paresis of, **5:**262
Multidrug-resistant infections, tuberculosis (MDRTB),
  1:24, 49, **9:**195
Multifactorial inheritance, **2:**191, 273–275
Multifocal ablation, for presbyopia, **13:**174–175, 174*i*
Multifocal choroiditis
  in HIV infection/AIDS, **9:**257–258
  and panuveitis syndrome (MCP), **9:**177*t*, 185, 185*i*,
    12:174*t*, 178–179, 179*i*
Multifocal cornea, retinoscopy in detection of, **8:**49

Multifocal electroretinogram, **5:**102, 102*i*, **12:**32, 32*i*
Multifocal lenses, **3:**150–164. *See also* Bifocal lenses
  intraocular, **3:**225–229, **11:**146–147, **13:**163–164, 163*i*
    clinical results of, **3:**228–229
      for presbyopia, **13:**173
  occupation and, **3:**163–164
  power of, determining bifocal add for, **3:**150–152
  Prentice's rule and, **3:**155–162, 160*i*
  types of, **3:**152, 153*i*, 155
Multi-infarct dementia, **1:**284
Multinucleated cells
  cytologic identification of, **8:**68–69, 69*i*
  giant cells, **4:**13
Multiplanar incisions, for clear corneal incision,
  11:124, 125*i*
Multiple endocrine neoplasia, **1:**230–231, **8:**309*t*
  corneal nerve enlargement in, **8:**357, 357*i*, 358*t*
Multiple evanescent white dot syndrome (MEWDS),
  5:107, 108*i*, **9:**177*t*, 181–182, 182*i*, **12:**174*t*,
  175–176, 176*i*
Multiple overlapping thin slab acquisition, for
  magnetic resonance angiography, **5:**66
Multiple sclerosis, **5:**317–325
  chiasmal/retrochiasmal abnormalities in, **5:**321
  clinical course/presentation of, **5:**318–320
  diagnosis of, **5:**323*t*, 324
  epidemiology of, **5:**317
  fundoscopic abnormalities in, **5:**321
  genetics of, **5:**317
  HLA association in, **5:**317, **9:**94*t*
  intermediate uveitis and, **9:**152
  laboratory evaluation of, **5:**322, 323*t*
  neuroimaging in, **5:**322
  ocular flutter caused by, **5:**253
  ocular motility disturbances in, **5:**321–322
  optic nerve involvement and, **4:**205, 205*i*, **5:**143,
    320–321
    in children, **6:**366
    treatment of, **5:**143–144
  pathology of, **5:**318, 319*i*
  prognosis of, **5:**318
  treatment of, **5:**324–325
  uveitis in children differentiated from, **6:**320*t*
Multiple sulfatase deficiency, **8:**340–341
Multiple-zone intraocular lenses, **3:**226–227, 227*i*
Multizone keratectomies, **13:**25–26, 26*i*
Mumps virus
  immunization against, **1:**306
  ocular infection caused by, **8:**163
    conjunctivitis, **6:**228
Munchausen syndrome, **5:**303
Munchausen syndrome by proxy, ocular trauma and,
  6:442
Munnerlyn's formula, **3:**234
Mural cells, retinal blood vessel, **2:**84
Muscarinic agents, **2:**394–402
  antagonists, **2:**400–402, 401*t*, 402*i*
  direct-acting agonists, **2:**394–398, 397*i*, 398*t*, 399*i*
  indirect-acting agonists, **2:**398–400, 399*i*
Muscarinic receptors
  in iris–ciliary body, **2:**308, 308*t*
  signal transduction and, **2:**311, 312*i*
  in tear secretion, **2:**292, 292*i*
Muscle capsule, of rectus muscles, **6:**22
  surgery and, **6:**23

Muscle cone, **6:**19*i*, 22
Muscle physiology, **6:**31–33
Muscle relaxants
  for benign essential blepharospasm, **7:**227
  tear production affected by, **8:**81*t*
Muscle of Riolan, **2:**22, 24, 24*i*
Muscle-weakening procedures. *See* Weakening
  procedures
Muscles. *See specific muscle and* Extraocular muscles
Muscular artery, inferior/superior, **5:**15
Muscular dystrophy, Duchenne
  mutation rate of, **2:**256
  retinal degeneration and, **12:**236
Mustardé flap, for eyelid repair, **7:**189, 191*i*, 192
Mutagens, **2:**256, **8:**282
Mutamycin. *See* Mitomycin
Mutation, **2:**191, 214–215, 255–259, **8:**307. *See also*
  specific type
  base pair, **2:**214
    conserved, **2:**214
  carcinogenesis and, **1:**252, 253
  carrier of, **2:**183
  disease-producing, **2:**214–215
  dominant negative, **2:**185
  frameshift (framing error/frameshift), **2:**186
  gain of function and, **2:**214
  knockout, **2:**234–237, 236*i*
  missense, **2:**191
  nonsense, **2:**191
  null, **2:**214
  point, **2:**255–256
  screening for, **2:**230–231, 232*i*, 233–234*i*
Mutton-fat keratic precipitates, **9:**104, 104*i*
  in sarcoidosis, **9:**104*i*, 198, 199*i*
  in sympathetic ophthalmia, **4:**153
  in uveitis, **9:**104, 104*i*, 136
Myasthenia gravis, **2:**403, **5:**224, **6:**151–152, 151*i*, 153*t*,
  7:218
  clinical presentation of, **5:**325–326
  diagnosis of, **5:**326–328, 327*i*, **6:**151–152, 151*i*
    edrophonium in, **2:**403, **5:**326–327, **6:**151, 151*i*,
    153*t*, **7:**213
  eyelid fissure changes in, **2:**23*i*
  Graves ophthalmopathy and, **7:**54
  neuro-ophthalmic signs of, **5:**325–328
  ptosis in, **5:**274*i*, 275, **7:**213, 218
  strabismus in, **6:**151–152, 151*i*, 153*t*
  treatment of, **5:**328
Mycelex. *See* Clotrimazole
Mycelium, **8:**129
Mycobacterium (mycobacteria), **1:**23–25, **8:**127
  avium/avium-intracellulare, **1:**49, **5:**361
  chelonei, **8:**127
  fortuitum, **8:**127
  in HIV infection/AIDS, **1:**23, 49–50
  kansasii, **1:**49
  leprae, **8:**127
  nontuberculous (atypical) infection caused by, **1:**23,
    49–50, **8:**127, 185
  ocular infection/inflammation caused by, **8:**127
  stains and culture media for identification of, **8:**137*t*
  tuberculosis, **1:**23–25, **8:**127. *See also* Tuberculosis
    choroidal infection caused by, **12:**184, 184*i*
    in HIV infection/AIDS, **5:**361
    screening/testing for, **1:**23–24, 301–302

Mycology, **8:**119*t*, 128–131, 129*i*, 129*t*, 130*i*. *See also* Fungi
Mycophenolate mofetil, **1:**200
  for uveitis, **9:**119*t*
    in children, **6:**321
Mycoplasma pneumoniae, **1:**22
Mycostatin. *See* Nystatin
Mycotic (fungal) keratitis, **4:**66, 66*i*, **8:**185–187, 186*i*
Mydfrin. *See* Phenylephrine
Mydriacyl. *See* Tropicamide
Mydriasis/mydriatics, **2:**309–310, 401*t*
  adrenergic agents, **2:**309–310, 405
  benign episodic, **5:**270–271
  blunt trauma causing, **5:**265
  after cataract surgery in children, **6:**302
  cholinergic agents, **2:**310, 400
  congenital, **6:**268
  cycloplegia/cycloplegic agents and, **3:**141–142
  drug-induced, **5:**266
  multifocal IOLs and, **13:**164, 173
  for retinal examination, **12:**17
  seizures and, **1:**283–284
  traumatic injury and, **8:**397
  for uveitis, **9:**114–115, 128
Myectomy, **6:**175*t*
  for benign essential blepharospasm, **7:**227
Myelinated (medullated) nerve fibers, **4:**121, 121*i*, **6:**360, 360*i*
Myelitis, optic nerve involvement and, **4:**205
Myeloid stem cells, **1:**160
Myeloma, monoclonal antibody and, **9:**56
Myeloperoxidase, oxygen radicals produced by, **9:**86
Myeloproliferative disorders, hypercoagulability and, **1:**171
Myiasis, ocular, **8:**133–134
Mykrox. *See* Metolazone
MYO7A gene, **2:**221
MYOC mutation, **6:**271, **10:**14
Myocardial contractility, **1:**129
  enhancement of in heart failure management, **1:**130–131
  reduction of in angina management, **1:**120–121
Myocardial infarction, **1:**113–115. *See also* Acute coronary syndrome; Ischemic heart disease
  ECG changes in, **1:**116
  heart failure and, **1:**128
  hypertension management and, **1:**91*t*
  management of, **1:**122–125
    cardiac-specific troponins and, **1:**117, 118*i*
    percutaneous coronary intervention for, **1:**111
  pericarditis after (post-MI/Dressler syndrome), **1:**115
  stroke and, **1:**102
Myocardial oxygen requirements, reducing
  for acute coronary syndrome, **1:**122
  for angina, **1:**121
Myocardial scintigraphy, thallium-201, **1:**119
Myocilin, **10:**12
  gene for. *See* TIGR/myocilin (TIGR/MYOC) gene
  in glaucoma, **10:**12, 14
Myoclonic epilepsy with ragged red fibers (MERRF), mitochondrial DNA mutations and, **2:**218, 219*i*
Myoclonus, cherry-red spot in, **6:**436*t*, **12:**243
Myofibromas, of orbit, **6:**380
Myogenic ptosis, **7:**214–215, 214*i*, 217*t*

Myoglobin
  in immunohistochemistry, **4:**37
  serum, in myocardial infarction, **1:**117–118
Myoid
  of cone, **2:**79, 82*i*
  of rod, **2:**79, 82*i*
Myokymia
  facial, **5:**287*t*, 289
  superior oblique, **5:**254, **6:**156–157
Myomyous junctions, **2:**23
Myopathies
  extraocular, in thyroid ophthalmopathy, **5:**329*i*, 330, **6:**149, **7:**48, 53
  mitochondrial, **12:**245
    with encephalopathy/lactic acidosis/strokelike episodes (MELAS), **5:**297, **12:**245
      mitochondrial DNA mutation and, **2:**211, 218, 219*i*
  neuro-ophthalmic signs of, **5:**334–335
Myopia, **3:**116, 116*i*
  with achromatopsia, racial and ethnic concentration of, **2:**260
  adult-onset, **3:**120–121
  age of onset of, **3:**120–121, **6:**200
  amblyopia and, **6:**70
  in childhood glaucoma, **6:**284
  choroidal neovascularization in, **12:**71–72*t*, 85–86
  congenital, **3:**121, 146
  congenital stationary night blindness with, ocular findings in carriers of, **2:**270*t*
  contact lens-corrected aphakia and, **3:**176*i*, 178–179
  developmental (juvenile-onset), **3:**120–122, 146
  diverging lens for correction of, **3:**143, 144*i*
  etiology of, **3:**121
  high (pathologic/degenerative). *See* High (pathologic/degenerative) myopia
  in infants and children, **3:**120–122, 146
  instrument, in automated refraction, **3:**312
  intermittent exotropia and, **6:**112
  juvenile-onset (developmental), **3:**120–122, 146
  lattice degeneration and, **12:**258
  lenticular, **11:**45
  muscarinic agents causing, **2:**398
  pathologic (malignant/progressive/degenerative). *See* High (pathologic/degenerative) myopia
  physiologic (simple/school), **3:**120
  prevalence of, **3:**120–121
  primary open-angle glaucoma and, **10:**88
  residual
    after intrastromal corneal ring segment placement, **13:**81
    after radial keratotomy, **13:**62–63, 64
  retinal reflex in, **3:**126, 127*i*
  retinopathy of prematurity and, **6:**332
  societal cost of, **3:**120–121
  in Stickler syndrome, **6:**341
  surgical correction of
    bioptics for, **13:**143, 155–156, 157*t*
    clear lens extraction/refractive lens exchange for, **13:**158
    epikeratoplasty (epikeratophakia) for, **13:**75–76
    incisional corneal surgery for, **13:**59–66
    intrastromal corneal ring segments for, **13:**77–84, 78*i*, 79*t*

LASIK for
with astigmatism, **13**:117–118
high myopia, **13**:117
low myopia, **13**:116
moderate myopia, **13**:116–117
light-adjustable IOLs for, **13**:165–166
monovision for, **13**:172
phakic IOLs for, **13**:144–146
PRK/LASEK for, **13**:98. *See also* Photorefractive
keratectomy
radial keratotomy for, **13**:59–66. *See also* Radial
keratotomy
retinal detachment and, **13**:191–192, 203
wavefront-guided laser ablation for, **13**:133–135
vitreous changes associated with, **2**:338
wavefront aberration produced by (positive defocus),
13:15, 15*i*
Myopic astigmatism
LASIK for, **13**:117–118
wavefront-guided laser ablation for, **13**:133–135
Myopic shift, in cataracts, **11**:76–77
Myopic spherical photorefractive keratectomy, **13**:98.
See also Photorefractive keratectomy
Myosin, mutations in gene for, in Usher syndrome,
12:235
Myosin VIIA, mutations in, **2**:350
Myositis, orbital, **4**:190, 191*i*, **5**:219, **6**:385
Myotomy, **6**:175*t*
marginal, **6**:175*t*
Myotonic dystrophy, **5**:335
lens disorders/cataracts in, **11**:62–63, 63*i*
in children, **6**:288*t*
retinal degeneration and, **12**:232*t*, 234
Mysoline, **1**:283*t*
Myxedema, **1**:225, 226
pretibial. *See* Infiltrative dermopathy
Myxedema coma, **1**:226
Myxedema madness, **1**:226
MZM. *See* Methazolamide

N

Na. *See* Sodium
Na$^+$,K$^+$-ATPase (sodium-potassium pump)
in Fuchs endothelial dystrophy, **8**:325
in lens active transport, **11**:19–20
pump-leak theory and, **11**:20, 21*i*
in lens ionic balance, **2**:329
in retinal pigment epithelium, **2**:358, 361
in rods, **2**:342, 344*t*
Na$^+$/K$^+$-Ca exchanger, in rods, **2**:342, 344*t*
NAAT (nucleic acid amplification test). *See* Polymerase
chain reaction
Nabumetone, **1**:197*t*
Nadbath block, adverse reactions to, **1**:336
Nadolol, **1**:88*t*, 90*t*
NADP, in lens carbohydrate metabolism, **11**:14, 15*i*
NADPH
in free radical generation, **2**:366, 371
in lens carbohydrate metabolism, **11**:14, 15*i*
Nafcillin, **1**:55*t*, 67, **2**:429
for endophthalmitis, **9**:218*t*
Nail-patella syndrome, **8**:352*t*

NAION. *See* Nonarteritic anterior ischemic optic
neuropathy
Nalfon. *See* Fenoprofen
Nalidixic acid, **1**:72–73
Naloxone, for narcotic reversal, **1**:335
Namenda. *See* Memantine
Naming-meshing system, for uveitis differential
diagnosis, **9**:109, 110–111*t*
Nanophthalmos, **2**:126, 163, **4**:89, **8**:287–288, 289
angle-closure glaucoma and, **10**:15, 145
cataract surgery in patients with, **11**:213, 214*i*
Naphazoline, **2**:423, 424*t*, 451
Naphazoline/antazoline, **2**:423, 424*t*
Naphazoline/pheniramine, **2**:423, 424*t*
Naphcon-A. *See* Naphazoline/pheniramine
Naprosyn. *See* Naproxen
Naproxen, **1**:197*t*, **2**:421*t*
Alzheimer disease prevention and, **1**:288
ocular effects of, **1**:324*t*
for uveitis in children, **6**:320
NARP. *See* Neuropathy, with ataxia and retinitis
pigmentosa
Narrow complex tachycardias, **1**:136
Nasal cavity, **7**:20
Nasal chondritis, in relapsing polychondritis, **1**:187
Nasal conchae (turbinates), **5**:10, **7**:20
infracture of, for congenital tearing/nasolacrimal
duct obstruction, **6**:245–246, **7**:263, 265*i*
Nasal CPAP, **1**:156
Nasal endoscopy, for acquired tearing evaluation, **7**:271
Nasal mucocele, congenital, **6**:221
Nasal radiating fibers, **5**:111
Nasal septum, **7**:20
NASCET (North American Symptomatic Carotid
Endarterectomy Trial), **1**:108, **5**:181–182, 182*t*,
12:152
Nasociliary nerve, **2**:115, **5**:52, 53*i*, **7**:15
terminal branches of, **5**:54
Nasolacrimal canal, **7**:11, 256
balloon catheter dilation of, for congenital tearing/
nasolacrimal duct obstruction, **6**:246, **7**:264–265
Nasolacrimal duct, **2**:10, 35, 35*i*, **5**:10, **6**:239, **7**:20, 255*i*,
256
development of, **6**:200
irrigation of
for acquired tearing evaluation, **7**:270–271, 270*t*,
271*i*
for congenital tearing management, **7**:262–263,
264*i*
obstruction of. *See also* Tearing
acquired, **7**:278
examination in evaluation of, **7**:267–268, 268*i*
irrigation in evaluation of, **7**:270–271, 270*t*,
271*i*
probing in evaluation of, **7**:271
congenital, **6**:200, 241–247, 242*i*, **7**:258, 261–265
balloon catheter dilation (balloon dacryoplasty)
for, **6**:246, **7**:264–265
in dacryocystocele, **7**:260–261, 260*i*
irrigation for, **7**:262–263, 264*i*
lacrimal sac massage for, **6**:242
nonsurgical management of, **6**:242
probing for, **6**:243, 243–245, 244*i*, 245*i*, **7**:261,
262–265, 263*i*

silicone intubation for, **6:**246–247, **7:**263–264, 266*i*
surgical management of, **6:**242–247, 244*i*, 245*i*
turbinate infracture for, **6:**245–246, **7:**263, 265*i*
in dacryocystitis, **7:**278–279
occlusion of, **2:**35
ocular medication absorption and, **2:**382, 382*i*, 383*i*
trauma to, **7:**284
Naso-orbital-ethmoidal fractures, **7:**101, 101*i*
Nasopharyngeal carcinoma, Epstein-Barr virus associated with, **1:**30, 254
Natacyn. *See* Natamycin
Natalizumab, for multiple sclerosis, **5:**324
Natamycin, **2:**437, 438*t*
for fungal keratitis, **8:**186, 187
Nateglinide, **1:**212*t*, 213
Natural (innate) immunity, **9:**9, 10. *See also* Innate immune response
Natural killer cells, **9:**70
tumor immunology and, **8:**249
in viral conjunctivitis, **9:**35
Nausea and vomiting, postoperative
management of, **1:**338
after strabismus surgery, **6:**191
NCL. *See* Neuronal ceroid lipofuscinosis
Nd:YAG laser, **3:**22, 23. *See also* Lasers
for LASIK flap creation, **13:**109–110
mechanical light damage caused by, **12:**307
Nd:YAG laser therapy
capsulotomy, **11:**187–191, 189*i*
in children, **11:**197
complications of, **11:**190–191
contraindications to, **11:**188
indications for, **11:**188
lens-particle glaucoma and, **11:**67–68
procedure for, **11:**188–190, 189*i*
retinal detachment and, **11:**175, 190, **12:**334
for corneal epithelial basement membrane dystrophy, **8:**313
cycloablation, for childhood glaucoma, **6:**281
intrastromal photodisruption, **13:**29
keratectomy, **13:**21*t*
for orbital lymphangioma, **7:**69
phacolysis, **11:**138
Nd:YLF laser, for intrastromal photodisruption, **13:**29
ND-1 gene, in Leber hereditary optic neuropathy, **2:**219, 219*i*
ND-4 gene, in Leber hereditary optic neuropathy, **2:**218, 219*i*
ND-6 gene, in Leber hereditary optic neuropathy, **2:**219–220, 219*i*
Near blindness, **3:**245*t*, 252. *See also* Low vision; Visual loss/impairment
Near-normal vision, **3:**245*t*, 251
magnifiers for reading and, **3:**258
spectacles for reading and, **3:**255
Near point of accommodation, measuring, **3:**150–151
Near point of convergence, **6:**87
Near reflex
assessment of, **6:**87
pathways for, **2:**111
spasm of, **3:**148, **5:**313
esotropia and, **6:**98*t*, 106
Near response, in pupillary examination, **5:**258

Near visual acuity
in low vision, magnification for, **3:**255–258
testing
in children, **6:**80
nystagmus and, **6:**161
distance for, **3:**111–112
Nebcin. *See* Tobramycin
Neck, cosmetic/rejuvenation surgery on, **7:**244–247, 245*i*, 246*i*, 247*i*
liposuction, **7:**245–246, 246*i*
Necrosis, definition of, **8:**247*t*
Necrotizing encephalopathy, Leigh (Leigh syndrome), **2:**262*t*
mitochondrial DNA mutations and, **2:**219*i*, 220
Necrotizing fasciitis, of orbit, **7:**44–45
Necrotizing keratitis, **8:**29
herpes simplex causing, **8:**147–148, 148*i*, 150
Necrotizing retinitis
atypical, diagnosis of, **9:**63
herpetic (acute retinal necrosis), **4:**123, 124*i*, **9:**140, 154–156, 155*i*, 156*i*, **12:**185–186, 185*i*
Necrotizing scleritis, **4:**90, 90*i*, **8:**25*t*, 29, 236–239, 236*t*
with inflammation, **8:**236*t*, 237, 238*i*
without inflammation (scleromalacia perforans), **8:**236*t*, 238–239, 238*i*
in Wegener granulomatosis, **9:**62
Nedocromil, **1:**157*t*, **2:**424*t*, 425
Needle penetration/perforation of globe
during retrobulbar anesthesia, **12:**296
during surgery, **12:**336, 337*i*
Needle sticks
HIV transmission by, **1:**39
chemoprophylaxis for, **1:**45, 46–47*t*
prevention of, **8:**50
Nefazodone, **1:**276
Negative angle kappa, **6:**86, 87*i*
Negative defocus, **13:**15
Negative predictive value (NPV), of screening/diagnostic test, **1:**354
Negative staining (fluorescein), **8:**20
Negative thin lenses, **3:**72–74, 73*i*
Neglect, elder, **1:**236–237
Neisseria, **1:**12–14, **8:**125
gonorrhoeae (gonococcus), **1:**13–14, **8:**125, 125*i*
conjunctivitis caused by, **8:**119*t*, 171–172, 172*i*
in children, **6:**225
in neonates, **6:**222, 222*i*, **8:**172, 173
invasive capability of, **8:**116
resistant strains of, **1:**13–14
meningitidis (meningococcus), **1:**12–13, **8:**125
conjunctivitis in children caused by, **6:**225
immunization against, **1:**13, 309
invasive capability of, **8:**116
Nelfinavir, **1:**42
for postexposure HIV prophylaxis, **1:**46–47*t*
Nematodes, diffuse unilateral subacute neuroretinitis caused by, **6:**318, **12:**189, 190
Neo-Synephrine. *See* Phenylephrine
Neoantigen, **9:**59
Neocerebellum, **5:**39
Neomycin, **2:**428*t*, 435
in combination preparations, **2:**431*t*, 432*t*
ototoxicity of, mitochondrial DNA mutations and, **2:**220

Neonatal adrenoleukodystrophy, 12:233*t*, 234, 236, 242, 242*i*
Neonatal hemangiomatosis, diffuse, 6:377
Neonatal ophthalmia. *See* Ophthalmia, neonatorum
Neonates. *See also* Infants
  conjunctivitis in, 6:221–224, 222*i*, 8:51*t*, 172–174.
    See also Ophthalmia, neonatorum
  corneal transplantation in, 8:470–471
  electroretinogram in, 12:31
  hemorrhagic disease of newborn in, 1:169
  herpes simplex infection in, 1:27, 8:140
  normal ocular flora in, 8:115
  ocular infections in, 6:215–221. *See also specific type*
    ophthalmia neonatorum, 6:221–224, 222*i. See also*
    Ophthalmia, neonatorum
  screening eye examinations in, 6:292–294
Neoplasia. *See also specific type or structure involved and*
  Cancer; Intraocular tumors; Tumors
  classification of, 4:16–17, 17*i*, 17*t*
  clinical approach to, 8:253–278
  cytologic identification of, 8:70, 70*i*
  definition of, 4:16–17, 8:246, 247*t*
  diagnostic approaches to, 8:250, 251*i*
  facial pain associated with, 5:301
  histopathologic features of, 8:246, 247*t*
  management of, 8:252
  masquerade syndromes and, 9:228–233
  ocular flutter caused by, 5:253
  oncogenesis and, 8:248–249, 248*t*
  tumor cell biology and, 8:245–252
Neoral. *See* Cyclosporine
Neosporin, 2:431*t*
Neostigmine, 2:309, 396*i*, 403
  for myasthenia gravis diagnosis, 5:327, 6:151–152
Neo-Synephrine. *See* Phenylephrine
Neovascular glaucoma, 10:132–136, 133*t*, 134*i*, 135*i*
Neovascular membrane, subretinal, in age-related
  macular degeneration, 4:139
Neovascularization
  of anterior chamber angle, in diabetic patients,
    12:111
  in branch retinal vein occlusion, 12:138
    photocoagulation for, 12:138–140, 140*i*
  in central retinal artery occlusion, 12:150
  in central retinal vein occlusion, 12:141, 142,
    144–145
  choroidal. *See* Choroidal neovascularization
  corneal
    contact lenses causing, 3:208–209, 8:108
    inflammation and, 8:29
    after pediatric corneal transplantation, 8:470
    stem cell deficiency and, 8:109
  of iris (rubeosis iridis), 2:40, 61, 4:155–156, 155*t*
    in branch retinal vein occlusion, 12:139
    in central retinal artery occlusion, 12:150
    in central retinal vein occlusion, 5:107, 12:142,
      144–145
    in diabetic patients, 12:111
    disorders predisposing to, 10:132, 133*t*, 134*i*, 135*i*
    in ocular ischemic syndrome, 12:150, 151
  in ocular ischemic syndrome, 12:150–151, 151*i*
  in pars planitis, 9:148, 151, 240, 12:182
  pupillary reactivity affected by, 5:259
  in radiation retinopathy, 12:305, 306*i*

retinal. *See also* Retinal disease, vascular
  in age-related macular degeneration, 4:139
  ischemia causing, 4:130–133, 132*i*
  peripheral, 12:124, 125*t*
    vitreous hemorrhage and, 12:287
  in retinopathy of prematurity, 4:137, 6:325–332,
    12:124–136
    screening for, 6:328–329, 329*t*, 330*i*, 331*i*,
      351–356, 354*i*
  sea fan, in sickle cell disease, 12:122, 122*i*, 123*i*
  stromal, contact lenses causing, 8:108
  in uveitis, 9:240
Nepafenac, 1:197
Nephritis
  lupus, 1:179
  tubulointerstitial, and uveitis, 6:315–316
Nephroblastoma. *See* Wilms tumor
Nephronophthisis, juvenile, retinal degeneration and,
  12:236
Nephropathy
  diabetic, 1:217–218
  HIV-associated, 1:37–38
Nephrotoxicity, of aminoglycosides, 1:70
Neptazane. *See* Methazolamide
Nerve fiber bundle defect, in glaucoma, 10:60
Nerve fiber layer, 2:80–81*i*, 83, 85, 4:118, 118*i*, 12:10*i*,
  11–12, 11*i*
  defects of, in optic atrophy, 5:87–88, 88*i*
  in glaucoma, 10:47–48
    quantitative measurement of, 10:55–56
  homonymous, 5:164
  imaging of, 5:69
  infarcts of. *See* Cotton-wool spots
  optic nerve, 2:98
    blood supply of, 2:103
  in papilledema, 5:112, 115–116, 115*i*
  peripapillary, gliosis of, 5:116, 116*i*
  transient, of Chievitz, 2:140, 144
Nerve fibers, 5:111, 112*i. See also* Nerve fiber layer
  diffuse loss of, examination of, 10:55
  distribution of, 10:46, 46*i*
  medullated (myelinated), 4:121, 121*i*, 6:360, 360*i*
Nerve loops, 2:50, 51*i*
Nerve (neural) sheath tumors
  of orbit, 4:200, 201*i*
  of uveal tract, 4:165
Nerves, cranial. *See specific nerve and* Cranial nerves
Nervus intermedius, 2:117
NES. *See* Nonepileptic seizures
Netilmicin, 1:61*t*, 70
Netromycin. *See* Netilmicin
Nettleship-Falls X-linked ocular albinism, 6:345, 347*t*
  ocular findings in carriers of, 2:270*t*, 271*i*, 272
Neural crest cells, 2:127, 131–132, 133*t*, 137*i*, 138*i*, 8:6
  corneal endothelium derived from, 2:47
  ocular structures derived from, 2:131–132, 133*t*
Neural folds, 2:127, 136
Neural plate, 2:136, 137*i*
Neural reflex arc, immune response arc compared
  with, 9:17, 18*i*
Neural rim, 10:51, 53*i*
Neural tube, 2:127, 131, 136, 137*i*, 142*i*
Neural tumors
  nystagmus caused by, 6:159*t*

orbital, 7:72–79, 73*i*, 76*i*, 77–78*i*
  in children, 6:381
Neuralgia
  glossopharyngeal, 5:300
  postherpetic, 1:28, 5:301, 8:153, 155–156
  trigeminal (tic douloureux), 5:299
Neurilemoma (neurinoma, schwannoma)
  conjunctival, 8:269, 270*i*
  of orbit, 4:200, 201*i*, 6:381, 7:79
  of uveal tract, 4:165, 283
Neuritis, optic. *See* Optic neuritis
Neuroblastic layers, inner and outer, 2:140
Neuroblastoma
  in children, 6:374–375, 374*i*
    nystagmus caused by, 6:159*t*
    of orbit, 6:374–375, 374*i*
  of orbit, 6:374–375, 374*i*, 7:94, 94*i*
Neurocristopathy, 2:127, 132, 168. *See also* Anterior
    segment, dysgenesis of; Axenfeld-Rieger syndrome
  definition of, 6:206
  glaucoma associated with, 6:271
Neurocutaneous syndromes. *See* Phakoma/
    phakomatosis
Neuroectoderm, 2:127, 136
  ocular structures derived from, 2:133*t*, 8:6
  tumors arising in, 8:263–269, 263*t*
Neuroendocrine peptides, in aqueous humor, 2:317,
    320
Neurofibrillary tangles, in Alzheimer disease, 1:285,
    286
Neurofibromas
  acoustic (NF2), 5:337, 6:408–409. *See also*
    Neurofibromatosis, bilateral acoustic (type 2)
  conjunctival, 8:269
  discrete, 7:75
  nodular cutaneous and subcutaneous, 6:404
  of orbit, 4:192, 200, 201*i*, 7:26, 75, 76*i*
  plexiform, 6:381, 405, 405*i*
    glaucoma and, 6:405, 408
    of orbit, 6:381
  of uveal tract, 4:165, 283
Neurofibromatosis
  bilateral acoustic (type 2), 5:337, 6:401, 403, 408–409
  von Recklinghausen (type 1), 5:336*t*, 337–338, 338*i*,
    6:401–409, 402*t*, 7:75
    in children, 6:401–409, 402*t*
    choroidal lesions in, 6:404, 407
    expressivity in, 2:258–259
    glaucoma and, 6:278, 405, 408, 10:32, 154, 156
    glial cell lesions in, 6:404–407, 405*i*, 406*i*
    iris mamillations associated with, 6:265
    Lisch nodules associated with, 4:219*t*, 221*i*, 6:264,
      264*i*, 403–404, 404*i*, 408
    melanocytic lesions in, 6:403–404, 404*i*
    miscellaneous manifestations of, 6:407–409
    mutation rate of, 2:256
    nodular neurofibromas in, 6:404
    optic pathway/optic nerve gliomas and, 4:208,
      5:149, 6:381, 406–407, 406*i*, 7:72–74, 75
    orbital involvement in, 4:200, 201*i*, 7:75
    plexiform neurofibromas in, 6:381, 405, 405*i*
    ptosis in, 5:274*i*
Neurogenic ptosis, 7:215–219, 218*i*
Neurogenic tumors, conjunctival, 8:269, 270*i*
Neuroglial choristoma, 8:277

Neuroimaging, 5:61–81. *See also specific modality*
  in Alzheimer disease, 1:287
  choice of
    clinical location and, 5:71*t*
    clinical situation and, 5:72*t*
  in cranial nerve palsy/paralysis, 5:74, 74*i*
  critical questioning in, 5:71–78
    how to order, 5:78
    what to order, 5:75–78, 75*t*, 76*i*, 77*t*
    when to order, 5:71–75, 73*i*, 74*i*
  in drusen versus papilledema, 5:132, 133*i*
  in epilepsy, 1:282
  glossary of terms in, 5:78–81
  history of, 5:61
  localization and, 5:70, 71*t*, 72*t*
  metabolic and functional, 5:68–69
  in multiple sclerosis, 5:322
  negative studies in, 5:78, 79*i*, 80*i*, 81*i*
  noninvasive techniques of, 5:69
  in optic nerve hypoplasia, 6:454
  in optic neuritis, 5:73
  vascular, 5:65–69
  in visual field defects, 5:73, 73*i*
Neuroleptic malignant syndrome (NMS), 1:272
Neuroleptics (antipsychotic drugs), 1:271–273, 272*t*
  atypical, 1:263, 271–272, 272*t*
  idiosyncratic reaction to, 5:212
  ocular side effects of, 1:272–273
Neurologic disorders, 1:278–289. *See also specific type*
  Alzheimer disease/dementia, 1:284–289
  cerebrovascular disease, 1:101–109
  epilepsy, 1:280–284, 283*t*
  in Lyme disease, 1:19
  Parkinson disease, 1:278–280
  recent developments in, 1:263
  in systemic lupus erythematosus, 1:180, 181*t*, 182
Neuroma
  acoustic, of cerebellopontine angle, 5:284, 285*i*
  conjunctival, 8:269
Neuromuscular abnormalities. *See also specific type*
  constant exotropia and, 6:116
  retinal degeneration and, 12:235–236
Neuromuscular blocking agents, 2:402*i*, 403
Neuronal ceroid lipofuscinosis, 6:437*t*, 438, 12:233*t*,
    234, 236, 241, 241*i*
Neurontin. *See* Gabapentin
Neuro-ophthalmology
  anatomy in
    afferent visual pathways, 5:23–31
    bony anatomy of head, 5:5–10
    efferent visual (ocular motor) pathways, 5:32–49
    facial motor and sensory anatomy, 5:49–56
    ocular anatomic pathways, 5:56–60
  neuroimaging in, 5:61–81. *See also* Neuroimaging
  systemic conditions important in, 5:317–368
    cerebrovascular disorders, 5:345–358
    immunologic disorders, 5:317–332
    infectious disorders, 5:358–368
    inherited disorders, 5:334–343
    pregnancy and, 5:343–345
    sarcoidosis and, 5:332–333
Neuropathy
  with ataxia and retinitis pigmentosa, 12:245
    mitochondrial DNA mutations and, 2:218, 219*i*,
      220

diabetic, 1:218
 neurotrophic keratopathy/persistent corneal
  epithelial defect and, 8:102
 hereditary sensory and autonomic. *See* Familial
  dysautonomia
 mental, 5:301
 optic. *See* Optic neuropathy
Neuropeptide-processing enzymes, in aqueous humor,
 2:317
Neuropeptide Y, in tear secretion, 2:287, 290
Neuropeptides, 8:198t, 9:82t
Neuroretinal rim, 10:51, 53i
Neuroretinitis, 5:125, 126i
 cat-scratch disease causing, 5:368
 diffuse unilateral subacute (DUSN), 6:318,
  9:172–173, 172i, 173i, 12:189–190, 189i
 Leber idiopathic stellate, 6:366, 366i
 in syphilis, 9:190
Neuroretinopathy, acute macular, 9:182
Neurosensory retina, 2:79–85, 80–81i, 4:118–119, 118i,
 12:7–12, 8i, 9t, 10–11i. *See also* Retina
 anatomy of, 2:79–85, 80–81i, 82i, 83i
 biochemistry and metabolism of, 2:341–351
 development of, 2:138–142, 143i
 glial elements of, 2:83–84
 neuronal elements of, 2:79–83, 82i, 83i
 stratification of, 2:80–81i, 84–85
 vascular elements of, 2:84. *See also* Retinal blood
  vessels
Neurosyphilis
 treatment of, 1:18
 VDRL tests in, 1:16, 17t
Neurotoxin complex, purified, 2:449
Neurotransmitters
 in iris–ciliary body, 2:308–310, 308t
 in tear secretion, 2:287, 290
Neurotrophic keratopathy, 8:102–104, 103i
 diabetic neuropathy and, 8:102
 esthesiometry in evaluation of, 8:35
 herpetic eye disease and, 8:102–103, 103i, 151, 153,
  154
Neurotrophic ulcers, herpetic keratitis and, 8:103, 103i,
 151
Neutral-density filter effect, in strabismic amblyopia,
 6:69
Neutral zone, in congenital motor nystagmus, 6:163
Neutrality, 3:127, 127i
 with correcting lens, 3:128–129, 129i
 finding, 3:129, 130i
Neutralization, antibody, 9:58, 58i
Neutrophil chemotactic factor, 8:200t
Neutrophil elastase inhibitor, in vitreous, 2:337
Neutrophil rolling, 9:48, 49i
Neutrophils (polymorphonuclear leukocytes), 9:13
 in chemical burns, 8:392
 cytologic identification of, 8:65t, 66, 67i
  in immune-mediated keratoconjunctivitis, 8:203t
 in external eye, 8:196t
 in inflammation, 4:13–14, 14i
  granule products of, 9:86
 innate mechanisms for recruitment and activation
  of, 9:48–50, 49i
 tumor immunology and, 8:249
Nevanac. *See* Nepafenac

Nevirapine, 1:41
 for HIV chemoprophylaxis during pregnancy, 1:45
Nevoxanthoendothelioma. *See* Juvenile
 xanthogranuloma
Nevus
 anterior chamber/trabecular meshwork affected by,
  4:84
 blue, 7:171, 8:264
 of choroid, 4:157–158, 159i, 216–217, 216i, 6:390
  in children, 6:390
  melanoma differentiated from, 4:216–217,
   229–230
 of ciliary body, 4:216–217
 compound, 7:170
  of conjunctiva, 4:56, 56i
  of eyelid, 4:183, 183i
 congenital, 2:175–176, 4:182, 182i
 conjunctival, 4:55–56, 56i, 56t, 8:265–266, 266i, 267t
  in children, 6:387, 387i
 dysplastic, 4:184
 of eyelid, 4:182–185, 182i, 183i, 7:170, 170i
 flammeus (port-wine stain), 6:380, 8:270, 270t,
  10:154. *See also* Vascular malformations
  of orbit, 6:380
  in Sturge-Weber syndrome, 5:340, 341i, 6:278,
   380, 414–415, 415i
  in von Hippel–Lindau disease, 6:412
 intradermal, 4:183, 184i, 7:170
 iris, 4:156–157, 215–216, 215i, 219t, 6:389
  diffuse nodular (iris mamillations), 6:264–265,
   265i
   central (pupillary) cyst rupture and, 6:265
 junctional, 4:182, 183i, 7:170
 "kissing," 4:182, 182i
 macular, 4:182
 magnocellular. *See* Melanocytoma
 melanocytic, 4:182–185
  of anterior chamber/trabecular meshwork, 4:84
  giant congenital, 4:182
 nevocellular, 4:182, 182i
  congenital, 6:387, 388i
 of Ota (oculodermal melanocytosis/congenital
  oculomelanocytosis), 2:175, 4:56t, 7:171, 172i,
  8:264, 267t
  in children, 6:387–388, 388i
  glaucoma associated with, 10:32
  of iris, 4:220t
 Spitz, 4:184
 stromal, 4:56
 subepithelial, 4:56
 uveal tract, 4:157–158, 159i
Nevus cells, 8:245
 tumors arising from, 7:170–171, 8:263t. *See also*
  Nevus
Newborn. *See also* Neonates
 hemorrhagic disease of, 1:169
NF. *See* Neurofibromatosis
NF1 gene, 6:403
NF2 gene, 6:403
NFL. *See* Nerve fiber layer
NFT. *See* Neurofibrillary tangles
Niacin (nicotinic acid)
 discontinuing before surgery, 1:334
 for hypercholesterolemia, 1:149t
Niaspan. *See* Nicotinic acid

Nicardipine
for angina, 1:120
for hypertension, 1:89*t*, 94
Nicotinamide-adenine dinucleotide phosphate, in lens
carbohydrate metabolism, 11:14, 15*i*
Nicotine, 2:402*i*
Nicotinic acid (niacin)
discontinuing before surgery, 1:334
for hypercholesterolemia, 1:149*t*
Nicotinic agents, 2:403
Nicotinic receptors, in iris–ciliary body, 2:308*t*
NIDDM (non–insulin-dependent diabetes mellitus).
See Diabetes mellitus, type 2
Nidogen-1, in vitreous, 2:333
Niemann-Pick disease, 2:262*t*, 6:436*t*, 438
racial and ethnic concentration of, 2:259
retinal degeneration and, 12:243, 245*i*
Nifedipine
for angina, 1:120
contraindications to in non-ST-segment elevation
acute coronary syndrome, 1:122–123
for hypertension, 1:89*t*
Night blindness, 12:198–202
in choroideremia, 12:224
congenital
with normal fundi, 12:198–200, 199*i*, 200*i*
with prominent fundus abnormality, 12:200–202,
201*i*, 202*i*
stationary, 6:336–337, 12:198–200, 199*i*, 200*i*
electroretinogram patterns in, 12:30*i*, 198–200,
199*i*, 200*i*
with myopia, ocular findings in carriers of,
2:270*t*
dark adaptometry in evaluation of, 12:41–42, 42*i*
in gyrate atrophy, 12:225
in hypovitaminosis A, 8:92
Night vision, abnormalities of, 12:198–202. *See also*
Night blindness
after PRK, 13:102
after radial keratotomy, 13:63
Nisoldipine, 1:89*t*
Nitrates
for angina, 1:120
for diastolic dysfunction, 1:131
for non-ST-segment elevation acute coronary
syndrome, 1:122
Nitric oxide, 9:85–86
Nitric oxide synthase, 9:85–86
Nitrogen bases, 2:191
Nitrogen mustard (mechlorethamine), 1:258*t*
Nitrogen radicals, as inflammatory mediators, 9:85–86
Nitroglycerin
for angina, 1:120
for heart failure, 1:130
for hypertensive emergency, 1:94
for non-ST-segment elevation acute coronary
syndrome, 1:122
Nitroprusside
for heart failure, 1:130
for hypertensive emergency, 1:94
Nitrosureas, in cancer chemotherapy, 1:260*t*
Nizoral. *See* Ketoconazole
NK cells. *See* Natural killer cells
NKHHC. *See* Nonketotic hyperglycemic-hyperosmolar
coma

NLD. *See* Nasolacrimal duct
NMS. *See* Neuroleptic malignant syndrome
NNOS gene, 10:13*t*, 15
NNRTIs. *See* Non-nucleoside reverse transcriptase
inhibitors
NO. *See* Nitric oxide
No light perception (NLP). *See* Blindness
Nocardia/Nocardia asteroides, 8:128
endophthalmitis caused by, 9:223, 223*i*
Nodal points, 3:31–32, 31*i*
for calculation of retinal image size, 3:105–108, 108*i*
Nodular anterior scleritis, 8:236, 236*t*, 237*i*
Nodular basal cell carcinoma, 7:174–175, 175*i*
Nodular episcleritis, 4:89, 8:29, 235, 235*i*
in children, 6:388
Nodular fasciitis, 8:271
episcleral tumor caused by, 4:92
Nodular neurofibromas, cutaneous and subcutaneous,
in neurofibromatosis, 6:404
Nodules. *See specific type*
Nodulus, 5:33
Nolvadex. *See* Tamoxifen
Nonaccommodative esotropia, 6:98*t*, 104–107
Nonarteritic anterior ischemic optic neuropathy,
5:121*t*, 122–124, 123*i*, 124*t*
Nonaxial displacement of globe, in orbital disorders,
7:23
Noncoding strand of DNA (antisense DNA), 2:182,
202
Noncomitant deviations. *See* Incomitant
(noncomitant) deviations
Noncompliance with therapy, behavioral/psychiatric
disorders and, 1:277
Non–contact lenses, for retinal examination, 12:17
Noncontact (air-puff) tonometers, 10:28–29
Noncycloplegic (manifest) refraction, 3:141–142
before refractive surgery, 13:42–43
PRK/LASEK, 13:91, 92
Noncystic retinal tufts, 12:259, 261*i*
Non-dihydropyridines, for hypertension, 1:89*t*, 93
Nondisjunction, 2:191
aneuploidy caused by, 2:245*i*, 249
in Down syndrome, 2:250
in mosaicism, 2:252
Nonepileptic seizures, 1:281
Nonexperimental (observational) studies, 1:345
Non-field testing, in functional visual disorder
evaluation, 5:310
Nongranulomatous uveitis, 9:104, 108, 127–141, 127*i*,
128*i*
Nonhistone proteins, 2:204
Non–Hodgkin lymphomas
of CNS (intraocular lymphoma/reticulum cell
sarcoma/histiocytic [large cell] lymphoma),
4:277–279, 277*i*, 279*i*, 9:228–231, 228*i*, 230*i*,
12:182–183, 182*i*
uveitis in children differentiated from, 6:320*t*
vitreous involvement and, 4:114–115, 115*i*
conjunctival, 8:274–275, 274*i*
orbital, 4:194, 195*i*
Nonhomologous chromosomes, independent
assortment and, 2:244–245
Noninfectious (sterile) endophthalmitis, cataract
surgery and, 11:176

Non–insulin-dependent diabetes mellitus (NIDDM). *See* Diabetes mellitus, type 2
Noninvasive pressure support ventilation, 1:156
Nonketotic hyperglycemic-hyperosmolar coma, 1:216
Nonnecrotizing keratitis, 8:146–147, 146*i*, 147*i*
Nonnecrotizing scleritis, 8:25*t*, 29
Non-nucleoside reverse transcriptase inhibitors (NNRTIs), 1:41–42, 9:246, 247*t*
Nonoptic reflex systems, 6:39
Nonoptical visual aids, 3:260–263
Nonorganic/nonphysiologic visual loss. *See* Functional visual loss
Nonpenetrant gene, 8:307
Nonpeptide protease inhibitors, for HIV infection/AIDS, 1:42
Nonperfusion, capillary. *See* Retinal capillary nonperfusion
Nonpigmented epithelium, ciliary body, 2:66, 68*i*
Non–Q wave infarction, 1:114, 116. *See also* Acute coronary syndrome
    management of, 1:122–124
Non–Q wave, nontransmural infarction, 1:114, 116
Nonrefractive accommodative esotropia (high accommodative convergence/accommodative esotropia), 6:98*t*, 102–104
Nonrhegmatogenous retinal detachment. *See* Retinal detachment
Nonsense mutation, 2:191
Nonseptate filamentous fungi, 8:130–131. *See also* Fungi
Non–Sjögren syndrome aqueous tear deficiency, 8:72*t*, 80
Nonspherical optics, 3:224–225
Nonsteroidal anti-inflammatory drugs (NSAIDs), 1:196–198, 197*t*, 2:417*t*, 420–423, 421*i*, 9:96
    adverse reactions to topical use of, 8:101
    Alzheimer disease and, 1:288
    COX-1/COX-2 inhibition by, 1:196, 2:306, 9:96
    for headache, 5:296
    for ocular allergy, 6:236
        allergic conjunctivitis, 8:208–209
    ocular side effects of, 1:197–198, 324*t*
    platelet function affected by, 1:168
    after PRK/LASEK, 13:96
        overcorrection and, 13:100
    prostaglandin synthesis affected by, 2:306, 420–421
    for rheumatic disorders, 1:196–198, 197*t*
    for rheumatoid arthritis, 1:174
    for scleritis, 8:240
    for uveitis, 6:320, 9:118
Non-T, Non-B effector lymphocytes (null cells), 9:15, 25, 70
Nontranslated strand of DNA (sense DNA), 2:195, 201–202
Nontreponemal tests, for syphilis, 1:16–17, 302
Nontuberculous (atypical) mycobacteria, 1:23, 8:127, 185
    in HIV infection/AIDS, 1:23, 49–50
Nonvisual assistance, for low-vision patient, 3:260–263
Nonvisual tasks, in functional visual disorder evaluation, 5:305
Norepinephrine
    adrenergic agents/receptor response and, 2:404–405, 404*i*, 405–409, 406*i*
    dilator muscle affected by, 2:309, 309–310, 405–407

in iris–ciliary body, 2:308, 308*t*
in tear secretion, 2:290, 292, 292*i*, 293, 293*i*
Norfloxacin, 1:62*t*, 73
Normal distribution, clinical relevance of research and, 1:344
Normal flora, ocular, 8:114–115, 115*t*
Normal incidence, 3:46–47
Normal retinal correspondence, 6:41–43, 42*i*
Normal-tension glaucoma. *See* Glaucoma, normal-tension
Normal vision, 3:245*t*, 251
Normality of field, in perimetry interpretation, 10:68–69, 69*i*
Normodyne. *See* Labetalol
Noroxin. *See* Norfloxacin
Norrie disease, 6:342
    gene for, X-linked familial exudative retinopathy and, 12:284
North American Symptomatic Carotid Endarterectomy Trial (NASCET), 1:108, 5:181–182, 182*t*, 12:152
North Carolina macular dystrophy, 12:226–227, 227*i*
Northern blot analysis, 2:191, 230
Norvasc. *See* Amlodipine
Norvir. *See* Ritonavir
NOS. *See* Nitric oxide synthase
Nose, 7:20–21. *See also under* Nasal
    inferior meatus of, 5:10
    orbital tumors originating in, 7:92–93
Nosema, stromal keratitis caused by, 8:190
Nosocomial (hospital-acquired) infections, treatment of, 1:77–78
Nothnagel syndrome, 5:227
Notochord, 2:136, 137*i*
Nougaret disease, rod transducin mutation causing, 2:34
Novolog. *See* Aspart insulin
NPDR. *See* Diabetic retinopathy, nonproliferative
NPH insulin, 1:209, 209*t*
NPPIs. *See* Nonpeptide protease inhibitors
NPS gene, 10:13*t*
NPV. *See* Negative predictive value
NPY. *See* Neuropeptide Y
NR2E3 gene, in Goldmann-Favre syndrome, 12:229
NRC. *See* Normal retinal correspondence
NSAIDs. *See* Nonsteroidal anti-inflammatory drugs
nt. *See* Nucleotides
NtRTIs. *See* Nucleotide reverse transcriptase inhibitors
Nuclear cataracts, 4:102–103, 11:45–46, 47*i*
    in children, 6:289, 289*i*, 292*t*
    congenital, 11:37, 38*i*
Nuclear envelope, 2:203
Nuclear flip techniques, 11:135
Nuclear inclusions, cytologic identification of, 8:69
Nuclear lesions, diplopia and, 5:226
Nuclear matrix, 2:203
Nuclear pores, 2:203
Nuclear splitting techniques, 11:131–132, 132*i*
    phaco fracture technique, 11:131–132, 132*i*
    small capsulorrhexis and, 11:126
Nucleic acid amplification test. *See* Polymerase chain reaction
Nucleic acids. *See also* DNA; RNA
    in retinal pigment epithelium, 2:358
    viral, 8:118–119

Nucleofractis. *See also* Nuclear splitting techniques
  4-quadrant, 11:131–132, 132*i*
  with small capsulorrhexis, 11:126
Nucleolus, 2:203
Nucleoside, 2:191
Nucleoside analogues, 1:3, 41, 9:246, 247*t*
  in HAART, 1:43
Nucleosome, 2:191, 204
Nucleotide reverse transcriptase inhibitors (NtRTI),
  1:41
Nucleotides, 2:191, 199, 200–201, 8:306
  disorders of metabolism of, corneal changes in,
    8:354–355
Nucleus, cell, 2:203–204
Nucleus, lens. *See* Lens (crystalline), nucleus of
Nucleus of Darkschewitsch, 5:39
Nucleus prepositus hypoglossi, 5:39, 202
Nucleus raphe interpositus, 5:34
Nucleus reticularis tegmenti pontis, 5:34
Null allele, gene therapy and, 2:237
Null-cell adenomas, 1:229
Null cells (non-T, non-B effector lymphocytes), 9:15,
  25, 70
Null hypothesis, 1:342
Null mutations, 2:214
Null point, 6:160
  in congenital motor nystagmus, 6:163
  nystagmus surgery and, 6:168–170, 170*i*
"Numb chin" syndrome, 5:301
Numbness, facial, pain associated with, 5:301
Nursing (breast feeding)
  fluorescein dye transmission to breast milk and,
    12:21
  glaucoma medications and, 10:176
  refractive surgery contraindicated during, 13:41
Nutrapore, PermaVision lens made from, 13:72–73,
  175
Nutritional deficiency
  cataract formation and, 11:63–64
  dry eye syndrome and, 8:92–94
  optic neuropathy and, 5:152, 153*i*
Nutritional supplements. *See also specific type*
  in age-related macular degeneration management,
    12:60–61
  in retinitis pigmentosa management, 12:212–213
Nyctalopia. *See also* Night blindness
  in hypovitaminosis A, 8:92
  rod-specific mutations causing, 2:348, 349
Nystagmus, 5:239–256, 6:159–171, 159*t*
  acquired, 5:239, 6:165–168, 169*i*
    pendular, 5:250–251
  in albinism, 6:345–348
  Alexander's law for, 5:244, 246, 248
  amplitude of, 5:240
  in aniridia, 6:162, 262
  Bruns, 5:248
  central vestibular, 5:247–248
  childhood (early-onset), 5:241–243, 6:159–171,
    333–334, 334*t*
    types of, 6:162–168
  in color blindness, 12:196
  congenital, 5:241–242, 6:160, 161, 162–165, 163*i*,
    164*t*
  convergence-retraction, 5:254, 6:167
  in decreased vision, 6:452

definition of, 6:159
differential diagnosis of, 6:168, 169*i*
dissociated (disconjugate/disjunctive), 5:240, 251,
  6:168
downbeat, 5:248–249, 248*i*, 6:167
with esotropia, 6:98*t*, 101, 164
evaluation of, 6:160–162, 163*i*, 163*t*
funduscopic evaluation in, 6:162, 163*t*
gaze-evoked, 5:39, 224, 225*i*, 244, 245*i*
gaze positions affecting, 6:160, 160*i*
head-shaking, 5:200
in hereditary retinal disorders, 6:333–334, 334*t*
history in, 6:160–161, 161*t*
in infants, 6:334, 334*t*
in internuclear ophthalmoplegia, 5:224, 225*i*, 6:155
intracranial tumors causing, 6:159*t*
introduction to, 5:239–240, 240*i*, 241*i*
jerk, 5:239, 6:159, 160, 165, 166*i*
latent/manifest latent, 5:242–243, 6:165, 166*i*
monocular, 5:243, 6:167
in multiple sclerosis, 5:322
nomenclature associated with, 6:159–160
ocular examination in, 6:161–162, 163*i*, 163*t*
ocular motility testing in, 6:162
oculopalatal, 5:251
opsoclonus and, 6:167
optokinetic, 5:167, 198, 6:161, 451
  assessment of, 5:201–202, 6:451
  in congenital motor nystagmus, 6:164
  dysfunction of, 5:205–206
  in functional visual disorder evaluation, 5:305
patterns of, 5:241*i*
pediatric cataracts and, 6:294, 11:195
pendular, 5:239, 240*i*, 6:159
  acquired, 5:250–251
periodic alternating, 5:250, 6:165
peripheral vestibular, 5:245–247, 246*t*
prisms for, 6:168
pupil assessment in, 6:162, 163*t*
rebound, 5:244
retractorius, 6:167
saccadic intrusions and, 5:252–254, 252*i*
see-saw, 5:251, 6:166–167
seizures causing, 1:284
sensory defect, 6:164
spasmus nutans, 5:243, 6:165–166
spontaneous, 5:200
with strabismus, 6:162, 164, 171
surgery for, 6:168–171, 170*i*, 170*t*
torsional, 5:249–250
treatment of, 5:255, 6:168–171, 170*i*
upbeat, 5:249
vestibular, 5:245–250
  central, 5:247–250, 247*t*
  peripheral, 5:245–247, 246*t*
voluntary, 5:253–254, 312
Nystagmus blockage syndrome, 6:164
  surgery for, 6:171
Nystatin, 1:64*t*, 76

O

OAT (ornithine amino transferase) mutations, 2:351
  in gyrate atrophy, 2:351, 12:225

OAV. *See* Oculoauriculovertebral (OAV) spectrum/
    sequence
Obesity
    cataract surgery and, **11**:205–206
    in diabetes mellitus type 2, **1**:201, 202, 205
        weight reduction and, **1**:201, 207, 208–209
    hypertension and, **1**:85, 95
Object agnosia, **5**:192
Object beam, in optical coherence tomography, **3**:322,
    324*i*
Objective angle, in amblyoscope testing, **6**:64
Objective lens
    of operating microscope, **3**:296, 297*i*
    of slit-lamp biomicroscope, **3**:281, 283*i*
    of telescope, **3**:82, 83*i*
Objective refraction, **3**:125–134, 125*i*, 127*i. See also*
    Retinoscopy
    automatic, **3**:313
    in children, **3**:146
    manual, **3**:313
Objective visual space, **6**:41
Objects (optics)
    characteristics of, **3**:30
    at infinity, **3**:74–75
    real, **3**:30
    virtual, **3**:30, 67–69, 69*i*
Obligatory suppression, **6**:55
Oblique astigmatism, **3**:118
Oblique axes, combining cylinders at, **3**:100–101, 101*i*
Oblique muscles, **2**:8, 15*i*, 17*i*, 18*t*, 19*i*, **5**:41, 42, 42*i*,
    6:14*i*, 15–16, 17*t*, 18*i*, **7**:12, 140*i*, 141*i. See also*
    Inferior oblique muscles; Superior oblique muscles
    action of, **6**:15–16, 17*t*, 28–29, 30–31, 30*t*, 34*i*, 35*i*
    anatomy of, **6**:14*i*, 15–16, 17*t*, 18*i*
        surgery and, **6**:23, 24*i*
    field of action/activation of, **6**:29
    insertions of, **2**:16, 17*i*, 18*t*
    origins of, **2**:16, 18*t*
    overaction of, **6**:127–130, 128*i*, 129*i*
        A-pattern deviations associated with, **6**:119, 121*i*
        V-pattern deviations associated with, **6**:119, 120*i*
        vertical deviations caused by, **6**:127–130, 128*i*,
            129*i*
    palsy of, **6**:132–136, 133*i*, 136*i*, 137*t*
    weakening procedures for, **6**:180–181
        for A- and V-pattern deviations, **6**:122–123, 124,
            124–125, 180, 181
        for vertical deviations, **6**:128–129, 130
Oblique myokymia, superior, **5**:254, **6**:156–157
Oblique subnucleus, inferior, **5**:45
Oblique tenotomy
    for Brown syndrome, **6**:146, 181
    for third nerve (oculomotor) palsy, **6**:148
Observational studies, **1**:345
Obstetric history
    in infant with decreased vision, **6**:452
    infantile corneal opacities and, **6**:255, 256*t*
    nystagmus and, **6**:161
Obstructive pulmonary disease, **1**:143–144
    ocular surgery in patients with, **1**:329, **11**:203–204
Obstructive shock, **1**:317. *See also* Shock
OCA1 albinism, **2**:362
OCA1A albinism, **6**:346*t*
OCA1B albinism, **6**:346*t*
OCA1MP albinism, **6**:347*t*

OCA1TS albinism, **6**:347*t*
OCA2 albinism, **2**:362, **6**:346*t*
OCA3 albinism, **6**:346*t*
Occipital association cortex, near reflex initiated in,
    2:111
Occipital bone, **5**:9
Occipital (primary visual/calcarine/striate) cortex,
    2:108, **5**:28–29, 30*i*, 31, 31*i*, **6**:44, 45, 45*i*, 47*i*
    development of, **6**:46, 48*i*
        abnormal visual experience affecting, **6**:49–52, 50*i*,
            51*i*, 67–68
    disorders of, **5**:191–196, 193*t*
        hallucinations and, **5**:170
        object recognition problems and, **5**:192, 193*i*, 194
        vision or vision deficit awareness in, **5**:195–196
        visual-spatial relationships in, **5**:194–195
Occipital ischemia, transient visual loss caused by,
    5:185–186
Occipital lobe lesions
    hallucinations and, **5**:190–191
    retrochiasmal, **5**:167–170, 168*i*, 169*i*, 170*i*
    transient visual loss caused by, **5**:185
Occipital seizures, transient visual loss caused by, **5**:186
Occluding zonules, corneal, **2**:45
Occlusion, in phacoemulsification, **11**:115
Occlusion amblyopia, **6**:70, 73
    eye trauma and, **6**:441–442
Occlusion therapy. *See also* Patching
    for amblyopia, **6**:72–73
        cataract surgery and, **6**:302
        compliance issues and, **6**:74
        complications of, **6**:73
Occlusive retinal disease. *See also specific type*
    arterial, **12**:145–152
        branch retinal artery occlusion, **4**:133, **12**:146–148,
            146*i*, 147*i*
        central retinal artery occlusion, **4**:133–134,
            5:105–106, 106*i*, **12**:148–150, 148*i*, 149*i*
        ocular ischemic syndrome, **12**:150–152, 151*i*
        precapillary retinal arteriole occlusion,
            12:145–146, 146*i*
    venous, **12**:136–145
        branch retinal vein occlusion, **4**:134–135, 135*i*,
            12:136–141, 137*i*, 139*i*, 140*i*
        carotid occlusive disease and, **12**:145
        central retinal vein occlusion, **4**:133–134, 134*i*,
            5:106–107, 106*i*, **12**:141–145, 142*i*
        photocoagulation for, wavelength selection and,
            12:315*t*
Occupation
    bifocal segment and, **3**:163–164
    light toxicity and, **12**:309
Occupational therapist, in vision rehabilitation, **3**:264
OCD. *See* Optical chamber depth
Ochronosis, **2**:263
    corneal pigmentation in, **8**:377*t*
OCT. *See* Optical coherence tomography
Octopus 1-2-3, **10**:70, 71*i*
Octopus perimeters, **10**:65, 70, 71*i*
Ocu-Chlor. *See* Chloramphenicol
Ocufen. *See* Flurbiprofen
Ocuflox. *See* Ofloxacin
Ocular (eyepiece), of telescope, **3**:82, 83*i*
Ocular adnexa. *See also specific structure*
    anatomy of, **2**:5–12

benign lesions of, 7:166–169
in children, 6:200
in craniosynostosis syndromes, 6:429–430
definition of, 7:166
glands of, 2:29*t*
in glaucoma evaluation, 10:32
infections of in children, 6:230–232, 232*i*, 233*i*
Kaposi sarcoma of, 9:258–259, 258*i*, 259*i*
radiation affecting, 1:255–256
in systemic malignancies, 1:262
Ocular albinism, 2:176, 362, 6:347*t*, 12:239–240, 240*i*
autosomal recessive, 6:347*t*
ocular findings in carriers of, 2:176, 270*t*, 271*i*
X-linked (Nettleship-Falls), 6:345, 347*t*
ocular findings in carriers of, 2:270*t*, 271*i*, 272
Ocular alignment
in infant with decreased vision, 6:452
tests of. *See also specific type*
in children, 6:80–86
confounding factors and, 6:86
Vernier acuity and, 3:111
unsatisfactory, after strabismus surgery, 6:184
Ocular allergy. *See also* Allergic reactions
in children, 6:233–236
Ocular autonomic pathways, 5:56–60
parasympathetic, 5:57, 59–60, 59*i*, 60*i*
sympathetic, 5:56–57, 58*i*
Ocular biometrics. *See* Biometry/biometrics
Ocular bobbing, 5:208, 256
reverse, 5:256
Ocular cytology. *See* Cytology
Ocular development. *See* Eye, development of
Ocular deviation
conjugate, in comatose patients, 5:256
tonic, 5:211–212
Ocular dipping, 5:256
Ocular dominance columns, 5:29, 6:46, 47*i*
Ocular examination. *See* Examination
Ocular flutter, 5:253
Ocular hemorrhage. *See* Hemorrhages
Ocular histoplasmosis syndrome, 9:160–163, 160*i*, 161*i*,
162*i*, 177*t*, 12:72*t*, 79–82, 80*i*
histo spots in, 9:160, 160*i*, 161
HLA association in, 9:94*t*, 160
management of, 12:72*t*, 80–82
Ocular history. *See also* History
keratorefractive surgery and, 13:41
Ocular hypertelorism, 6:207, 424
Ocular hypertension. *See* Elevated intraocular pressure
Ocular Hypertension Treatment Study (OHTS), 10:28,
86, 87*t*, 97–98, 157
Ocular hypotension. *See* Hypotony
Ocular immunology/immune response. *See* Immune
response; Immune response arc
Ocular infection. *See* Infection
Ocular inflammation. *See* Inflammation; Uveitis
Ocular ischemia (ocular ischemic syndrome),
5:183–184, 184*i*, 9:221–222, 12:150–152, 151*i*
Ocular larval migrans, 8:133. *See also Toxocara*
(toxocariasis)
Ocular lateropulsion, 5:205
Ocular media. *See* Optical medium
Ocular melanocytosis (melanosis oculi), 8:264–265,
265*i*, 267*t*
in children, 6:387–388, 388*i*

Ocular microbiology. *See* Microbiology
Ocular migraine, 5:184. *See also* Migraine headache
Ocular motility. *See also* Eye movements; Ocular motor
pathways
assessment of, 5:197–212
before cataract surgery, 11:81
in children, 6:80–95
binocular sensory cooperation tests in, 6:93–94
convergence and, 6:87–88
cycloplegic refraction in, 6:94–95
fusional vergence and, 6:88–89
ocular alignment tests in, 6:80–86
positions of gaze and, 6:86–87, 88*i*
prism adaptation test in, 6:92
special motor tests in, 6:89–92
convergence in, 5:203–204
eye movement assessment in, 5:199–204. *See also*
Eye movements, assessment of
in functional visual disorder evaluation, 5:311–313
optokinetic nystagmus in, 5:201–202
pursuit system in, 5:203
before refractive surgery, 13:44
saccadic system in, 5:202–203
stability in, 5:199
vestibulo-ocular reflex in, 5:200–201
disorders of, 5:204–212
in ataxia-telangiectasia, 5:342, 6:417
in blowout fractures, 7:102–104, 103*i*
surgery and, 7:104–105
conditions causing, 7:26
in Graves ophthalmopathy, 7:26
history/presenting complaint in, 6:77–78
in inborn errors of metabolism, 6:436–437*t*
in multiple sclerosis, 5:321–322
nystagmus/spontaneous, 5:239–256, 6:162. *See also*
Nystagmus
after orbital surgery, 7:117
pursuit, 5:210
saccadic, 5:206–209
gaze palsy and, 5:208–209, 209*i*, 210*i*
ocular motor apraxia and, 5:207–208
stability, 5:204–212
tonic eye deviation and, 5:211–212
vergence, 5:210–211
vestibulo-ocular, 5:205
efferent visual system and, 5:197
after evisceration, 7:123
examination of, 5:239–240
extraocular muscles controlling, 7:12
fundamental principles of, 5:197–199
infranuclear pathways in, 5:197
supranuclear pathways in, 5:197
Ocular motor apraxia, 5:207–208
acquired, 5:194, 207–208
congenital, 5:207, 6:156
Ocular motor pathways, 5:32–49
cranial nerves and, 5:42–43, 44*i*, 45–49, 45–49*i*
extraocular muscles and, 5:41–42, 42*i*
infranuclear, 5:197
supranuclear, 5:197
Ocular movements. *See* Eye movements
Ocular myasthenia gravis, 7:218. *See also* Myasthenia
gravis
Ocular pain. *See* Pain

Ocular pharmacology, 2:393–458. *See also specific agent and* Drugs, ocular
    age/aging and, 1:235–236
    legal aspects of, 2:393–394
    principles of, 2:379–392
Ocular prostheses, 7:122
Ocular stability
    assessment of, 5:199
    dysfunction of, 5:204–212
Ocular surface. *See also* Conjunctiva; Cornea; Epithelium
    blood supply of, 8:59
    definition of, 8:55, 423
    disorders of. *See also* Dry eye syndrome
        contact lens wear and, 8:106–108
        diagnostic approach to, 8:61–70
        factitious, 8:105–106, 106*i*
        immune-mediated
            diagnostic approach to, 8:202–203
            patterns of, 8:201–202
        infectious. *See* Infection
        limbal stem cell deficiency, 8:58
        neoplastic, 8:255*t*
            diagnostic approaches to, 8:250, 251*i*
            histopathologic processes and conditions and, 8:246–247, 247*t*
            management of, 8:252
            neuroectodermal, 8:263–269, 263*t*
            oncogenesis and, 8:248–249, 248*t*
        ocular cytology in, 8:63–70
        scleral contact lenses in management of, 3:202
        tear deficiency states, 8:61–63, 62*i*, 62*t*
    immunologic features of, 8:195–196, 196*t*
    inflammatory conditions in children affecting, 6:388
    maintenance of, 8:424–425
    mechanical functions of, 8:59–60
    microanatomy of, 8:245
    physiology of, 8:55–60
    surgery of, 8:423–425, 423*t*, 427–443. *See also specific procedure*
        indications for, 8:423*t*
    wound healing/repair and, 8:383–386, 424. *See also* Wound healing/repair
        response to, 8:424–425
Ocular (intraocular) surgery, 13:143–166. *See also specific procedure*
    anterior segment trauma caused by, 8:418–420
    after arcuate keratotomy, 13:69
    cystoid macular edema after, 12:154
    in elderly patients, 1:237–238
    endophthalmitis after, 9:207, 208*t*, 209–211, 12:328–331. *See also* Endophthalmitis
        acute-onset, 9:210–211, 210*i*, 211*i*, 12:329, 330*i*
        bleb-associated, 9:207, 208*t*, 212–213, 12:331, 332*i*
        chronic (delayed-onset), 9:211, 212*i*, 12:329–331, 331*i*
    after limbal relaxing incisions, 13:69
    for melanoma, 4:238
    needle penetration of globe and, 12:336, 337*i*
    ocular surface, 8:423–425, 423*t*, 427–443
    perioperative management for, 1:327–338
        intraoperative complications and, 1:334*t*, 335–337
        medication management and, 1:332*t*
        postoperative care and, 1:337–338

preoperative assessment/management and, 1:327–335, 328*t*, 332*t*. *See also* Preoperative assessment/preparation for ocular surgery
    after radial keratotomy, 13:64–66
    for refractive errors, 13:143–166. *See also* Bioptics
    retinal detachment after, 12:334–336, 334*i*
    suprachoroidal hemorrhage and, 12:332–334, 333*i*
    for uveitis, 6:322, 9:121
    vitrectomy for complications of, 12:328–340
Ocular tilt reaction, 5:205
Ocular toxoplasmosis. *See* Toxoplasma (toxoplasmosis)
Ocular trauma. *See* Trauma
Ocular tumors. *See* Intraocular tumors; Tumors
Oculinum. *See* Botulinum toxin
Oculoauriculovertebral (OAV) spectrum/sequence, 6:431–432, 432*i*, 433*i*, 8:352*t*. *See also* Goldenhar syndrome
Oculocardiac reflex, 6:191
    atropine affecting, 2:402
Oculocerebral hypopigmentation (Cross syndrome), 6:346*t*
Oculocerebrorenal syndrome (Lowe syndrome), 2:172, 6:348–349
    childhood glaucoma and, 6:278–279, 348, 10:155*t*
    congenital corneal keloids in, 8:299
    ocular findings in carriers of, 2:270*t*
    pediatric cataract and, 6:288*t*, 348
Oculocutaneous albinism, 2:176, 177*i*, 362, 6:345, 347*t*, 12:239–240, 240*i*
    racial and ethnic concentration of, 2:260
Oculodentodigital dysplasia/syndrome (Meyer-Schwickerath and Weyers syndrome)
    childhood glaucoma and, 10:155*t*
    retinal degeneration and, 12:232*t*
Oculodentoosseous dysplasia, 8:352*t*
Oculodermal melanocytosis (nevus of Ota), 6:387–388, 8:264, 267*t*
Oculodigital reflex, 6:451
    in Leber congenital amaurosis, 12:211
Oculoglandular syndrome, Parinaud, 4:49, 8:178–179, 12:184–185
    in children, 6:229, 230*i*
Oculogyric crisis, 5:212
Oculomandibulodyscephaly, 8:352*t*. *See also* Hallermann-Streiff syndrome
Oculomasticatory myorhythmia, 5:255
Oculomotor foramen, 7:14
Oculomotor nerve. *See* Cranial nerve III
Oculomotor nerve palsy. *See* Third nerve (oculomotor) palsy
Oculopalatal nystagmus, 5:251
Oculopharyngeal dystrophy, 5:334–335
Oculorenal syndromes, familial, 6:348–349
Ocupress. *See* Carteolol
Ocusert. *See* Pilocarpine
Ocusert Delivery System, 2:390. *See also* Pilocarpine
OcuvitePreserVision, 2:454
OD. *See* Optical density
ODD. *See* Optic disc (optic nerve head), drusen of
Odds ratio, 1:361
Off-bipolars, 2:352, 352*i*
"Off pump bypass surgery," 1:122
Off retinal ganglion cells, 2:352–353, 353*i*, 354*i*
Ofloxacin, 1:62*t*, 73, 2:430–433, 431*t*
    for bacterial keratitis, 8:183

for gonococcal conjunctivitis, 8:172
OGTT. *See* Oral glucose tolerance test
Oguchi disease, 6:336, 12:200–201, 201*i*
  arrestin mutation causing, 2:227, 349
  racial and ethnic concentration of, 2:260
  rhodopsin kinase mutations causing, 2:349
OHS. *See* Ocular histoplasmosis syndrome
Oil droplet appearance
  in galactosemia, 11:61, 62*i*
  in lenticonus and lentiglobus, 6:289, 11:31
Oil glands, of eyelid, lesions of, 7:166–167
Oil red O stain, 4:36
Ointments, ocular, 2:386
  lubricating, 5:286. *See also* Lubricants
OIS. *See* Orbital inflammatory syndrome
OKN. *See* Optokinetic nystagmus
Olanzapine, 1:271, 272
Older patients. *See* Age/aging; Geriatrics
Oleate, in vitreous, 2:337
Olfactory bulb, 2:93, 95*i*
Olfactory nerve. *See* Cranial nerve I
Olfactory tract, 2:93, 95*i*
Oligemic shock, 1:317. *See also* Shock
Oligoarticular (pauciarticular) onset juvenile idiopathic
  arthritis, 1:178, 6:313–314, 313*t*
  eye examination schedule for children with, 6:316*t*
  uveitis in, 6:313–314, 313*t*
Oligodendrocytes, 4:203
Oligodendroglia, retinal, 2:353
Oligonucleotide hybridization, in mutation screening,
  2:231, 233*i*
Oligonucleotides
  allele-specific, 2:182
    in mutation screening, 2:231, 233*i*
  antisense
    in gene therapy, 2:238, 238*i*
    for glaucoma, 10:177
Oligosaccharide antibiotics, 1:75
Olivary nucleus
  inferior, 5:40
  superior, 5:43
Olivopontocerebellar atrophy, retinal degeneration and,
  12:232*t*, 235
Olmesartan, 1:88*t*
Olopatadine, 2:424*t*, 425
Omega-3 fatty acid supplements, for meibomian gland
  dysfunction, 8:83
OMIM. *See* Online Mendelian Inheritance in Man
Omnicef. *See* Cefdinir
Omniflox. *See* Temafloxacin
OMP. *See* Ophthalmic medical personnel
On-bipolars, 2:352, 352*i*
On retinal ganglion cells, 2:352–353, 353*i*, 354*i*
Onchocerca volvulus (onchocerciasis), 8:51*t*, 132,
  9:195–197
Oncocytoma, 8:261
Oncogenes/oncogenesis, 1:252, 2:192, 215, 8:248–249,
  248*t*
Oncovin. *See* Vincristine
Ondansetron, perioperative, 1:332*t*, 338
One-and-a-half syndrome, 5:225, 226*i*
100-hue test (Farnsworth-Munsell), 12:43
  in low vision evaluation, 5:96
One-piece bifocals, 3:152, 153*i*

One toy, one look rule, for pediatric examination, 6:3,
  4*i*
ONH. *See* Optic nerve (cranial nerve II), hypoplasia of
Onlays, corneal, 13:71–85
  alloplastic, 13:77
Online Mendelian Inheritance in Man (OMIM), 2:222
Online search, 1:340
Onychoosteodysplasia, 8:352*t*
OPA1 gene, 5:136
Opacities
  fundus evaluation with, 11:84
  vitreous
    amyloidosis causing, 12:286–287
    in asteroid hyalosis, 12:285, 286*i*
    in toxoplasmosis, 9:166, 166*i*, 239
    in uveitis, 9:239
Opcon-A. *See* Naphazoline/pheniramine
Open-angle glaucoma, 10:83–117. *See also* Glaucoma
  central retinal vein occlusion and, 12:143
  childhood (congenital/infantile/juvenile). *See also*
    Glaucoma, childhood
    clinical manifestations and diagnosis of,
      6:272–273, 273*i*, 274*t*
    genetics of, 6:271
    juvenile, 6:271, 272
    natural history of, 6:277
    pathophysiology of, 6:272
    primary
      congenital, 6:271, 272–277, 273*i*, 274*t*, 275*i*,
        276*i*, 277*i*
      juvenile, 6:271, 272
    secondary, 6:277–280
    treatment of, 6:280–283
  classification of, 10:5, 6*t*, 7*i*
    mechanisms of outflow obstruction in, 10:9*t*
  cornea plana and, 8:291
  cycloplegic use in, 2:401
  without elevated intraocular pressure, 10:92–96, 94*t*.
    See also Glaucoma, normal-tension
  genetics of, 10:14
  management of
    medical, 10:174–175
    surgical, 10:180–197, 181*i*, 187–191*i*, 193*i*, 193*t*,
      195*i*. *See also specific procedure*
      cataract and filtering surgery combined,
        10:195–197
      full-thickness sclerectomy in, 10:194–195, 195*i*
      incisional, 10:183–194, 187–191*i*, 193*i*, 193*t*
      laser trabeculoplasty in, 10:180–183, 181*i*
  microcornea and, 8:289
  pars planitis and, 9:151
  peripheral anterior synechiae in, 10:5, 7
  pigment dispersion syndrome and, 4:84, 85*i*
  primary, 10:82–93
    adult-onset diabetes and, 10:10–11
    age and, 10:7–8, 86, 91*t*
    cardiovascular disease and, 10:89
    central retinal vein occlusion and, 10:90
    characteristics of, 10:6*t*
    clinical features of, 10:83–87, 85*t*, 91*t*
    clinical trials of, 10:85*t*, 87–90*t*
    congenital, 6:271, 272–277, 273*i*, 274*t*, 275*i*, 276*i*,
      277*i*
    demographics in, 10:10
    described, 10:83

diabetes mellitus and, 10:88–89
disorders associated with, 10:87–90
epidemiology of, 10:7–11
family history and, 10:87
intraocular pressure in, 10:83–84
juvenile, 6:271, 272
myopia and, 10:88
optic disc appearance in, 10:84–86, 85t, 87–90t
prevalence of, 10:7–8
prognosis of, 10:91–92
race and, 10:86, 91t
refractive surgery in patients with, 13:189–191, 190i
risk factors for, 10:7, 10–11, 86–87, 91t
visual field loss in, 10:84–86, 85t, 87–90t
secondary, 10:99–117
  characteristics of, 10:6t
  in children, 6:277–280
  drug use in, 10:116–117
  episcleral venous pressure elevation and, 10:108–109, 108t, 109i
  hyphema and, 10:110–112, 111i
  intraocular tumors causing, 10:106
  lens-induced, 10:103–106, 104i, 104t, 105i
  ocular inflammation and, 10:106–108, 108i
  penetrating keratoplasty and, 8:460–461, 10:116, 116t
  pigmentary, 10:101–103, 101–103i
  trauma causing, 4:81–82, 82i
    accidental, 10:109–114, 110–113i
    surgical, 10:114–115, 115i
  in Sturge-Weber syndrome, 5:340
  uveitis and, 9:237
Open-loop trackers, 13:98
Open reading frame, 2:192, 202
Operating microscope, 3:296–297, 296i, 297i
  phototoxicity and, 2:459, 11:171–172, 12:308
Operation/reoperation techniques, 6:176
Operculated holes, 12:253, 254, 255i
  treatment of, 12:265, 265–266, 266t, 267t
Ophthacet. See Sulfacetamide
Ophthaine. See Proparacaine
Ophthalmia
  neonatorum, 6:221–224, 222i, 8:51t, 172–174
    chemical, 6:223
    chlamydial, 6:222–223, 8:173, 174
    gonococcal, 6:222, 222i, 8:172, 173
    herpes simplex causing, 1:27, 6:223. See also Conjunctivitis, herpes simplex virus causing
    prophylaxis for, 6:223–224
  nodosum, 8:395
  sympathetic, 4:152–153, 153i, 154i, 9:67–68, 200–203, 200i, 201i, 202t, 12:300–301
    enucleation for prevention of, 7:119–120, 8:410–411
    HLA association in, 9:94t
    surgical procedures/injuries leading to, 9:202t
Ophthalmic artery, 2:39i, 41i, 5:10, 13, 15, 178i, 7:14i, 15
  development of, 2:155
  extraocular muscles supplied by, 2:16–18, 6:16
  eyelids supplied by, 7:147, 8:7
  occlusion of, 12:148, 149i
    chronic, ocular ischemic syndrome and, 12:150
  optic nerve supplied by, 2:102, 4:204

terminal, 5:15
Ophthalmic Devices Panel, 13:31, 36–37
Ophthalmic echography. See Ultrasonography
Ophthalmic examination. See Examination
Ophthalmic instrumentation. See also specific type
  phototoxicity from, 2:459–465, 460t, 12:308–309
    cataract surgery and, 11:171–172
Ophthalmic irrigants, 2:451. See also Irrigation
  endothelial changes caused by, 8:420
Ophthalmic lenses, 3:62–84. See also Lenses
  afocal systems of, 3:81–84
  Badal principle and, 3:80–81
  combinations and, 3:67
  concave, 3:72–74, 73i
  focal lengths of, 3:79
  focal planes/points and, 3:69–71, 70i
  Knapp's law and, 3:80–81, 81i
  lensmeters and, 3:80–81
  objects/images at infinity and, 3:74–75
  paraxial ray tracing
    through concave spherical lenses, 3:74, 74i, 75i
    through convex spherical lenses, 3:71–72, 71i, 72i
  principal/planes points and, 3:75–76
  reduced vergence, 3:62–65, 63i, 64i
  thick, 3:78–79, 78i
  thin-lens approximation, 3:66–67
  transverse magnification, for simple spherical refracting surface, 3:65–66, 66i
  vergence, 3:62–65, 63i, 64i
  virtual images/objects and, 3:67–69, 68i, 69i
Ophthalmic medical personnel (OMP), in vision rehabilitation, 3:264–265
Ophthalmic nerve. See Cranial nerve V (trigeminal nerve), V₁
Ophthalmic pathology, 4:9–210
  of anterior chamber and trabecular meshwork, 4:77–85
  communication among health care team members and, 4:31–32
  congenital anomalies and, 4:12
  of conjunctiva, 4:43–59, 44i
  of cornea, 4:61–76
  degeneration and dystrophy and, 4:15–16
  diagnostic electron microscopy in, 4:40
  of eyelids, 4:167–185
  fine-needle aspiration biopsy for, 4:40–41
  flow cytometry in, 4:38–39, 38i
  frozen section for, 4:41
  history of, 4:5–8
  immunohistochemistry in, 4:37–38, 37i
  inflammation and, 4:12–15, 13i, 14i, 15i, 16i
  of lens, 4:93–104
  molecular pathologic techniques in, 4:39–40, 39i
  neoplasia and, 4:16–17, 17i, 17t
  of optic nerve, 4:203–210
  of orbit, 4:187–202, 201i, 7:35
  organizational paradigm for, 4:11–19, 19t
  of retina, 4:117–147
  of sclera, 4:87–92
  special procedures in, 4:37–41
  specimen handling for, 4:31–36, 36t
  topography and, 4:12
  of uveal tract, 4:149–166
  of vitreous, 4:105–115
  wound repair and, 4:19–29, 20i

Ophthalmic prisms. *See* Prisms
Ophthalmic vein, **4:**204, **5:**20, 22*i*, **7:**15, **12:**15
    eyelids drained by, **8:**7
Ophthalmic wound healing/repair. *See* Wound healing/
    repair
Ophthalmometry. *See* Keratometry
Ophthalmomyiasis, **8:**133–134
Ophthalmopathy, thyroid (Graves/dysthyroid). *See*
    Thyroid ophthalmopathy
Ophthalmoplegia
    chronic progressive external, **6:**150–151, 153*t*,
        12:236, 245, 246*t*, 247*i*
        mitochondrial DNA deletions and, **2:**218
    internuclear, **5:**39, 210, 224–225, 225*i*, 226*i*, **6:**155
        myasthenia gravis and, **5:**224
        nystagmus in, **5:**224, 225*i*, **6:**155
        unilateral, **5:**225, 226*i*
        wall-eyed bilateral, **5:**224, 225*i*
Ophthalmoplegic migraine, **5:**231. *See also* Migraine
    headache
Ophthalmoscopy
    before cataract surgery, **11:**83
    in choroidal/ciliary body melanoma, **4:**224
    direct, **3:**269–271, 269*i*, 270*i*
        fundus illumination in, **3:**270, 271*i*
        viewing system for, **3:**269–270, 270*i*
    indirect, **3:**272–275, 272*i*, 275*i*
        aerial image in, **3:**272, 273*i*, 277*i*, 279*i*
            binocular observation and, **3:**275, 276*i*, 279*i*
        binocular observation and, **3:**275, 276*i*
        in choroidal/ciliary body melanoma, **4:**224
        fundus illumination in, **3:**272, 275, 279*i*
        fundus image formation and, **3:**272, 273*i*
        illumination source for, **3:**272
        in ocular trauma, **12:**290
        in optic disc evaluation, **10:**51
        in posterior vitreous detachment, **12:**258
        pupil conjugacy and, **3:**272–275, 274*i*
        in retinal examination, **12:**17
        in retinopathy of prematurity, **12:**125
    laser, **3:**279
        in optic nerve head evaluation, **10:**55
        in retinal examination, **12:**24–25
    video, **3:**279
Ophthetic. *See* Proparacaine
Opiates, abuse of, **1:**268*t*, 269
OPL. *See* Optical path length; Outer plexiform layer
Opportunistic infections, **8:**118. *See also specific type*
    candidiasis, **9:**163–164, 223–224
    cryptococcosis, **9:**163, 257
    cytomegalovirus retinitis, **4:**123, 124*i*, **9:**71, 156–157,
        249–250
    in HIV infection/AIDS, **1:**37–38, **9:**248, 260, 260*i*.
        See also specific type
    treatment of, **1:**45–51
Opsins (cone), **2:**345, **12:**10
    genes for, **2:**347
Opsoclonus (saccadomania), **5:**253, **6:**167
    in neuroblastoma, **6:**374
Opsoclonus-myoclonus syndrome, **5:**253
Opsonization, antibody, **9:**58, 58*i*
Optic
    of intraocular lens, **3:**213
    of scleral contact lens, **3:**200, 201*i*
Optic ataxia, **5:**194

Optic atrophy, **4:**206, 207*i*, **5:**87–88, 88*i*, 123,
    6:364–365, 365*t*, 454
    ascending, **4:**206
    Behr, **6:**364
    cavernous, of Schnabel, **4:**206, 207*i*
    in children, **6:**364–365, 365*t*, 454
    in craniosynostosis, **6:**429
    descending, **4:**206
    dominant, **5:**136–137, 137*i*, **6:**364
    in inborn errors of metabolism, **6:**436–437*t*
    Leber hereditary, **5:**134–136, 135*i*, **6:**364–365
    in onchocerciasis, **9:**196
    retrochiasmal lesions causing, **5:**164, 166*i*
Optic canal, **2:**102, **5:**5, 10, 26, **7:**11–12
    decompression of, for traumatic visual loss, **7:**108
Optic cap (apical zone), **3:**174, 205, **8:**38
Optic chiasm. *See* Chiasm
Optic cup, **2:**96, 127
    development of, **2:**137–138, 141*i*, 142*i*, **11:**25
    enlargement of, **2:**98. *See also* Cupping of optic disc
Optic disc (optic nerve head). *See also* Optic nerve
    anatomy of, **2:**76, 95–101, 98*i*, 99*i*, 100*i*
    aplasia of, **6:**363
    atrophy of. *See* Optic atrophy
    avulsion of, **12:**302, 303*i*
    blood supply of, **2:**103, 104*i*, 105*i*
    cavernous hemangioma of, **12:**163
    coloboma of, **2:**171*i*, **4:**204–205, **6:**359–360, 360*i*
    congenital/developmental abnormalities of,
        2:173–175, 174*i*, 176*i*, **5:**138–141, **6:**359–364
        in fetal alcohol syndrome, **6:**433–434
    cupping of. *See* Cupping of optic disc
    in diabetic papillopathy, **5:**127, 127*i*
    differentiation of, **2:**145
    disorders of in children, **6:**359–368
    drusen of, **4:**206–208, 208*i*, **5:**115, 115*i*, 129–134,
        131*i*
        astrocytic hamartoma differentiated from,
            5:132–134, 133*i*
        in children, **5:**133–134, **6:**368, 368*i*
        papilledema differentiated from, **5:**130–132, 132*i*,
            133*i*
        pseudopapilledema and, **5:**115, 115*i*, **6:**368, 368*i*
    edema of, **5:**26, 88–89, 89*i*, 89*t*. *See also* Papilledema
        in acute papilledema, **5:**112–113
        in anterior optic neuropathy, **5:**111–113, 115–129
        in children, **6:**366
            in craniosynostosis, **6:**429
            in leukemia, **6:**344, 344*i*
        in cystoid macular edema, **12:**154
        in papillitis, **5:**125–126
    evacuated anomalies of, **5:**140–141
    evaluation of, in glaucoma, **10:**51
        clinical, **10:**51–57, 52*t*, 53*i*, 54*i*
        quantitative measurement in, **10:**55–56
    in Foster Kennedy syndrome, **5:**123, 123*i*
    in glaucoma, **10:**53–54, 54*i*, 84–86, 85*t*, 87–90*t*
    hypoplasia of, **2:**173–175, 174*i*, 176*i*, **5:**138–139,
        139*i*, **6:**362–363, 362*i*, 453–454
    in leukemia, **6:**344, 344*i*
    in megalopapilla, **6:**361
    melanocytoma (magnocellular nevus) of, **4:**208, 209*i*
        melanoma differentiated from, **4:**230, 232*i*
    morning glory, **6:**359, 359*i*

nerve fiber layer of
  examination of, **10**:54
    diffuse loss in, **10**:55
  focal abnormalities of, **10**:54–55
  perimetry changes correlated with, **10**:78
  retinal nerve fibers entering, **5**:111, 112*i*
  tilted (Fuchs coloboma), **5**:139–140, 140*i*, **6**:360–361, 361*i*
  vasculitis of (papillophlebitis), **4**:133–134, **5**:128, 128*i*
    in central retinal vein occlusion, **12**:141
Optic disc pit, acquired, **10**:52
  formation of, **10**:52–53, 53*i*
Optic foramen, **2**:9, 10*i*, 11*i*
Optic gliomas. *See* Optic nerve (optic pathway) glioma
Optic nerve (cranial nerve II). *See also* Optic disc
  anatomy of, **2**:93–98, 94*i*, 95*i*, **5**:25–27, **10**:44, 46–49, 46*i*, 47*i*
  anterior/anterior zone of, **10**:47–48, 47*i*
    vascular anatomy/vasculature of, **10**:47, 47*i*, 48
  aplasia of, **6**:363, 453
  atrophy of. *See* Optic atrophy
  avulsion of, **12**:302, 303*i*
  blood supply of, **2**:102–104, 104*i*, 105*i*, 106*i*, **4**:204, **10**:47, 47*i*, 48
  coloboma of, **2**:175, **6**:359–360, 360*i*
  congenital abnormalities of, **2**:173–175, 174*i*, 176*i*, **4**:204–205, **6**:359–364
    in fetal alcohol syndrome, **2**:161
  degenerations of, **4**:206–208, 207*i*, 208*i*
  described, **10**:44
  development of, **2**:143*i*, 144–145
  disorders of, **4**:203–210. *See also specific type*
    in children, **6**:359–368
    in craniosynostosis, **6**:429
    illusions and, **5**:189
    neoplastic, **4**:208–210, 209*i*, 210*i*
    radiation causing, **1**:256
    relative afferent pupillary defect in, **5**:86–87
  distribution of nerve fibers in, **10**:46, 46*i*
  evaluation of
    before cataract surgery, **11**:84
    in glaucoma, **10**:44, 46–49, 46*i*, 47*i*
    in nystagmus, **6**:162
    recording findings in, **10**:56–57
  in glaucoma, **10**:4, 44, 46–49, 46*i*, 47*i*. *See also* Optic neuropathy, in glaucoma
    examination of, **10**:44, 46–49, 46*i*, 47*i*
    primary congenital glaucoma and, **6**:276, 277*i*
    refractive surgery and, **13**:189, 190*i*
    theories of damage and, **10**:50–51
  glioma of. *See* Optic nerve (optic pathway) glioma
  in Graves ophthalmopathy, **7**:48, 53
  hypoplasia of, **2**:173–175, 174*i*, 176*i*, **5**:138–139, 139*i*, **6**:362–363, 362*i*, 453–454
    in fetal alcohol syndrome, **2**:161
  infection/inflammation of, **4**:205, 205*i*, 206*i*
  intracanalicular portion of, **2**:93, 97*t*, 102
    blood supply of, **2**:103
    compressive lesions of, **5**:145–151
  intracranial portion of, **2**:93, 97*t*, 102, 103*i*
    blood supply of, **2**:103
  intraocular portion of, **2**:93, 95–101, 95*t*, 98*i*, 99*i*, 100*i*

intraorbital portion of, **2**:93, 97, 97*t*, 101–102, 101*i*, **5**:26, **7**:12
  blood supply of, **2**:103, 104*i*
  compressive lesions of, **5**:145–151
  length of, **7**:7*t*, 12
laminar portion of, **2**:99, **10**:48, 49
in leukemia, **6**:344, 344*i*
pathology of, **10**:44, 46–49, 46*i*, 47*i*
prelaminar portion of, **2**:98, 98*i*, 99*i*, **10**:48, 49. *See also* Optic disc
  blood supply of, **2**:103
regional differences in, **2**:93, 95*t*, 96*i*, 97*i*
retinal ganglion cell axons in, **10**:44, 46
retinoblastoma involving, **4**:144, 145*i*, 254–255, 264
retrolaminar portion of, **2**:99–101, 100*i*, **10**:49
secondary tumors of, **4**:284–285
superficial nerve fiber layer of, **10**:48–49
topography of, **4**:203–204, 203*i*, 204*i*
trauma to, **5**:153–155, 154*i*, **7**:107
in uveitis, **9**:103*t*
Optic nerve glioblastoma (malignant optic glioma), **4**:209, **5**:151, **7**:72
Optic nerve (optic pathway) glioma (pilocytic astrocytoma), **4**:208–209, 209*i*, **5**:148–151, 149*i*, 150*t*, **7**:72–75, 73*i*
  in children (juvenile), **4**:208, 209*i*, **6**:381, 406–407, 406*i*
  malignant (glioblastoma), **4**:209, **5**:151, **7**:72
  in neurofibromatosis, **5**:149, **6**:381, 406–407, 406*i*, **7**:72–74, 75
  orbital involvement in, **6**:381
Optic nerve head. *See* Optic disc
Optic nerve sheath decompression surgery, for nonarteritic anterior ischemic optic neuropathy, **5**:124
Optic nerve sheath fenestration, for idiopathic intracranial hypertension, **5**:119
Optic nerve sheath meningioma, **5**:130*i*, 145–148, 147*i*, 148*t*, **7**:77
  in children, **5**:148
  optic glioma differentiated from, **6**:406
Optic neuritis, **5**:298
  atypical, tests for, **5**:143
  in children, **6**:365–366, 365*i*, 366*i*
  contrast sensitivity affected by, **3**:115
  hallucinations and, **5**:190
  in multiple sclerosis, **5**:320–321
  neuroimaging in evaluation of, **5**:73
  nonarteritic anterior ischemic optic neuropathy differentiated from, **5**:124*t*
  postviral, **5**:141
  retrobulbar, **5**:141–144, 142*i*
    contrast sensitivity affected by, **3**:115
    treatment of, **5**:143–144
Optic neuropathy, **5**:111–157
  anterior
    ischemic, **5**:120–124, 121*t*, 347
      arteritic, **5**:120–122, 121*i*, 121*t*
      nonarteritic, **5**:121*t*, 122–124, 123*i*, 124*t*
    with optic disc edema, **5**:111–113, 115–129
    without optic disc edema, **5**:129–141
  compressive
    intraorbital/intracanalicular, **5**:145–151
    in thyroid-associated orbitopathy, **5**:330, 330*i*
    described, **10**:51

in giant cell arteritis, 1:190
in glaucoma, 10:3, 49–57, 50i, 52t, 53i, 54i
    theories of damage and, 10:50–51
in Graves ophthalmopathy, 5:145, 7:48, 53
hypertensive, 12:98–99, 100i
of increased intracranial pressure. *See* Papilledema
infiltrative, 5:156
Leber hereditary, 5:134–136, 135i, 6:364–365
    mitochondrial DNA mutations and, 2:218–220,
        219i, 5:134–135, 6:365
nutritional, 5:152, 153i
posterior, 5:141–156
    ischemic, 5:155
radiation-induced, 1:256
    MR imaging of, 5:65i
in sarcoidosis, 5:129, 130i, 333
thyroid-related, 5:145, 7:48, 53
toxic, 1:271, 5:152
traumatic, 5:153–155, 154i, 7:107
    direct, 5:153, 154i
    indirect, 2:102, 5:154
visual field patterns in, 5:111, 112i, 113t, 114i
Optic pits (optic holes), 2:127, 136, 175, 4:204, 5:140,
    6:363, 363i
Optic radiations, 2:107–108, 460, 460t, 5:28
Optic stalks, 2:136, 141i, 142i, 144–145
Optic sulcus/sulci, 2:127, 136, 140i
Optic tract, 2:104–105, 107i, 5:27–28, 28i, 6:45i, 46
    retrochiasmal lesions of, 5:164–165, 165i, 166i
Optic tract syndrome, 5:16, 164
Optic ventricle, 2:137
Optic vesicle, 2:127, 136, 142i, 8:6
    lens development and, 2:137, 145–146, 147i, 11:25,
        26i
Optic zone, of contact lens, 3:175
Optical axis, 3:29–30, 29i, 6:29–30, 11:5, 7i
Optical chamber depth, in IOL selection, 3:218
Optical coherence tomography (OCT), 3:322–323,
    324i, 5:69, 8:33, 12:24
    in central serous chorioretinopathy, 12:52
    in cystoid macular edema, 12:154
    in epiretinal membrane, 12:87, 324
    in idiopathic macular hole, 12:89, 91
    in optic nerve head evaluation, 10:56
    in posterior vitreous detachment, 12:280
    in retinal nerve fiber evaluation, 10:56
    in vitreomacular traction syndrome, 12:324
Optical conjugacy, pupil, in indirect ophthalmoscopy,
    3:272–275, 274i
Optical constants, of schematic eye, 3:106i
Optical cross, 3:95–98. *See also* Cylinder power
Optical degradation, for amblyopia, 6:73
Optical density, 3:14
Optical doubling, in pachymetry, 3:293
Optical feedback, in lasers, 3:19, 22, 22i
Optical focusing, in pachymetry, 3:293
Optical interfaces, 3:41–42
    light propagation at, 3:41–42, 42i, 43i
    reflection at, 3:13–14, 13i
Optical medium
    abnormalities of, 5:103–104
    clear, traumatic visual loss with, 7:106–108
    opaque. *See* Cataract; Opacities

refractive index of, 3:39–41, 40t. *See also* Refractive
    index
    definition of, 3:6
Optical path difference OPD-Scan, 8:49
Optical path length (OPL), 3:52–53, 53i
Optical performance, IOL, standards for, 3:225
Optical pocket, for endoscopic brow and forehead lift,
    7:239
Optical system
    afocal, 3:81–84, 83i
    approximation for analysis of, 3:55–56. *See also*
        specific type and First-order optics
    eye as, 3:105–123
    Gaussian reduction and, 3:80
    graphical image analysis and, 3:76–78, 77i, 77–78i,
        78i
Optical zone, 8:39
    in radial keratotomy, 13:59, 60
    outcome affected by, 13:61, 62
Opticin, in vitreous, 2:333, 337
Opticrom. *See* Cromolyn
Optics
    of contact lenses, 3:177–183
    cosmetic, for anophthalmic socket, 7:127
    geometrical, 3:25–104. *See also* Geometrical optics
    physical, 3:3–24, 24i. *See also* Physical optics
    quantum, definition of, 3:3
Optineurin, gene for, in glaucoma, 10:14
OptiPranolol. *See* Metipranolol
Optisol GS, for donor cornea preservation, 8:449
Optivar. *See* Azelastine
OPTN gene, in glaucoma, 10:13t, 14
Optociliary shunt vessels, in papilledema, 5:116–117
Optokinetic nystagmus, 5:167, 198, 6:161, 451
    assessment of, 5:201–202, 6:451
    in congenital motor nystagmus, 6:164
    dysfunction of, 5:205–206
    in functional visual disorder evaluation, 5:305
Optometer principle, 3:81
    in automated refraction, 3:312, 314i
    in manual lensmeter operation, 3:81
Optotypes, 3:112
    evaluation of visual acuity in children and, 6:4, 71,
        79
OPV (Sabin vaccine), 1:304t, 307
OR. *See* Odds ratio
Ora bays, 12:8
    enclosed, 12:8–9, 262
Ora serrata, 2:77, 88, 89i, 12:8
    muscle insertion relationships and, 2:16
Oral contraceptives
    central retinal vein occlusion and, 12:143
    hypercoagulability associated with, 1:171
    hypertension and, 1:96
    ocular effects of, 1:325t
    tetracycline use and, 2:433–434
Oral glucose tolerance test, 1:206, 207
Oral hypoglycemic agents, 1:211–214, 212t. *See also*
    specific type
    surgery in diabetic patient and, 1:220, 332
Oral medication, sustained-release preparations of,
    2:388
Oral ulcers
    in Behçet syndrome, 1:193
    in systemic lupus erythematosus, 1:179, 181t

Orbicularis oculi muscle, **2:**21, 23–24, 24*i*, 25*i*, 30*i*, **4:**168, **7:**139–140, 141*i*, 142*i*, 143*i*, **8:**6, 7*i*
  tear flow pumped by, **7:**256, 257*i*
  weakness of, in myasthenia gravis, **5:**326
Orbit
  amyloid deposits in, **4:**191, 192*i*
  anatomy of, **2:**5–12, **5:**9–10, 9*i*, **7:**7–22
    assessment of before refractive surgery, **13:**44
      PRK/LASEK, **13:**90
    bony, **5:**6–7*i*
    vascular
      arterial supply in, **5:**11–12*i*, 15
      venous drainage in, **5:**20, 21*i*
  anophthalmic socket and, **7:**119–129
  basal cell cancer involving, **7:**177–178
  bony, **2:**5, 6*i*, **4:**187–188
  cellulitis affecting. *See* Orbital cellulitis
  congenital disorders of
    anomalies, **4:**188, 188*i*, **7:**37–39, 38*i*, 39*i*
    tumors, **7:**63–64, 65*i*
  connective tissues of, **2:**20, 20*i*
  cysts of, **2:**165–167, 165*i*, 166*i*, **6:**381–382, 382*i*
    chocolate, **7:**68
    dermoid, **2:**178, **4:**188, 188*i*, **6:**381, 382*i*, **7:**63–64, 65*i*
    epidermoid, **6:**381, **7:**63
    epithelial, **4:**188
    with microphthalmos (colobomatous cyst), **6:**383, 383*i*, **7:**37–38
  degenerations of, **4:**191, 192*i*
  development of, **2:**156–158, **6:**200
  dimensions of, **6:**208, 208*i*, **7:**7, 7*t*
  disorders of, **4:**187–202, 201*i*. *See also specific type*
    compressive, **5:**128–129, 130*i*. *See also* Orbital decompression
    congenital, **6:**207–209, 209*i*
    evaluation of, **7:**23–36
    globe displacement and, **7:**23, 24
    imaging studies in
      primary, **7:**27–34, 28*i*
      secondary, **7:**34
    laboratory studies in, **7:**35–36
    neoplastic, **4:**192–202, 201*i*. *See also* Orbit, tumors of
    palpable masses and, **7:**24, 26–27
    pain and, **7:**23
    periorbital changes and, **7:**24, 25*t*
    proptosis and, **7:**23–24
    pulsation and, **7:**24, 26–27
    rate of progression of, **7:**24
    Th1 delayed hypersensitivity and, **9:**68*t*
  dysmorphic, **6:**207–209, 208*i*, 209*i*
  emphysema of, in blowout fractures, **7:**101–102, 104
  in external eye defense, **8:**114
  fascial system of, **6:**19–23, 19*i*
  fissures in, **2:**10–12, **7:**10*i*, 11, 21–22
  floor of, **2:**8, 9*i*, **7:**10, 10*i*
    fractures of, **2:**8, **7:**21, 102–106, 103*i*
      in children, **6:**138–140, 139*i*
      vertical deviations and, **6:**138–140, 139*i*
  foramina in, **2:**9–10, 11*i*, 12*i*
  foreign bodies in, **7:**106
  fossae of, **7:**21–22

  fractures of, **2:**8, **7:**21, 97–106, 99*i*, 101*i*, 103*i*
    in children, **6:**138–140, 139*i*, 449–450, 449*i*
      esodeviation and, **6:**98*t*
      vertical deviations and, **6:**138–140, 139*i*
    diplopia and, **5:**218–219
  hemorrhages in, **7:**72, 106
    after blepharoplasty, visual loss and, **7:**232–233
    from orbital lymphangioma, **7:**67–68
  infection/inflammation of, **4:**188–190, 189*i*, 190*i*, 191*i*, **7:**41–61
    in children, **6:**230–233, 232*i*, 233*i*, 384–385, 384*i*, 385*i*
    idiopathic. *See* Orbital inflammatory syndrome
  infiltrative lesions of, **5:**129, 130*i*
  lacrimal gland neoplasia and, **4:**192–193, 193*i*, 194*i*, **7:**89–92, 90*i*
  lateralization of (orbital hypertelorism), **6:**207, 424
  leukemic infiltration of, **4:**194–196, **6:**345, 375, **7:**94–95
  lipodermoids of, **7:**64, 65*i*
  lymphoproliferative lesions of, **4:**194–196, 195*i*, **7:**81–89, 83*i*, 86*t*
  margin of, **2:**5, 7*i*
  myositis affecting, **5:**219, **6:**385
    idiopathic orbital inflammation presenting as, **4:**190, 191*i*
  nerves of, **7:**14*i*, 15, 19*i*
  optic nerve in, **2:**93, 97, 97*t*, 101–102, 101*i*, **7:**12
    blood supply of, **2:**103, 104*i*
    length of, **7:**7*t*, 12
  paranasal sinuses and, **7:**7, 20–21, 21*i*
  periorbital structures and, **7:**12, 20–22, 21*i*
  retinoblastoma affecting, **4:**254–255, 255*i*
  roof of, **2:**5–6, 7*i*, **7:**8
    bony anatomy of, **5:**6*i*
    fractures of, **7:**100
      in children, **6:**449, 449*i*
  sensory nerves of, anatomy of, **5:**49–56, 53*i*
  septum of, **2:**24–26, 24*i*, 27*i*, **7:**6, 7, 140–141, 140*i*, 141*i*, **8:**7*i*, 8
    lacerations of, **7:**184–185
  soft tissues of, **4:**187–188, **7:**12–19
  surgery of, **7:**109–117. *See also specific procedure*
    for blowout fractures, **7:**105–106
      indications for, **7:**104–105
    complications of, **7:**117
    incisions for, **7:**109, 111*i*
    postoperative care and, **7:**116
    special techniques in, **7:**116–117
    surgical spaces and, **7:**12–13, 109, 110*i*
    for volume expansion in craniosynostosis, **6:**428, 430
  teratomas of, **2:**166, **7:**64
  tight, **7:**107
  topography of, **4:**187–188, **7:**7–10, 8*i*, 9*i*, 10*i*
  trauma to, **7:**97–108
    foreign bodies, **7:**106
    hemorrhages, **7:**72, 106
    midfacial (Le Fort) fractures, **7:**97, 98*i*
    orbital fractures, **2:**8, **7:**21, 97–106, 99*i*, 101*i*, 103*i*
    septal disruption and, **7:**12–13
    visual loss with clear media and, **7:**106–108
  tuberculosis affecting, **7:**47

tumors of, 4:192–202, 201*i*, 7:63–96. *See also specific type*
  adipose, 4:201
  benign, 6:376–385
  bony, 6:380
  in children, 6:369–385, 370–371*t*
    differential diagnosis of, 6:369–372
  congenital, 7:63–64, 65*i*
  connective tissue, 6:380
  ectopic tissue masses, 6:381–384
  enucleation for, 7:119–122
  exenteration for, 7:127–129, 128*i*
  with fibrous differentiation, 4:199–200, 199*i*
  inflammatory disorders simulating, 6:384–385
  lymphoproliferative, 4:194–196, 195*i*, 7:81–89, 83*i*, 86*t*
  malignant
    metastatic, 6:374–376
    primary, 6:372–374
  mesenchymal, 7:79–81, 79*i*, 82*i*
  metastatic, 4:202, 6:374–376, 7:94–96
    in adults, 7:95–96, 95*i*
    in children, 6:374–376, 7:94, 94*i*
    management of, 7:96
  MR imaging of, 5:64*i*
  with muscle differentiation, 4:198, 199*i*
  nerve sheath, 4:200, 201*i*
  neural, 7:72–79, 73*i*, 76*i*, 77–78*i*
    in children, 6:381
  pain caused by, 5:298–299
  palpable, 7:24, 26–27
  pathologic examination of, 7:35
  primary, 6:372–374
  secondary, 4:202, 5:219, 7:92–93, 92*i*
    eyelid carcinoma and, 7:177–178
  staging of, 4:293*t*
  vascular, 4:195–196, 197*i*, 7:64–69, 66*i*, 68*i*
    in children, 6:376–380, 377*i*, 378*i*, 379*i*
    masquerading conditions and, 7:69–70, 71*i*, 72*i*
vascular system of, 7:15, 16–18*i*
  anatomy of, 2:38–41, 39*i*, 40*i*, 41*i*
  development of, 2:155–156
volume of, 2:5, 7:7*t*
walls of
  apertures in, 7:8*i*, 9*i*, 10*i*, 11–12
  bony anatomy of, 5:7*i*
  lateral, 2:8–9, 10*i*, 7:8–9
  medial, 2:6, 8*i*, 7:9–10, 9*i*
    fracture of, 7:101–102, 101*i*
    length of, 7:7*t*
  wound healing/repair and, 4:24
Orbital apex fractures, 7:100
Orbital apex syndrome, 5:236
  in orbital cellulitis, 7:42
  in phycomycosis, 7:45–46
Orbital canal, 5:10
Orbital cellulitis, 7:20, 42–44, 43*i*, 44*t*, 45*i*
  in children, 6:231–233, 232*i*, 7:42
  fungal (mucormycosis), 6:233, 233*i*, 7:45–46
    exenteration in management of, 7:45–46, 128
  after strabismus surgery, 6:185–186, 186*i*
Orbital decompression, 7:115, 116*i*
  complications of, 7:117
  for lymphangioma, 7:69

for thyroid/Graves ophthalmopathy/orbitopathy, 5:331–332, 7:54, 115
  for traumatic visual loss, 7:107, 108
Orbital fat, 7:13, 141
  aging affecting, 7:236
  dermatochalasis and, 7:228
  eyelid lacerations and, 7:184–185
Orbital fissures, 2:10–12, 5:10, 7:10*i*, 11, 21–22
  inferior, 2:12, 5:8*i*, 10, 7:10*i*, 11, 21–22, 22
  superior, 2:10–12, 11*i*, 12*i*, 5:8*i*, 7:11, 21
    cranial nerve VI in, 5:43, 45–49*i*
    lesions of, 5:236
Orbital hypertelorism, 6:207, 424
Orbital implants, 7:121–122
  in children, 7:121
  exposure and extrusion of, 7:125, 125*i*
  for superior sulcus deformity, 7:124
Orbital inflammatory syndrome (idiopathic orbital inflammation/orbital pseudotumor), 4:190, 191*i*, 5:298, 7:56–59, 57*i*
  in children, 6:384, 385*i*
  orbital lymphoma differentiated from, 4:195–196
  plasma cell–rich, 7:88
  in Wegener granulomatosis, 1:192
Orbital lacrimal gland, 2:31, 34*i*, 289
Orbital muscle, 5:56
Orbital orbicularis muscles, 7:140, 140*i*, 143*i*
Orbital pseudotumor. *See* Orbital inflammatory syndrome
Orbital rim, anatomy of, 5:10
Orbital varices, 6:379, 7:70–71, 72*i*
  glaucoma associated with, 10:32
Orbital vein, 6:16
  eyelids drained by, 7:147
  thrombophlebitis of, 7:61
Orbitectomy, for lacrimal gland tumors, 7:91
Orbitis, sclerosing. *See* Orbital inflammatory syndrome
Orbitomeatal line, definition of, 5:80
Orbitopathy, thyroid/thyroid-related immune/Graves. *See* Thyroid ophthalmopathy
Orbitotomy
  anterior, 7:109–114
    inferior approach for, 7:110–111, 112*i*, 113*i*
    medial approach for, 7:111–114
    superior approach for, 7:109
  for cavernous hemangioma, 7:67
  lateral, 7:114–115
  in orbital evaluation, 7:35
ORC. *See* Origin replication/recognition complex
ORF. *See* Open reading frame
Orf virus, ocular infection caused by, 8:121
Organ culture storage techniques, for donor cornea, 8:449
Organ transplantation. *See also* Transplantation
  for enzyme deficiency disease, 2:281
Organic mental syndromes. *See* Mental disorders due to general medical condition
Organogenesis
  definition of, 2:127
  in eye, 2:136–158, 139*t*. *See also specific structure*
Orientation and mobility specialist, in vision rehabilitation, 3:264–265
Origin of replication, 2:192, 212
Origin replication/recognition complex, 2:192
Orinase. *See* Tolbutamide

Ornithine, elevated serum levels of, in gyrate atrophy, 12:225
Ornithine aminotransferase (OAT) mutation/defect, 2:351
  in gyrate atrophy, 2:351, 12:225
Orthokeratology, 3:203–205, 13:84–85
Orthomyxoviruses, ocular infection caused by, 8:122
Orthophoria, 6:9
Orthoptics
  fusional vergences and, 6:89
  for intermittent exotropia, 6:113
  for suppression, 6:55
  for undercorrection of intermittent exotropia, 6:114
Orthostatic hypertension, 1:96
Orudis. See Ketoprofen
Oruvail. See Ketoprofen
Oscillations
  disconjugate/disjunctive, 5:240
  macrosaccadic, 5:204, 252–253, 252i
Oscillatory potentials, in electroretinogram, 12:27, 28i, 29
  vascular disease and, 12:35
Oscillopsia, 5:239
Oseltamivir, 1:65t, 77, 291, 305
Osler-Weber-Rendu disease (hereditary hemorrhagic telangiectasia), 1:166, 8:91
Osmitrol. See Mannitol
Osmoglyn. See Glycerin
Osmolarity, tear film, 8:63
Osmotic agents, 2:415–416, 415t
Osmotic hypothesis, of "sugar" cataract formation, 2:331
Osseous choristoma, 8:277
Ossifying fibroma, of orbit, 4:200, 6:380
Osteoblasts, 1:241
Osteoclasts, 1:241
Osteocutaneous ligaments, 7:135
Osteocytes, 1:241
Osteodystrophy, Albright hereditary, 8:351t
Osteogenesis imperfecta, 8:288, 352t
  bleeding disorders in, 1:166
  blue sclera in, 8:288
Osteoid, 1:241
Osteoma
  choroidal, 4:164–165, 6:390
    melanoma differentiated from, 4:230–233, 233i
  of orbit, 7:81
  secondary, 7:93
Osteomyelitis, maxillary, 6:233
Osteopenia, definition of, 1:243
Osteoporosis, 1:240–247
  bone density levels in, 1:242–243
  bone physiology and, 1:241
  clinical features of, 1:242
  corticosteroid use and, 1:195
  definition of, 1:243
  diagnosis of, 1:242–244, 243t
  in men, 1:246–247
  risk factors for, 1:241, 242t
  testing for, 1:243–244
  treatment of, 1:244–246, 245t
Osteosarcoma
  of orbit, 6:274, 7:81
  retinoblastoma associated with, 4:265t
Ota, nevus of. See Nevus, of Ota

Otitic hydrocephalus, 5:358
Ototoxicity
  of aminoglycosides, 1:70
  mitochondrial DNA mutations and, 2:220
Outcome/outcome measures, 1:362
  baseline probability of, 1:361
  in clinical research, 1:342
    case series and, 1:346–347
Outer eye. See External (outer) eye
Outer ischemic retinal atrophy, 4:128, 129i
Outer neuroblastic layer, 2:140
Outer nuclear layer, 2:80–81i, 82i
Outer plexiform layer, 2:80–81i, 82i, 84
Outer segments. See Cone outer segments;
  Photoreceptor outer segments; Rod outer segments
Outpatient visits, geriatric patient and, 1:236
Overactivity disorders, of cranial nerve VII, 5:286–290, 287t
Overdepression in adduction, 6:129
Overelevation in adduction, 6:128
Overlap syndromes (mixed connective tissue disease), 1:185
Overrefraction, 3:142–143, 314
  acuity testing in corneal abnormalities and, 8:15
  in aphakia, 3:164–165
  with automated refractors, 3:314
Overwear syndromes (contact lens), metabolic epithelial damage in, 8:106–107
Ovoid bodies, in neurofibromatosis, 6:407
Oxacarbazepine, 1:283t
Oxacillin, 1:67, 2:429
Oxaprozin, 1:197t
Oxazolidinones, 1:63t, 74–75
Oxidoreductases, taxon-specific crystallins as, 2:327
Oxitropium, 1:157–158, 157t
Oxivent. See Oxitropium
Oxycephaly, 6:421
Oxychloro complex, as ocular medication preservative, 2:381
Oxygen
  in aqueous humor, 2:322
  corneal supply of, contact lenses and, 3:185
  reduction of myocardial requirements for
    for acute coronary syndrome, 1:122
    for angina, 1:121
Oxygen radicals. See Free radicals
Oxygen-regulated protein, mutations in, 2:350
Oxygen tension
  in lens
    energy production and, 2:330
    free radical reactions and, 11:16–17
  in retina, free radical reactions and, 2:370
Oxygen therapy
  for anaphylaxis, 1:319
  hyperbaric, for nonarteritic anterior ischemic optic neuropathy, 5:124
  for malignant hyperthermia, 6:192, 193t
  for pulmonary diseases, 1:156
  retinopathy of prematurity and, 6:326, 12:126, 132
  for shock, 1:318
Oxygen transmissibility, 3:185
  of rigid contact lenses, 3:185
Oxymetazoline, 2:451
Oxyradicals, 2:366. See also Free radicals

Oxytetracycline, **2**:433–434
  with polymyxin B, **2**:431*t*

P

p7 nucleocapsid zinc finger inhibitors, for HIV
  infection/AIDS, **1**:42
p21, in carcinogenesis, **1**:253
p24 antigen testing, in HIV infection/AIDS, **1**:39, **9**:246
p53 gene
  in carcinogenesis, **1**:253
  in DNA repair, **2**:213
  in pterygium, **8**:366
p arm, **2**:192, 205
P cells (parvocellular neurons/system), **5**:24, **6**:44,
    45–46, 47*i*, **10**:44, 46
  development of, **6**:46
    abnormal visual experience affecting, **6**:49
P gene, defects of in albinism, **2**:243, **6**:345
P-selectin, in neutrophil rolling, **9**:48, 49*i*
P value, **1**:344
PA. *See* Polyacrylamide
Pacchionian granulations, **5**:20
Pacemakers
  for heart failure, **1**:132
  laser surgery in patient with, **13**:41
Pacerone. *See* Amiodarone
PACG. *See* Angle-closure glaucoma, primary
Pachymetry (pachymeter), **3**:293–294, 293*i*, **8**:31–34,
    33*i*
  before cataract surgery, **11**:87
  in Fuchs endothelial dystrophy, **8**:325
  infection control and, **8**:50
  for intrastromal corneal ring segment placement,
    13:80
  before LASIK, **13**:111
  before phakic intraocular lens insertion, **13**:146
  before refractive surgery, **13**:47–48
Pachyonychia congenita, **8**:309*t*
Paclitaxel, **1**:257, 259*i*
PACs. *See* Premature atrial complexes
Paecilomyces, ocular infection caused by, **8**:130
PAF. *See* Platelet-activating factors
Paget disease of bone, angioid streaks in, **12**:83
Pagetoid spread
  in primary acquired melanosis, **4**:57
  of sebaceous carcinoma, **4**:180, 181*i*
PAHX gene, Refsum disease caused by mutations in,
    2:351
Pain. *See also specific type*
  facial, **5**:299–301
    atypical, **5**:299
  icepick, idiopathic stabbing headache and, **5**:297
  ocular causes of, **5**:298, 298–299
  orbital, **7**:23
    in blowout fractures, **7**:102
    in idiopathic orbital inflammation, **7**:56–57
  orbital causes of, **5**:298–299
  periorbital, **5**:298
    in optic neuritis, **5**:141
  postoperative, management of, **1**:338
    after PRK/LASEK, **13**:96–97
  in recurrent corneal erosion, **5**:298, **8**:98
  somatoform, **1**:266

in traumatic hyphema, **8**:401
in uveitis, **9**:102, 102*t*, 127
  with visual loss, **5**:83–84
"Painless" (subacute lymphocytic) thyroiditis, **1**:226
Palatine bone, **5**:10, **7**:7, 8*i*, 10*i*
Paleocerebellum, **5**:39
Palinopsia, **5**:191
  hallucinatory, **5**:190–191
Palisades of Vogt, **8**:8
Pallidotomy, for Parkinson disease, **1**:280
Palmitate/palmitic acid
  in retinal pigment epithelium, **2**:358
  in vitreous, **2**:337
Palpation, orbital, **7**:24, 26–27
Palpebral artery, **2**:39*i*
Palpebral conjunctiva, **2**:29, 30*i*, 32*i*, 36, **4**:43, 168, **8**:8.
    See also Conjunctiva
Palpebral fissures, **2**:21, 22*i*, 23*i*
  in infants and children, **6**:200
    congenital widening of (euryblepharon), **6**:211,
      7:154, 155*i*
    slanting of, **6**:212–213
      A- and V-pattern deviations and, **6**:119, 122*i*
    surgery affecting, **6**:23, 25*i*
    vertical height of, in ptosis, **7**:209, 210*i*
Palpebral lacrimal gland, **2**:31, 33*i*, 34*i*, 289
Palpebral muscle, **5**:56
Palpebral vernal conjunctivitis/keratoconjunctivitis,
    6:234, 235*i*, **8**:209, 209*i*
Palsy. *See specific type or structure affected and* Paralysis
PAM. *See* Potential acuity meter; Primary acquired
  melanosis
2-PAM. *See* Pralidoxime
PAN. *See* Periodic alternating nystagmus; Polyarteritis
  nodosa
Pancoast syndrome, **5**:263
Pancreas
  beta (β) cells in, in diabetes mellitus, **1**:202
    genetic defects and, **1**:204*t*
  cancer of, **1**:297
  exocrine, disorders of in diabetes mellitus, **1**:204*t*
  transplantation of, for diabetes, **1**:214
Pancreatitis, Purtscher-like retinopathy and, **12**:94
Pancuronium, **2**:402*i*, 403
Panel D-15 (Farnsworth) test, **3**:254, **12**:44, 45*i*
Panel tests, of color vision, **12**:43–44, 45*i*
Panencephalitis, subacute sclerosing, **8**:162–163
  posterior uveitis caused by, **9**:159–160
Panfundoscope contact lens, **3**:288, 289*i*
Panic disorder, **1**:267
Panipenem, **1**:69
Pannus/micropannus, **4**:68, 69*i*, **8**:29, 32*i*
  contact lens wear causing, **8**:108
  subepithelial fibrovascular, **4**:68
  in trachoma, **8**:175, 176*i*
Panophthalmitis, tuberculous, **12**:184
Panretinal photocoagulation. *See also*
  Photocoagulation; Scatter laser treatment
    for branch retinal vein occlusion, **12**:140, 140*i*
    for central retinal artery occlusion, **12**:150
    for central retinal vein occlusion, **12**:144–145
    for diabetic retinopathy, **12**:107–111, 108*i*, 110*i*
    lenses for, **12**:318*t*
    for ocular ischemic syndrome, **12**:151
Panum's area of single binocular vision, **6**:42*i*, 43, 52

Panuveitis, **9:**107, 187–204. *See also specific cause and Uveitis*
  in Behçet syndrome, **9:**132–133
  causes of, **9:**112*t*
    immunologic and granulomatous diseases, **9:**197–206
    infectious diseases, **9:**187–197
  in children, **6:**311
  differential diagnosis of, **9:**109*t*
  multifocal choroiditis and (MCP), **9:**177*t*, 185, 185*i*, **12:**178
  sarcoid, **12:**180, 180*i*
  signs of, **9:**106
  subretinal fibrosis and uveitis syndrome (SFU), **9:**177*t*, 184, 184*i*, 185*i*
  sympathetic ophthalmia and, **4:**152–153, 153*i*, 154*i*, **9:**67–68, 200–203, 200*i*, 201*i*, 202*t*
  in Vogt-Koyanagi-Harada syndrome, **9:**203–205, 204*i*, 205*i*, 206*i*, **12:**181
Papanicolaou test (Pap smear), for cancer screening, **1:**294, 295*t*
  in HIV infection/AIDS, **1:**41
Papillae
  Bergmeister, **2:**91, 175, **4:**107, **6:**361, **12:**280
  conjunctival, **8:**23–26, 24*t*, 25*t*, 26*i*, 27*i*
    in atopic keratoconjunctivitis, **8:**212, 212*i*
    in floppy eyelid syndrome, **8:**95, 96*i*
    in giant papillary (contact lens–induced) conjunctivitis, **8:**215, 215*i*
    in palpebral vernal keratoconjunctivitis, **8:**209, 209*i*
  dermal (dermal ridges), **8:**245, 246*i*
  limbal, **4:**45–46
Papillary carcinoma, of thyroid gland, **1:**227
Papillary conjunctivitis, **4:**45–46, 47*i*, **8:**23–26, 24*t*, 25*t*, 26*i*, 27*i*
  giant (contact lens–induced), **3:**210, **4:**45, **8:**214–216, 215*i*
  in reactive arthritis/Reiter syndrome, **8:**228
Papilledema. *See also* Optic disc (optic nerve head), edema of
  acute, **5:**112–113, 115–116, 115*i*, 116*i*
  in children, **6:**366
  chronic, **5:**116–117, 116*i*, 117*i*
  in craniosynostosis, **6:**429
  in cryptococcal meningitis, **5:**368
  drusen differentiated from, **5:**130–132, 132*i*, 133*i*
  in leukemia, **6:**344
  pseudopapilledema and, **5:**113, 115, **6:**367–368, 367*t*
  pseudotumor cerebri and, **6:**365–366
  transient visual loss and, **5:**174–175
Papillitis, **5:**125–126, 126*i*
Papillomacular bundle, **5:**25, 25*i*
Papillomacular fibers, **5:**111, 114*i*
Papillomas, **8:**162, 246
  conjunctival, **4:**51, 52*i*, **8:**162, 255–256, 255*t*, 256*i*
  eyelid, **4:**170–171, **7:**163–164, 164*i*
    in children, **6:**385
  lacrimal sac, squamous cell, **7:**284
Papillomatosis, definition of, **4:**169
Papillomaviruses. *See* Human papillomaviruses
Papillopathy, diabetic, **5:**127, 127*i*
Papillophlebitis, **4:**133–134, **5:**128, 128*i*
  in central retinal vein occlusion, **12:**141
Papovaviruses, ocular infection caused by, **8:**121

Papule, of eyelid, **8:**24*t*
Paracallosal branch, of cerebral artery, **5:**16
Paracentesis, in cataract surgery, **11:**122–123
Paracentral scotoma, **10:**60, 61
  in age-related macular degeneration, **12:**63
Paracentral zone, **8:**38, 39*i*
Paracrine actions, of cytokines, **9:**80
Paradoxical diplopia, **6:**56, 56*i*
Paradoxical pupillary phenomena, **5:**270, **6:**162, 163*t*, 452
Paraflocculus, **5:**39
Parafollicular (C) cells, **1:**221
Parafovea/parafoveal zone, **2:**87, **4:**119, **12:**8, 8*i*, 9*t*
Parafoveal/juxtafoveal retinal telangiectasis, **4:**121–122, **12:**157–158, 158*i*, 159*i*
Parakeratosis, definition of, **4:**168, **8:**247*t*
Parallel prisms, for nystagmus in low-vision patient, **3:**260
Paralysis (paresis/paretic syndromes). *See also specific type or structure affected*
  diplopia caused by, **5:**221, 222*i*
    restrictive syndromes differentiated from, **5:**217, 218*i*
Paralysis accommodation, for refraction in infants and children, **3:**146
Paralytic ectropion, **7:**196*i*, 199–200, 200*i*
Paralytic strabismus, Hering's law and, **6:**36
Paramedian pontine reticular formation, **2:**116, 116*i*, **5:**34, 202
Paramyxoviruses, ocular infection caused by, **8:**122
Paranasal sinuses, **2:**12, 13*i*, **5:**9, 9*i*, **7:**7, 20–21, 21*i*
  Aspergillus causing infection of, **7:**46–47
  orbital cellulitis caused by infections of, **6:**231, 232*i*, **7:**42, 44*t*
  orbital tumors originating in, **7:**92–93, 93*i*
  preseptal cellulitis caused by infection of, **6:**230, **7:**41–42
  tuberculous infection of, orbital involvement and, **7:**47
Paraneoplastic disorders
  bilateral diffuse uveal melanocytic proliferation, **12:**165–166, 165*i*
  retinopathies, **5:**101, 108–109, **12:**237–239, 238*i*
Paranoia, in elderly, **1:**239–240
Paraprotein, corneal deposition of, **8:**349–350
Parasellar region, **5:**5
  chiasm affected in lesions of, **5:**160–163, 162*i*
  tumors of
    drugs for, **5:**163
    meningioma, **5:**162
Parasites
  ocular infection caused by, **8:**119*t*, 131–134. *See also specific organism or type of infection*
    eyelid margin involvement and, **8:**168–169
  orbital infection caused by, **4:**189, **7:**47
Parasol retinal ganglion cells, **6:**44–45
Parastriate cortex (Brodmann area 18), **5:**29, 31. *See also* Visual (calcarine/occipital) cortex
Parasympathetic ganglia/nerves/pathway, **5:**57, 59–60, 59*i*, 60*i*
  cholinergic drug action and, **2:**394, 395*i*
  in ciliary ganglion, **2:**14, 14*i*
  cranial nerve III and, **2:**110
  cranial nerve VII and, **2:**118–119
  orbit supplied by, **7:**15

in tear secretion, 2:292–293, 292*i*, 293*i*
Parasympatholytic agents, accommodation affected by, 11:22
Parasympathomimetic agents
   accommodation affected by, 11:22
   for glaucoma, 10:161–162*t*, 166–168
Paravertebral sympathetic plexus, 5:56
Paraxial rays, approximation of, 3:56–58, 57*i*, 58*i*, 59
Paraxial raytracing
   through concave spherical lenses, 3:74, 74*i*, 75*i*
   through convex spherical lenses, 3:71–72, 71*i*, 72*i*
Paredrine. *See* Hydroxyamphetamine
Paremyd. *See* Hydroxyamphetamine
Parental age, chromosomal aberrations and, in Down syndrome, 2:250
Paresis. *See specific type and* Paralysis
Pareto chart, 1:368, 370*i*
Parietal bone, 5:9
Parietal lobe lesions
   hallucinations and, 5:190
   retrochiasmal, 5:166–167
Parieto-occipital artery, 5:20, 20*i*
Parinaud oculoglandular syndrome, 4:49, 8:178–179, 12:184–185. *See also* Cat-scratch disease
   in children, 6:229, 230*i*
Parinaud (dorsal midbrain) syndrome, 5:208–209, 210*i*
   eyelid retraction in, 5:279, 7:224
   nystagmus in, 6:167
PARK. *See* Photoastigmatic keratectomy
Parkinson disease/parkinsonism, 1:278–280
   medications for, tear production affected by, 8:81*t*
   postencephalitis, oculogyric crisis in, 5:212
   recent developments in, 1:263
   saccadic disorders in, 5:206
Parks-Bielschowsky 3-step test, for fourth nerve palsy, 5:232–233
Parlodel. *See* Bromocriptine
Parotidomasseteric fascia, 7:137
Paroxysmal atrial tachycardia, 1:136–137
Paroxysmal nocturnal hemoglobinuria, 1:162
   hypercoagulability and, 1:171
   screening test for, 1:159, 162
Parry-Romberg syndrome, 8:353*t*
Pars plana, 2:66, 4:150
   cryoablation of, for pars planitis, 9:150
   in uveitis, 9:103*t*
Pars plana lensectomy, 11:138–139
   juvenile rheumatoid arthritis–associated uveitis and, 9:235
Pars plana magnet extraction, of foreign body, 12:298
Pars plana vitrectomy, 12:323, 324*i*. *See also* Vitrectomy
   for *Aspergillus* endophthalmitis, 12:189, 189*i*
   for branch retinal vein occlusion, 12:140–141
   for capsular rupture during phacoemulsification, 11:179
   cataract surgery after, 11:224
   for choroidal neovascularization, 12:327, 328*i*
   complications of, 12:342, 342*t*
   for cystoid macular edema, postoperative, 12:154, 332, 333*i*
   in diabetic patients, 12:111–112, 112*t*, 116–117
      macular edema and, 12:116
      for tractional retinal detachments, 12:341
   for endophthalmitis, 9:217, 219, 226
      acute-onset, 12:329, 330

      bleb-associated, 12:331, 332*i*
      chronic (delayed-onset), 12:329–331, 331*i*
      postoperative, 11:177
   endophthalmitis after, 9:207
   for epiretinal membranes, 12:88, 323–324, 325*i*
   for foreign-body removal, 12:298
   for idiopathic macular hole, 12:325–326, 327*i*
   for intraocular lymphoma diagnosis, 4:278
   for macular diseases, 12:323–327
   for pars planitis, 9:150, 12:182
   for retained lens fragments after phacoemulsification, 11:183, 12:338–339, 338*t*, 339*i*
   for retinal detachment, 12:272, 340, 341
      in cytomegalovirus retinitis, 9:253
   for specimen collection, 9:216
   for submacular hemorrhage, 12:326, 328*i*
   for uveal lymphoid infiltration diagnosis, 4:280
   for vitritis, 9:121
Pars planitis, 9:147–152, 148*i*, 12:182. *See also* Intermediate uveitis
   in children, 6:311, 312*t*, 316–317, 317*i*
      diagnosis of, 6:321*t*
   clinical characteristics of, 9:147–148, 148*i*
   complications of, 9:151–152
   cystoid macular edema and, 12:154
   diagnosis/differential diagnosis of, 6:312*t*, 321*t*, 9:148–149
   prognosis of, 9:149
   treatment of, 9:149–150
Pars plicata, 2:66, 4:150
Pars reticulata, 5:54
Partial (bridge) conjunctival flap, 8:437
Partial polarization, 3:10
   metallic reflection and, 3:14
Partial seizures, 1:281, 320
Partial thromboplastin time (PTT), 1:165
Partially accommodative esotropia, 6:98*t*, 104
Particle characteristics of light, 3:3, 6*i*, 7
Particle-wave duality, 3:7
Partition coefficient, drug lipid solubility and, 2:384
Parvocellular neurons (P cells/system), 5:24, 6:44, 45–46, 47*i*, 10:44, 46
   development of, 6:46
      abnormal visual experience affecting, 6:49
PAS. *See* Periodic acid–Schiff stain
Passive immunization, 1:303
PAT. *See* Paroxysmal atrial tachycardia
Patanol. *See* Olopatadine
Patching
   for amblyopia, 6:72
      after cataract surgery, 6:302
      compliance issues and, 6:74
      complications of, 6:73
   for corneal abrasion, 8:407
      in children, 6:445
   for dissociated vertical deviation, 6:131
   for esotropia in sixth nerve palsy, 6:107
   for intermittent exotropia, 6:113
   occlusion amblyopia caused by, 6:70
   orbital surgery and, 7:116
   for overcorrection of intermittent exotropia, 6:113
   for perforating injury, 8:410
   for undercorrection of intermittent exotropia, 6:114
Path, optical, length of, 3:52–53, 53*i*

Pathergy, in Behçet syndrome, 1:193
Pathologic myopia. *See* High (pathologic/degenerative) myopia
Pathology, ophthalmic. *See* Ophthalmic pathology
Patient database, monitoring systems and, 1:364–365
Patient selection
  for clear lens extraction/refractive lens exchange, 13:156–158
  for conductive keratoplasty, 13:140–141
  for intrastromal corneal ring segments, 13:78–79
  for LASIK, 13:110–112
  for monovision, 13:172
  for multifocal IOLs, 13:163–164
  for phakic intraocular lenses, 13:144–147
  for PRK/LASEK, 13:90–91
  for radial keratotomy, 13:61
Pattern dystrophies, 12:222–223, 222*i*
  age-related macular degeneration differentiated from, 12:59, 67
Pattern electroretinogram, 5:101–102, 12:33, 33*i*
Pauciarticular (oligoarticular) onset juvenile idiopathic arthritis, 1:178, 6:313–314, 313*t*
  eye examination schedule for children with, 6:316*t*
  uveitis in, 6:313–314, 313*t*
Paving-stone (cobblestone) degeneration, 4:128, 129*i*, 12:263, 264*i*
PAX genes, 2:130, 159, 181, 188. *See also specific type*
  in aniridia, 2:255, 6:261–262, 277
  in posterior embryotoxon, 4:78
PAX2 gene, 2:159
  mutation in, 2:206
PAX3 gene, mutation in, 2:206, 265
PAX6 gene, 2:131, 159, 8:308
  in aniridia, 2:254, 255, 265, 6:261–262, 271, 277
  mutation in, 2:206
  in Peters anomaly, 8:294
  in posterior embryotoxon, 4:78
PCA. *See* Posterior cerebral artery
PCD. *See* Programmed cell death
PCI. *See* Percutaneous coronary intervention
PCNSL. *See* Primary central nervous system lymphomas
PCO. *See* Posterior capsular opacification
Pcom. *See* Posterior communicating artery
PCP. *See Pneumocystis carinii (Pneumocystis jiroveci)* infections, pneumonia
PCPIOL (posterior chamber phakic intraocular lenses). *See* Phakic intraocular lenses, posterior chamber
PCR. *See* Polymerase chain reaction
PCV (pneumococcal vaccine), 1:291, 304*t*, 308
PDGF. *See* Platelet-derived growth factors
PDP. *See* Product Development Protocol
PDR. *See* Diabetic retinopathy, proliferative
PDT. *See* Photodynamic therapy
Pearl cyst, of iris, 4:219*t*
Pearson marrow-pancreas syndrome, mitochondrial DNA deletions and, 2:218
Peau d'orange, in pseudoxanthoma elasticum, 12:83, 83*i*, 237
Pediatric cataract. *See* Cataract
Pediatric electroretinogram, 12:35, 35*i*
Pediatric glaucoma. *See* Glaucoma
Pedicle, of cone, 2:80, 83*i*
Pedicle flap, for canthal repair, 7:192

Pediculosis (lice), ocular infection caused by, 8:133, 169
  cholinesterase inhibitors for, 2:400
Pedigree analysis, 2:275–276, 275*i*, 8:308
PEG-400, in demulcents, 2:450
Pegaptanib, for age-related macular degeneration, 12:71–72, 76–78
Peginterferon alfa-2a/peginterferon alfa-2b. *See also* Interferons
  for hepatitis C, 1:31
Pelizaeus-Merzbacher disease, retinal degeneration and, 12:233*t*
Pelli-Robson chart, 3:114, 252, 5:97
Pellucid marginal degeneration, 8:332–333, 333*i*, 334*i*, 334*t*, 13:11–12, 47, 48*i*
  refractive surgery contraindicated in, 8:46–47, 47*i*
Pelopsia, 5:189
Pelvic examination, for cancer screening, 1:295*t*
Pemirolast, 2:424, 424*t*
Pemphigoid
  cataract surgery in patients with, 11:207
  cicatricial, 8:200, 217*t*, 219–223, 221*i*, 222*i*
    drug-induced (pseudopemphigoid), 8:219–220, 394, 395
    mucous membrane grafting for, 8:439
Pemphigus, vulgaris, 8:220
Pen-Vee K. *See* Penicillin V
Penalization
  for amblyopia, 6:73
  for dissociated vertical deviation, 6:131
Penbutolol, 1:88*t*
Penciclovir, 2:442
  for herpes simplex virus infections, 8:142*t*
Pencil, of light, 3:26, 41–42, 43*i*
Pendular nystagmus, 5:239, 240*i*, 6:159
  acquired, 5:250–251
Penetrance/penetrant gene, 2:192, 258, 8:307
  familial, 2:264–265
  incomplete (skipped generation), 2:266
Penetrating injuries, 12:295–296. *See also* Trauma
  canthal soft tissue, 7:184–186
  in children, 6:446–447, 446*i*
  definition of, 8:407
  endophthalmitis after, 9:212, 12:300
  eyelid, 7:184–186, 185*i*. *See also* Lacerations, eyelid
  lens damage caused by, 11:55, 57*i*, 58*i*
    glaucoma and, 10:109–114, 110–113*i*, 11:67–68
  retinal breaks caused by, 12:254
  tractional retinal detachment and, 12:273–274
Penetrating keratoplasty. *See* Keratoplasty, penetrating
Penetrex. *See* Enoxacin
Penicillamine, for Wilson disease, 2:281, 8:356
Penicillin G, 1:55*t*, 67, 2:428*t*, 429
Penicillin-resistant *N gonorrhoeae*, 8:172
Penicillin V (phenoxymethyl penicillin), 1:55*t*, 67, 2:429
Penicillinase, 2:427, 429
Penicillinase-resistant penicillins, 1:67, 2:429
Penicillins, 1:54, 55–57*t*, 67–68, 2:427–428, 427*i*, 428*t*, 429. *See also specific agent*
  allergic reaction to, 1:67–68, 2:428
  broad-spectrum, 2:429
  for Lyme disease, 5:364
  penicillinase-resistant, 1:67, 2:429
  semisynthetic, 1:55–57*t*
  structure of, 2:427, 427*i*

for syphilis, **1**:17–18, 18*t*, **9**:190
  in infants and children, **6**:221
Pentagonal resection, for trichiasis, **7**:208
Pentam 300. *See* Pentamidine
Pentamidine, **1**:63*t*
  for *Pneumocystis carinii (Pneumocystis jiroveci)*
    choroiditis, **9**:257
  for *Pneumocystis carinii (Pneumocystis jiroveci)*
    pneumonia, **1**:45
Pentavac. *See* DTacP-IPV-Hib vaccine
Pentolair. *See* Cyclopentolate
Pentose phosphate pathway (hexose monophosphate
    shunt)
  in corneal glucose metabolism, **2**:297–299, 298*i*
  in lens glucose/carbohydrate metabolism, **2**:330,
    11:14, 15*i*
Penumbra, **1**:102
Pen-Vee K. *See* Penicillin V
Peptide fusion inhibitors, for HIV infection/AIDS, **1**:42
Peptide hormones
  in aqueous humor, **2**:317, 320
  in tear secretion, **2**:293–294
Peptidoglycan, in bacterial cell wall, **8**:123
Perceptual distortion. *See* Metamorphopsia
Percheron artery, **5**:18
Percutaneous coronary intervention (PCI), **1**:111, 115
Percutaneous transluminal coronary angioplasty
    (PTCA/balloon angioplasty)
  for angina, **1**:121
  for ST-segment elevation acute coronary syndrome,
    1:125
  troponin levels in determining need for, **1**:117
Perennial allergic conjunctivitis, **6**:234, **8**:207–209
Perfluoropropane (C₃F₈)
  for submacular hemorrhage, **12**:326
  for tamponade in retinal detachment, **12**:340, 341
Perforating injuries. *See also* Trauma
  anterior segment, **8**:407–418
    ancillary tests in, **8**:409*t*
    evaluation of, **8**:407–408, 408*t*, 409*t*
    examination in, **8**:408, 409*t*
    history in, **8**:407–408, 408*t*
    management of, **8**:409–418, 441–442
      nonsurgical, **8**:410, 441–442
      postoperative, **8**:416–417
      preoperative, **8**:409–410
      surgical, **8**:410–416, 411*i*, 412*t*, 413*i*, 414*i*, 415*i*,
        417*i*, 418*i*
    ocular signs of, **8**:409*t*
    penetrating injury differentiated from, **8**:407
    wound healing/repair and, **8**:385
  definition of, **8**:407
  lens damage caused by, **11**:55, 57*i*, 58*i*
  posterior segment, **12**:296
    retinal breaks caused by, **12**:254
Perforin, **9**:68, 69*i*
Perfusion-weighted magnetic resonance imaging, in
    cerebral ischemia/stroke, **1**:104
PERG. *See* Pattern electroretinogram
Pergolide, for Parkinson disease, **1**:279
Periarteritis nodosa, infantile (Kawasaki syndrome/
    mucocutaneous lymph node syndrome), **1**:189*t*,
    6:238

Peribulbar anesthesia
  for cataract surgery, **11**:94, 96*i*
    anticoagulation therapy and, **11**:201, 202
  for phakic IOL insertion, **13**:147
Pericallosal branch, of cerebral artery, **5**:16
Pericanalicular connective tissue, **2**:57, 58*i*
Pericarditis, after myocardial infarction, **1**:115
Pericytes, retinal blood vessel, **2**:84, 354
Perifovea/perifoveal zone, **2**:87, **4**:119, **12**:8, 8*i*, 9*t*
Perifoveal vitreous detachment, posterior, **12**:280
Perimacular folds, in shaking injury, **6**:443–444
Perimetry, **5**:90–96
  Armaly-Drance screening, **10**:78, 79*i*
  automated
    achromatic, **10**:57
    in functional visual disorder evaluation, **5**:310,
      311*i*
    short-wavelength, **10**:58
    standard, in glaucoma, **10**:57
    static, **5**:92–93, 93*i*, 94*i*, 95*i*, 96, **10**:59, 65–68, 66*i*,
      68*i*
      artifacts seen on, **10**:70–71, 72*i*, 73*i*
      in glaucoma, **10**:57
      learning effect and, **10**:74, 75*i*
      screening tests, **10**:67
      testing strategy in, categories of, **10**:65–67
  in choroidal/ciliary body melanoma, **4**:226
  definitions of terms used in, **10**:59–60
  described, **10**:57
  frequency-doubling technology, **10**:58–59
  full-threshold, **10**:66–67
  in glaucoma, purposes of, **10**:57
  Goldmann, **5**:91–92, 93*i*
    in functional visual disorder evaluation, **5**:310,
      312*i*
    in hereditary retinal/choroidal degenerations,
      12:205
    nodal point concept used in, **3**:105–108
    in vision rehabilitation, **3**:252
  high-pass resolution, **10**:58
  interpretation in
    artifacts and, **10**:70–71, 72*i*, 73*i*
    optic disc correlation and, **10**:78
    progression and, **10**:74–78, 76*i*, 77*i*
    series of fields, **10**:72, 74–78, 75*i*
    single field, **10**:68–71, 69*i*, 71–73*i*
      comparison of techniques, **10**:70
      normality versus abnormality, **10**:68–69, 69*i*
      quality in, **10**:68
  kinetic, **3**:252, **5**:90–91, **10**:57, 58*i*
    in glaucoma, **10**:57, 58*i*
    in vision rehabilitation, **3**:252
  manual, **10**:78–79, 79*i*, 80*i*
    kinetic, **10**:59
  static, **5**:90–91, **10**:59
    automated. *See* Perimetry, automated, static
    in vision rehabilitation, **3**:252
  suprathreshold, **10**:65–66
  Swedish interactive thresholding algorithm testing,
    10:67
  tangent screen in, **5**:91
  threshold, **10**:66, 67–68, 68*i*
  threshold-related, **10**:66, 66*i*
  types of, **10**:59–60

variables in, 10:60–65, 72*i*
  background luminance, 10:63
  background wavelength, 10:65
  fixation, 10:62–63
  patient, 10:60
  perimetrist, 10:61
  presentation time, 10:64–65
  pupil size, 10:65
  refractive errors, 10:65, 72*i*
  stimulus luminance, 10:63
  stimulus movement speed, 10:65
  stimulus size, 10:64
  stimulus wavelength, 10:65
  in vision rehabilitation, 3:252
Perinatal ocular infection, 6:215–221. *See also specific
  type*
Perindopril, 1:88*t*
Perineuritis, radial, *Acanthamoeba* keratitis and, 8:187
Periocular drug administration, 2:386
  for pars planitis, 9:149–150
  for toxoplasmosis, 9:168
  for uveitis, 9:115*t*, 116–117, 117*i*
Periocular hemangiomas, 7:66
Periocular tissues, development of, 2:156–158
Periodic acid–Schiff stain (PAS), 4:35, 36*t*
Periodic alternating gaze deviation, in comatose
  patients, 5:256
Periodic alternating nystagmus, 5:250, 6:165
Periorbita (periorbital structures), 7:12, 20–22, 21*i*. *See
  also specific structure*
  capillary hemangiomas involving, 7:65
  cellulitis affecting, 7:41–44. *See also* Orbital cellulitis;
    Preseptal cellulitis
  ecchymosis of
    in child abuse, 6:442
    in neuroblastoma, 6:374, 374*i*
  innervation of, 7:14*i*, 15–16, 19*i*
  involutional changes in, 7:228–229
  orbital diseases causing changes in, 7:24, 25*t*
Periorbital sinuses, 2:12, 13*i*
Peripapillary atrophy, examination of, 10:55
Peripapillary fibers, 2:98
Peripapillary staphyloma, 6:364
Peripapillary vascular loops, 4:107
Peripheral airway disease, 1:154
Peripheral anterior synechiae (PAS), in glaucoma, 10:5,
  7
  gonioscopy in identification of, 10:39
Peripheral arterial arcade, 2:24*i*, 27*i*, 29, 32*i*
Peripheral corneal guttae (Hassall-Henle bodies/warts),
  2:47, 8:362, 375
Peripheral curve, of contact lens, 3:174*i*, 175
Peripheral cystoid degeneration, 4:126, 126*i*, 12:264
  reticular, 12:264, 275, 275*i*
  typical, 12:264, 275, 275*i*
Peripheral fusion, in monofixation syndrome, 6:57
Peripheral iridectomy
  for angle-closure glaucoma, 10:200
  for ICCE, 11:106–107
Peripheral iridoplasty, for angle-closure glaucoma,
  10:199–200
Peripheral keratitis, 8:32*t*
  scleritis and, 8:239
  ulcerative, 8:362
    differential diagnosis of, 8:230*t*

Mooren ulcer and, 8:231, 232–234, 233*i*, 234*i*
  in systemic immune-mediated diseases, 8:203,
    229–232, 230*t*, 232*i*
  in Wegener granulomatosis, 1:192
Peripheral lymphoid structures, 9:16
Peripheral nervous system disorders, Sjögren syndrome
  and, 8:79
Peripheral neurofibromatosis, 6:403. *See also*
  Neurofibromatosis, von Recklinghausen (type 1)
  developmental glaucoma and, 10:154, 156
Peripheral retinal excavations, 12:262
Peripheral retinal neovascularization, 12:124, 125*t*. *See
  also* Neovascularization
  vitreous hemorrhage and, 12:287
Peripheral retinal tufts, 12:259–260, 261*i*, 262*i*
Peripheral (anterior) retina, 12:8
Peripheral suppression, 6:54
Peripheral surgical space (extraconal fat/surgical space),
  7:13, 109, 110*i*
Peripheral uveitis. *See* Intermediate uveitis; Pars
  planitis
Peripheral vascular disease
  in diabetes, 1:216–217
  hypertension and, 1:96
Peripheral vascular resistance, reduction of in heart
  failure management, 1:130
Peripheral zone, 8:38–39, 39*i*
Peripherin, 2:344, 344*t*
  mutations in gene for, 2:349–350
Peripherin-*RDS* gene mutations, 2:349–350, 12:204
  in adult-onset vitelliform lesions, 12:219
  in pattern dystrophies, 12:219, 222
  in retinitis pigmentosa, 12:207, 210
  in Stargardt disease, 12:216
Periphlebitis
  in multiple sclerosis, 9:152
  in sarcoidosis, 4:126, 155, 8:88, 9:199
Peristaltic pump, for phacoemulsification aspiration,
  11:119, 119*i*
  vacuum rise time for, 11:120*i*, 121
Peritomy incision, for extraocular muscle surgery,
  6:184
Periungal fibroma, in tuberous sclerosis, 5:338
Periventricular leukomalacia, 6:363
PERK (Prospective Evaluation of Radial Keratotomy)
  study, 13:60
Perkins tonometer, in children, 6:274
Perls' Prussian blue stain, 4:36*t*
PermaVision lens, 13:72–73, 73*i*, 175
Permax. *See* Pergolide
Pernicious anemia, 1:162
Peroxidase, 8:200*t*
Peroxidation, lipid, 2:366–368, 367*i*, 368*i*
  in lens opacification, 11:16
Peroxisomal disorders, retinal degeneration and,
  12:234, 236, 242
Peroxy radicals, 2:366. *See also* Free radicals
PERRLA mnemonic, 5:257
Persantine. *See* Dipyridamole
Persistence, as microbial virulence factor, 8:117
Persistent corneal epithelial defect, 8:101–104, 103*i*
  after penetrating keratoplasty, 8:461
  after PRK/LASEK, 13:104

Persistent fetal vasculature (persistent hyperplastic primary vitreous), 2:175, 177*i*, 4:106, 106*i*, 6:290–291, 292*i*, 292*t*, 324–325, 324*i*, 11:42, 12:280–283, 283*i*
  Bergmeister papillae and. *See* Bergmeister papillae
  cataract and, 4:106, 11:42, 197, 12:282, 283*i*
  glaucoma and, 6:279
  retinoblastoma differentiated from, 4:256–257, 256*t*
  secondary angle-closure glaucoma and, 10:145
Persistent hyaloid artery/system, 2:147, 156, 156*i*, 175, 176*i*, 177*i*, 4:107, 12:280, 281. *See also* Persistent fetal vasculature
Persistent pupillary membranes, 6:267–268, 268*i*
Personality disorders, 1:267
Pes anserinus, 2:118
PET. *See* Positron emission tomography
Petechiae, 1:166
Peters anomaly, 2:168, 169, 170*i*, 6:254–255, 254*i*, 278, 8:292–294, 293*i*, 310*t*, 10:152–153, 153*t*, 11:32. *See also* Axenfeld-Rieger syndrome
Petit mal seizures, 1:282
Petroclinoid (Gruber's) ligament, 2:117, 5:43
Petrosal nerve, greater superficial, 2:119, 5:55
Petrosal sinuses, inferior/superior, 5:23
PEX1 gene, Refsum disease caused by mutations in, 2:351
PFL. *See* Posterior focal length
PFV. *See* Persistent fetal vasculature
PG. *See* Prostaglandins; Proteoglycans
PG analogs. *See* Prostaglandin analogs
PG/PGH synthetase (prostaglandin synthetase/prostaglandin G/H synthetase). *See* Cyclooxygenase
PGI₂. *See* Prostacyclin
pH, of ocular medication, absorption affected by, 2:384–385
PHACE(S) syndrome, 6:377
Phaco burn, 8:420
Phaco chop technique, 11:132–134, 133*i*
Phaco fracture technique, 11:131–132, 132*i*
Phaco tip, 11:115–118, 116*i*, 117*i*
Phacoanaphylaxis. *See* Phacoantigenic endophthalmitis
Phacoantigenic endophthalmitis (lens-induced granulomatous/phacoanaphylactic endophthalmitis/phacoanaphylaxis), 4:96, 96*i*, 97*i*, 9:64, 135–136, 135*i*, 136*i*, 10:105–106, 11:64, 67
Phacoemulsification, 11:93, 112–137
  anterior capsulotomy for, 11:126–127
  in anterior chamber, 11:128
  aspiration system for, 11:118–121, 119*i*, 120*i*
    settings for, 11:135*t*, 136–137
  capsular opacification and contraction and, 11:164*t*, 186–191
    Nd:YAG laser capsulotomy for, 11:187–191, 189*i*
  capsular rupture during, 11:164*t*, 179–180
  in clear lens extraction/refractive lens exchange, 13:159
  corneal complications of, 8:420, 11:167–168
  endolenticular, 11:129
  expulsive hemorrhage risk and, 11:216
  flat or shallow anterior chamber and, 11:163–166
    intraoperative complications, 11:163–165
    postoperative complications, 11:165–166
    preoperative considerations, 11:82
  fluidics of, 11:118–121
    terminology related to, 11:115

foldable intraocular lenses for, 11:145–146
globe exposure for, 11:121
in high refractive error patient, 11:221–222
hydrodelineation in, 11:127
hydrodissection in, 11:127
incisions for, 11:121–126. *See also* Incisions, for cataract surgery
instrumentation for, 11:113–121
  settings for, 11:135–137, 135*t*, 136*i*
at iris plane, 11:128
irrigation in, 11:118
  toxic solutions exposure and, corneal edema caused by, 11:168
location of, 11:128–129
nucleus removal in
  chopping techniques for, 11:132–134, 133*i*
  nuclear flip techniques for, 11:135
  splitting techniques for, 11:131–132, 132*i*
  small capsulorrhexis and, 11:126
  whole, 11:129–131, 129*i*, 130*i*
patient preparation for, 11:121
patient selection for, 11:113
in posterior chamber, 11:128
procedure for, 11:121–137
retained lens fragments after, 11:182–183, 12:337–339, 338*t*, 339*i*
retinal detachment and, 11:175
supracapsular, 11:128–129, 134
surgeon's transition to, 11:112–113
terminology related to, 11:114–115
ultrasound for, 11:115–118, 116*i*, 117*i*, 118*i*
  terminology related to, 11:114
in uveitis, 9:135*i*, 235–237
in zonular dehiscence/lens subluxation or dislocation, 11:226–227, 227*i*, 228*i*
Phacoemulsification handpiece, 11:115–118, 116*i*, 117*i*
Phacolysis, 11:138
Phacolytic glaucoma, 4:81, 82*i*, 96, 101, 9:52, 136, 10:104, 104*i*, 104*t*, 105*i*, 11:67
Phacomorphic glaucoma, 10:122, 128–129, 130*i*, 131*i*, 11:68, 68*i*
Phacotoxic uveitis, 9:135. *See also* Phacoantigenic endophthalmitis
Phagocytosis, 9:50
Phagolysosomes/phagosomes, in retinal pigment epithelium, 2:79
Phakic intraocular lenses, 11:147–148, 13:50*t*, 143–155, 145*t*
  advantages of, 13:144
  ancillary preoperative tests for, 13:146–147
  anterior chamber, 11:148, 13:147–148, 148*i*
    complications of, 13:151, 153*t*
    results of, 13:152*t*
  background of, 13:143–144
  complications of, 13:150–155, 153*t*
  contraindications to, 13:146
  decentration of, 13:151, 154–155, 155*i*
  disadvantages of, 13:144
  indications for, 13:144–146
  informed consent for, 13:146
  iris-fixated, 13:148, 149*i*
    complications of, 13:153*t*, 154
  with LASIK (bioptics), 13:143, 155–156, 157*t*
  outcomes of, 13:149, 152*t*
  patient selection for, 13:144–147

penetrating keratoplasty and, 13:204
posterior chamber, 13:148–149, 149i, 150i
   complications of, 13:153t, 154–155, 155i
   with LASIK (bioptics), 13:143, 155–156, 157t
   results of, 13:152t
   preoperative patient evaluation and, 13:146
   retinal detachment and, 13:151, 192
   risks/benefits of, 13:50t, 144
   surgical technique for insertion of, 13:147–149
Phakic Refractive Lens (PRL), 13:149, 150i. See also
      Phakic intraocular lenses, posterior chamber
Phakinin, 2:327
Phakoma/phakomatosis, 5:335, 336t, 337–343,
      12:160–164, 161i, 162i, 164i. See also specific type
   in children, 6:401–420, 402t
   retinal, in tuberous sclerosis, 6:410–412, 411i
Phakomatous choristoma (Zimmerman tumor), 4:169,
      8:277
Pharmacodynamics, 2:380, 392
Pharmacogenetics, 2:192, 278–279
Pharmacokinetics, 2:380, 381–391
   age-related changes in, 1:235–236, 2:381
Pharmacologic anisocoria, 5:262, 266
Pharmacologic testing, for Horner syndrome,
      5:262–263
Pharmacology, ocular, 2:393–458. See also specific agent
      and Drugs, ocular
   age/aging and, 1:235–236
   legal aspects of, 2:393–394
   principles of, 2:379–392
Pharmacotherapeutics, 2:380, 393–458. See also specific
      agent and Drugs, ocular
Pharyngoconjunctival fever, 6:226, 8:157–158
Phase separation, drug lipid solubility and, 2:384, 385i
Phasic cells, 2:353, 354i
Phenethicillin, 2:429
Pheniramine/naphazoline, 2:423, 424t
Phenobarbital, for seizures, 1:283t
Phenocopy, 2:192, 256–257, 8:307
Phenol red–impregnated cotton thread test, of tear
      secretion, 8:63
Phenothiazines
   lens changes caused by, 11:53, 54i
   retinal degeneration caused by, 12:248–249, 249i
Phenotype, 2:192, 256, 8:307
   alleles and, 2:243
Phenoxybenzamine, 2:309
Phenoxymethyl penicillin. See Penicillin V
Phentolamine, 2:309
   for hypertension, 1:94
Phenylalkanoic acids, 2:421. See also Nonsteroidal anti-
      inflammatory drugs
Phenylbutazone, 1:197t
Phenylephrine, 2:310, 400, 401t, 405, 451
   for fundus examination in premature infant, 6:326
Phenylketonuria, enzyme defect in, 2:263
Phenytoin, 1:283t, 284
Pheochromocytoma
   hypertension in, 1:83, 84t
   in multiple endocrine neoplasia, 1:230
   in von Hippel–Lindau disease, 6:412
Phialophora, ocular infection caused by, 8:130
Philadelphia practical classification, for retinoblastoma,
      6:396, 397t
Phleboliths, orbital varices and, 7:70

Phlyctenular keratoconjunctivitis, in children, 6:388
Phlyctenules/phlyctenulosis, 8:24t
   in staphylococcal blepharoconjunctivitis, 8:166, 167i,
      168
PHMB. See Polyhexamethylene biguanide
PHN. See Postherpetic neuralgia
-phoria (suffix), definition of, 6:10
Phorias. See Heterophorias
Phoropter refraction, 3:142–143
Phosphate, in aqueous humor, 2:317
Phosphatidyl-inositol-4,5-bisphosphate (PIP$_2$), in
      signal transduction in iris–ciliary body, 2:311, 313i
Phosphatidylcholine, in retinal pigment epithelium,
      2:358
Phosphatidylethanolamine, in retinal pigment
      epithelium, 2:358
Phosphodiesterase, rod (rod PDE), 2:343, 344t
   mutations in, 2:349
Phosphodiesterase inhibitors, for heart failure, 1:130
Phosphofructokinase, in lens carbohydrate metabolism,
      11:14, 15i
Phospholine. See Echothiophate
Phospholipase A$_2$, 9:80
   in eicosanoid synthesis, 2:305, 306i
   nonsteroidal anti-inflammatory drug derivation and,
      2:420–421
   in tear film, 2:290
Phospholipase C
   in signal transduction in iris–ciliary body, 2:311,
      313i
   in tear secretion, 2:292, 292i
Phospholipid antibody syndrome (antiphospholipid
      antibody syndrome), 1:171, 182–184
Phospholipids. See also Lipids
   in retinal pigment epithelium, 2:358
   in tear film, 2:289. See also Lipid layer of tear film
Phosphonoformic acid. See Foscarnet
Photic damage/phototoxicity, 2:459–465, 460t, 3:167
   age-related macular degeneration and, 12:61
   ambient exposure to ultraviolet or visible light and,
      12:309
   cataract surgery and, 11:171–172
   free radical damage and, 2:370–371, 459
   occupational, 12:309
   ophthalmic instrumentation causing, 2:459–465,
      460t, 12:308–309
   retinal, 2:459, 12:307–309
   in retinitis pigmentosa, 12:210, 213
   retinopathy of prematurity and, 6:326, 12:132
Photoablation, 3:23–24, 13:29, 87–135, 88–89i. See also
      specific procedure
   custom/multifocal, for presbyopia, 13:174–175, 174i
   for melanoma, 4:238
   for retinoblastoma, 4:262
   types of lasers for, 13:30
   wavefront-guided, 13:30, 49, 90
Photoastigmatic keratectomy, 13:98–99. See also
      Photorefractive keratectomy
Photochemical injury, 2:459, 12:307
Photochromic lenses, 3:166
Photocoagulation, 3:23, 12:313–320
   for age-related macular degeneration, 12:61–62,
      70–73, 71–72t, 73i, 74i
   anesthesia for, 12:317

for branch retinal vein occlusion, **12**:138–140, 139*i*, 140*i*
for central retinal artery occlusion, **12**:150
for central retinal vein occlusion, **12**:144–145
for central serous chorioretinopathy, **12**:53–54
for choroidal hemangioma, **4**:164, 245
for choroidal neovascularization, **12**:70–73, 71–72*t*, 73*i*, 74*i*
in myopia, **12**:71–72*t*, 85–86
in ocular histoplasmosis, **12**:72*t*, 80–81
for Coats disease, **12**:157
complications of, **12**:318–320
for diabetic macular edema, **12**:113–116, 115*i*, 116*t*
for diabetic retinopathy, **4**:136, 136*i*, **12**:106–111, 108*i*, 110*i*, 117–118
indications for, **12**:317–318
laser wavelengths used in, **12**:313–317, 315–316*t*
for macroaneurysms, **12**:159
for melanoma, **4**:238
for myopia, **12**:71–72*t*, 85–86
for ocular histoplasmosis, **9**:161, **12**:72*t*
for ocular ischemic syndrome, **12**:151
for parafoveal (juxtafoveal) retinal telangiectasis, **12**:158
for pars planitis, **9**:150
practical aspects of, **12**:317
prophylactic, in acute retinal necrosis, **9**:155–156
for retinal angiomas, **6**:413, **12**:163
for retinal breaks, **12**:265
for retinal capillary hemangioma, **4**:247
for retinoblastoma, **4**:262
for retinopathy of prematurity, **6**:330, **12**:134, 135*i*
for sickle cell retinopathy, **12**:123–124
thermal light injury caused by, **12**:307
for von Hippel–Lindau syndrome/disease (retinal angiomatosis), **6**:413, **12**:163
Photodisruption, **3**:23
intrastromal, **13**:21*t*, 29
Photodynamic reactions, **2**:459
Photodynamic therapy, **2**:391, 454
for choroidal hemangioma, **4**:245
for choroidal neovascularization, **12**:71–72*t*, 73–76, 320–322
in age-related macular degeneration, **12**:71–72*t*, 73–76, 320–322
in central serous chorioretinopathy, **12**:54
complications of, **12**:321–322
in myopia, **12**:71–72*t*, 85, 320–322
ocular histoplasmosis syndrome and, **12**:72*t*, 82
for von Hippel–Lindau syndrome/disease (retinal angiomatosis), **12**:163
Photographic keratoscope/photokeratoscopy, **3**:302–303, **8**:41
Photometric quantities, phototoxicity and, **2**:462
Photometry, **3**:14–15
terms used in, **3**:16*t*
Photomicroscopy, specular, **3**:294–295, 295*i*, **8**:18, 36–37, 36*i*
before cataract surgery, **11**:87
in optical focusing technique for pachymetry, **3**:293
before phakic intraocular lens insertion, **13**:146
Photomydriasis, multifocal IOLs and, **13**:164
Photon characteristics of light, **3**:3, 6*i*, 7
Photons, **3**:7

Photo-oxidation, **2**:366–367
in retina, **2**:370–371
Photophobia, **5**:299
in cone dystrophy, **5**:104
in congenital/infantile glaucoma, **6**:272
in uveitis, **9**:127
Photopic/light adapted electroretinogram, **12**:28*i*, 29, 205, 206*t*
in hereditary retinal/choroidal degenerations, **12**:205, 206*t*
Photopsias
in posterior vitreous detachment, **12**:257
in rhegmatogenous retinal detachment, **12**:268
Photoreceptor dystrophies, **12**:205–215. *See also* Retinitis, pigmentosa
Photoreceptor inner segments, **2**:79, 80*i*, 82*i*. *See also* Photoreceptors
Photoreceptor outer segments, **2**:79, 80*i*, 82*i*. *See also* Photoreceptors
shed, retinal pigment epithelium phagocytosis of, **2**:360–361
Photoreceptor-specific guanylate cyclase (*RETGC1*) gene, in Leber congenital amaurosis, **6**:335
Photoreceptors, **2**:79–80, 80*i*, 83*i*. *See also* Cones; Rods
in age-related macular degeneration, **12**:58
atrophy of, in macular degeneration, **4**:139
biochemistry and metabolism of, **2**:341–351
development of, **2**:141
genetic approaches to function/dysfunction of, **2**:347–348, 347*i*, 348*i*
Photorefractive keratectomy (PRK), **13**:21*t*, 23, 23*i*, 50*t*, 87, 90–106
ablation techniques and, **13**:95–96, 96*i*
Bowman's layer and, **2**:299–300
calibration of excimer laser for, **13**:91
cataract surgery after, **11**:211
intraocular lens power calculation and, **11**:151
central islands after, **13**:101–102, 101*i*
centration techniques and, **13**:95–96, 96*i*
in children, **13**:195
CLAPIKS after, **13**:207–208
complications of, **13**:100–105
contact lens fitting after, **13**:206
corneal biomechanics affected by, **13**:23, 23*i*, 24–25
corneal haze and, **13**:103–104, 103*i*
corneal wound healing/repair and, **13**:28
corticosteroid-induced complications after, **13**:105, 189, 208
decentered ablation and, **13**:102–103, 102*i*
dry eye and, **8**:80, **13**:105
elevated intraocular pressure after, **13**:105, 189, 208
endothelial effects of, **13**:105
enhancements/reoperation and, **13**:99–100
epithelial debridement for, **13**:93–94, 93*i*
herpetic keratitis after, **13**:185
hyperopic, **13**:26, 27*i*, 99
hyperopic astigmatic, **13**:99
for keratoconus, **8**:332
laser centration/ablation for, **13**:95–96, 96*i*
lasers approved for, **13**:32*t*, 33*t*, 34*t*
for LASIK enhancement, **13**:119
mixed astigmatic, **13**:99
myopic, **13**:98
optical aberrations after, **13**:102
outcomes of, **13**:97–100

overcorrection after, 13:100
patient selection for, 13:90–91
after penetrating keratoplasty, 8:465t, 466,
    13:187–188
penetrating keratoplasty after, 13:203–204
persistent epithelial defect after, 13:104
postablation measures for
    immediate, 13:96
    operative day, 13:96–97
    subsequent postoperative care, 13:97
preoperative patient preparation for, 13:92–93
preoperative planning/laser programming for, 13:92
after radial keratotomy, 13:64–65
retinal detachment and, 13:192
risks/benefits of, 13:50t
spherical aberration after, 3:102
stromal infiltrates after, 13:104, 104i
surgical techniques for, 13:91–95
toric, 13:98–99
tracking devices for, 13:98
undercorrection after, 13:101
wavefront-guided, 13:21t, 90, 133–135
Photoscreening, for amblyopia, 6:67
Photosensitivity, in systemic lupus erythematosus,
    1:179, 181t
Photostress recovery test
    before cataract surgery, 11:86
    in low vision evaluation, 5:97
Phototherapeutic keratectomy (PTK), 8:440
    for calcific band keratopathy, 8:374
    for corneal epithelial basement membrane
        dystrophy, 8:313
    lasers approved for, 13:32t, 33t
    for recurrent corneal erosions, 8:100
Photothermal injury, 2:459
Photothermal laser therapy, 13:29
Phototransduction
    cone, 2:345
    rod, 2:341–344, 342i, 343i
PHPV (persistent hyperplastic primary vitreous). See
    Persistent fetal vasculature
Phthiriasis palpebrum (Phthirus pubis infection), 8:133,
    133i, 169
    cholinesterase inhibitors for, 2:400
Phthirus pubis (crab/pubic louse), 8:133, 133i
    ocular infection (phthiriasis palpebrum) caused by,
        8:133, 169
    cholinesterase inhibitors for, 2:400
Phthisis bulbi (phthisical eye), 4:28, 29, 29i, 31, 31i
    after penetrating injury, 12:295
    retinoblastoma regression and, 6:392
Phycomycetes (phycomycosis). See Mucor
    (mucormycosis)
Physical drug dependence, 1:267
Physical examination, preoperative assessment and,
    1:327, 328t
Physical optics, 3:3–24, 24i
    absorption and, 3:14
    coherence and, 3:7–9, 8i, 9i
    definition of, 3:3
    diffraction and, 3:11–12, 12i
    illumination and, 3:14–17, 15i, 16t, 17t
    interference and, 3:7–9, 8i, 9i
    laser fundamentals and, 3:17–24, 20t, 22i, 24i
    photon (particle) aspects of light and, 3:3, 6i, 7

polarization and, 3:10–11
reflection and, 3:13–14, 13i
scattering and, 3:12–13
transmission and, 3:14
wave theory and, 3:3–7, 4i, 5i
Physiologic (simple/essential) anisocoria, 5:260, 261i,
    262
Physiologic cup/physiologic cupping, 2:96, 98. See also
    Optic cup
Physiologic (simple/school) myopia, 3:120
Physostigmine, 2:309, 396i, 398t, 399, 401–402
    for atropine intoxication, 6:95
Phytanic acid storage disease. See Refsum disease/
    syndrome
Pia mater, optic nerve, 2:101–102, 101i, 4:203, 204i
PIC. See Punctate inner choroiditis/choroidopathy
PICA. See Posterior inferior cerebellar artery
Picornaviruses, ocular infection caused by, 8:121
Picosecond laser, for photodisruption, 13:29
Pie in the sky defects, 5:166
Pierre Robin sequence (anomaly/deformity), 6:205,
    433, 8:353t
    Stickler syndrome and, 6:341, 433, 12:284
Piezoelectric transducer, in ultrasonic handpiece,
    11:114, 115
Piggybacking
    with corneal contact lenses, for keratoconus, 3:200
    with intraocular lenses, 3:214, 221, 11:153
        in children, 11:200
        clear lens extraction/refractive lens exchange and,
            13:160
Pigment, visual. See Pigments, visual
Pigment dispersion syndrome, 10:101–103, 101–103i
    after anterior chamber phakic IOL insertion, 13:153t
    anterior chamber and trabecular meshwork affected
        in, 4:84, 85i
    cornea affected in, 4:73, 76i, 8:375
    glaucoma and, 4:84, 85i
    after iris-fixated phakic IOL insertion, 13:153t
    after posterior chamber phakic IOL insertion,
        13:153t, 154
Pigment epithelial detachment. See Retinal pigment
    epithelium (RPE), detachment of
Pigment epithelium. See Ciliary epithelium, pigmented;
    Iris pigment epithelium; Retinal pigment
    epithelium
Pigment epithelium–derived factor, in aqueous humor,
    2:317, 320
Pigment granules
    cytologic identification of, 8:69–70, 69i
    in retinal pigment epithelium, 2:362
    in vitreous ("tobacco dust"/Shafer's sign), 12:268,
        276, 288
Pigment spot of sclera, 8:263
Pigmentary glaucoma, 10:101–103, 101–103i
Pigmentary retinopathy, 12:207, 231, 233t. See also
    Retinitis, pigmentosa
    hearing loss and, 12:235. See also Usher syndrome
    systemic diseases with, 12:231, 232–233t
Pigmentations/pigment deposits, 12:231
    congenital abnormalities and, 2:175–178, 177i, 178i
    corneal, 4:73–74, 76i, 8:375
        drug-induced, 8:376–378, 377t
    iris, 2:62, 63i
        development of, 2:154–155

latanoprost and, 2:414
after laser skin resurfacing, 7:238
lens, drugs causing, 11:52
retinal pigment epithelium and, 2:362
in age-related macular degeneration, 12:58
trabecular meshwork, 4:80, 10:41–42
Pigmented lesions, 8:267t
benign, 8:263–265, 263t
malignant, 8:263t, 268–269, 268i
preinvasive, 8:263t, 266–268, 267t
Pigments, visual
absorption spectra of, 12:313, 314i
regeneration of, retinal pigment epithelium in,
2:359, 360i, 361i
Pilagan. See Pilocarpine
Pilar (trichilemmal) cyst, 7:166
Pili, bacterial, 8:123
Pilocar. See Pilocarpine
Pilocarpine, 2:309, 395–397, 396i, 398t
accommodation affected by, 11:22
in Adie's tonic pupil diagnosis, 5:266
in anisocoria diagnosis, 5:262
cataracts caused by, 11:53–54
for dry eye, 8:75
for glaucoma, 2:397, 10:161–162t, 166–167, 167
in children, 6:283
sustained release device for administration of, 2:390
systemic side effects of, 2:398, 399i
Pilocytic astrocytoma, optic. See Optic nerve (optic
pathway) glioma
Pilomatrixomas, 7:169
Pilopine. See Pilocarpine
Pilopine gel. See Pilocarpine
Piloptic. See Pilocarpine
Pilostat. See Pilocarpine
Pindolol, 1:88t
Pinealoblastoma/pineoblastoma, 4:260
Pinealoma, retinoblastoma associated with, 4:265t
Pinguecula, 4:49–50, 49i, 8:365
Pinhole imaging, 3:25–27, 25i, 28i, 33–34, 34i
image quality and, 3:36–38, 37i, 38i
visual acuity and, 3:109–110
Pinhole visual acuity, 3:109–110
Pink puffers, 1:154
Pioglitazone, 1:212t, 213–214
PIOL. See Phakic intraocular lenses
PION (posterior ischemic optic neuropathy). See
Posterior optic neuropathy, ischemic
PIP₂. See Phosphatidyl-inositol-4,5-bisphosphate
Piperacillin, 1:56t, 67, 2:429
with tazobactam, 1:57t, 70
Pipracil. See Piperacillin
Pirbuterol, 1:157t
Piroxicam, 1:197t, 2:421t
ocular effects of, 1:324t
Piston, wavefront aberrations and, 13:15
Pits
foveal, 2:144
optic (optic holes), 2:127, 136, 175, 4:204, 5:140,
6:363, 363i
Pituitary adenoma, 1:228–229
chiasmal syndromes caused by, 5:161–162, 162i
MR imaging of, 1:229, 5:73i
in pregnancy, 5:344
Pituitary apoplexy, 1:229–230

Pituitary hormones, hypothalamic hormones and,
1:227–230, 229t
Pituitary necrosis, postpartum (Sheehan syndrome),
5:345
PITX2 gene
in Axenfeld-Rieger syndrome, 6:253, 272
in glaucoma, 10:13t
in Peters anomaly, 8:294
Pixel, definition of, 5:80
PJCs. See Premature junctional complexes
PK (penetrating keratoplasty). See Keratoplasty,
penetrating
PL. See Preferential looking
PLA₂. See Phospholipase A₂
Placido-based topography/Placido disk, 3:302–303,
303i, 304i, 8:41, 13:6, 7, 8, 47
computerized, 8:41–46, 42i, 43i, 44i, 45i, 46i, 13:6
in keratoconus, 8:331, 331i
Placode, 2:127
lens, 2:136–137, 145–146
Plagiocephaly, 6:421, 423i
in Saethre-Chotzen syndrome, 6:426
V-pattern deviations associated with, 6:429
Planck's constant, 3:7
Plane of incidence and reflection, 3:42, 43i
Plane of incidence and transmission, 3:44, 45i
Plane (plano) mirror
retinoscopy settings and, 3:125i, 126
vergence calculations for, 3:92, 92i
Plane parallel plate, 3:84, 85i
Plane-polarized light, 3:10
Planes of unit magnification, 3:75
Planoconcave lenses, for slit-lamp delivery of
photocoagulation, 12:317
Planocylindrical lenses, 3:94, 96i
Plant alkaloids, in cancer chemotherapy, 1:257, 259t
Plants/vegetation, ocular injuries caused by, 8:395–396
Plaque radiotherapy. See Radioactive plaque therapy
Plaquenil. See Hydroxychloroquine
Plaques
Hollenhorst (cholesterol emboli)
in branch retinal artery occlusion, 4:133, 12:146,
147i
in central retinal artery occlusion, 12:149
transient visual loss and, 5:173, 173i
optic nerve, 4:205
senile scleral, 8:378, 379i
Plasma, 1:159
Plasma cell tumors, of orbit, 7:88
Plasma cells, 4:15, 16i
cytologic identification of, 8:65t, 68, 68i
in external eye, 8:196t
monoclonal proliferation of, corneal deposits and,
8:349–350
Plasma proteins, in aqueous humor, 2:317, 318–320
Plasmacytoma, of orbit, 7:88
Plasmid-liposome complexes, as gene therapy vectors,
2:237
Plasmid resistance, 1:66
Plasmids, 2:192
bacterial, 8:123
for gene therapy, 2:237
Plasminogen
antifibrinolytic agents affecting, 2:453
in aqueous humor, 2:319

in ligneous conjunctivitis, 8:213, 214
Plasminogen activator
in aqueous humor, 2:319
tissue. *See* Tissue plasminogen activator
Plastic spectacle lenses, 3:168
bifocal, 3:152
reverse slab-off and, 3:161
prism calibration for, 3:85, 86*i*
Plateau iris, 10:128, 129*i*, 130*i*
Plateau iris configuration, 10:128
Plateau iris syndrome, 10:128, 130*i*
characteristics of, 10:6*t*
Platelet-activating factors, 8:200*t*, 9:77, 78*i*, 79–80
Platelet count, 1:165
Platelet-derived growth factors, 2:456, 9:82*t*
Platelet-fibrin embolus, transient visual loss and, 5:175, 176*i*, 177*t*
Platelet glycoprotein IIb/IIIa receptor antagonists. *See* Glycoprotein IIb/IIIa receptor antagonists
Platelets, 1:159
aspirin affecting, 2:422
disorders of, 1:166–168
drugs causing, 1:167–168, 331–332
of function, 1:167–168
of number, 1:167
in hemostasis, 1:164
Platinol. *See* Cisplatin
Platinum eyelid weights, for exposure keratopathy, 8:95
Platysmaplasty, 7:247, 247*i*
Plavix. *See* Clopidogrel
Pleiotropism, 2:192, 222, 259, 8:307
Plendil. *See* Felodipine
Pleomorphic adenoma (benign mixed tumor)
of eyelid, 7:167
of lacrimal gland, 4:192–193, 193*i*, 7:89–90, 90*i*
Pleomorphic rhabdomyosarcoma, 6:373, 7:80
Pleomorphism, specular photomicroscopy in evaluation of, 8:37
Plexiform layer
inner, 2:80–81*i*, 85
outer, 2:80–81*i*, 82*i*, 84
Plexiform neurofibromas, 6:381, 405, 405*i*
glaucoma and, 6:405, 408
of orbit, 4:192, 200, 201*i*, 6:381, 7:26, 75–76, 76*i*
Plica semilunaris, 2:22*i*, 30–31, 4:43
incorporation of during strabismus surgery, 6:187–188, 188*i*
Plume theory, of central islands, 13:101
Plurihormonal adenomas, 1:229
Pluripotent, definition of, 2:127
Pluripotential stem cells, 1:160
Plus cylinder refraction, 3:136
Plus disease, 4:137, 6:326, 327*t*, 329*i*, 12:129, 130*i*
Plus (convex) lenses, anophthalmic socket camouflage and, 7:127
PMA. *See* Premarket approval
PML. *See* Progressive multifocal leukoencephalopathy
PMMA. *See* Polymethylmethacrylate
PMNs (polymorphonuclear leukocytes). *See* Neutrophils
PMPA. *See* Tenofovir
Pneumatic retinopexy, for retinal detachment, 12:272, 335
Pneumatic tonometer (pneumatonometry), 10:28–29
after LASIK, 13:208

after PRK/LASEK, 13:105, 108
Pneumocandins, 1:76
for *Pneumocystis carinii (Pneumocystis jiroveci)* pneumonia, 1:47
Pneumococcal vaccine, 1:291, 304*t*, 308
Pneumococcus. *See Streptococcus, pneumoniae*
Pneumocystis carinii (Pneumocystis jiroveci) infections, 1:45–47, 8:131
choroiditis, 9:256–257, 256*i*, 257*i*
in HIV infection/AIDS, 1:45–47
pneumonia, 1:45–47, 9:247, 256
Pneumolysin, 8:124
Pneumonia
in HIV infection/AIDS, 1:45–47, 9:247. *See also Pneumocystis carinii (Pneumocystis jiroveci)* infections
pneumococcal, 1:6–7, 308
immunization against, 1:291, 304*t*, 308
PO (pupil–optic nerve) section, 4:33–34, 34*i*
POAG. *See* Open-angle glaucoma, primary
Podophyllin/podophyllotoxins, in cancer chemotherapy, 1:257, 259*t*
POHS. *See* Presumed ocular histoplasmosis syndrome
Point mutations, 2:255–256
Point source of light, in geometric optics, 3:26
Point spread function (PSF), 3:38
keratorefractive surgery and, 3:232–234
Poison ivy toxin, immune response arc in response to, 9:29–30
Poker spine, in ankylosing spondylitis, 1:176
Poland syndrome, Möbius syndrome and, 6:154
Polar cataracts, 11:34–35, 36*i*
in children, 6:288, 288*i*
hereditary factors in, 6:287*t*
surgery for removal of, 11:212–213
Polarimetry, scanning laser, in retinal nerve fiber evaluation, 10:55–56
Polarity, abnormal, definition of, 8:247*t*
Polarization, 3:10–11. *See also* Polarizing sunglasses
applications of, 3:10–11
of laser light, 3:18
reflection and, 3:13–14, 13*i*
Polarizing projection charts, 3:11
Polarizing sunglasses (polarized/Polaroid lenses), 3:10, 13*i*, 165
Polaroid slide test, in functional visual disorder evaluation, 5:307, 308*i*
Polio, immunization against, 1:307
Poliosis
in staphylococcal blepharitis, 8:164
in Vogt-Koyanagi-Harada syndrome, 9:203, 204*i*
PolyA tail, 2:209
Polyacrylamide, 2:452
as viscoelastic, 11:160
Polyallelism, 2:243
Polyangiitis, microscopic, 1:189*t*, 192
Polyarteritis nodosa, 1:189*t*, 191–192, 7:60, 9:175, 176*i*
eyelid manifestations of, 4:173*t*
refractive surgery contraindicated in, 13:198
Polyarthritis
in Behçet syndrome, 1:193
in systemic lupus erythematosus, 1:179, 181*t*
Polyarticular onset juvenile idiopathic arthritis, 1:178–179, 6:313*t*, 314
eye examination schedule for children with, 6:316*t*

rheumatoid factor (RF)-negative, uveitis in, 6:313*t*, 314
Polycarbonate spectacle lenses, 3:168–169
Polycarbophil, for dry eye, 2:450
Polychondritis, relapsing, 1:187–188
    eyelid manifestations of, 4:173*t*
Polycillin. *See* Ampicillin
Polyclonal antibodies, 9:56
Polycoria, 2:170, 6:269
Polycystic kidney disease, hypertension in, 1:83, 84*t*
Polydystrophy, pseudo–Hurler, 6:436*t*, 8:342
Polyene antibiotics, 2:437, 438*t*
Polygenic inheritance, 2:192, 273–275, 274*t*
Polyhexamethylene biguanide, for *Acanthamoeba* infection, 2:444, 8:189
Polymegethism, specular photomicroscopy in evaluation of, 8:37
Polymerase chain reaction (PCR), 2:193, 227–230, 229*i*, 4:39–40, 39*i*
    in *Chlamydia trachomatis* infection, 1:22
    in *Haemophilus influenzae* infection, 1:11
    in herpes simplex infection, 1:27
    in HIV infection/AIDS, 9:245
    for HIV RNA, 1:43
    in infection diagnosis, 1:3
    in Lyme disease, 1:20
    in mutation screening, 2:233*i*, 234*i*
    in toxoplasmosis, 1:26
    in tuberculosis, 1:23, 302
Polymers, contact lens
    for flexible contact lenses, 3:184–185
    for rigid (hard) contact lenses, 3:183–185
Polymethylmethacrylate (PMMA)
    contact lenses made from, 3:173, 175, 183–184, 201
    intraocular lenses made from, 3:213, 11:139–142, 143
        for children, 6:298, 301, 11:157
        instrumentation for handling, 11:152
        phakic IOLs and, 13:144
    refractive index of, 3:40*t*
Polymorphic amyloid degeneration, 8:370
Polymorphisms, 2:193, 215, 256, 8:307
    denaturing gradient gel electrophoresis in identification of, 2:230
    restriction fragment length (RFLP), 2:195, 222–223, 224*i*
    single-stranded conformational, 2:230
Polymorphonuclear leukocytes. *See* Neutrophils
Polymorphous dystrophy, posterior, 8:310*t*, 327–329, 328*i*
Polymyalgia rheumatica, 1:190
Polymyositis, 1:186–187
Polymyxin, 1:54
Polymyxin B, 2:437
    in combination preparations, 2:431*t*, 432*t*
Polyneuropathy, familial amyloid, vitreous involvement in, 4:111, 111*i*
Polyol (sorbitol) pathway, in lens glucose/carbohydrate metabolism, 2:331, 331*i*, 11:14–16, 15*i*
    diabetic retinopathy and, 2:354
Polyopia, in cataracts, 11:77
Polyphosphoinositide turnover, 2:311–312, 312*i*, 313*i*
Polyploidy, 2:249

Polypoidal choroidal vasculopathy (posterior uveal bleeding syndrome), age-related macular degeneration differentiated from, 12:67–68, 69*i*
Polyposis, familial adenomatous (Gardner syndrome), retinal manifestations of, 2:173, 4:122–123, 230, 6:390, 12:236–237, 237*i*
Polyps, colorectal cancer and, 1:297–298
"Polypseudophakia, temporary," 11:200
Polysaccharide encapsulation, as microbial virulence factor, 1:4
Polysorbate, in demulcents, 2:450
Polysporin. *See* Polymyxin B
Polysulfone, for intracorneal implant, 13:72, 175
Polytetrafluoroethane, for frontalis suspension, 7:222
Polythiazide, 1:88*t*
Polytrim. *See* Polymyxin B
Polyvinyl alcohol, for dry eye, 2:450
Ponstel. *See* Mefenamic acid
Pontine cistern, lateral, 2:118
Pontine nuclei, dorsolateral, 5:34
Pontine reticular formation, paramedian, 2:116, 116*i*, 5:34, 202
Pontocaine. *See* Tetracaine
Pontomedullary junction, 2:116
Pooling, fluorescein, 12:21, 22*i*. *See also* Hyperfluorescence
    in central serous chorioretinopathy, 12:22*i*, 52
    in cystoid macular edema, 12:154, 155*i*
Population, measurement systems and, 1:364
Population inversion, 3:21–22, 22*i*
Pores, nuclear, 2:203
Pork tapeworm *(Taenia solium)*, 8:133, 9:171
    orbital infection caused by, 7:47
PORN. *See* Progressive outer retinal necrosis
Porphyria/porphyria cutanea tarda, 8:355
Porro-Abbe prism, 3:280, 282*i*, 297*i*
PORT. *See* Punctate outer retinal toxoplasmosis
Port-wine stain (nevus flammeus), 6:380, 8:270, 270*t*, 10:154. *See also* Vascular malformations
    of orbit, 6:380
    in Sturge-Weber syndrome, 5:340, 341*i*, 6:41, 278, 380, 414–415, 415*i*
    in von Hippel–Lindau disease, 6:412
Portable electronic applanation devices, 10:28–29
POS. *See* Parinaud oculoglandular syndrome
Posaconazole, 1:76
Position, in schematic eye, 3:106*i*
Position maintenance system, 6:39
Position of rest, 6:31
Positional candidate gene screening, 2:227
Positional cloning, 2:225–226
Positions of gaze. *See* Gaze, positions of
Positive angle kappa, 6:86, 87*i*
    in retinopathy of prematurity, 6:86, 331, 331*i*
Positive defocus, 13:15, 15*i*
Positive predictive value (PPV), of screening/diagnostic test, 1:354
Positive staining (fluorescein), 8:20
Positron emission tomography (PET), 5:69
    in ischemic heart disease, 1:119
Posner-Schlossman syndrome (glaucomatocyclitic crisis), 9:107, 135, 10:107
Post-traumatic stress disorder (PTSD), 1:267
Post-cataract extraction restriction, 5:219

Postcentral gyrus (primary sensory cortex), **5**:50, 50*i*, 51*i*

Postencephalitis parkinsonism, oculogyric crisis in, **5**:212

Posterior aqueous diversion syndrome. *See* Aqueous misdirection

Posterior capsular opacification (PCO), **11**:186–187
in children, **11**:198
IOLs and, **3**:213
Nd:YAG laser capsulotomy for, **11**:186–187, 187–191, 189*i*

Posterior capsular rupture, phacoemulsification and, **11**:164*t*, 179–180

Posterior cerebral artery, **5**:11, 16, 18, 20*i*

Posterior chamber, **2**:43–44, 43*i*, 55*i*
phacoemulsification in, **11**:128
whole nucleus emulsification and, **11**:129–131, 129*i*
in uveitis, **9**:103*t*, 106. *See also* Posterior uveitis

Posterior chamber intraocular lenses. *See* Intraocular lenses

Posterior chiasmal syndrome, **5**:158, 161*i*

Posterior ciliary arteries, **2**:38–40, 39*i*, 40*i*, 67, **5**:15, 16*i*

Posterior ciliary nerves, **2**:38, 297

Posterior clinoid process, **2**:117

Posterior collagenous layer (retrocorneal fibrous membrane), **2**:301–302, **8**:33–34

Posterior commissure, **2**:110, **5**:39

Posterior communicating artery, **5**:20

Posterior conjunctival arteries, **2**:36

Posterior corneal defects/depression . *See* Keratoconus, posterior; Peters anomaly

Posterior corneal dystrophies
amorphous, **8**:297
polymorphous, **8**:310*t*, 327–329, 328*i*

Posterior embryotoxon, **2**:127, 168, 168*i*, **4**:78, 78*i*, **6**:251–252, 251*i*, **8**:291, 292*i*. *See also* Anterior segment, dysgenesis of; Neurocristopathy
in Axenfeld-Rieger syndrome, **6**:251*i*, 252, 253, **8**:292

Posterior ethmoidal air cells, **5**:9, 9*i*

Posterior ethmoidal artery, **5**:13, 15

Posterior ethmoidal foramen, **5**:10

Posterior fixation suture (fadenoperation), **6**:175*t*

Posterior focal length (PFL), **3**:79

Posterior focal plane, **3**:71

Posterior focal point, **3**:71

Posterior inferior cerebellar artery, **5**:18, 19*i*

Posterior infusion syndrome, **11**:164–165

Posterior keratoconus. *See* Keratoconus, posterior

Posterior lacrimal crest, **2**:5, 7*i*

Posterior lamella, **2**:27*i*

Posterior lamellar keratoplasty, **8**:475–476

Posterior lenticonus/lentiglobus, **4**:97, 98*i*, **11**:30, 31
in children, **6**:289–290, 291*i*, 292*t*

Posterior nonbanded zone, of Descemet's membrane, **2**:47, 48*i*

Posterior optic neuropathy, **5**:141–156
ischemic, **5**:155

Posterior pigmented layer, of iris, **2**:62*i*, 64, 65*i*
development of, **2**:154–155

Posterior pole, **2**:86

Posterior segment
assessment of before refractive surgery, **13**:46
childhood glaucoma associated with abnormalities of, **6**:279

complications of anterior segment surgery and, vitrectomy for, **12**:328–340
metastatic tumors of, **4**:269–271, 270*i*, 271*i*, 272*i*
trauma to, **12**:289–303. *See also* Trauma
blunt, **12**:290–295
child abuse and, **12**:301–302, 302*i*
endophthalmitis and, **12**:300
evaluation of patient after, **12**:289–290
foreign bodies, **12**:296–299, 297*i*, 299*t*
lacerating and penetrating injuries, **12**:295–296
optic disc avulsion and, **12**:302, 303*i*
perforating injuries, **12**:296
shaken baby syndrome and, **12**:301–302, 302*i*
sympathetic ophthalmia and, **12**:300–301

Posterior subcapsular (cupuliform) cataract, **4**:99, 99*i*, **11**:48–49, 53*i*
in children, **6**:291, 292*t*
corticosteroids causing, **11**:50–52
in myotonic dystrophy, **11**:62–63

Posterior sutures, **11**:9

Posterior synechiae
anisocoria and, **5**:262
in children, **6**:270
mydriasis in prevention of, **2**:400
in sarcoidosis, **6**:270, **9**:198
in uveitis, **9**:104*i*, 105*i*

Posterior uveal bleeding syndrome (polypoidal choroidal vasculopathy), age-related macular degeneration differentiated from, **12**:67–68, 69*i*

Posterior uveal melanoma, **4**:159–163, 222–241. *See also* Choroidal/ciliary body melanoma
staging of, **4**:289–290*t*

Posterior uveitis, **9**:107, 153–185. *See also specific cause and* Choroiditis; Retinitis; Uveitis
causes of, **9**:112*t*
in children, **6**:311, 312*t*, 317–319, 318*i*
differential diagnosis of, **6**:312*t*
diffuse unilateral subacute neuroretinitis and, **6**:318
familial juvenile systemic granulomatosis (Blau syndrome) and, **6**:318
laboratory tests for, **6**:321*t*
masquerade syndromes and, **6**:320*t*
toxocariasis and, **6**:317–318, 318*i*
toxoplasmosis and, **6**:317
Vogt-Koyanagi-Harada syndrome and, **6**:318
differential diagnosis of, **6**:312*t*, **9**:111*t*
immunologic, **9**:175–185
infectious, **9**:154–173
signs of, **9**:103*t*, 106

Posterior vascular capsule, **11**:29, 29*i*
remnant of (Mittendorf dot), **2**:91, 175, 177*i*, **4**:107, **6**:361, **11**:29–30, 31, **12**:280

Posterior vestibular artery, **5**:18

Posterior vitreous detachment, **2**:89, 90*i*, 338, **4**:111, 112*i*, **12**:256–258, 256*i*, 257*i*, 279–280
idiopathic macular holes and, **12**:89, 92*i*

Postexposure prophylaxis
hepatitis B, **1**:305
HIV, **1**:45, 46–47*t*
measles, **1**:306

Postganglionic Horner syndrome, **5**:264–265
isolated, **5**:264

Postganglionic nerves, **2**:110
cholinergic drug action and, **2**:394, 395*i*

iris sphincter supplied by, 2:66
Postherpetic neuralgia, 1:28, 8:153, 155–156
Postictal paralysis (Todd's paralysis), 1:282
Postictal period, 1:282
Post-MI syndrome, 1:115
Postoperative (2-stage) adjustment, after strabismus
    surgery, 6:176
Postoperative care of ophthalmic surgery patient,
    1:337–338
  cataract surgery and, 11:80, 108, 112
    in children, 11:198
  LASIK and, 13:115
  PRK/LASEK and
    immediate postablation measures for, 13:96
    operative day postablation treatment and,
        13:96–97
    subsequent postoperative care and, 13:97
Postoperative chest physiotherapy, 1:156
Postoperative endophthalmitis, 9:207, 208t, 209–211,
    12:328–331
  acute-onset, 9:210–211, 210i, 211i, 12:329, 330, 330i
  bleb-associated, 9:207, 208t, 212–213, 12:331, 332i
  after cataract surgery, 9:207, 208t, 209, 11:164t,
        176–178, 176i
    prevention of, 11:97
  chronic (delayed-onset), 9:211, 212, 12:329–331,
        331i
  after strabismus surgery, 6:186, 186i
    scleral perforation and, 6:185, 186i
  vitrectomy for, 12:329–331
Postoperative state, hypercoagulability and, 1:171
Postpartum pituitary necrosis (Sheehan syndrome),
    5:345
Postpartum thyroiditis, 1:227
Poststroke dementia, 1:285
Posttarsal venous drainage, of eyelid, 7:147
Posttest probability, 1:358
Posttransfusion hepatitis, transfusion-transmitted virus
    (TTV) causing, 1:32
Posttransfusion isoantibody production, 1:167
Posttranslational modification, 2:193
  of lens proteins, 2:328
Posttraumatic angle recession, 4:25, 25i, 10:42–43, 43i
  glaucoma and, 4:82–84, 83i
Posttraumatic endophthalmitis, 9:207, 208t, 211–212,
    12:300
Posttraumatic macular hole, 12:292, 294i
Postural hypertension, 1:96
Potassium
  in aqueous humor, 2:316t, 317
  in lens, 2:328
  in tear film, 2:290
  transport of, 2:361
  in vitreous, 2:337
Potassium balance, in lens, pump-leak theory of
    maintenance of, 11:20–21, 21i
Potassium channels, in lens, 2:329
Potassium-sparing diuretics, 1:87, 88t
Potential acuity meter (PAM), 3:316–317, 316i, 8:15
  in low vision evaluation, 5:97–98
  for patient evaluation before cataract surgery, 11:85
Potentials, cortical, 12:39–41
  electrically evoked, 12:41
  visually evoked. See Visually evoked cortical
      potentials

Povidone-iodine, 2:437
  for ophthalmia neonatorum prophylaxis, 6:223
Power
  for medical lasers, 3:18–19, 18t
  in phacoemulsification, 11:114, 117–118
  radiant, 2:460, 460t
Power (optical)
  of bifocal add, determining, 3:150–152
  candle (luminous intensity), 3:16t
  contact lens, 3:174, 177, 194
  curve, 3:177
  cylinder, 3:95–98
    combined lenses and, 3:100–101, 101i
    finding, 3:132–133
    refinement of, cross-cylinder refraction for,
        3:136–139, 138i
  dioptric, of bifocal segment, occupation and, 3:163
  of fluid lens, 3:180, 181i
  intraocular lens
    determination of, 3:216–221, 218i, 220t
      in adults, 11:148–152
      in children, 6:301, 11:157
    clear lens extraction/refractive lens exchange
        and, 13:160
    refractive surgery and, 3:221–222, 11:82,
        150–152, 13:65, 160, 199–203, 201t
    triple procedure and, 11:209
  incorrect, 11:193–194
  reflecting, of mirrors, 3:90
  refractive, 3:61–62
    of cornea, 8:39–40, 13:5–6
      keratometry in measurement of, 8:40–41, 13:5
    of schematic eye, 3:107t
  sphere, fogging in determination of, 3:141
  of tear lens, 3:180, 181i
Power cross, 3:95–98, 98i, 99i. See also Power (optical),
    cylinder
Power curve, contact lens, 3:174i, 177
Power maps, 8:43, 43i, 44i, 45i, 13:6–7, 47
Power prediction formulas, for IOLs, 3:218–219, 218i,
    220i, 11:149–150
Power readings, on lasers, 3:18–19, 18t
Poxviruses, ocular infection caused by, 8:121, 160–162
PPD test. See Purified protein derivative (PPD) test
PPM. See Persistent pupillary membranes
PPMD. See Posterior corneal dystrophies,
    polymorphous
PPRF. See Paramedian pontine reticular formation
PPV. See Positive predictive value
Prader-Willi syndrome
  childhood glaucoma and, 10:155t
  imprinting abnormalities causing, 2:210
Pralidoxime, 2:396i, 400
Pramipexole, for Parkinson disease, 1:279
Pramlintide, for diabetes, 1:214
Prandin. See Repaglinide
Pravachol. See Pravastatin
Pravastatin, for hypercholesterolemia, 1:149t, 150t
Prazosin
  for heart failure, 1:130
  for hypertension, 1:89t
pRB protein, retinoblastoma and, 6:394
Prealbumin. See Transthyretin
Preauricular lymph nodes, eyelids drained by, 8:7

Precancerous lesions
    definition of, 8:246–247
    eyelid, 7:172–173, 172i, 173i
Precancerous melanosis (lentigo maligna/Hutchinson's
    melanotic freckle), 7:174
Precapillary retinal arteriole obstruction, 12:145–146,
    146i. See also Cotton-wool spots
Precentral gyrus, 5:54
Precorneal tear film, 2:44, 287, 288i. See also Tear film
    (tears)
Precose. See Acarbose
Precursor cytotoxic T lymphocytes, 9:68, 69i
Pred Forte/Pred Mild. See Prednisolone
Prediabetic states, 1:206
Prednisolone, 2:394, 417t
    anti-inflammatory/pressure-elevating potency of,
        2:419t
    in combination preparations, 2:432t
    for corneal graft rejection, 8:469
    for endophthalmitis, 9:218t
    for hyphema, 6:448
    for stromal keratitis, 8:148, 149t
    for uveitis, 9:115t, 116
Prednisone
    cataracts caused by, 11:51
    for cluster headaches, 5:297
    for endophthalmitis, 9:218t
    for giant cell arteritis, 1:190, 5:122
    for optic neuritis, 5:143
    for rheumatoid arthritis, 1:174–175
    for Stevens-Johnson syndrome, 8:218
    for thyroid-associated orbitopathy, 5:331
    for toxoplasmosis, 6:217, 12:187, 187t
    for uveitis, 9:115t
Preeclampsia, 1:96, 5:343, 344i. See also Eclampsia
Preferential looking, for visual acuity testing in
    children, 6:69, 69i, 78t, 79, 202–203, 451
Preferred retinal locus (PRL), 3:246, 247i, 253
Preganglionic autonomic nerves, cholinergic drug
    action and, 2:394, 395i
Preganglionic Horner syndrome, 5:263
Pregnancy. See also under Congenital
    alcohol use during (fetal alcohol syndrome), 1:270,
        2:160–161, 161i, 162i
        childhood glaucoma and, 10:155t
        craniofacial malformations and, 6:433–434, 434i
    antiphospholipid antibody syndrome and, 1:171,
        182, 183, 184
    cocaine abuse during, 1:271
    cytomegalovirus infection during, 1:29, 6:218–219,
        219i
    diabetes during (gestational diabetes mellitus),
        1:203t, 205t, 206
    diabetic retinopathy affected by, 12:105
        timetable for ophthalmic examination and,
            12:119, 119t
    fluorescein angiography during, 12:21
    glaucoma medications during, 10:176
    herpes simplex virus infection during, 1:27,
        6:219–220, 8:139–140
    history of
        in infant with decreased vision, 6:452
        infantile corneal opacities and, 6:255, 256t
        nystagmus and, 6:161
    HIV during, chemoprophylaxis and, 1:45

hypertension/hypertension management and,
    1:96–97
immunization during, 1:303, 305, 307
maternally transmitted eye infection and, 6:215–221
    ophthalmia neonatorum and, 6:221–224, 222i
neuro-ophthalmic disorders associated with,
    5:343–345, 344i, 345i
phenytoin use during, 1:284
radiation exposure during, 1:255
refractive surgery contraindicated during, 13:41
rubella during, 6:217–218, 218i, 8:163
syphilis during, 1:15, 6:220–221
thyroiditis after, 1:227
toxemia of. See Eclampsia; Preeclampsia
toxoplasmosis during, 1:26, 6:215–217, 217i, 9:165,
    167, 168, 168i
transient visual loss in, 5:343–344, 344i, 345i
Pregnancy diagnosis, 8:282–283
Pregnancy history
    in infant with decreased vision, 6:452
    infantile corneal opacities and, 6:255, 256t
    nystagmus and, 6:161
Prehypertension, 1:81, 82, 82t, 292
    in children and adolescents, 1:97
Prelaminar nerve/prelaminar portion of optic nerve,
    2:98, 98i, 99i, 10:48, 49
    blood supply of, 2:103
PRELEX procedure (presbyopic refractive lensectomy),
    13:163–164
Preload, 1:129
    manipulation of in heart failure, 1:130, 131
Premarket approval (PMA), 13:36
    delays in, 13:37–38
Premarket Notification 510(k) application, 13:35
Premature atrial complexes, 1:135
Premature contractions, 1:135–136
Premature junctional complexes, 1:135
"Premature presbyopia" (accommodative
    insufficiency), 3:147
Premature ventricular complexes, 1:135–136
Prematurity, retinopathy of. See Retinopathy, of
    prematurity
Premelanosomes, in retinal pigment epithelium, 2:79,
    144
Prenatal diagnosis, 2:247t, 278
Prentice position, 3:85i, 86
Prentice's rule, 3:87–88, 88i, 155, 157i
    with automated lensmeter, 3:307
    bifocal design and, 3:155–162
Preocular tear film, 2:287
    tear dysfunction and, 2:294
Preoperative assessment/preparation for ocular surgery,
    1:327–335, 328t, 332t
    in adults, 1:327–328, 328t
    cataract surgery, 11:79–80
        in children, 11:195–196
    in elderly patients, 1:237
    fasting and, 1:331
    LASIK, 13:112
    medication management and, 1:331–334, 332t
    in pediatric patients, 1:328–329
    phakic intraocular lens insertion, 13:146–147
    PRK/LASEK, 13:90–93
    refractive surgery, 13:39–56, 40t
    sedation and, 1:335

specific concerns and, 1:329–331
testing recommendations and, 1:327–328
Prepapillary vascular loops, 12:280, 282*i*
Preperiosteal SOOF lift, 7:241, 242*i*
Preretinal macular fibrosis, 12:87
Presbyopia, 3:147, 11:22, 23, 13:167–180
catenary (hydraulic support) theory of
accommodation and, 13:171
in contact lens wearers, correction of, 3:182–183
Helmholtz theory of accommodation and, 13:168
"premature" (accommodative insufficiency), 3:147
Schachar theory of accommodation and, 13:169–170
surgical correction of, 13:167–180
accommodating IOLs for, 13:178–180, 179*i*
accommodative, 13:176–180
clear lens extraction/refractive lens exchange for,
13:158
conductive keratoplasty for, 13:173
corneal inlays for, 13:175–176
custom/multifocal ablations for, 13:174–175, 174*i*
monovision and, 13:171–172
multifocal IOLs for, 13:163–164, 163*i*, 173
nonaccommodative, 13:171–176
refractive surgery and, 13:42
scleral surgery for, 13:176–177, 177*i*
Presbyopic refractive lensectomy (PRELEX procedure),
13:163–164
Preschool children. *See also* Children
low vision in, 3:266
Presentation time, perimetry affected by, 10:64–65
Preseptal cellulitis, 4:170, 170*i*, 7:41–42
in children, 6:230–231
after strabismus surgery, 6:185–186
Preseptal orbicularis muscles, 7:140, 140*i*, 143*i*
Preseptal palpebral muscle, 5:56
Preseptal tissues, 7:139
Preservatives
in contact lens solutions, allergic/sensitivity reactions
and, 3:210, 8:107, 107*i*
in ocular medications
allergic/adverse reactions to, 2:381, 450,
8:101–102, 375–376
demulcents, 2:450, 8:75
irrigating solutions, 2:451
persistent corneal defects caused by (toxic
ulcerative keratopathy), 8:101–102, 375–376
toxic keratoconjunctivitis caused by, 8:393–395
Press-on prism, 3:89–90, 160
for basic (acquired) esotropia, 6:104–105
for esotropia in sixth nerve palsy, 6:107
for nystagmus, 6:168
for overcorrection of intermittent exotropia, 6:113
for thyroid-associated orbitopathy, 5:331
Pressure, episcleral venous, 10:22–23
Pressure-independent outflow, 10:22
Presumed ocular histoplasmosis syndrome, 12:79–81,
80*i*. *See also* Ocular histoplasmosis syndrome
PresVIEW scleral expansion bands, 13:176, 177*i*
Pretarsal orbicularis muscles, 7:139–140, 143*i*
Pretarsal palpebral muscle, 5:56
Pretarsal space, 2:27*i*
Pretarsal tissues, 7:139, 140*i*
venous drainage of, 7:147

Pretectal (Parinaud/dorsal midbrain) syndrome,
5:208–209, 210*i*
eyelid retraction in, 5:279, 7:224
nystagmus in, 6:167
Pretectum/pretectal nuclei, 2:110, 5:27
vertical gaze palsy caused by, damage to, 5:209, 210*i*
Pretest probability, 1:357–359, 358*t*
Pretibial myxedema. *See* Infiltrative dermopathy
Pretrichial brow lift, 7:241
Preventive medicine, 1:291–311
immunization in, 1:302–311
ophthalmology practices and, 8:50–51
recent developments in, 1:291
screening procedures in, 1:291–302. *See also*
Screening/diagnostic tests
Preveon. *See* Adefovir
Prevnar. *See* Pneumococcal vaccine
Primacor. *See* Milrinone
Primaquine, for *Pneumocystis carinii (Pneumocystis
jiroveci)* pneumonia, 1:45
Primary acquired melanosis, 4:56–59, 56*t*, 57*i*, 58*i*,
8:266–268, 267*i*, 267*t*
Primary angle-closure glaucoma. *See* Angle-closure
glaucoma, primary
Primary antiphospholipid antibody syndrome, 1:182
Primary central nervous system lymphomas,
9:228–231, 228*i*
Primary congenital glaucoma, 10:147
Primary dye test (Jones I test), 7:268, 269*t*
Primary endothelial failure, after penetrating
keratoplasty, 8:461
Primary glaucoma. *See* Glaucoma
Primary HIV infection (retroviral syndrome), 1:38
Primary lens fibers, 2:146
development of, 11:26–27, 27*i*
Primary open-angle glaucoma (POAG). *See* Open-
angle glaucoma, primary
Primary position of gaze, 6:13, 28, 86, 88*i*
Primary sensory cortex (postcentral gyrus), 5:50, 50*i*,
51*i*
Primary visual (striate/occipital) cortex. *See* Visual
(calcarine/occipital) cortex
Primary vitreous, persistent hyperplasia of (persistent
fetal vasculature), 4:106, 106*i*, 11:42, 12:280–283,
283*i*
retinoblastoma differentiated from, 4:256–257, 256*t*
Primaxin. *See* Imipenem-cilastin
Primers, in polymerase chain reaction, 2:193, 229*i*, 230
Priming
of effector lymphocytes, 9:25
of macrophages, 9:51*i*, 52
Primitive streak, 2:136
Primitive zone, 2:138–140
Primordium (anlage), 2:125, 127
Prince rule, 3:151
Principal meridians
alignment of, combination of spherocylindrical
lenses and, 3:99–100
of astigmatic surface or lens, 3:95–98, 98*i*
locating axes of, in retinoscopy, 3:130–132, 131*i*,
132*i*
Principal planes, 3:75–76
Principal points, 3:75–76
Prinivil. *See* Lisinopril
Prinzide. *See* Lisinopril

Prinzmetal (variant) angina, 1:113
Prions, 8:134
Prism adaptation test, 6:92
Prism and cover test (alternate cover test), 6:82, 83i
    for intermittent exotropia evaluation, 6:111
    simultaneous, 6:82
Prism diopter, 3:85–86, 86i
Prism dissociation, for binocular balance testing, 3:141
Prism power, 3:31. See also Transverse magnification
Prisms, 3:84–90, 84i
    aberrations of, 3:89
    angle of deviation and, 3:84–85, 85i
    anophthalmic socket camouflage and, 7:127
    for basic (acquired) esotropia, 6:104–105
    effect of lens on (Prentice's rule), 3:87–88, 88i, 155,
        157i
    for esotropia in sixth nerve palsy, 6:107
    Fresnel. See Fresnel prisms
    in functional visual disorder evaluation, 5:307
    for homonymous hemianopia, 3:260
    image displacement and, 3:86–87, 86i
    for induced tropia test, 6:79
    for intermittent exotropia, 6:113
    inverting
        in operating microscope, 3:296, 297i
        in slit-lamp biomicroscope, 3:280, 282i
    for low-vision patients, 3:260
    methods for using, 3:170
    for monofixation syndrome evaluation, 6:61–63, 63i
    for nystagmus, 3:260, 6:168
    for overcorrection of intermittent exotropia, 6:113
    parallel, for low-vision patients, 3:260
    partial, for low-vision patients, 3:260
    plane parallel plate, 3:84, 85i
    Porro-Abbe, 3:280, 282i, 297i
    Prentice's rule and, 3:87–88, 88i, 155, 157i
        bifocal design and, 3:155–162
    Risley, 3:89
    rotary, 3:89
    in slit-lamp biomicroscope, 3:280, 282i
    therapeutic use of, 3:169–170
    for thyroid-associated orbitopathy, 5:331
    for undercorrection of intermittent exotropia, 6:114
    vector addition of, 3:88–89, 88i
    wavefront aberrations and, 13:15, 16i
Private sequence variations, 2:214
PRK. See Photorefractive keratectomy
PRL. See Phakic Refractive Lens; Preferred retinal locus
PRNG. See Penicillin-resistant N gonorrhoeae
Probability of outcome, baseline, 1:361
Proband, 2:193, 275, 8:308
Probing of lacrimal system
    for acquired nasolacrimal duct/canalicular
        obstruction, 7:271, 275
    for congenital dacryocele, 6:241
    for congenital nasolacrimal duct obstruction, 6:243,
        243–245, 244i, 245i, 7:261, 262–265, 263i
Procaine, 2:445t
Procaine penicillin, 1:55t
Procardia. See Nifedipine
Procerus muscle, 7:140, 143i
Process (content of care), 1:362
Processing phase of immune response arc, 9:22–24, 23i
    response to poison ivy and, 9:29, 30
    response to tuberculosis and, 9:30–31

Prodrugs, 2:389
Product Development Protocol (PDP), 13:36
Profenal. See Suprofen
Progenitor cell, 2:127
Prograf. See Tacrolimus
Programmed cell death (PCD/apoptosis), 2:125, 181,
        182, 6:206, 8:247t, 248
    by cytotoxic T lymphocytes, 9:68, 69i
    in DNA repair, 2:213
    Fas ligand in, 9:38, 68, 69i
Progressive addition lenses, 3:152–155, 154i, 156i
Progressive external ophthalmoplegia, chronic,
        6:150–151, 153t, 12:236, 245, 246t, 247i
    mitochondrial DNA deletions and, 2:218
Progressive facial hemiatrophy, 8:353t
Progressive multifocal leukoencephalopathy, in HIV
        infection/AIDS, 5:362, 363i
Progressive myopia. See High (pathologic/degenerative)
        myopia
Progressive outer retinal necrosis (PORN), 9:155, 156i
    in HIV infection/AIDS, 9:155, 253–254, 254i
Progressive supranuclear palsy, 5:199
    slowed saccades in, 5:206
Progressive systemic sclerosis (scleroderma), 1:185–186
    eyelid manifestations of, 4:173t
Project-O-Chart slide, 6:94
Projection charts, polarizing, 3:11
Prokaryotes/prokaryotic cells, 2:193, 8:122–123. See
        also Bacteria
Prolactinomas (lactotroph adenomas), 1:228
Prolate cornea, 13:6
    intrastromal corneal ring segments and, 13:77
Prolixin. See Fluphenazine
Promoter, 2:193, 202, 202i
Propagation of light, 3:39–54
    curved surfaces and, 3:51, 52i
    Fermat's principle and, 3:51–53, 53i
    law of reflection and, 3:42–44
    law of refraction and, 3:44–46, 46i
    normal incidence and, 3:46–47
    optical interfaces and, 3:41–42, 42i
    optical media and, 3:39–41, 40t
    rectilinear, law of, 3:41, 42i
    refractive index and, 3:39–41, 40t
    specular reflection and, 3:42–44, 42i, 43i
    specular transmission and, 3:44–46, 45i, 46i
    stigmatic imaging and, 3:53–54, 54i
    total internal reflection and, 3:47–49, 48i, 50i
Propamidine, for Acanthamoeba keratitis, 8:189
Proparacaine, 2:446t, 447–448
Prophylactic Treatment of AMD Trial (PTAMD),
        12:61–62
Propine. See Dipivefrin
Propionibacterium acnes, 8:126, 126i
    as normal ocular flora, 8:115, 115t, 126
    ocular infection caused by, 8:126
        endophthalmitis, 4:97, 98i, 9:53, 208t, 209,
            210–211, 212i, 12:329
Propofol, perioperative, 1:332t, 335
Proposita/propositus, 2:193, 275
Propranolol, 1:88t, 90t, 2:404i
Proptosis (exophthalmos/exorbitism), 4:187, 6:207,
        7:23–25
    bilateral, 7:23–24, 26
    in craniosynostosis, 6:426

evaluation checklist for, 7:27
exposure keratopathy and, 8:95
in Graves ophthalmopathy (thyrotoxic), 4:189–190,
190i, 5:329, 7:26, 48, 48i, 53. *See also* Thyroid
ophthalmopathy
in children, 6:149, 149i, 384, 384i
eyelid retraction differentiated from, 7:223–224
in orbital cellulitis, 6:231, 232i
in orbital phycomycosis, 7:45–46
in orbital tumors, 7:23–24
lymphangioma, 6:379
neuroblastoma, 6:374
rhabdomyosarcoma, 6:373
teratoma, 6:382, 382i
in retinoblastoma, 4:254–255, 255i
unilateral, 7:26
in uveal lymphoid infiltration, 4:279–280
Propulsid. *See* Cisapride
Propylene glycol, for dry eye, 2:450
Propylthiouracil, for Graves hyperthyroidism, 1:225
Prosom. *See* Estazolam
Prosopagnosia, 5:192
Prospective Evaluation of Radial Keratotomy (PERK)
study, 13:60
Prostacyclin, 2:305, 306i
Prostaglandin analogs, 2:413–414, 414t, 10:163t,
171–172
Prostaglandin G/H synthase. *See* Cyclooxygenase
Prostaglandin inhibitors, for cystoid macular edema,
12:155
Prostaglandins, 2:305–306, 306i, 8:200t, 9:78–79, 78i
for childhood glaucoma, 6:283
modes of action of, 2:314t
nonsteroidal anti-inflammatory drugs and, 9:96
receptors for, 2:307
in signal transduction, 2:312, 314t
synthesis of, 2:305–306, 306i
anti-inflammatory drugs affecting, 2:306–307
Prostamides, for glaucoma, 10:163t, 171–172
Prostate cancer, 1:296
orbital metastases in, 7:95i, 96
screening for, 1:296
Prostate-specific antigen, in cancer screening, 1:296
Prostheses, ocular, 7:122
Prostigmin. *See* Neostigmine
Protan defects, 12:43, 195, 196t
ocular findings in carriers of, 2:270t
Protease inhibitors, 1:3, 42, 9:246, 247t
antituberculous drug interactions and, 1:49
in HAART, 1:43
Protease-sparing regimen, in HAART, 1:43
Proteases
corneal, as inflammatory mediators, 8:198t
microbial, in ocular infections, 8:117
PMN-derived, 9:86
Protein AF, 8:348
Protein AP, 8:348
Protein C (activated protein C), 1:164, 165
deficiency of, 1:170
resistance to, 1:170
Protein kinase C, diabetes complications and, 1:217
Protein kinase C/Ca²⁺–dependent signal transduction,
in tear secretion, 2:292–293, 292i
Protein kinase C inhibitors, in diabetes management,
1:201, 217

Protein S, 1:164, 165
deficiency of, 1:170
Proteinaceous degeneration, 8:368–369. *See also*
Spheroidal degeneration
Proteinase-3, scleritis/retinal vasculitis in Wegener
granulomatosis and, 1:192, 9:62
Proteinase inhibitors
in aqueous humor, 2:319
in cornea, 2:301
Proteinases
in aqueous humor, 2:317, 319
in cornea, 2:301
Proteins
in aqueous humor, 2:304, 305, 316–317, 318–320
breakdown of blood–aqueous barrier and, 2:322
dynamics and, 2:305
disorders of metabolism of, corneal changes in,
8:345–349
lens. *See* Lens proteins
in retinal pigment epithelium, 2:358
in rod outer segments ("rim" proteins), 2:344, 344t
mutations of, 2:347, 347i
synthesis of, 2:210–212, 211i
in tear film, 2:290
vitreous, 2:337
Proteoglycans
corneal, 2:300, 8:10
scleral, 8:14
Proteus, 8:126
postoperative endophthalmitis caused by, 9:211
Prothrombin, mutation in gene for, 1:170
Prothrombin time (PT), 1:165
international normalized ratio and, 1:165
Proton density MRI, 5:62, 63i, 64i, 7:30
parameters of, 5:64t
signal intensity on, 5:65t
Proto-oncogene, 2:193
Protoplasmic astrocytes, 2:84
Protozoal infection
gastrointestinal, in HIV infection/AIDS, 1:48–49
ocular, 8:131–132, 131i, 9:164–169
Protractors, eyelid, 7:139–140, 143i
Proventil. *See* Albuterol
Provera. *See* Medroxyprogesterone
Proximal (instrument) convergence, 6:38
Proximal fusion, tenacious, in intermittent exotropia,
6:111
Proximal illumination, for slit-lamp biomicroscopy,
8:18
Prozac. *See* Fluoxetine
PRP. *See* Panretinal photocoagulation
Prussian blue stain, Perls, 4:36t
PSA. *See* Prostate-specific antigen
PSC. *See* Posterior subcapsular (cupuliform) cataract
Pseudoadenomatous hyperplasia (Fuchs adenoma),
4:146, 241–242
Pseudocholinesterase, defective, succinylcholine effects
and, 2:279
Pseudocolobomas, in Treacher Collins syndrome, 6:432
Pseudocryptophthalmos, 8:285, 286
Pseudocyst, foveal, 12:91
Pseudodementia, in elderly, 1:240
Pseudodominance, 2:194, 264
Pseudoepiphora, 7:274

Pseudoepitheliomatous hyperplasia, **7:**164, **8:**255*t*, 256–257
Pseudoesotropia, **6:**86, 97, 97*t*
Pseudoexfoliation (exfoliation syndrome), **4:**80, 81*i*, 97–98, 98*i*, **10:**42, 99–101, 99*i*, 100*i*, **11:**65–66, 66*i*
    zonular incompetence and, cataract surgery in patient with, **11:**226–227, 227*i*, 228*i*
Pseudoexotropia, **6:**109
    in retinopathy of prematurity, **6:**331, 331*i*
Pseudo Foster Kennedy syndrome, **5:**123
Pseudogene, **2:**194
Pseudoglands of Henle, **4:**45
Pseudogliomas, **4:**140
    in incontinentia pigmenti, **6:**419
Pseudoguttae, inflammatory, **8:**29
Pseudohermaphrodites, **2:**252
Pseudo–Hurler polydystrophy, **6:**436*t*, **8:**342
Pseudohypopyon, retinoblastoma causing, **4:**253–255, 254*i*
Pseudoisochromatic plates, for color vision testing, **12:**43, 44*i*
    in low vision evaluation, **5:**96
Pseudomelanoma, **4:**229
Pseudomembrane, **4:**45, **8:**24*t*, 25*t*
Pseudomembranous enterocolitis, *Clostridium difficile* causing, **1:**8
Pseudomonas
    aeruginosa, **1:**14–15, **8:**126, 127*i*
        resistant strains of, **1:**14, 15
    ocular infection/inflammation caused by, **8:**126
        keratitis, **8:**179–180, 180*i*
        postoperative endophthalmitis, **9:**211
Pseudopapilledema, **5:**113, 115, **6:**367–368, 367*t*
    drusen and, **5:**115, 115*i*, **6:**368, 368*i*
Pseudopemphigoid, **8:**219–220, 394, 395
Pseudophakia, prophylactic treatment of retinal breaks and, **12:**267
Pseudophakic bullous edema, after cataract surgery, **8:**419–420
Pseudophakic bullous keratopathy, after cataract surgery, **8:**419–420, **11:**164*t*, 192–193, 193*i*
Pseudophakic glaucoma, **10:**132
    in children, **6:**280
Pseudoplasticity, of viscoelastic substance, **11:**158
Pseudopolycoria, **6:**269, 269*i*
Pseudoproptosis, **6:**372, **7:**26
Pseudoptosis, **5:**278, **7:**219, 220*i*
Pseudoretinitis pigmentosa
    in congenital rubella, **6:**218
    in congenital syphilis, **6:**220
Pseudo-Roth spots, in leukemia, **4:**281
Pseudostrabismus, **6:**86
    in epicanthus, **7:**156
    in retinopathy of prematurity, **6:**331, 331*i*
Pseudotumor
    cerebri (idiopathic intracranial hypertension), **5:**118–120, 118*t*, **6:**366–367
    orbital. *See* Orbital inflammatory syndrome
Pseudoxanthoma elasticum, **1:**166
    angioid streaks in, **12:**83, 83*i*, 237
    peau d'orange fundus changes in, **12:**83, 83*i*, 237
PSF. *See* Point spread function
Psoriasis, **1:**178
Psoriatic arthritis, **1:**178, **9:**132, 133*i*
    uveitis in children and, **6:**313*t*, 314

PSR. *See* Sickle cell retinopathy, proliferative
Psychiatric disorders. *See* Behavioral/psychiatric disorders
Psychic paralysis of gaze, **5:**194
Psychomotor seizures, **1:**281
Psychophysical testing, **12:**41–47. *See also specific test*
Psychotic disorder. *See also* Schizophrenia
    brief, **1:**265
Psychotropic drugs
    dependence and, **1:**267
    tear production affected by, **8:**81*t*
PT. *See* Prothrombin time
PTAMD (Prophylactic Treatment of AMD Trial), **12:**61–62
PTC. *See* Pseudotumor, cerebri
PTCA. *See* Percutaneous transluminal coronary angioplasty
Pterygium, **4:**50, 50*i*, **8:**309*t*, 366, 366*i*
    conjunctival transplantation for, **8:**429, 430*i*, 431–432
    excision of, **8:**429, 430*i*
        bacterial scleritis after, **8:**191, 191*i*
Pterygoid process, of sphenoid bone, **5:**5, 9
Pterygoid venous plexus, **5:**20, 22*i*
    eyelids drained by, **7:**147
Pterygomaxillary area, **5:**9, 10
Pterygopalatine fossa, **5:**11, **7:**21
Pterygopalatine ganglion/nerves, **2:**119, **5:**52
PTK. *See* Phototherapeutic keratectomy
Ptosis (blepharoptosis), **5:**276–279, **6:**153*t*, 213–214, 213*t*, **7:**208–223
    acquired, **5:**277–278, 278*t*, **6:**213–214, 213*t*, **7:**208
        aponeurotic, **7:**215, 216*i*
        eyelid position in downgaze and, **7:**211–212
        myogenic, **7:**214
        neurogenic, **7:**217–218
    anophthalmic, **7:**127
    aponeurotic, **7:**215, 216*i*, 217*t*
    apparent (pseudoptosis), **7:**219, 220*i*
    bilateral, **5:**226
    in blepharophimosis syndrome, **6:**213, 213*i*
    in blowout fractures, **7:**103
    botulinum toxin causing, **5:**277, **6:**196
    botulinum toxin for, **7:**226
    brow, **7:**234–235, 234*i*
    cerebral, **5:**277
    in children, **6:**153*t*, 213–214, 213*t*
    in chronic progressive external ophthalmoplegia, **5:**334, 334*i*, **6:**153*t*
    classification of, **6:**213*t*, **7:**208–209, 213–219
    congenital, **5:**276, 277*i*, **6:**213–214, 213*t*, **7:**208, 214
        amblyopia in, **7:**211
        aponeurotic, **7:**215
        eyelid fissure changes in, **2:**23*i*
        eyelid position in downgaze and, **7:**211–212
        myogenic, **7:**214, 214*i*, 217*t*
        neurogenic, **7:**215–218, 218*i*
    enucleation and, **7:**123
    essential, **7:**226
    evaluation of, **7:**208–209
        in children, **6:**213–214
    in Graves eye disease (thyroid ophthalmology), **6:**153*t*
    in Horner syndrome, **7:**217
        pharmacologic testing for, **7:**212–213, 212*i*

induction of, botulinum toxin in, 5:286
levator aponeurotic defects causing, 5:278
lower eyelid, 7:217
Marcus Gunn jaw-winking, 5:276, 277i, 279, 281, 6:214, 7:217, 218i
synkinesis in, 6:214, 7:211, 217, 218i
mechanical, 5:278, 7:219, 8:23
in myasthenia gravis, 5:274i, 275, 327, 327i, 6:143t, 151, 151i, 7:213, 218
edrophonium chloride (Tensilon) test and, 7:213
myogenic, 7:214, 214i, 217t
in neurofibromatosis, 5:274i
neurogenic, 7:215–219, 218i
nonphysiologic causes of, 5:314
in orbital rhabdomyosarcoma, 6:373, 373i
physical examination of patient with, 7:209–213, 211i, 212i
steroid-induced, 5:278
surgical repair of, 7:220–223, 221i
synkinesis in, 6:214, 7:211, 217, 218i
traumatic, 5:278, 7:219
treatment of, 7:187, 220–223, 221i
in children, 6:213–214
visual field testing in, 7:212
Ptosis data sheet, 7:210, 210i
PTSD. See Post-traumatic stress disorder
PTT. See Partial thromboplastin time
Pubic louse (Phthirus pubis), 8:133, 133i
ocular infection caused by, 8:133, 169
cholinesterase inhibitors for, 2:400
Public health ophthalmology, 8:51, 51t
PUK. See Peripheral keratitis, ulcerative
Pulfrich phenomenon, 5:189
Pull-over (stay) sutures, 6:176
Pulley system, rectus muscle, 6:21
Pulmicort. See Budesonide
Pulmonary diseases, 1:153–158
evaluation of, 1:155
obstructive, 1:153–154
ocular surgery in patients with, 1:329, 11:203–204
preoperative and postoperative considerations in patient with, 1:158
recent developments in, 1:153
restrictive, 1:154
treatment of, 1:155–158, 157t
Pulmonary function tests, 1:155
Pulsation, orbital, 7:24, 26–27
Pulse pressure, in shock, 1:318
Pulsed-dye laser therapy, for capillary hemangiomas, 7:66
Pulseless disease (Takayasu arteritis), 1:189t, 191
Pump-leak theory, 11:20–21, 21i
Pumping, for lasers, 3:19, 21–22, 22i
Punch (incisional) biopsy, 7:171, 176i
Puncta, 2:22, 34, 6:239, 7:254, 255i
atresia of, 6:239–240
disorders of
acquired, 7:274
congenital, 6:239–240, 7:257–258
agenesis and dysgenesis, 7:257–258, 265–267
malposition of, 7:274
supernumerary, 6:240
Punctal occlusion
for cicatricial pemphigoid, 8:223
for dry eye, 7:274, 8:75t, 76–77

Punctate epithelial defects/erosions
conjunctival, 8:24t
corneal, 8:24t, 30i, 32t
refractive surgery and, 13:44, 45i
Punctate epithelial keratitis/keratopathy, 8:24t, 29, 30i, 32t
contact lens wear and, 3:208
exposure causing, 8:95
microsporidial, 8:190
staphylococcal blepharoconjunctivitis and, 8:165, 166i, 168
superficial Thygeson, 8:224–225, 225i
topical anesthetic abuse causing, 8:105–106
Punctate inner choroiditis/choroidopathy (PIC), 9:177t, 182, 183i, 12:174t, 179, 179i
Punctate outer retinal toxoplasmosis (PORT), 9:166, 167i
Punctate staining patterns (fluorescein), 8:20, 21t
Pupil. See Pupils
Pupil–optic nerve (PO) section, 4:33–34, 34i
Pupil size, perimetry affected by, 10:65
Pupil-sparing third nerve (oculomotor) palsy, 5:230–231
Pupillary block
in angle-closure glaucoma, 10:120–121, 121i
angle closure without, 10:121–122, 121t
after cataract surgery, flat anterior chamber and, 11:166
microspherophakia causing, 11:33
secondary angle-closure glaucoma without, 10:132–146
secondary angle closure with, 10:128–132, 129i, 131i, 131t
Pupillary capture, after cataract surgery, 11:184–185, 185i
Pupillary (central) cysts, 6:265
Pupillary defects, 5:257–271
afferent. See also Relative afferent pupillary defect
in traumatic optic neuropathy, 7:107
in ptosis, 7:212
Pupillary light-near dissociation, 5:269–270, 269t
Pupillary light reflex (pupillary response to light), 5:57, 59i, 85, 86i. See also Pupils, examination of
consensual response in, 5:258
direct response in, 5:258
disorders of, 5:269–270, 269t
evaluation of before cataract surgery, 11:81
in functional visual disorders, 5:305
in infant with decreased vision, 6:452
midbrain lesions affecting, 5:270
in newborn, 6:201, 451
in nystagmus evaluation, 6:162, 163t
paradoxical, 5:270, 6:162, 163t, 452
pathways for, 2:110–111
Pupillary membrane (anterior vascular capsule), 2:155, 11:29, 29i
persistent, 6:267–268, 268i
Pupillary ruff, 2:64
Pupilloplasty, for cataracts, 11:77
trauma and, 11:225
Pupils
abnormalities of, 5:257–271. See also specific type
examination of, 5:258–259
rare, 5:270–271
size/shape/location and, 6:261, 268–269, 269i

accommodation and, **5:**313–314
Adie's. *See* Pupils, tonic
Argyll-Robertson, **5:**270
  in syphilis, **9:**190
Argyll-Robertson-like, **5:**270
constriction of, in near reflex, **2:**111
deformed (corectopia), **2:**170, **6:**269
  midbrain, **5:**260
dilation of. *See* Mydriasis/mydriatics
displaced (ectopia), **2:**170
distance between, bifocal segment decentration and, **3:**163
in ectopia lentis et pupillae, **11:**42
entrance, **3:**110
examination of, **5:**258–259
  before cataract surgery, **11:**81
  in glaucoma, **10:**33
  in infant with decreased vision, **6:**452
  in nystagmus, **6:**162, 163*t*
  PERRLA mnemonic in, **5:**257
  in ptosis, **7:**212
  before refractive surgery, **13:**43
    PRK/LASEK, **13:**90
fixed and dilated, **5:**313–314
in infants and children, **6:**200–201
irregularity of, **5:**259–260
keyhole (iris coloboma), **2:**171, 171*i*, **6:**262–264, 263*i*
Marcus Gunn. *See* Marcus Gunn pupil
ovalization of
  after anterior chamber phakic IOL insertion, **13:**151, 153*t*
  after iris-fixated phakic IOL insertion, **13:**153*t*
position of, wavefront aberration as function of, **3:**102, 103*i*
reactivity/response of to light. *See* Pupillary light reflex
size of
  abnormalities in, **6:**268
  baseline, **5:**259
  change in, **5:**314
  contrast sensitivity affected by, **3:**115
  evaluation of, **5:**258
  perimetry affected by, **10:**65
  refractive surgery and, **3:**235–236
  visual resolution affected by, **3:**109–110
small, in glaucoma patient, cataract surgery and, **11:**219
springing, **5:**270–271
tadpole, **5:**259–260
in third nerve palsy, **5:**228–230, 229*i*
tonic (Adie's pupil/syndrome), **5:**266–267, 267*i*, 268*i*
  testing for, **2:**395–396
white. *See* Leukocoria
Purified neurotoxin complex, **2:**449
Purified protein derivative (PPD) test, **1:**23–24, **9:**194–195. *See also* Tuberculin skin test
  immune response arc and, **9:**31
Purine antagonists, in cancer chemotherapy, **1:**258*t*
Purine bases/purines, **2:**191, 194, 199, 200*i*, **8:**306
  hyperuricemia caused by disorders of metabolism of, **8:**354–355
Purite. *See* Oxychloro complex
Purkinje cells, **5:**40
Purkinje-Sanson image, **3:**293

Purkinje's entoptic phenomenon, evaluation of, before cataract surgery, **11:**86
Purpura, **1:**166
  Henoch-Schönlein, **1:**189*t*
  idiopathic thrombocytopenic, **1:**167
  thrombotic thrombocytopenic, **1:**167
    choroidal perfusion abnormalities and, **12:**166
Pursuit eye movements/pursuit pathways/system, **5:**198, **6:**39
  assessment of, **5:**203
  dysfunction of, **5:**210
  smooth, **5:**34, 35–36*i*, **6:**39
Purtscher/Purtscher-like retinopathy, **12:**94–95, 94*i*, 95*t*
Pustule, of eyelid, **8:**24*t*
PVCs. *See* Premature ventricular complexes
PVD. *See* Posterior vitreous detachment
PVL. *See* Periventricular leukomalacia
PVR. *See* Vitreoretinopathies, proliferative
PXE. *See* Pseudoxanthoma elasticum
Pyoceles, orbital invasion by, **7:**93
Pyogenic granuloma, **8:**270*t*, 271, 271*i*
  in children, **6:**388
Pyramidal tract, **2:**116
Pyrazolones, **2:**421. *See also* Nonsteroidal anti-inflammatory drugs
Pyridoxine (vitamin B$_6$)
  for gyrate atrophy, **12:**225–226
  for homocystinuria, **2:**281, **6:**438
Pyrimethamine, **2:**433
  for toxoplasmosis, **6:**216, **9:**168, **12:**187, 187*t*
Pyrimidine antagonists
  in cancer chemotherapy, **1:**258*t*
  for rheumatic disorders, **1:**199
Pyrimidine bases/pyrimidines, **2:**191, 194, 199, 200*i*, **8:**306
Pythagorean theorem, review of, **3:**32–33, 33*i*

Q

q arm, **2:**194, 205
Q/D. *See* Quinupristin/dalfopristin
Q factor, corneal shape and, **3:**231–232
Q formula, Hoffer, for IOL power selection, **13:**202
  clear lens extraction/refractive lens exchange and, **13:**160
Q value, **13:**8–9
Q wave infarction, **1:**114, 116. *See also* Acute coronary syndrome
  management of, **1:**124–125
Q waves, in myocardial infarction, **1:**114, 116
QCT. *See* Dual-energy quantitative computed tomography
Quadrafoil, **13:**17, 19*i*
Quality, of field, in perimetry interpretation, **10:**68
Quality improvement, continuous, **1:**370, 371*i*
Quantum optics, definition of, **3:**3
Quetiapine, **1:**272
Quibron. *See* Theophylline
Quickert sutures, for involutional entropion, **7:**204
Quinapril, **1:**88*t*, 90*t*
Quinolones, **1:**54, 62*t*, 72–73. *See also specific agent*
Quinupristin/dalfopristin, **1:**63*t*, 74
Quxin. *See* Levofloxacin

R

RA. *See* Rheumatoid arthritis
Rab escort protein 1 *(REP 1/CHM)* gene mutation,
    2:351
    in choroideremia, 2:351, 12:224
Rabies vaccination, 1:310
Rabies virus, ocular infection caused by, 8:163
Raccoon ascarid *(Baylisascaris procyonis),* diffuse
    unilateral subacute neuroretinitis caused by, 9:172,
    12:190
Race
    angle closure/angle closure glaucoma and, 10:11,
        122–123
    cancer and, 1:252, 253, 254
    genetic disorders and, 2:259–260
    hypertension and, 1:97
    open-angle glaucoma and, 10:10, 86, 91t
Racemose angioma/hemangioma (Wyburn-Mason
    syndrome), 4:248, 249i, 5:336t, 342–343, 343i,
    6:402t, 419–420, 420i, 12:163
Racquet (single pedicle) flaps, 8:438
rad (R/roentgen), radiation dose measurement, 1:255
Radial incisions
    for keratorefractive surgery, corneal biomechanics
        affected by, 8:13, 13:19
    for radial keratotomy, 13:61, 62i
        depth affecting outcome and, 13:61
Radial keratotomy (RK), 13:21t, 59–66
    cataract surgery after, 11:211, 13:65, 202
        intraocular lens power calculation and, 11:151
    complications of, 13:60, 63–64, 64i, 65i
    contact lens fitting after, 3:202, 13:205–206
    corneal topography and, postoperative, 13:10, 10i, 63
    difference map and, 13:10, 10i
    efficacy and predictability of, 13:62–63
    history of, 13:59, 60i
    hyperopic shift and, 13:60, 63, 64
    iron lines associated with, 8:378
    ocular surgery after, 13:64–65
    patient selection for, 13:61
    penetrating keratoplasty after, 13:65, 203
    refraction after, 13:63
        stability of, 13:63
    retinal detachment and, 13:192
    surgical techniques for, 13:61
    in United States, 13:60–61
    variables affecting outcome of, 13:61–63, 62i
    visual acuity after, 13:63
Radial perineuritis, *Acanthamoeba* keratitis and, 8:187
Radial perivascular lattice degeneration, 4:127–128
Radial thermal keratoplasty, 13:137–138
Radiance (brightness), 2:460, 460t, 3:15, 16t. *See also*
    Intensity
    as image characteristic, 3:39
    for medical lasers, 3:18, 18t
Radiant energy, for medical lasers, 3:18, 18t
Radiant energy density, for medical lasers, 3:18, 18t
Radiant exposure, 2:460, 460t
    effective, 2:462
Radiant flux, 3:16t
Radiant intensity, 3:16t
    for medical lasers, 3:18t
Radiant power, 2:460, 460t
    for medical lasers, 3:18, 18t

Radiation. *See also* Radiation therapy; Ultraviolet light
    anterior segment injury caused by, 8:388–389
    carcinogenic effects of, 1:253
    cataracts caused by, 11:55–57
    eye and adnexa affected by, 1:255–256
    fetal exposure and, 1:255
    in free radical generation, 2:366
    retina affected by, 12:305–309, 306i
    tissue damage from, 2:459–465, 460t
Radiation optic neuropathy, 1:256
    MR imaging of, 5:65i
Radiation retinopathy, 1:256, 12:305, 306i
Radiation therapy, 1:255–256, 5:69–70
    for basal cell carcinoma of eyelid, 7:179
    for capillary hemangiomas, 7:66
    for choroidal hemangioma, 4:245
    complications of, 5:70
    for Graves ophthalmopathy, 5:331, 7:54–55
    increased sensitivity to, in ataxia-telangiectatsia,
        6:417
    for lacrimal gland tumors, 7:91
    for lacrimal sac tumors, 7:284
    for lymphoma, 4:278
    for lymphoproliferative lesions of orbit, 7:87
    for melanoma, 4:237–238
    for metastatic eye disease, 4:273–275
    for optic nerve glioma, 5:151, 7:74–75
    for optic nerve sheath meningioma, 5:148, 7:78
    optic neuropathy after, 1:256
    for parasellar tumors, 5:163
    for retinal capillary hemangioma, 4:247
    for retinoblastoma, 4:263, 6:396
    retinopathy after, 1:256, 12:305, 306i
    for rhabdomyosarcoma, 7:80
    for uveal lymphoid infiltration, 4:280
Radiculitis, herpes, 5:360
Radioactive iodine
    for thyroid (Graves) ophthalmopathy, 1:225, 7:54
    for thyroid scanning, 1:223
Radioactive iodine uptake, 1:223
Radioactive plaque therapy (brachytherapy)
    for choroidal hemangioma, 4:245
    for melanoma, 4:237
        of iris, 4:218
    for metastatic eye disease, 4:273–275
    for retinoblastoma, 4:263
Radiofrequency
    for conductive keratoplasty, 13:139, 140i, 141i
    for punctal occlusion, 8:77
Radiofrequency catheter ablation, for atrial fibrillation/
    flutter, 1:138
Radiography
    chest, in pulmonary diseases, 1:155
    for foreign-body identification, 12:297–298
    in orbital evaluation, 7:27–28, 28i
Radiometric quantities/units, 2:460, 460t
Radiometry, 3:14
    terms used in, 3:16t
Radionuclide scintigraphy/scans
    for acquired tearing evaluation, 7:272, 273i
    in ischemic heart disease, 1:119
Radius of curvature, 8:9, 41
    instantaneous (tangential power), 8:43, 43i, 44i, 13:7,
        7i
    keratometry in measurement of, 8:40–41

in schematic eye, **3**:107*t*
Radiuscope, **3**:175, 195
Raeder paratrigeminal syndrome, **5**:265
RAIU. *See* Radioactive iodine uptake
Raloxifene, for osteoporosis, **1**:245*t*, 246
Rami oculares, **2**:119
Ramipril
  for heart failure, **1**:130
  for hypertension, **1**:88*t*
  for non-ST-segment elevation acute coronary
    syndrome, **1**:123
Ramsay Hunt syndrome, **5**:284
Ranbezolid, **1**:75
Random-Dot E test, **6**:93
Random dot stereopsis tests, **6**:93–94
Randomization, in clinical trials, **1**:351, 351*i*
Randot test, **6**:93
Range of accommodation, **3**:119
  measuring, **3**:151
Ranitidine, preoperative, **1**:331
RANTES, **8**:198*t*
RAPD. *See* Relative afferent pupillary defect
Rapid plasma reagin (RPR) test, **1**:16–17, 302,
  9:189–190, **12**:190
ras oncogene, **2**:215
Ravuconazole, **1**:76
Ray, **3**:26
  exact tracing of, **3**:55–56, 55*i*. *See also* Raytracing
  paraxial, approximation of, **3**:56–58, 56*i*, 57*i*
Ray model of light, **3**:3
Rayleigh criterion, **3**:12
Rayleigh scattering, **3**:12
Raynaud phenomenon
  in scleroderma, **1**:185
  in systemic lupus erythematosus, **1**:179, 180*i*
Raytracing
  paraxial
    through concave spherical lenses, **3**:74, 74*i*, 75*i*
    through convex spherical lenses, **3**:71–72, 71*i*, 72*i*
  retinal, **3**:320
RB. *See* Reticulate body; Retinoblastoma
Rb locus, **2**:253
RB1 (retinoblastoma) gene, **2**:253–254, **4**:141, 213, 252,
  6:394
  secondary malignancies and, **4**:144
RBBB. *See* Right bundle branch block
RBCs. *See* Red blood cells
RBP. *See* Retinol-binding protein
RCFM. *See* Retrocorneal fibrous membrane
RDS-peripherin gene mutations, **2**:349–350, **12**:204
  in adult-onset vitelliform lesions, **12**:219
  in pattern dystrophies, **12**:219, 222
  in retinitis pigmentosa, **12**:207, 210
  in Stargardt disease, **12**:216
Reactive arthritis (Reiter syndrome), **1**:176–177,
  8:227–228, **9**:130–131, 131*i*, 132*i*
  HLA association in, **9**:94*t*, 129
Reactive hyperplasia/reactive lymphoid hyperplasia. *See*
  Lymphoid hyperplasia
Reactive nitrogen products, as inflammatory mediators,
  9:85
Reactive oxygen intermediates, as inflammatory
  mediators, **9**:83–85, 84*i*

Reading
  magnification for in low vision, **3**:255–259
    with magnifiers, **3**:258–260
    with spectacles, **3**:255–256
  position of, prismatic effects of bifocal lenses and,
    3:155, 156*i*, 158*i*
  vision rehabilitation and, **3**:255–259
Reading cards, for near visual acuity testing, in
  children, **6**:80
Reading glasses, single-vision, for induced anisophoria,
  3:162
REAL (Revised European-American) classification, for
  lymphomas, **4**:194–195, **7**:85, 86*t*
Reattachment surgery. *See* Retinal detachment, surgery
  for
Rebleeding
  after cerebral aneurysm rupture, **5**:352
  after traumatic hyphema, **8**:399–401, 400*i*, 401*i*
Rebound headache, analgesic, **5**:296
Rebound hypertension, **1**:97–98
Rebound nystagmus, **5**:244
Recall bias, **1**:349
Receiver operating characteristics (ROC) curve, **1**:355,
  356*i*, 357, 357*i*
Receptor activation, in immune response, adaptive
  versus innate immunity and, **9**:10
Receptor agonist, **2**:392
Receptor antagonist, **2**:392
Receptor–effector coupling, **2**:311
Receptors, **2**:308–310, 308*t*, 312–313, 314*t*
  in iris–ciliary body, **2**:308–310, 308*t*
  ocular drug interactions and, **2**:392
  in signal transduction, **2**:310–311, 312*i*, 313*i*
Recess-resect procedures
  monocular
    for esodeviation, **6**:179, 179*t*
    for exodeviation, **6**:179, 181*t*
  for nystagmus (Kestenbaum-Anderson procedure),
    5:255, **6**:168–170, 170*i*
Recession (extraocular muscle), **6**:23, 175*t*. *See also*
  specific muscle
  and anteriorization, **6**:175*t*
Recessive inheritance (recessive gene/trait), **2**:194, 260,
  8:307
  autosomal, **2**:261–265, 262*t*, 265*t*
  disorders associated with, **2**:194, 261–265
    gene therapy for, **2**:237
  X-linked, **2**:267–268, 268*t*
Recessive optic atrophy, **6**:364
Recessive tumor-suppressor gene, Rb locus as, **2**:253
Recipient eye, preparation of
  for lamellar keratoplasty, **8**:474
  for penetrating keratoplasty, **8**:455–456
Reciprocal innervation, Sherrington's law of, **6**:35
Recognition, minimum angle of (MAR), **3**:112, 112*t*
  logarithm of (logMAR), **3**:112, 112*t*
Recognition receptors, in immune response, adaptive
  versus innate immunity and, **9**:10, 11
Recognition threshold, **3**:112
Recombinant, definition of, **2**:194
Recombinant DNA, **2**:194, 227, 229*i*
Recombinant tissue plasminogen activator. *See* Tissue
  plasminogen activator
Recombination, **2**:184, 194, 204, 227
  T- and B-cell antigen receptor diversity and, **9**:87

Recombivax HB. *See* Hepatitis B vaccine
Reconstructive surgery
  for craniofacial malformation, 6:430–431
  eyelid, 7:188–193
    after basal cell carcinoma surgery, 7:178–179
    for blepharophimosis syndrome, 7:153
    for epicanthus, 7:156
    for euryblepharon, 7:154
    for eyelid defects involving eyelid margin,
      7:189–192, 191*i*
    for eyelid defects not involving eyelid margin,
      7:188–189
    for lower eyelid defects, 7:189–192, 191*i*
    after Mohs' micrographic surgery, 7:178–179
    for upper eyelid defects, 7:188–190, 190*i*
  socket, 7:126
Recoverin (CAR antigen), 2:344*t*, 5:109
  cancer-associated retinopathy and, 9:61
Recruitment, 6:32
Rectal examination, in cancer screening, 1:295*t*
Rectilinear propagation, law of, 3:41, 42*i*
Rectus muscles, 2:15*i*, 17*i*, 18*t*, 19*i*, 5:41, 42, 42*i*,
    6:13–14, 14*i*, 17*t*, 7:13, 140*i*. *See also specific muscle*
  action of, 6:17*t*, 18*i*, 28, 30, 30*t*, 31*i*, 32*i*, 33*i*
  anatomy of, 6:13–14, 14*i*, 17*t*
    in infants, 6:202
    surgery and, 6:23–26, 24*i*, 25*i*
  fascial capsules of, 6:22
    surgery and, 6:23
  field of action/activation of, 6:29
  horizontal, 6:13–14, 14*i*, 17*t*, 18*i*
    A-pattern deviations associated with dysfunction
      of, 6:119
    action of, 6:13–14, 17*t*, 28, 30, 31*i*, 32*i*
    anatomy of, 6:13–14, 14*i*, 17*t*, 18*i*
    surgery of
      for A- and V-pattern deviations, 6:123–124,
        123*i*, 124, 182
      for nystagmus, 6:168–171, 170*i*, 170*t*
    V-pattern deviations associated with dysfunction
      of, 6:119
  insertion relationships of, 2:15–16, 17*i*, 18*t*, 6:16, 18*i*
  intermuscular septum of, 6:21
    surgery and, 6:23
  origins of, 2:16, 18*t*
  pulley system for, 6:21
  surgery of, 6:181–183
    for A- and V-pattern deviations, 6:123–124, 123*i*,
      124, 182
    anatomy and, 6:23–26, 24*i*, 25*i*
    for classic congenital (essential infantile)
      esotropia, 6:100
    for constant exotropia, 6:114
    for Duane syndrome, 6:143–144
    for esodeviation, 6:107–108, 178–179, 179*t*
    eyelid position changes after, 6:189–190, 190*i*
    for hypotropia and hypertropia, 6:181–182
    for intermittent exotropia, 6:113–114
    for nystagmus, 6:168–171, 170*i*, 170*t*
    for overcorrection of intermittent exotropia, 6:114
    for sixth nerve paralysis, 6:107–108
    for third nerve (oculomotor) palsy, 6:148
    for undercorrection of intermittent exotropia,
      6:114

vertical, 6:14, 14*i*, 17*t*, 18*i*
    A-pattern deviations associated with dysfunction
      of, 6:119
    action of, 6:14, 17*t*, 28, 30
    anatomy of, 6:14, 14*i*, 17*t*, 18*i*
    surgery of
      for A- and V-pattern deviations, 6:124
      eyelid position changes after, 6:189–190, 190*i*
      for hypotropia and hypertropia, 6:181–182
    V-pattern deviations associated with dysfunction
      of, 6:119
Rectus subnucleus
  inferior, 5:45
  superior, 5:45–46
Recurrent corneal erosion, 8:98–100, 100*i*
  pain caused by, 5:298, 8:98
  posttraumatic, 8:407
Red blood cells, 1:159
  cytologic identification of, 8:68
  development of, 1:160
Red eye. *See also* Conjunctivitis
  contact lenses causing, 3:209–210
Red filter (glass/lens) test
  in eye movement assessment, 6:85
  in suppression/anomalous retinal correspondence
    evaluation, 6:58–60, 59*i*
Red-green color vision, 2:345–346
  defects in, 12:195
    gene defects causing, 2:346–347, 346*i*, 350
    ocular findings in carriers of, 2:270*t*
    testing for, 12:43–44, 44*i*, 45*i*. *See also* Red-green
      test
Red-green test
  duochrome/bichrome, 3:140
    before refractive surgery, 13:43
      PRK/LASEK, 13:91
  in functional visual disorder evaluation, 5:307
  Lancaster, 6:85–86
Red lasers, 12:314, 315–316*t*
Red reflex, 3:126–127. *See also* Retinal reflex
  in cataract, 11:38
  in keratoconus, 8:330
  in lenticonus and lentiglobus, 6:289, 11:31
  in pediatric cataract, 6:292
  poor, cataract surgery and, 11:210
Reduced schematic eye, 3:106–108, 108*i*
Reduced vergence, 3:62–65
Reduction division, in meiosis, 2:190
Reese-Ellsworth classification of retinoblastoma,
    4:258–259, 258*t*, 6:394–396, 396*t*
Reference beam, in optical coherence tomography,
    3:322, 324*i*
Reference sphere, wavefront analysis and, 3:238
Refixation movements, microsaccadic, 5:199
Reflecting power, of mirrors, 3:90
Reflection, light, 3:13–14, 13*i*
  angle of, 3:43*i*, 44
  at curved surfaces, 3:51, 52*i*
  diffuse, 3:41–42, 43*i*
  law of, 3:42–44, 43*i*, 44*i*
  metallic, 3:13
  polarizing sunglasses in reduction of glare from,
    3:10, 13*i*, 165
  specular, 3:42–44, 43*i*, 44*i*
    for slit-lamp biomicroscopy, 8:17–18, 18*i*

total internal (TIR), **3**:14, 47–49, 48*i*, 50*i*
  gonioscopy and, **3**:47–49, 50*i*
Reflection coefficient, **3**:44
Reflex. *See specific type*
Reflex arc, neural, immune response arc compared
  with, **9**:17–19, 18*i*
Reflex blepharospasm, **5**:290
Reflex secretors, **2**:292
Reflex tear arc, **7**:253, **8**:57
  non–Sjögren syndrome disorders of, **8**:80
  in Sjögren syndrome, **8**:78–79
Reflex tearing, **2**:118*i*, 119
  absorption of ocular medication affected by,
    2:381–382, 385
Reflexive saccades, in Parkinson syndromes, **5**:206
Refractile bodies/spots
  in papilledema, **5**:117, 117*i*
  in sickle cell retinopathy, **12**:121
Refracting power, **3**:31. *See also* Transverse
  magnification
Refraction. *See also* Refractive errors
  angle of, **3**:44, 46*i*
  before cataract surgery, **11**:87
    IOL power determination and, **11**:148–150
  clinical, **3**:125–171. *See also* Visual acuity
    absorptive lenses and, **3**:165–167
    accommodative problems and, **3**:147–150, 148*t*
    aphakic lenses and, **3**:164–165
    automated, **3**:312–314, 313*i*, 314*i*, 315*i*
    corneal abnormalities affecting, **8**:15
    cycloplegic, **3**:141–142, 142*t*
      in children, **6**:94–95, 94*t*
    in glaucoma evaluation, **10**:31–32
    high-index glass lenses and, **3**:168
    impact-resistant lenses and, **3**:168
    monocular diplopia and, **3**:170–171
    multifocal lenses and, **3**:150–164
    noncycloplegic (manifest), **3**:141–142
      before refractive surgery, **13**:42–43
      PRK/LASEK, **13**:91, 92
    objective (retinoscopy), **3**:125–134. *See also*
      Retinoscopy
    overrefraction and, **3**:142–143, 164–165
    plastic lenses and, **3**:168
    polycarbonate lenses and, **3**:168–169
    prescribing for children, **3**:145–147
    prisms and, **3**:169–170
    spectacle correction of ametropias and, **3**:143–145,
      144*i*
    subjective, **3**:134–141, 313
  at curved surfaces, **3**:51, 52*i*
  law of (Snell's law), **3**:44–46, 46*i*, 47, 47*i*, **8**:39–40
    contact lens power and, **3**:174
    Fermat's principle and, **3**:51–52
    small-angle approximation and, **3**:59–60
  before PRK/LASEK, **13**:91, 92
  after radial keratotomy, **13**:63
    stability of, **13**:63
  refractive surgery and, **13**:42–43
    IOL power calculation and, **13**:200–201, 201*t*
Refractive accommodative esotropia, **6**:98*t*, 101–102
Refractive ametropia, **3**:116
Refractive astigmatism, contact lenses and, **3**:182

Refractive errors. *See also specific type and* Ametropia
  amblyopia caused by
    ametropic, **6**:70
    anisometropic, **6**:69–70
  changes in after strabismus surgery, **6**:184
  in children, **6**:199–200, 201*i*
  correction of. *See also* Contact lenses; Spectacle
    lenses (spectacles)
    in amblyopia treatment, **6**:72
    intraocular lenses for, **11**:147–148
    surgical. *See* Refractive surgery
  in craniofacial syndromes, **6**:429
  developmental models of, **3**:121
  high, cataract surgery in patient with, **11**:221–222
  after penetrating keratoplasty, **13**:187–189, 187*i*
  perimetry affected by, **10**:65, 72*i*
  prevalence of, **3**:120–121, 122
  in primary angle closure/angle-closure glaucoma,
    10:12, 124
  in ptosis, **7**:211
Refractive index, **3**:39–41, 40*t*
  of cornea, **8**:8, 40
  definition of, **3**:6, 39
  of lens, **11**:6
  reflection magnitude and, **3**:13
  in schematic eye, **3**:106*i*, 107*t*
  of tear (fluid) lens, **3**:180–181
Refractive keratotomy. *See* Keratotomy
Refractive lens exchange, **13**:156–161
  advantages of, **13**:161
  complications of, **13**:160–161
  disadvantages of, **13**:161
  indications for, **13**:156
  informed consent for, **13**:158
  IOL calculations for, **13**:160
  patient selection for, **13**:156–158
  retinal detachment and, **13**:158, 160, 161, 192
  surgical planning/techniques for, **13**:158–160
Refractive lensectomy. *See also* Refractive lens exchange
  presbyopic (PRELEX procedure), **13**:163–164
Refractive power, **3**:61–62
  of cornea, **8**:39–40, **13**:5–6
    keratometry in measurement of, **8**:40–41, **13**:5
  of schematic eye, **3**:107*t*
Refractive states of eye, **3**:115–119. *See also* Refractive
  errors
  emmetropization and, **3**:120
Refractive surgery, **13**:50*t*. *See also specific procedure
  and* Keratorefractive surgery
  adjustable (ARS), **13**:156, 157*t*. *See also* Bioptics
  astigmatism after, corneal topography in detection/
    management of, **8**:46, 48
  basic science of, **13**:5–30
  cataract/cataract surgery and, **11**:211, **13**:173
    intraocular lens power calculation and, **11**:82,
      150–152, 211
    planning and, **11**:82, 102–103
  classification of, **13**:19, 20–22*t*
  contact lens use after, **13**:204–208
  corneal topography and, **8**:46–48, 47*i*, 48*i*, **13**:6–12,
    47, 48*i*
  indications for, **13**:9–10, 9*i*
  corneal transplant after, **13**:203–204
  corneal wound healing and, **13**:28–29
  glaucoma after, **13**:208–209

in glaucoma patient, **13**:189–191, 190*i*
intraocular lens power calculations after, **3**:221–222,
  13:65, 160, 199–203, 201*t*
keratorefractive procedures, **13**:5. *See also*
  Keratorefractive surgery
laser biophysics and, **13**:29–30
lenticular procedures, **13**:5
in ocular hypertension patient, **13**:189–191, 190*i*
in ocular and systemic disease, **13**:183–198. *See also*
  specific disorder
optical considerations in, **3**:231–242, **13**:5–30
  corneal shape, **3**:231–235, 235*i*
  pupil size, **3**:235–236
patient expectations and, **13**:39–40
after penetrating keratoplasty, **13**:187–189, 187*i*
penetrating keratoplasty after, **13**:203–204
postoperative considerations and, **13**:199–209
preoperative evaluation for, **13**:39–56, 40*t*
retinal detachment after, **13**:203
risks/benefits of, discussion of with patient,
  13:49–50, 50*t*. *See also* Informed consent
strabismus after, **6**:157
wavefront-aberrations after, **13**:13–17
Refsum disease/syndrome (phytanic acid storage
  disease), **12**:233*t*, 234, 236, 242, 242*i*, 243*i*
  gene defects causing, **2**:351
  ichthyosis and, **12**:237
  infantile, **2**:262*t*, **6**:437*t*, **12**:242
    gene defects causing, **2**:351
    Leber congenital amaurosis and, **6**:335
Regan chart, **3**:114
Regeneration, **4**:19. *See also* Wound healing/repair
Regional anesthesia, **2**:445–449, 445*t*
Regional enteritis (Crohn disease), **1**:177, **9**:131–132
Regional gigantism, **6**:405
Regional immunity, **9**:28
Reglan. *See* Metoclopramide
Regressed drusen, **12**:58
Regression formulas, for IOL power determination,
  3:218–219, 218*i*, **11**:149–150
Regular astigmatism, **3**:93–98, 94*i*, 117–118
  retinoscopy of, **3**:129–133, 131*i*, 132*i*
  wavefront aberration produced by, **3**:102, **13**:15, 16*i*
Regular insulin, **1**:209, 209*t*
Regulatory regions, of gene, **2**:202
Rehabilitation. *See* Vision rehabilitation
Rehabilitation teachers, **3**:265. *See also* Vision
  rehabilitation
Reid's line, definition of, **5**:80
Reis-Bücklers dystrophy, **8**:310*t*, 315, 316*i*
Reiter syndrome (reactive arthritis), **1**:176–177,
  8:227–228, **9**:130–131, 131*i*, 132*i*
  HLA association in, **9**:94*t*, 130
Rejection (graft), **8**:448, 449, 466–470, 468*i*, 469*i*
  corneal allograft, **8**:448, 449, 466–470, 468*i*, 469*i*,
    9:39, 40*i*, 41
  after lamellar keratoplasty, **8**:475
  after penetrating keratoplasty, **8**:466–470, 468*i*, 469*i*
  transplantation antigens and, **8**:447, **9**:93–94
Rejuvenation surgery, facial, **7**:237–248. *See also specific
  procedure and* Facial surgery
Relafen. *See* Nabumetone
Relapsing polychondritis, **1**:187–188
  eyelid manifestations of, **4**:173*t*

Relative afferent pupillary defect (Marcus Gunn pupil)
  cataract surgery and, **11**:81
  in central retinal artery occlusion, **5**:106
  in central retinal vein occlusion, **5**:107, **12**:143
  in multiple evanescent white dot syndrome, **5**:107
  retrochiasmal lesions causing, **5**:165
  testing for, **5**:84–87, 86*i*
    in functional visual disorder evaluation, **5**:307
    practical tips in, **5**:85–86
Relative risk/risk ratio (RR), **1**:292, 360–361
Relatives, first-degree/second-degree, **2**:194
Relaxation time, in MRI, **5**:80, 81, **7**:30–31
Relaxing incisions
  for corneal astigmatism after penetrating
    keratoplasty, **8**:466
  limbal, **13**:21*t*, 66, 67*i*, 68–69, 69*t*
    cataract surgery and, **11**:103
Relenza. *See* Zanamivir
Reliability, **1**:363
Remicade. *See* Infliximab
Reminyl. *See* Galantamine
Remodeling pathway, platelet-activating factors in, **9**:80
Remote-controlled conventional refractors, **3**:313
Renal cell carcinoma, in von Hippel–Lindau disease,
  6:412
Renal disease
  chronic, in children, **6**:349
  congenital, retinal degeneration and, **12**:236
  hypertension management and, **1**:91*t*, 95
  in scleroderma, **1**:185
  in systemic lupus erythematosus, **1**:179, 181*t*
  uveitis in children and, **6**:315–316
Renal–retinal dysplasia/dystrophy, familial, **6**:349,
  12:236
Renal transplantation, ocular disorders following, **6**:349
Rendu-Osler-Weber disease (hereditary hemorrhagic
  telangiectasia), **1**:166, **8**:91
Renese. *See* Polythiazide
Renin-angiotensin-aldosterone system, in hypertension,
  1:83, 83*i*
Renovascular hypertension, **1**:83, 84*t*
Reoperation
  adjustable sutures and, **6**:176
  surgical planning and, **6**:177
ReoPro. *See* Abciximab
REP 1 (Rab escort protein 1/*CHM*) gene mutation,
  2:351
  in choroideremia, **2**:351, **12**:224
Repaglinide, **1**:212*t*, 213
Repair, **4**:19. *See also* Wound healing/repair
Reparative (stimulated) macrophages, **9**:50, 51*i*, 52–53
Repeat element/sequence, L1, **2**:189, 203
Reperfusion
  for angina, **1**:121–122
  for ST-segment elevation acute coronary syndrome,
    1:124–125
Replication
  DNA, **2**:194, 212
    origin, **2**:192, 212
    segregation and, **2**:195, 217
    slippage, **2**:195
  microbial, as virulence factor, **8**:117
Replicative segregation, **2**:195, 217
Reproducibility, **1**:363
Requip. *See* Ropinirole

Rescriptor. *See* Delavirdine
Rescue breathing, 1:314
Rescula. *See* Unoprostone
Research studies. *See* Clinical research/studies;
   Experimental (interventional) studies
Resection (extraocular muscle), 6:23, 174
Reserpine, 1:89*t*, 90*t*
Residence time (of medication), 2:382
Resistance (drug). *See also specific agent and specific*
   organism
   antibiotic, 1:3, 66
      new drug classes and, 1:74–75
   antiretroviral, 1:41, 43, 44
Resolution
   diffraction affecting, 3:11–12
   minimum angle of (MAR), 3:112, 112*t*
      logarithm of (logMAR), 3:112, 112*t*
   pupil size affecting, 3:109–111
Resolution threshold, 3:112
Resolving power, 3:31. *See also* Transverse
   magnification
Respbid. *See* Theophylline
Respimat. *See* Fenoterol, with ipratropium
Respiratory disorders. *See* Pulmonary diseases
Response accommodative convergence/accommodation
   ratio, 6:88
Rest, position of, 6:31
Restasis. *See* Cyclosporine A, topical
Restimulation, of effector lymphocytes, 9:25
Resting macrophages, 9:51–52, 51*i*
Resting neutrophils, 9:48
Restoril. *See* Temazepam
Restriction endonucleases, 2:185, 222–223
   for mutation screening, 2:222–223, 231, 233*i*
Restriction fragment length polymorphisms (RFLPs),
   2:195, 222–223, 224*i*
Restrictive pulmonary diseases, 1:154
Restrictive syndromes
   diplopia caused by, 5:217–221
      paretic syndromes differentiated from, 5:217, 218*i*
   posttraumatic, 5:218–219
Resuscitation (cardiopulmonary), 1:313–317
   medications used in, 1:316*t*
   for ventricular fibrillation, 1:140
RET oncogene, amyloidosis and, 8:347*t*
RETAANE (anecortave acetate), 2:455, 12:77*t*, 78
Retained lens material, cataract surgery and,
   11:182–183, 12:337–339, 338*t*, 339*i*
Retavase. *See* Reteplase
Rete ridges, 8:245, 246*i*
Reteplase, for ST-segment elevation acute coronary
   syndrome, 1:124
RETGC1 gene, in Leber congenital amaurosis, 6:335
Reticular degenerative retinoschisis, 4:126, 12:276
Reticular dystrophy, 12:222, 222*i*
Reticular formation, paramedian pontine, 2:116, 116*i*,
   5:34
Reticular peripheral cystoid degeneration, 4:126, 126*i*,
   12:264, 275, 275*i*
Reticulate body, *Chlamydia*, 8:128
Reticulum cell sarcoma, 9:228–231, 228*i*, 230*i*,
   12:182–183, 182*i*. *See also* Lymphomas, intraocular
   uveitis in children differentiated from, 6:320*t*

Retina. *See also under* Retinal
   anatomy of, 2:43*i*, 44, 76–85, 5:23–25, 25*i*, 12:7–12,
      8*i*, 9*t*, 10–11*i*
   angiography in examination of, 12:18–23, 20*i*, 22*i*.
      See also Fluorescein angiography; Indocyanine
      green angiography
   anterior (peripheral), 12:8
   antioxidants in, 2:369*i*, 371–373, 373*i*, 374*i*
   arteriovenous anastomoses in, in Takayasu arteritis,
      1:191
   arteriovenous malformations of, 12:164
   astrocytic hamartoma of, optic disc drusen
      differentiated from, 5:132–134, 133*i*
   atrophy of, ischemia causing, 4:128, 129*i*. *See also*
      Retinal ischemia
   in branch retinal artery occlusion, 4:133
   biochemistry and metabolism of, 2:341–355
   blood supply of. *See* Retinal blood vessels
   capillary hemangioma of. *See* Retinal angiomatosis
   cavernous hemangioma of, 4:247, 248*i*, 12:163–164,
      164*i*
   coloboma of, 2:171
   congenital disorders of, 2:173, 4:119–123, 121*i*, 122*i*,
      123*i*, 12:195–202
   contrast sensitivity affected by disorders of, 3:115
   degenerations of. *See* Retinal degenerations
   detachment of. *See* Retinal detachment
   development of, 2:138–142, 143*i*, 6:47–48, 200
   diabetes affecting. *See* Diabetic retinopathy
   disorders of. *See* Retinal disease; Retinopathy
   dysplasia of, congenital, 2:173
   dystrophies of. *See* Retinal dystrophies
   edema of. *See* Retinal edema
   electromagnetic energy affecting, 12:305–309, 306*i*
   electrophysiology of, 2:354–355, 355*i*, 12:27–41. *See*
      also specific test
   emboli in. *See also* Emboli
      clinical aspects/implications and, 5:177*t*, 180–181
   equatorial, 12:8
   examination of, 12:17–18
      before cataract surgery, 11:83, 84
   fleck, of Kandori, 12:200
   free radicals affecting, 2:370–371
   gliosis of, 4:134, 134*i*, 147
   gyrate atrophy of, 2:262*t*, 12:225–226
   hamartomas of, 4:146, 242, 242*i*, 6:390
   in HIV infection/AIDS, 9:248, 249*i*. *See also* Retinitis
   in children, 6:219
      progressive outer retinal necrosis and, 9:155,
         253–254, 254*i*
   immune response in, 9:34*t*, 40–41
   infection/inflammation of, 4:123–126, 124*i*, 125*i*. *See*
      also Retinitis
   pain caused by, 5:298
   layers of, 12:9, 10*i*
   in leukemia, 4:281
   mechanical injury of, light causing, 12:307
   necrosis of
      acute (necrotizing herpetic retinitis), 4:123, 124*i*,
         9:140, 154–156, 155*i*, 156*i*, 12:185–186, 185*i*
      progressive, 9:155, 156*i*
         in HIV infection/AIDS, 9:155, 253–254, 254*i*
   neovascularization of. *See also* Neovascularization
      disorders of in retinopathy of prematurity, 4:137,
         6:325–332, 12:124–136
      screening for, 6:328–329, 329*t*, 330*i*, 331*i*,
         351–356, 354*i*

ischemia causing, **4:**130–133, 132*i*
peripheral, **12:**124, 125*t*
vitreous hemorrhage and, **12:**287
neurosensory, **2:**79–85, 80–81*i*, **4:**118–119, 118*i*,
12:7–12, 8*i*, 9*t*, 10–11*i*
anatomy of, **2:**79–85, 80–81*i*, 82*i*, 83*i*
biochemistry and metabolism of, **2:**341–351
development of, **2:**138–142, 143*i*
glial elements of, **2:**83–84
neuronal elements of, **2:**79–83, 82*i*, 83*i*
stratification of, **2:**80–81*i*, 84–85
vascular elements of, **2:**84. *See also* Retinal blood
vessels
optical coherence tomography in examination of,
12:24
peripheral (anterior), **12:**8
phakoma of, in tuberous sclerosis, **6:**410–412, 411*i*
photic injury of, **12:**307–309
in retinitis pigmentosa, **12:**210, 213
in retinopathy of prematurity, **12:**132
photochemical injury of, **12:**307
photocoagulation causing lesions of, **12:**319
physiology and psychophysics of, **12:**27–47
pigment epithelium of. *See* Retinal pigment
epithelium
in primary central nervous system lymphoma, **9:**228,
228*i*, 230*i*
radiation affecting, **12:**305–309, 306*i*
regional differences in, **2:**78, 78*i*
scanning laser ophthalmoscopy in evaluation of,
12:24–25
splitting of, in shaking injury, **6:**444, 444*i*
systemic diseases affecting, in childhood, **6:**343–351
in systemic lupus erythematosus, **1:**182, **9:**61,
173–175, 174*i*
thermal injury of, light causing, **12:**307
thickness of, analysis of, **12:**25, 26*i*
topography of, **2:**43*i*, 44*i*, **4:**117–119, 118*i*, 120*i*
transplantation of, **9:**42
tumors of, **4:**139–147. *See also* Retinoblastoma
metastatic, **4:**273, 274*i*
in uveitis, **9:**103*t*
vascular abnormalities of. *See* Retina,
neovascularization of; Retinal disease, vascular
vascularization of. *See* Retina, neovascularization of;
Retinal disease, vascular
vitreous interface with, **12:**7
abnormalities of, **12:**87–93. *See also specific type*
in von Hippel–Lindau disease, **6:**402*t*, 412–413, 413*i*
wound healing/repair and, **4:**24
Retinal adhesion, retinal pigment epithelium in
maintenance of, **2:**362
Retinal angiography, **12:**18–23, 20*i*, 22*i*. *See also*
Fluorescein angiography; Indocyanine green
angiography
Retinal angiomatosis (angiomatosis retinae, von Hippel
syndrome/disease), **4:**246–247, 246*i*, **5:**336*t*, 340,
342*i*, **6:**402*t*, 412–413, 413*i*, **12:**160–163, 161*i*, 162*i*
with hemangioblastomas (von Hippel–Lindau
disease/syndrome), **5:**336*t*, 340, 342*i*, **6:**402*t*,
412–413, 413*i*
retinoblastoma differentiated from, **6:**394
photocoagulation for, **12:**163
wavelength selection and, **12:**316*t*

Retinal arterioles
constriction of, in hypertensive retinopathy, **12:**97
obstruction of, **12:**145–146, 146*i*. *See also* Cotton-
wool spots
Retinal artery
central, **2:**84, 102, 103, 104, 104*i*, 105*i*, **5:**11–12*i*, 15,
16*i*, **12:**12
macroaneurysms of, **12:**158–160, 160*i*
age-related macular degeneration differentiated
from, **12:**67, 68*i*
microaneurysms of
in HIV infection/AIDS, **9:**248
ischemia causing, **4:**131, 132*i*
in nonproliferative diabetic retinopathy, **12:**103,
104*i*
occlusion of *See* Retinal artery occlusion
Retinal artery occlusion
branch, **4:**133, **12:**146–148, 146*i*, 147*i*
central, **4:**133–134, **5:**105–106, 106*i*, **12:**148–150,
148*i*, 149*i*
in sickle cell hemoglobinopathies, **12:**121
Retinal blood vessels, **2:**80*i*, 84, **4:**118–119, **12:**10*i*, 12.
See also specific vessel
anomalies of, **4:**121–122, 122*i*
development of, **2:**156
disease of. *See* Retinal disease, vascular
ischemia and, **4:**130–133, 131*i*, 132*i*
Retinal breaks, **12:**253–256. *See also* Retinal tears
in acute retinal necrosis (herpetic necrotizing
retinitis), **9:**155, 156*i*
asymptomatic, treatment of, **12:**266, 267*t*
in herpetic retinitis (acute retinal necrosis), **12:**185
lattice degeneration and, **12:**258
treatment of, **12:**265, 266–267, 266*t*, 267*t*
paving-stone (cobblestone) degeneration and, **12:**263
photocoagulation for, **12:**265
wavelength selection and, **12:**316*t*
in posterior vitreous detachment, **12:**256, 257*i*, 258
prophylactic treatment of, **12:**264–268, 266*t*, 267*t*
retinal detachment and, **12:**253, 268, 269*t*, 270*i*
prophylaxis of, **12:**264–268, 266*t*, 267*t*
symptomatic, treatment of, **12:**265–266, 266*t*
traumatic, **12:**254–256, 255*i*
Retinal capillary nonperfusion
in Coats disease, **12:**156, 157*i*
in diabetic retinopathy, **12:**116
in radiation retinopathy, **12:**305, 306*i*
Retinal correspondence
anomalous, **6:**41, 53, 54*i*, 55–57
harmonious, **6:**60, 64, 65*i*
testing for, **6:**56–57, 58–65
unharmonious, **6:**60, 65, 65*i*
normal, **6:**41–43, 42*i*
Retinal degenerations, **4:**126–140. *See also specific type
and* Retinal dystrophies
gene defects causing, **2:**347–348, 347*i*, 348*i*, 351
hearing loss and, **12:**235. *See also* Usher syndrome
lattice, **4:**127–128, 127*i*
radial perivascular, **4:**127–128
paving-stone (cobblestone), **4:**128, 129*i*, **12:**263, 264*i*
peripheral and reticular cystoid, **4:**126, 126*i*
systemic disease and, **12:**231–251
Retinal detachment, **2:**78, **4:**111–112, 112*i*, 113*i*,
12:268–274
in acute retinal necrosis (herpetic necrotizing
retinitis), **9:**155, 156*i*

after anterior chamber phakic IOL insertion, 13:151, 192
after anterior segment trauma repair, 8:417
after blunt trauma, in young patient, 12:254–255
in branch retinal vein occlusion, 12:138
after cataract surgery, 11:104, 164*t*, 175–176, 175*i*, 12:334–336, 334*i*, 13:192
    in children, 11:198
    retained lens material and, 12:337, 338–339
in central serous chorioretinopathy, 12:22*i*, 51, 52
in child abuse, 6:442
choroidal hemangioma and, 4:164, 243–246
after clear lens extraction/refractive lens exchange, 13:158, 160, 161, 192
in Coats disease, 4:121–122, 122*i*, 12:156, 157*i*
complex, vitrectomy for, 12:340, 341
in cytomegalovirus retinitis, 9:157, 157*i*, 253, 12:193
in diabetic retinopathy, 12:112, 273
    vitrectomy for, 12:341
differential diagnosis of, 12:275–277
enclosed ora bays and, 12:262
exudative, 12:274, 274*i*
    in Coats disease, 12:156, 157*i*
    photocoagulation causing, 12:320, 321*i*
in familial exudative vitreoretinopathy, 12:284
fellow eye in patient with, 12:267
in herpetic retinitis (acute retinal necrosis), 12:185–186
high myopia and, 13:191–192, 203
after LASIK, 13:192, 203
lattice degeneration and, 12:258–259, 259*i*, 260*i*
    treatment of, 12:265, 266–267, 266*t*, 267*t*
lesions not predisposing to, 12:263–264
lesions predisposing to, 12:258–262
in leukemia, 4:281–282
management of, 12:271–273, 272*i*
meridional folds and, 12:262, 263*i*
muscarinic therapy and, 2:398
after Nd:YAG laser capsulotomy, 11:175, 190, 12:334
nonrhegmatogenous (secondary), 12:269*t*
    angle-closure glaucoma and, 10:141
in pars planitis, 9:148, 151
peripheral retinal excavations and, 12:262
persistent fetal vasculature and, 6:324
pneumatic retinopexy for, 12:272, 335
posterior vitreous detachment and, 12:258
postoperative, 12:334–336, 334*i*
proliferative vitreoretinopathy in, 12:268–271, 270*i*, 271*t*
in punctate inner choroidopathy, 12:179, 179*i*
refractive surgery and, 13:191–193, 203
retinal pigment epithelial maintenance of adhesion and, 2:362
in retinopathy of prematurity, 6:330, 12:129, 129*i*, 130*i*, 136
retinoschisis and, 12:276–277, 277*t*
rhegmatogenous, 4:112, 113*i*, 9:222, 12:268–273, 269*t*, 270*i*, 271*t*
    diagnostic features of, 12:269*t*
    management of, 12:271–273, 272*i*
    posterior vitreous detachment and, 2:89, 90*i*, 91*i*
in sarcoidosis, 8:88
scleral buckle for, 12:272, 272*i*, 336
sickle cell retinopathy and, 12:124

scleral perforation during strabismus surgery and, 6:185
secondary (nonrhegmatogenous), 12:269*t*
    angle-closure glaucoma and, 10:141
in sickle cell retinopathy, vitreoretinal surgery for, 12:124
subclinical, 12:268
surgery for, 12:271–273
    anatomic reattachment, 12:273
    after LASIK, 13:203
    refractive surgery after, 13:193
    in retinopathy of prematurity, 6:331
    secondary angle-closure glaucoma and, 10:143–144
    strabismus and, 6:157
    visual acuity after, 12:273
tractional, 12:7, 269*t*, 273–274
    in diabetic retinopathy, 12:112, 273
        vitrectomy for, 12:341
    after penetrating injury, 12:273, 295
    in retinopathy of prematurity, 12:129
traumatic, in young patient, 12:254–255
in uveal lymphoid infiltration, 4:279
in uveitis, 9:240
uveitis in children differentiated from, 6:329*t*
vitrectomy for, 12:272, 336
    in diabetic patients, 12:112, 116–117, 341
vitreoretinal tufts and, 12:259–260, 261*i*, 262*i*
in Vogt-Koyanagi-Harada syndrome, 9:203, 204*i*, 12:181
in von Hippel–Lindau disease, 12:160
in young patient, 12:254–255
Retinal dialyses, 4:26, 27*i*, 12:253, 254, 255*i*
    treatment of, 12:266*t*, 267*t*
Retinal disease, 4:117–147. *See also specific type and Macula, disease of; Retinitis; Retinopathy*
    angiography in, 12:18–23, 20*i*, 22*i*. *See also Fluorescein angiography; Indocyanine green angiography*
    cataract surgery in patients with, 11:224
    in children, 6:323–357, 452
    color vision testing in, 12:43–44, 44*i*, 45*i*
    congenital, 2:173, 4:119–123, 121*i*, 122*i*, 123*i*, 12:195–202
    contrast sensitivity testing in, 12:45–47, 46*i*
    cortical evoked potentials in, 12:39–41, 40*i*
    dark adaptation testing in, 12:41–42, 42*i*
    decreased vision with, 5:104
    in diabetes. *See Diabetic retinopathy*
    diagnostic approach to, 12:17–26
    electrically evoked potentials in, 12:41
    electrooculogram in, 12:36–38, 37*i*, 38*i*
    electrophysiologic testing in, 12:27–41. *See also specific test*
    electroretinogram in, 12:30–31, 30*i*, 33–36, 34*i*, 35*i*
    evoked cortical potentials in, 12:39–41, 40*i*
    hallucinations caused by, 5:189–190
    hereditary, 6:333–337
    hydroxychloroquine toxicity and, 1:198, 12:247–248, 248*i*
    illusions caused by, 5:188
    in infant with decreased vision, 6:452
    optical coherence tomography in, 12:24
    peripheral, 12:253–277
    photocoagulation causing, 12:319

photocoagulation for, wavelength selection and, **12**:313–317, 315–316*t*

psychophysical testing in, **12**:41–47

refractive surgery in patient with, **13**:191–193

retinal thickness analyzer in assessment of, **12**:25, 26*i*

scanning laser ophthalmoscopy in, **12**:24–25

stationary, **12**:195–202

Th1 delayed hypersensitivity and, **9**:68*t*

vascular, **12**:97–164. *See also specific type*

  antiphospholipid antibody syndrome and, **1**:184

  arterial occlusion and, **12**:145–152

  Behçet syndrome and, **12**:181

  Coats disease and, **6**:332–333, 333*i*, **12**:156–157, 157*i*

  congenital, **4**:121–122, 122*i*

  cystoid macular edema and, **12**:154–156, 155*i*

  in diabetes. *See* Diabetic retinopathy

  in incontinentia pigmenti, **6**:419, 419*i*

  macroaneurysms, **12**:158–160, 160*i*

    age-related macular degeneration differentiated from, **12**:67, 68*i*

  microaneurysms, in nonproliferative diabetic retinopathy, **12**:103, 104*i*

  parafoveal (juxtafoveal) telangiectasis, **4**:121–122, **12**:157–158, 158*i*, 159*i*

  peripheral neovascularization and, **12**:124, 125*t*

  phakomatoses, **12**:160–164, 161*i*, 162*i*, 164*i*

  in retinopathy of prematurity, **6**:325–332, **12**:124–136

    screening for, **6**:328–329, 329*t*, 330*i*, 331*i*, 351–356, 354*i*

  secondary angle-closure glaucoma and, **10**:143–144

  in sickle cell hemoglobinopathies, **12**:119–124, 120*t*, 121*i*, 122*i*, 123*i*

  systemic hypertension and, **1**:98–99, 98*t*, **12**:97–99, 98*i*, 99*i*, 100*i*

  vasculitis and, **12**:152–154, 153*i*

  venous occlusion and, **12**:136–145

  in Wyburn-Mason syndrome, **6**:419–420, 420*i*

visually evoked potentials in, **12**:39–41, 40*i*

Retinal dystrophies. *See also specific type and* Retinal degenerations

electroretinogram in evaluation of, **12**:33–34, 34*i*

hereditary, **12**:203–229

  diagnostic and prognostic testing in, **12**:204–205, 206*t*

  inner, **12**:228–229

  photoreceptor, **12**:205–215

Retinal edema, **4**:130–131, 130*i*, 131*i*. *See also* Macular edema

in branch retinal vein occlusion, **12**:136

in central retinal artery occlusion, **12**:148, 148*i*

in central retinal vein occlusion, **12**:141, 142*i*

in clinically significant macular edema, **12**:114, 114*i*

Retinal excavations, peripheral, **12**:262

Retinal folds, in shaking injury, **6**:443–444

Retinal ganglion cells. *See* Ganglion cells, retinal

Retinal gene therapy, **9**:42

Retinal hemorrhages

in arterial macroaneurysms, **12**:158, 159

in branch retinal vein occlusion, **12**:136

in central retinal vein occlusion, **12**:141, 142*i*

dot-and-blot, **5**:183, 184*i*

in HIV infection/AIDS, **9**:248

ischemia causing, **4**:131, 132*i*

in leukemia, **4**:281, **6**:344

in nonproliferative diabetic retinopathy, **12**:103, 104*i*

in ocular ischemic syndrome, **12**:151, 151*i*

in shaking injury, **6**:433, 433*i*, 444, **12**:301, 302*i*

Retinal holes

atrophic, **12**:253

  treatment of, **12**:265, 266, 266*t*, 267*t*

operculated, **12**:253, 254, 255*i*

  treatment of, **12**:265, 265–266, 266*t*, 267*t*

Retinal illuminance, **3**:16*t*

Retinal image, size of

calculation of, **3**:106–108, 108*i*

contact lenses affecting, **3**:176*i*, 177–179

Retinal ischemia, **4**:128–135

cellular responses to, **4**:128–130, 129*i*

central and branch retinal artery and vein occlusions causing, **4**:133–135, 134*i*, 135*i*

inner ischemic retinal atrophy and, **4**:128, 129*i*, 133–134

outer ischemic retinal atrophy and, **4**:128, 129*i*

retinopathy of prematurity and, **4**:136–137

vascular responses to, **4**:130–133, 131*i*, 132*i*

Retinal locus, preferred, **3**:246, 247*i*, 253

Retinal migraine, **5**:184, 294–295. *See also* Migraine headache

Retinal neovascularization. *See also* Neovascularization; Retinal disease, vascular

ischemia causing, **4**:130–133, 132*i*

peripheral, **12**:124, 125*t*

  vitreous hemorrhage and, **12**:287

in retinopathy of prematurity, **4**:137, **6**:325–332, **12**:124–136

  screening for, **6**:328–329, 329*t*, 330*i*, 331*i*, 351–356, 354*i*

Retinal nerve fiber layer. *See* Nerve fiber layer

Retinal nerve fibers, **5**:111, 112*i*. *See also* Nerve fiber layer

diffuse loss of, examination of, **10**:55

distribution of, **10**:46, 46*i*

myelinated (medullated), **4**:121, 121*i*, **6**:360, 360*i*

Retinal pigment epithelium (RPE), **4**:117–118, **12**:12–14, 13*i*

adenomas/adenocarcinomas of, **4**:147, 241–242

age-related macular degeneration causing abnormalities of, **12**:57–58

anatomy of, **2**:71*i*, 77–79, 78*i*, 357, **5**:24, **12**:12–14, 13*i*

antioxidants in, **2**:369*i*, 371–373, 373*i*, 374*i*

atrophy of, **12**:57–58, 58*i*

biochemistry and metabolism of, **2**:357–363

central areolar atrophy of, **4**:139

in choroideremia, **12**:224, 225*i*

composition of, **2**:357–358

congenital abnormalities of, **2**:173, 176–178, 178*i*

  hypertrophy, **2**:173, 178, 178*i*, **4**:122–123, 123*i*, **6**:390, 391*i*, **12**:14, 264

    melanoma differentiated from, **4**:230, 231*i*, 232*i*

degeneration of, **12**:58

detachment of

  in age-related macular degeneration, **12**:55–56, 63, 64–66

  in central serous chorioretinopathy, **12**:22*i*, 51, 52

  drusenoid, **12**:220, 221*i*

  fibrovascular, **12**:64–66

development of, 2:143*i*, 144
dystrophies of, age-related macular degeneration
 differentiated from, 12:59, 67
electrooculogram and, 12:36–38, 37*i*, 38*i*
gene defects in, photoreceptor dysfunction/
 degeneration caused by, 2:347–348, 348*i*,
 350–351, 363
geographic atrophy of, 12:57–58, 58*i*
in gyrate atrophy, 12:225, 226*i*
hamartoma of, 4:146, 242, 242*i*, 6:390
hyperpigmentation of, in age-related macular
 degeneration, 12:58
hyperplasia of, 12:14, 263
hypertrophy of, 12:14, 264
 congenital, 2:173, 178, 178*i*, 4:122–123, 123*i*,
 6:390, 391*i*, 12:14, 264
immune response in, 9:34*t*, 40–41
inflammation of (acute retinal epitheliitis/ARPE/Krill
 disease), 9:177*t*, 178, 179*i*
lipids in, 2:358
nongeographic atrophy (degeneration) of, 12:58
phagocytosis by, 2:360–361
physiologic roles of, 2:359–362, 360*i*, 361*t*
pigment granules in, in age-related macular
 degeneration, 12:58
in primary central nervous system lymphoma, 9:229
proteins in, 2:358
regional differences in, 2:78, 78*i*
retinal adhesion maintained by, 2:362
in retinitis pigmentosa, 2:363
in Sorsby fundus dystrophy, 2:363
in Stargardt disease, 12:216, 216*i*, 217*i*
subretinal space maintenance by, 2:361–362
tests in evaluation of, 12:36–39, 37*i*, 38*i*, 39*i*
topography of, 4:117–118
transplantation of, 9:42
transport functions of, 2:361–362
tumors of in children, 6:390
Retinal raytracing, 3:320
Retinal reflex, 3:126–128, 127*i*, 128*i*
 aberrations of, 3:133
 in axis determination, 3:130–132, 131*i*, 132*i*
 characteristics of, 3:128, 128*i*
Retinal rivalry, 6:52, 53*i*
Retinal scar, formation of, 4:24
Retinal sheathing, in sarcoidosis, 9:199, 200*i*
Retinal striae, 12:87
Retinal tears, 4:112. *See also* Retinal breaks
 giant, 12:253
 vitrectomy for, 12:340, 341
 lattice degeneration and, 12:259, 260*i*
 treatment of, 12:265, 266–267, 266*t*, 267*t*
 meridional folds and, 12:262
 paving-stone (cobblestone) degeneration and, 12:263
 photocoagulation causing, 12:319
 in posterior vitreous detachment, 12:256, 257*i*, 258
Retinal telangiectasia/telangiectasis, 12:156–157, 157*i*.
 See also Coats disease
 parafoveal (juxtafoveal), 4:121–122, 12:157–158,
 158*i*, 159*i*
Retinal thickness analyzer, 12:25, 26*i*
Retinal tufts, peripheral, 12:259–260, 261*i*, 262*i*
Retinal vasculitis, 12:152–154, 153*i*
 in Behçet syndrome, 1:194, 9:133, 134*i*, 12:181
 benign, 5:128, 128*i*

 differential diagnosis of, 9:111*t*
 in herpetic disease, 9:140
 HLA association in, 9:94*t*
 in polyarteritis nodosa, 9:175, 176*i*
 in systemic lupus erythematosus, 9:61, 173–175, 174*i*
 in Wegener granulomatosis, 9:62, 175–176, 176*i*
Retinal vasospasm (migraine), 5:190, 294
Retinal vein
 arcade, 5:20, 21–22*i*
 central, 2:104, 104*i*, 5:16*i*, 20, 21–22*i*
Retinal vein occlusion
 branch, 4:134–135, 135*i*, 12:136–141, 137*i*, 139*i*, 140*i*
 intravitreal triamcinolone for, 12:141
 neovascularization in, 4:130–133, 12:138
 photocoagulation for, 12:138–139, 139–140, 139*i*,
 140*i*
 wavelength selection and, 12:315*t*
 vitrectomy for, 12:140–141
 central, 4:133–134, 134*i*, 5:106–107, 106*i*,
 12:141–145, 142*i*
 electroretinogram in, 12:34*i*, 35, 35*i*
 evaluation and management of, 12:143–144
 iris neovascularization in, 12:142, 144–145
 ischemic, 4:133–134, 12:141, 141–142
 nonischemic, 12:141
 papillophlebitis and, 12:141
 primary open-angle glaucoma and, 10:90
 hemispheric (hemicentral), 12:137, 137*i*
Retinaldehyde, in retinal pigment epithelium, 2:359,
 12:14
Retinitis, 9:107
 atypical necrotizing, diagnosis of, 9:63
 Candida, 9:163–164, 164*i*, 223–225, 223*i*
 cytomegalovirus, 1:3, 29, 4:123, 124*i*, 9:156–158,
 157*i*, 12:192–193, 192*i*
 antiviral immunity in, 9:71
 cidofovir for, 1:29, 48, 2:443–444, 9:252
 congenital (cytomegalic inclusion disease),
 6:218–219, 219*i*
 fomivirsen for, 1:48, 9:252
 foscarnet for, 1:29, 48, 2:443, 9:251
 ganciclovir for, 1:29, 2:443, 9:155, 250–252
 in HIV infection/AIDS, 1:3, 29, 47–48, 4:123,
 124*i*, 9:71, 156, 249–253, 251*i*
 in children, 6:219
 foveomacular (solar retinopathy/retinitis),
 12:307–308
 herpetic necrotizing (acute retinal necrosis), 4:123,
 124*i*, 9:140, 154–156, 155*i*, 156*i*, 12:185–186,
 185*i*
 measles, 9:159
 pigmentosa, 4:139–140, 140*i*, 9:221, 12:207–213
 autosomal dominant, 12:210
 rhodopsin mutations causing, 2:348
 autosomal recessive, 12:211
 rhodopsin mutations causing, 2:348
 rod cGMP gated channel mutations causing,
 2:349
 rod cGMP phosphodiesterase mutations
 causing, 2:349
 cataract surgery in patients with, 11:224
 central, 12:210
 clinical features of, 12:207–209, 208*i*

congenital (Leber congenital amaurosis),
     6:334–335, 335*i*, 452, 454–455, 12:211–212,
     233–234
     guanylate cyclase mutations causing, 2:349
     RPE65 gene defects causing, 2:350, 6:335
contrast sensitivity testing in, 12:46
counseling patients with, 12:212
cystoid macular edema and, 12:154, 212, 213*i*
decreased vision in, 5:110, 110*i*
definition of, 12:207
diagnosis of, 12:207–209, 208*i*
differential diagnosis of, 12:209
electroretinogram in, 12:34*i*, 208–209
genetics of, 12:210–211
hearing loss and, 12:235. *See also* Usher syndrome
management/therapy of, 12:212–213
with neuropathy and ataxia, 12:245
     mitochondrial DNA mutations and, 2:218, 219*i*,
     220
oxygen-regulated protein defects causing, 2:350
pericentral, 12:210
regional variants of, 12:209–210, 209*i*
retinal pigment epithelium in, 2:363
ROM1 gene mutations in, 2:350
sectorial, 12:210
simplex, 12:209
sine pigmento, 5:110, 12:207
unilateral, 12:210
uveitis in children differentiated from, 6:320
visual field testing in, 12:205–206, 207*i*
X-linked, 12:211
     ocular findings in carriers of, 2:270*i*, 270*t*
     retinal pigment epithelium in, 2:363
punctata albescens, 12:200, 207, 208*i*
     CRALBP defects causing, 2:351
rubella, 9:158–159, 159*i*
sclopetaria, 12:294–295, 294*i*
solar (solar retinopathy/foveomacular retinitis),
     12:307–308
in syphilis, 9:188, 189*i*, 190, 190*i*
in toxoplasmosis, 6:216, 217*i*, 9:165–166, 166*i*, 167*i*,
     254–255, 255*i*
in Wegener granulomatosis, 9:62, 175, 176*i*
Retinoblastoma, 4:140–144, 146*i*, 251–265, 265*t*,
     6:390–399, 393*i*, 9:232
associated tumors and, 6:396
classification of, 4:258–259, 258*t*, 287–288*t*,
     6:394–396, 396*t*, 397*t*
clinical evaluation/diagnosis of, 4:253–259, 253*t*,
     254*i*, 255*i*, 6:392–394, 393*i*
     differential diagnosis and, 4:255–258, 255*i*, 256*t*,
     257*i*
conditions associated with, 4:260
diffuse infiltrating, 4:253–254
endophytic, 6:392, 393*i*
enucleation for, 7:120
epidemiology of, 4:251, 251*t*
exenteration for, 7:128
exophytic, 6:392, 393*i*
extraocular, 6:398
fleurettes in, 4:143–144, 143*i*, 6:394
genetics of, 2:253–254, 4:141, 213, 252–253, 252*i*,
     6:295*i*, 394
     counseling and, 4:252–253, 252*i*, 6:394, 395*i*
glaucoma and, 6:279

histologic features of, 4:141–144, 141*i*, 142*i*
intracranial, 4:260
iris affected in, 4:220*t*, 221*i*
leukocoria in, 6:390–391, 393*i*
long arm 13 deletion syndrome and, 2:253–254
metastatic evaluation and, 4:254–255
monitoring patient with, 6:398–399
mutation rate of, 2:256
nonocular, 6:399
optic nerve affected in, 4:254–255
orbit affected in, 4:254–255, 255*i*
pathogenesis of, 4:140–141
persistent hyperplastic primary vitreous
     differentiated from, 12:282
presenting signs and symptoms of, 4:253, 253*t*
prognosis for, 4:264, 265*t*
progression of, 4:144, 145*i*, 146*i*
rosettes in, 2:173, 4:142–143, 143*i*, 260, 6:394
secondary malignancies and, 4:144, 264, 265*t*, 6:399
spontaneous regression of, 4:263, 6:392
staging of, 4:287–288*t*
strabismus in, 6:391
treatment of, 4:260–263, 263*i*, 6:396–398, 398*i*
trilateral, 4:260
uveitis in children differentiated from, 6:320*t*
vitreous seeding and, 4:253–254, 254*i*, 6:392, 393*i*
Retinoblastoma *(RB1)* gene, 2:253–254, 4:141, 213,
     252, 6:394
     secondary malignancies and, 4:144
Retinochoroidal collaterals (opticociliary shunt vessels),
     in papilledema, 5:116–117
Retinochoroiditis, 9:107
     in congenital herpes simplex, 6:219
     in cytomegalic inclusion disease, 6:218–219, 219*i*
     Toxoplasma causing, 9:164–169
          in HIV infection/AIDS, 9:254–255, 255*i*
Retinochoroidopathies, 9:176–185, 177*t*. *See also specific
     disorder*
     birdshot (vitiliginous chorioretinitis), 9:177*t*,
          180–181, 180*i*, 181*i*, 12:174*t*, 177–178, 178*i*
          HLA association in, 9:94*t*, 180–181
Retinocytoma (retinoma), 4:144, 146*i*, 259, 6:392
Retinogeniculocortical pathway, 6:44–45, 47*i*
     development of, 6:46–49
          abnormal visual experience affecting, 6:49–52, 50*i*,
          51*i*
Retinoic acid, ocular development/congenital
     anomalies and, 2:131, 160
Retinoic acid-binding protein, cellular, 2:361*t*
Retinoid-binding proteins, 2:361*t*
     interphotoreceptor, 2:359, 361*t*
Retinoids, for xerophthalmia/dry eye syndrome, 8:94
Retinol, 2:359, 360*i*
Retinol-binding protein, 2:361*t*
Retinopathy. *See also specific type and* Retinitis
     acute zonal occult outer (AZOOR), 5:107, 9:180,
          12:179–180, 180*i*
     in antiphospholipid antibody syndrome, 1:184
     cancer-associated, 5:101, 108–109, 9:61, 12:237–238,
          238*i*
     canthaxanthine, 12:249, 250*i*, 250*t*
     of carotid occlusive disease, 12:145
          central retinal vein occlusion differentiated from,
          12:143, 145
     central retinal artery occlusion and, 5:105–106, 106*i*

central retinal vein occlusion and, **5**:106–107, 106*i*
central serous, **5**:105, **12**:51–54
  age-related macular degeneration differentiated
    from, **12**:53, 59, 68–69, 69*i*
  fluorescein angiography in, **12**:22*i*, 52
in child abuse, **12**:301–302, 302*i*
chloroquine, **12**:247–248, 248*i*
in congenital rubella syndrome, **6**:218
in congenital syphilis, **6**:220
crystalline, drug toxicity causing, **12**:249, 250*i*
cytomegalovirus, in children, **6**:218–219, 219*i*
diabetic, in children, **6**:343
diabetic. *See* Diabetic retinopathy
drug-related, **12**:247–251
eclipse (solar retinopathy), **12**:307–308
exudative, retinopathy of prematurity and, **12**:131
HIV, **9**:248, 249*i*
hydroxychloroquine causing, **1**:198
hypertensive, **1**:98–99, 98*t*, **12**:97–98
  in renal disease in children, **6**:349
hyperviscosity, central retinal vein occlusion
  differentiated from, **12**:143
of incontinentia pigmenti, **6**:419, 419*i*
isotretinoin, **12**:250
in leukemia, **6**:343–344
melanoma-associated, **5**:101, 109, **12**:237–239
multiple evanescent white dot syndrome and, **5**:107,
  108*i*
paraneoplastic, **12**:237–239, 238*i*
pigmentary, **12**:207, 231, 233*t*. *See also* Retinitis,
  pigmentosa
  hearing loss and, **12**:235. *See also* Usher syndrome
  systemic diseases with, **12**:231, 232–233*t*
of prematurity, **4**:136–137, **6**:325–332, 351,
  12:124–136
  angle kappa and, **6**:86, 331, 331*i*
  cataract surgery in patients with, **11**:213
  classification of, **6**:326, 327*i*, 327*t*, 328*i*, 329*i*,
    12:127–130, 128*t*
  conditions associated with, **12**:131–132
  familial exudative vitreoretinopathy differentiated
    from, **12**:284
  glaucoma and, **6**:279
  management of, **6**:326–332, 329*i*, 330*i*, 331*i*,
    12:132–136, 133*i*, 134*i*, 135*i*
  natural course of, **12**:130–131
  pathogenesis of, **12**:126–132, 127*i*
  screening examinations for, **6**:328–329, 329*i*, 330*i*,
    331*i*, 351–356, 354*i*
  secondary angle-closure glaucoma and, **10**:145
  staging of, **12**:127–130, 128*i*, 128*t*, 129*i*, 130*i*, 131*i*
  terminology used with, **12**:127–130, 128*t*
Purtscher/Purtscher-like, **12**:94–95, 94*i*, 95*t*
radiation, **1**:256, **12**:305, 306*i*
retinitis pigmentosa and, **5**:110, 110*i*
in scleroderma, **1**:186
in shaken baby syndrome, **12**:301
sickle cell. *See* Sickle cell retinopathy
solar (foveomacular/solar retinitis), **12**:307–308
surface-wrinkling, **5**:105, **12**:87
tamoxifen, **12**:249, 250*i*, 250*t*
thioridazine, **12**:248–249, 249*t*
Valsalva, **12**:93–94
venous stasis, **5**:184, **12**:141, 145

Retinopexy, pneumatic, for retinal detachment, **12**:272,
  335
Retinoschisin, in X-linked retinoschisis, **12**:229
Retinoschisis, **12**:275–277, 275*i*, 276*i*, 277*t*
  foveal, **6**:340
  juvenile, **6**:340, 341*i*
  juvenile. *See* Retinoschisis, X-linked
  reticular degenerative, **4**:126, **12**:276
  retinal detachment and, **12**:276–277, 277*t*
  traumatic, in shaking injury, **6**:444, 444*i*
  typical degenerative, **12**:276, 276*i*
  X-linked (juvenile), **6**:340, 341*i*, **12**:228–229, 228*i*
    electroretinogram patterns in, **12**:30*i*, 228–229
Retinoscopes, **3**:125, 125*i*, 127*i*. *See also* Retinoscopy
Retinoscopic reflex. *See* Retinal reflex
Retinoscopy, **3**:125–134, **8**:49
  alignment in, **3**:126
  in children, **3**:146
    in cataract, **6**:292
  correcting lens in, **3**:128–129, 129*i*
  fixation in, **3**:126
  fogging and, **3**:126
  irregular astigmatism and, **3**:133
  neutrality in, **3**:129, 130*i*
  positioning in, **3**:126
  in regular astigmatism, **3**:129–133, 130*i*, 131*i*, 132*i*
  retinal reflex and, **3**:126–128, 127*i*, 128*i*
    aberrations of, **3**:133
    characteristics of, **3**:128, 128*i*
  steps in performance of, **3**:133–134
Retraction, eyelid, **4**:168, **5**:145, 279, 279*t*, **7**:223–225,
  224*i*
  after blepharoplasty, **7**:224, 233, 233*i*
  in Graves ophthalmopathy, **5**:274–275, 276*i*, 329,
    329*i*, **7**:26, 48–51, 48*i*, 53, 223–225, 224*i*
  proptosis differentiated from, **7**:223–224
  after strabismus surgery, **7**:224
  treatment of, **7**:224–225
Retractors, eyelid, **7**:141*i*, 142–145, 144*i*
  lower eyelid, **7**:140*i*, 144*i*, 145
    in involutional ectropion, repair of, **7**:198
    in involutional entropion, **7**:202–203
      repair of, **7**:203*i*, 204–205
  upper eyelid, **7**:142–144, 144*i*
Retrobulbar anesthesia. *See also* Anesthesia
  (anesthetics)
  adverse reactions to, **1**:322, 323, 335–336
  for cataract surgery, **11**:94, 95*i*
    anticoagulation therapy and, **11**:201, 202
  for extraocular muscle surgery, **6**:183
  needle perforation and, **12**:296
  for phakic IOL insertion, **13**:147
  strabismus after, **6**:157
Retrobulbar hemorrhage
  after blepharoplasty, visual loss and, **7**:232–233
  after cataract surgery, **11**:169
Retrobulbar optic neuritis, **5**:141–144, 142*i*
  contrast sensitivity affected by, **3**:115
  treatment of, **5**:143–144
Retrochiasmal lesions, **5**:164–170
  in multiple sclerosis, **5**:321
  of occipital lobe, **5**:167–170, 168*i*, 169*i*, 170*i*
  of optic tract, **5**:164–165, 165*i*, 166*i*
  of parietal lobe, **5**:166–167
  of temporal lobe, **5**:166, 167*i*

visual field loss patterns in, 5:164
Retrocorneal fibrous membrane (posterior collagenous layer), 2:301–302, 8:33–34
Retroillumination, for slit-lamp biomicroscopy, 8:19
Retrolaminar portion of optic nerve, 2:99–101, 100*i*, 10:49
  blood supply of, 2:103
Retrolental fibroplasia. *See* Retinopathy, of prematurity
Retro-orbicularis oculi fat (ROOF), 7:134
Retro-orbital plexus, 2:119
Retroposon, 2:195
Retrotransposition, 2:195
Retrovir. *See* Zidovudine
Retroviral syndrome (primary HIV infection), 1:38. *See also* HIV infection/AIDS
Retroviruses
  cancer association of, 1:254
  HIV as, 1:37
  ocular infection caused by, 8:122
Rev-Eyes. *See* Dapiprazole
Revascularization procedures. *See also* Coronary artery bypass graft; Percutaneous transluminal coronary angioplasty
  for angina, 1:121–122
  for ST-segment elevation acute coronary syndrome, 1:125
Reverse geometry designs, orthokeratology and, 3:203
Reverse ocular bobbing, 5:256
Reverse ocular dipping, 5:256
Reverse slab-off, for induced anisophoria, 3:161
Reverse telescopes, in slit-lamp biomicroscope, 3:280–281
Reverse transcriptase, 1:37, 8:122
  viral carcinogenesis and, 1:254
Reverse transcriptase inhibitors, 1:41
  in HAART, 1:43
  non-nucleoside (NNRTIs), 9:246, 247*t*
Reverse transcription, 2:195
Revised European-American (REAL) classification, for lymphomas, 4:194–195, 7:85, 86*t*
Reyataz. *See* Atazanavir
Rezulin. *See* Troglitazone
RF. *See* Rheumatoid factor
RFLPs (restriction fragment length polymorphisms), 2:195, 222–223, 224*i*
RGP contact lenses. *See* Rigid gas-permeable contact lenses
Rhabdomyomas, in tuberous sclerosis, 6:410
Rhabdomyosarcoma
  of orbit, 4:198, 199*i*, 6:372–373, 373*i*, 7:79–80, 79*i*
  retinoblastoma associated with, 4:265*t*
Rhegmatogenous retinal detachment. *See* Retinal detachment
Rheopheresis (differential membrane filtration), for nonneovascular AMD, 12:62
Rheumatic disorders, 1:173–200. *See also specific type*
  medical therapy for, 1:194–200, 197*t*
  recent developments in, 1:173
Rheumatoid arthritis, 1:173–175
  cataract surgery in patients with, 11:206–207
  juvenile. *See* Juvenile idiopathic (chronic/rheumatoid) arthritis
  peripheral ulcerative keratitis and, 8:203, 229, 232*i*
Rheumatoid factor, 1:174
  in aqueous tear deficiency, 8:73

in juvenile idiopathic (chronic/rheumatoid) arthritis, uveitis and, 6:313*t*, 314
in Sjögren syndrome, 8:73
testing for, 8:202*t*
Rheumatoid nodules, 1:174
Rheumatrex. *See* Methotrexate
Rhinocerebral mucormycosis, 5:366, 367*i*
Rhinophyma, in rosacea, 8:85–86
Rhinosporidium seeberi (rhinosporidiosis), 8:130
Rhinoviruses, ocular infection caused by, 8:121
Rhizopus infection, 8:130–131
  orbital, 7:45–46
Rhodopsin, 2:311, 341–344, 342*i*, 343*i*, 12:10
  in blue-green phototoxicity, 2:459
  gene for, 2:347
    mutations in, 2:227, 347, 348, 12:204
      in retinitis pigmentosa, 12:210
  light affecting, 2:342–344, 343*i*
  phosphorylation of, 2:342, 343
  regeneration of, retinal pigment epithelium in, 2:359, 360*i*, 361*i*
  in rods, 2:341–344, 342*i*, 343*i*, 344*t*
Rhodopsin kinase, 2:344*t*
  mutations in, 2:349
rhuFab, for age-related macular degeneration, 12:76, 77*t*
Rhytidectomy, 7:244–245, 245*i*, 246*i*
Ribavirin, 1:65*t*
  for hepatitis C, 1:31
Ribonucleic acid. *See* RNA
Ribosomal RNA (rRNA), 2:212
Ribosomes, protein synthesis in, 2:210
Ribozymes, for glaucoma, 10:177
Richner-Hanhart syndrome, 8:310*t*, 344–345
Riddoch phenomenon, 5:170, 196
Riders, 11:38
Ridley intraocular lens, 11:139–142, 140*i*
RIEG gene, 10:13*t*, 15
RIEG1 gene, 2:159, 10:13*t*
RIEG1/PITX2 gene. *See also PITX2* gene
  in Axenfeld-Rieger syndrome, 6:253
RIEG2 gene, 10:13*t*
Rieger anomaly/syndrome, 2:168, 169, 169*i*, 4:79, 6:278, 10:152, 153*t*. *See also* Axenfeld-Rieger syndrome
  gene for, 10:15
Rifabutin, 1:49
  protease inhibitor interactions and, 1:49
  uveitis caused by, 9:141, 12:250
Rifadin. *See* Rifampin
Rifampicin, protease inhibitor interactions and, 1:49
Rifampin, 1:24, 49, 54, 63*t*, 73
  ocular effects of, 1:324*t*
Right bundle branch block, 1:135
Right gaze (dextroversion), 6:36, 278
Rigid corneal contact lenses (hard contact lenses). *See also* Rigid gas-permeable contact lenses
  polymers used for, 3:183–185
Rigid gas-permeable contact lenses, 3:191–195
  adverse reactions to, 3:203
  base curve of, 3:174*i*, 177
  design of, 3:193*i*
  diameter of, 3:177, 193*i*
  edge profiles of, 3:193*i*
  fitting, principles for, 3:194–195

in giant papillary conjunctivitis patients, 8:216
materials for, 3:183–185
for myopia reduction (orthokeratology), 3:203–205,
13:84–85
parameters of, 3:192–195, 193*i*
power of, 3:177, 194
refractive surgery and, 13:205
after PRK, 13:206
after radial keratotomy, 13:205–206
tear (fluid) lens created by, 3:180–181, 181*i*
Riley-Day syndrome (familial dysautonomia), 2:262*t*,
6:260
neurotrophic keratopathy in, 8:103
racial and ethnic concentration of, 2:259
"Rim" proteins, 2:344, 344*t*. *See also specific type*
mutations in, 2:347, 347*i*
Rimantadine, 1:65*t*, 77
Rimexolone, 2:417*t*, 420
for uveitis, 9:115*t*, 116, 238
riMLF. *See* Rostral interstitial nucleus, of medial
longitudinal fasciculus
Ring melanoma, 4:157, 159, 161, 162*i*, 222
Ring of Schwalbe. *See* Schwalbe's line/ring
Ring scotoma, in retinitis pigmentosa, 5:110
Ring sign, in idiopathic orbital inflammation, 7:58
Riolan, muscle of, 2:22, 24, 24*i*
Rise time, in phacoemulsification, 11:115, 119–121,
120*i*
aspiration flow rate and, 11:121, 122*i*
Risedronate, for osteoporosis, 1:245*t*
Risk, relative, 1:292, 360–361
Risk difference, 1:360–361
Risk factor, 1:361. *See also specific type and* Ethnic
differences
in cross-sectional studies, 1:349–350
pretest probability of disease and, 1:357–359, 358*i*
Risley prism, 3:89
Risperdal. *See* Risperidone
Risperidone, 1:271
Ritipenem, 1:69
Ritonavir, 1:42
for postexposure HIV prophylaxis, 1:45, 46–47*t*
Rivalry pattern, 6:52, 53*i*
Rivastigmine, for Alzheimer disease, 1:288
River blindness (onchocerciasis), 8:51*t*, 132, 9:195–197
Rizzutti's sign, in keratoconus, 8:330, 330*i*
RK. *See* Radial keratotomy
RLF (retrolental fibroplasia). *See* Retinopathy, of
prematurity
RNA, 2:199, 8:306
amplification of, in polymerase chain reaction, 2:193
creation of from DNA, 2:209
heteronuclear/heterogeneous nuclear (hnRNA),
2:187, 209
messenger (mRNA), 2:126, 8:306
processing of, 2:209
in retinal pigment epithelium, 2:358
ribosomal (rRNA), 2:212
small interference (short interfering) (siRNA), 2:202
splicing of, 2:196, 209
alternative, 2:203
transfer (tRNA), 2:211–212, 8:306
RNA viruses, 8:118–119
cancer association of, 1:254

ocular infection caused by, 8:121–122, 162–163. *See
also specific virus*
ROC (receiver operating characteristics) curve, 1:355,
356*i*, 357, 357*i*
Rocephin. *See* Ceftriaxone
Rod cGMP phosphodiesterase (rod PDE), 2:343, 344*t*
mutations in, 2:349
Rod–cone dystrophies/degenerations. *See also* Retinitis,
pigmentosa
electroretinogram patterns in, 12:30*i*
Rod inner segments, 2:79, 82*i*. *See also* Rods
Rod monochromatism, 12:196. *See also* Achromatopsia
in children, 6:335–336, 455
Rod outer segments, 2:79, 82*i*, 341. *See also* Rods
energy metabolism in, 2:344
oxidative damage to, 2:370
phototransduction in, 2:341–344, 342*i*, 343*i*
Rod response, 2:355, 355*i*, 12:27, 28*i*, 29. *See also* Dark
adaptation testing
Rodenstock contact lens, for fundus biomicroscopy,
3:288, 289*i*
Rods, 2:79, 82*i*, 12:10. *See also* Rod outer segments
abnormalities of, 12:198–202
amacrine cells for, 2:352
electrophysiologic responses of, 2:354–355, 355*i*
gene defects in, photoreceptor dysfunction/
degeneration and, 2:347, 347*i*, 348–350
phototransduction in, 2:341–344, 342*i*, 343*i*
proteins in, 2:344, 344*t*
mutations of, 2:347, 347*i*
Rofecoxib, 2:307
removal of from market, 1:173, 196
Roferon-A. *See* Interferons (IFNs), α
Rohypnol. *See* Flunitrazepam
Rokitamycin, 1:75
ROM1 gene/ROM1 protein, 2:344, 344*t*
mutations in, 2:350
ROOF. *See* Retro-orbicularis oculi fat
ROP. *See* Retinopathy, of prematurity
Ropinirole, for Parkinson disease, 1:279
Rosacea, 8:84–86, 84*i*, 85*i*
cataract surgery in patients with, 11:206, 206*i*
meibomian gland dysfunction and, 8:82–83
Rose bengal stain, 2:451, 8:22
in tear-film evaluation, 8:22, 72, 73*i*
Rosengren-Doane tear pump, 7:256, 257*i*
Rosenmüller, valve of, 6:239, 7:254
Rosenthal, basilar vein of, 5:22
Rosenthal fibers, in optic nerve gliomas, 4:209, 209*i*
Rosette cataract, 11:55
Rosettes, 2:173
in retinal dysplasia, 2:173
in retinoblastoma, 2:173, 4:142–143, 143*i*, 260, 6:394
Rosiglitazone, 1:212*t*, 213–214
with metformin, 1:213
Rostral interstitial nucleus, of medial longitudinal
fasciculus, 5:34, 37*i*, 202
Rosuvastatin, for hypercholesterolemia, 1:149*t*, 150*t*
Rotary prism, 3:89
Rotation, center of, 6:27–28, 27*i*
Rotational corneal autograft, 8:472
Rotational flap
for eyelid repair, 7:190*i*, 191*i*, 192
for wound closure after pterygium excision, 8:429,
430*i*

Roth spots, 4:131
Rothmund-Thomson syndrome, 8:353*t*
Round segment one-piece bifocals, 3:152, 153*i*
Roxithromycin, 1:60*t*, 71
RP. *See* Retinitis, pigmentosa
RP12, 12:207
RPCD. *See* Reticular peripheral cystoid degeneration
RPE. *See* Retinal pigment epithelium
RPE65 gene/RPE65 protein, 2:358, 359
  mutations in, 2:350
    in Leber congenital amaurosis, 2:350, 6:335
RPED. *See* Retinal pigment epithelium (RPE), detachment of
RPG contact lenses. *See* Rigid gas-permeable contact lenses
RPR (rapid plasma reagin) test, 1:16–17, 302, 9:189–190, 12:190
RRD (rhegmatogenous retinal detachment). *See* Retinal detachment
rRNA. *See* Ribosomal RNA
RTA. *See* Retinal thickness analyzer
Rubella, 9:158–159, 159*i*
  congenital, 6:217–218, 218*i*, 8:163, 9:158–159, 159*i*
    cataracts and, 2:172–173, 4:95, 6:218, 11:38–39
  immunization against, 1:306–307
  posterior uveitis in, 9:158, 159*i*
Rubeola (measles) virus, 9:159
  immunization against, 1:304*t*, 306
  ocular infection caused by, 8:162–163
    conjunctivitis, 6:228
    posterior uveitis, 9:159
Rubeosis iridis (iris neovascularization), 2:40, 61, 4:155–156, 155*t*
  in branch retinal vein occlusion, 12:139
  in central retinal artery occlusion, 12:150
  in central retinal vein occlusion, 5:107, 12:142, 144–145
  in diabetic patients, 12:111
  disorders predisposing to, 10:132, 133*t*, 134*i*, 135*i*
  in ocular ischemic syndrome, 12:150, 151
Rubinstein-Taybi (broad-thumb) syndrome, childhood glaucoma and, 10:155*t*
Ruby laser, 3:22. *See also* Lasers
  photocoagulation with, for central serous chorioretinopathy, 12:53–54
Rudiment (anlage/primordium), 2:125, 127
Rufen. *See* Ibuprofen
Run diagrams, 1:368, 371*i*
Rush (plus) disease, 4:137, 6:326, 327*t*, 329*i*, 12:129, 130*i*
  retinopathy of prematurity and, 6:329
Russell bodies, 4:15, 16*i*, 54
Rust ring, iron foreign body causing, 8:406, 406*i*
Rx gene family, 2:131

S

S-100 protein, in immunohistochemistry, 4:37
S-3578, 1:68
S-cone opsin genes, 2:347
S cones, 2:345
  enhanced (Goldmann-Favre syndrome), 6:342, 12:201, 202*i*, 229
  horizontal cells for, 2:352

retinal ganglion cells for, 2:353
S-IgA. *See* Secretory IgA
SA node. *See* Sinoatrial (SA) node
SAARDs. *See* Slow-acting (disease-modifying) antirheumatic drugs
Sabin-Feldman dye test, for toxoplasmosis, 9:166–167
Sabin vaccine (OPV), 1:304*t*, 307
Sabril. *See* Vigabatrin
SAC. *See* Seasonal allergic conjunctivitis
Saccades/saccadic system, 5:198, 6:32–33, 39
  assessment of, 5:202–203
  dysfunction of, 5:206–209
    in Alzheimer disease, 1:288
    gaze palsy and, 5:208–209, 209*i*, 210*i*
    ocular motor apraxia and, 5:207–208
  hypermetric, 5:203, 207
  hypometric, 5:203, 207
  inability to initiate (ocular motor apraxia), 6:156
    in ataxia telangiectasia, 6:417
  intrusions in, 5:199, 204, 252–254
    with normal intersaccadic intervals, 5:252–253, 252*i*
    without normal intersaccadic intervals, 5:253
  reflexive, 5:206
  testing velocity of, 6:89
  visually guided, 5:34
Saccadomania (opsoclonus), 5:253, 6:167
  in neuroblastoma, 6:374
Saccular (berry) aneurysm, 1:105–106, 5:350
Saethre-Chotzen syndrome, 6:426, 428*i*
Sagittal depth (vault), of contact lens, 3:175, 176*i*
Sagittal sinus, superior, 5:20
  thrombosis of, 5:358
SAI (surface asymmetry index), 3:303
Salicylates, 1:197*t*, 2:421. *See also* Nonsteroidal anti-inflammatory drugs
Salk vaccine (IPV), 1:304*t*, 307
  in combination vaccines, 1:309
Salmeterol, 1:157, 157*t*
Salmon patches
  in sickle cell disease, 12:121, 122*i*
  in syphilitic keratitis, 6:260, 8:227, 299
Salmonella, 8:126
Salsalate, 1:197*t*
Salt-and-pepper fundus/retinopathy
  rubella and, 6:218, 9:158, 159*i*
  syphilis and, 9:188
    in infants and children, 6:220
Salzmann nodular degeneration, 8:372, 372*i*
SAM. *See* "Steeper add minus" rule
SAM (selective adhesion molecule) inhibitor, for multiple sclerosis, 5:324
Sampaolesi's line, 10:42
Sample size/sampling, 1:342, 365, 366
Sandhoff disease (GM$_2$ gangliosidosis type II), 2:262*t*, 6:350, 437*t*, 438
  retinal degeneration and, 12:243
Sandimmune. *See* Cyclosporine
Sands of the Sahara (diffuse lamellar keratitis/DLK), after LASIK, 13:127, 128*i*, 129*t*
Sanfilippo syndrome, 2:262*t*, 6:436*t*, 8:337*t*, 12:232*t*, 243
Sanger method, for DNA sequencing, 2:231, 232*i*
Saquinavir, 1:42
  for postexposure HIV prophylaxis, 1:46–47*t*

Sarcoid granuloma, **5**:333, **8**:271
Sarcoidosis, **5**:332–333, **8**:88, **9**:197–200, 197*i*, 198*i*,
    199*i*, 200*i*
  conjunctivitis and, **4**:47–49
  cranial nerve VII involvement in, **5**:285
  diagnosis and treatment of, **5**:333
  eyelid manifestations of, **4**:173*t*
  HLA association in, **9**:94*t*
  intraocular manifestations in, **5**:333
  neuro-ophthalmologic manifestations in, **5**:333
  numb chin associated with, **5**:301
  optic nerve affected in, **4**:205, 206*i*
  orbit affected in, **7**:59
  panuveitis in, **6**:315, **9**:107, 197–200, 197*i*, 198*i*, 199*i*,
    200*i*, **12**:180, 180*i*
  pediatric, **6**:270, 315
    iris nodules and posterior synechiae associated
      with, **6**:270
    uveitis in, **6**:315
  retina affected in, **4**:126, **8**:88
  uveal tract affected in, **4**:154–155, 154*i*. *See also*
      Sarcoidosis, panuveitis in
Sarcoma, **4**:17*i*
  Ewing, **6**:375
    retinoblastoma associated with, **4**:265*t*
  granulocytic (chloroma), **6**:375, **7**:94–95
  Kaposi. *See* Kaposi sarcoma
  orbital, **6**:372–374
    exenteration for, **7**:128
    secondary, **7**:94–95
    staging of, **4**:293*t*
  reticulum cell, **9**:228–231, 228*i*, 230*i*, **12**:182–183,
    182*i*. *See also* Lymphomas, intraocular
    uveitis in children differentiated from, **6**:320*t*
  soft tissue, retinoblastoma associated with, **4**:265*t*
SARS. *See* Severe acute respiratory syndrome
Satellite DNA, **2**:195, 203, 223
Satellite lesions, in toxoplasmosis, **6**:216
Sattler's veil (central epithelial edema), **8**:106
Saturation recovery (SR), definition of, **5**:81
SBE (subacute bacterial endocarditis). *See* Endocarditis
SCA. *See* Superior cerebellar artery
SCA7 gene, cone–rod dystrophy and, **12**:215
Scalp flap, coronal, for anterior orbitotomy, **7**:110
Scanning confocal microscope, **8**:37–38
Scanning laser ophthalmoscopy (SLO), **3**:246, 247*i*
  in retinal examination, **12**:24–25
Scanning laser polarimeter, in optic nerve head
    evaluation, **10**:55–56
Scanning-slit lasers, for photoablation, **13**:30
Scaphocephaly, **6**:424
Scar formation, wound repair and, **4**:19, 20*i*
Scatter diagram, **1**:368, 369*i*
Scatter laser treatment. *See also* Panretinal
    photocoagulation; Photocoagulation
  for branch retinal vein occlusion, **12**:140, 140*i*
  for central retinal artery occlusion, **12**:150
  for central retinal vein occlusion, **12**:144–145
  for diabetic retinopathy, **12**:107–111, 108*i*, 110*i*
  for ocular ischemic syndrome, **12**:151
  for retinopathy of prematurity, **12**:134, 135*i*
Scattering, light, **3**:12–13
  Rayleigh, **3**:12
  for slit-lamp biomicroscopy, **8**:19
Scavenging, **9**:51

Scavenging macrophages, **9**:51–52, 51*i*
SCD. *See* Sudden cardiac death
Schachar theory of accommodation, **11**:23, **13**:168–170,
    169*i*, 170*i*
  scleral expansion for presbyopia correction and,
    13:177
Schaumann's bodies, in sarcoidosis, **4**:155, **9**:198
Scheie Classification of Hypertension Retinopathy,
    Modified, **12**:97
Scheie syndrome, **2**:262*t*, **6**:436*t*, **8**:335–336, 337*t*
  congenital/infantile corneal opacities and, **6**:255,
    436*t*, **8**:298
  retinal degeneration and, **12**:232*t*
Scheiner double-pinhole principle, in automated
    refraction, **3**:312, 315*i*
Schematic eye, **3**:105–108, 106*i*, 107*t*
  optical constants of, **3**:106*i*, 107*t*
  reduced, **3**:108*i*
Schiøtz (indentation) tonometry, **10**:29
  HIV prevention precautions and, **9**:262
Schirmer tests, **5**:173, 298, **8**:62–63, 62*i*, 62*t*
  type I, **8**:62, 62*t*
    in pseudoepiphora, **7**:274
  type II, **8**:62, 62*t*
Schizoaffective disorder, **1**:265
Schizophrenia, **1**:264–265
  drugs for (antipsychotic drugs), **1**:271–273, 272*t*
Schizophreniform disorder, **1**:265
Schlemm's canal, **2**:53*i*, 54, 57*i*, 58, 58*i*, 59*i*, 60*i*, **4**:78,
    78*i*
  aqueous outflow through, **10**:17, 20–22, 21*i*
  development of, **2**:154
  gonioscopic visualization of, **10**:40, 41*i*
Schnabel, cavernous optic atrophy of, **4**:206, 207*i*
Schnyder crystalline dystrophy, **8**:310*t*, 321–323, 322*i*,
    338
School age children. *See also* Children
  low vision in, **3**:266
School (physiologic/simple) myopia, **3**:120
Schubert-Bornschein form of congenital stationary
    night blindness, **12**:198
Schwalbe's line/ring, **2**:51, 52*i*, 53*i*, **4**:78–79, 78*i*, 79*i*
  as angle landmark, **10**:39
  in Axenfeld-Rieger syndrome, **8**:292
  in posterior embryotoxon, **2**:168, 168*i*, **6**:251–252,
    251*i*, **8**:291, 292*i*
Schwann cells, retinal, **2**:353
Schwannoma (neurilemoma/neurinoma)
  conjunctival, **8**:269, 270*i*
  of orbit, **4**:200, 201*i*, **6**:381, **7**:79
  of uveal tract, **4**:165, 283
Schwartz-Matsuo syndrome, **10**:116
Schwartz syndrome, **9**:222, **10**:116
Scientific studies. *See* Clinical research/studies
Scintigraphy, lacrimal, for acquired tearing evaluation,
    7:272, 273*i*
Scissors reflex, **3**:133
Sclera, **2**:43*i*, 44*i*
  aging of, **8**:363, 378, 379*i*
  anatomy of, **2**:43*i*, 44*i*, 49–51, 50*i*, 51*i*, **8**:14
  bare, wound closure after pterygium excision and,
    8:429, 430*i*
  blue, **8**:288
    in Ehlers-Danlos syndrome, **8**:288
    in keratoglobus, **8**:334, 335

in Marfan syndrome, **8:**354
in osteogenesis imperfecta, **8:**288
congenital anomalies of, **4:**88–89, **8:**285–288
basic concepts of, **8:**281–283
causes of, **8:**281–282
diagnostic approach to, **8:**282–283
degenerations of, **4:**90*i*, 91–92, 91*i*, **8:**378, 378*i*
development of, **2:**152, **8:**6
disorders of, **4:**87–92, **8:**25*t. See also specific type and*
Episcleritis; Scleritis
degenerations, **8:**378, 378*i*
immune-mediated, **8:**202, 234–241
neoplastic, **4:**92
Th1 delayed hypersensitivity and, **9:**68*t*
in glaucoma, **10:**33
hypersensitivity reactions of, **8:**198–201, 199*i*, 199*t*
immunologic response/features of, **9:**34*t*
infection/inflammation of, **4:**89–91, 90*i*, **8:**25*t,*
29–31, 179–192. *See also* Episcleritis; Scleritis
perforation of
extraocular muscle/strabismus surgery and, **6:**26,
185
repair of, **8:**412
traumatic, **6:**446–447
pigment spot of, **8:**263
rupture of, in blunt trauma, **12:**295
stroma of, **2:**50, **4:**88, 88*i*
topography of, **2:**43*i*, 44*i*, **4:**87–88, 87*i*, 88*i*
wound healing/repair of, **4:**22, **8:**386
Scleral buckle
for retinal detachment, **12:**272, 272*i*, 336
refractive surgery after, **13:**193
sickle cell retinopathy and, **12:**124
in uveitis, **9:**240
for retinopathy of prematurity, **6:**331, **12:**136
Scleral contact lenses, **3:**200–202, 200*i*, 201*i*
in dry eye patients, **8:**76
for keratoconus, **3:**200
Scleral dellen, **8:**106
Scleral expansion, for presbyopia, **13:**176–177, 177*i*
Scleral plaques, senile, **8:**378, 379*i*
Scleral spur, **2:**53*i*, 54, 55*i*, 61
Scleral spur cells, **2:**54
Scleral sulcus, internal, **2:**54
Scleral support ring, for penetrating keratoplasty, **8:**455
in children, **8:**471
Scleral surgery. *See also specific procedure*
for presbyopia, **13:**176–177, 177*i*
Scleral tunnel incision, for cataract surgery, **11:**99–100,
100*i*, 121–123, 123*i*, 124*i*
in children, **11:**196
modification of preexisting astigmatism and, **11:**102
Sclerectomy, full-thickness, for open-angle glaucoma,
10:194–195, 195*i*
Scleritis, **4:**89–91, 90*i*, **5:**298, **8:**191–192, 191*i*, 234–241
anterior, **8:**236, 236*t*, 237*i*
complications of, **8:**239, 240*i*
in herpes zoster, **8:**154
immune components of, **8:**202, 234–241
laboratory evaluation of, **8:**239–240
management of, **8:**240–241
microbial, **8:**191–192, 191*i*
necrotizing, **8:**25*t*, 29, 236–239, 236*t*
with inflammation, **8:**236*t*, 237, 238*i*

without inflammation (scleromalacia perforans),
8:236*t*, 238–239, 238*i*
nonnecrotizing, **8:**25*t*, 29
posterior, **8:**236*t*, 239
subtypes and prevalence of, **8:**236*t*
in Wegener granulomatosis, **1:**192, **9:**62, 175
Sclerocornea, **4:**64, **6:**255, 256*t*, **8:**295–296, 295*i*, 310*t*
cornea plana and, **8:**290, 291, 295, 295*i*
intraocular lens implantation and, **11:**214, 216*i*
Sclerocorneal pocket approach, for lamellar
keratoplasty, **8:**476
Scleroderma, **1:**185–186
eyelid manifestations of, **4:**173*t*
Scleroderma renal crisis (scleroderma kidney), **1:**185
Sclerokeratitis, **8:**239, 240*i*
Scleromalacia, **8:**31
perforans, **4:**91, **8:**236*t*, 238–239, 238*i*
Sclerosing dacryoadenitis, **4:**190
Sclerosing inflammation of orbit/sclerosing orbitis,
4:190, 191*i*, **7:**57, 58. *See also* Orbital inflammatory
syndrome
orbital lymphoma differentiated from, **4:**195–196
Sclerosis, tuberous (Bourneville disease/syndrome),
5:336*t*, 338–340, 339*i*, **6:**402*t*, 409–412, 410*i*, 411*i*
glaucoma associated with, **10:**32
Sclerotic (gliotic) lesions, in multiple sclerosis, **5:**318
Sclerotic scatter, for slit-lamp biomicroscopy, **8:**19
Sclerotomy
anterior ciliary, for presbyopia, **13:**176
for expulsive suprachoroidal hemorrhage,
11:170–171
Sclerouveitis, **9:**106
in inflammatory bowel disease, **9:**132
Scopolamine, **2:**310, 401, 401*t*, 402*i*
for cycloplegia/cycloplegic refraction, **3:**142, 142*t,*
6:94, 94*t*
SCORE Study, **12:**141
Scotomata
in age-related macular degeneration, **12:**63
arcuate (Bjerrum), **10:**60, 62*i*
in cone–rod dystrophies, **12:**215
definition of, **5:**113*t*, **10:**60
in low vision, **3:**246, 247*i*, 253
of monofixation syndrome, **6:**57–58
4Δ base-out prism test in evaluation of, **6:**61–63,
63*i*
in multiple evanescent white dot syndrome, **5:**107
paracentral, **10:**60, 61
in retinitis pigmentosa, **5:**110, **12:**205–206, 207*i*
in Stargardt disease, **12:**217
suppression, diplopia after strabismus surgery and,
6:185
systemic hypoperfusion causing, **5:**170
Scotopic electroretinogram (dark-adapted
electroretinogram), **12:**27, 28*i*, 29, 206*t*. *See also*
Dark adaptation testing
Scraping, for specimen collection, **8:**63–64, 135
Screening/diagnostic tests, **1:**291–302, **6:**459. *See also*
specific test or disorder
interpretation of, **1:**353–360, 353*i*, 354*i*
clinical acceptance and, **1:**359
combination strategies and, **1:**359
continuous outcome and, **1:**355, 356*i*
criteria for diagnosis and, **1:**355–357, 357*i*
generalizability and, **1:**359

pretest probability and, 1:357–359, 358*t*
for neonates, 6:292–294
for retinopathy of prematurity, 6:328–329, 329*t*,
330*i*, 331*i*
Sculpting, instrument settings for, 11:135–136, 135*t*,
136*i*
Scurvy (vitamin C deficiency), 1:166, 8:94
SE (spin echo), definition of, 5:80
Sea-blue histiocyte syndrome. *See* Niemann-Pick
disease
Sea fan neovascularization, in sickle cell disease,
12:122, 122*i*, 123*i*
Seasonal allergic conjunctivitis, 6:234, 8:207–209
Sebaceous adenomas, 7:167
in tuberous sclerosis, 5:338, 339*i*, 6:410, 410*i*
Sebaceous carcinoma/adenocarcinoma, 4:180–182,
181*i*, 7:180–182, 180*i*, 181*i*, 8:261–263, 262*i*
medial canthal/lacrimal sac involvement and, 7:284
Sebaceous cysts (epidermal inclusion cysts), of eyelid,
7:164–166, 165*i*
Sebaceous glands, of eyelid, 4:168*t*, 7:166–167
tumors arising in. *See* Sebaceous adenomas;
Sebaceous carcinoma/adenocarcinoma
Sebaceous hyperplasia, of eyelid, 7:166–167
Seborrheic blepharitis, 8:86–87, 164*t*
Seborrheic keratosis, 4:174–175, 175*i*, 7:163, 165*i*
Second cranial nerve. *See* Optic nerve
Second-degree relatives, 2:194
Second messengers, in signal transduction, 2:311
Second-order neuron
dilator muscle innervation and, 2:65
lesions of, Horner syndrome caused by, 5:263, 263*i*,
264
Second sight, 11:45, 77
Secondary glaucoma. *See* Angle-closure glaucoma;
Glaucoma; Open-angle glaucoma
Secondary lens fibers, development of, 11:27*i*, 28
microspherophakia and, 11:32
Secondary positions of gaze, 6:28
Secretion, active, in aqueous humor formation,
10:18–19
Secretory IgA, in tear film, 2:290, 8:56, 198
in external eye defense, 8:113
Sectral. *See* Acebutolol
Sedative-hypnotics/sedation, 1:273–277, 274*t*
abuse and, 1:269
for benign essential blepharospasm, 7:227
preoperative, 1:335
See-saw nystagmus, 5:251, 6:166–167
Segregation (genetic), 2:195, 241, 244
replicative, 2:195, 217
Seidel test, 8:22, 22*i*
in flat anterior chamber, wound leak and, 11:165
Seizures, 1:280–284, 320–321. *See also* Epilepsy
facial weakness/paralysis caused by, 5:289
local anesthetics causing, 1:336
nonepileptic, 1:281
occipital, transient visual loss caused by, 5:186
Selectins, in neutrophil rolling, 9:48, 49*i*
Selection bias, 1:341
in case-control studies, 1:349
in case series, 1:346
Selective adhesion molecule (SAM) inhibitor, for
multiple sclerosis, 5:324

Selective estrogen receptor modulators, for
osteoporosis, 1:246
Selective laser trabeculoplasty, for open-angle
glaucoma, 10:182
Selective serotonin reuptake inhibitors, 1:274–276, 275*t*
Selegiline, for Parkinson disease, 1:279
Selenium, in retina and retinal pigment epithelium,
2:371–372
Selenoprotein P, in aqueous humor, 2:319
Self-antigens, tolerance to, 9:87–89
Self–blood-glucose monitoring, 1:215–216
Self-examination, breast, for cancer screening, 1:295*t*
Self-sealing incision, for cataract surgery
beveled/biplanar, clear corneal incision and,
11:124–125, 126*i*
scleral tunnel incisions and, 11:99
Sella turcica, 5:5
Semicircular flap, for eyelid repair, 7:189, 190*i*, 191*i*,
192
Semiconductor diode lasers, 3:23. *See also* Lasers
Semilunar fold, 8:8
Semilunar ganglion (Gasserian/trigeminal ganglion),
2:113*i*, 114, 5:52
Senescent cataracts, in diabetes, 11:61
Senile calcific plaques, 4:91, 91*i*
Senile furrow degeneration, 8:370
Senile lentigo (liver spots), 7:171
Senile macular degeneration. *See* Age-related macular
degeneration/maculopathy
Senile scleral plaques, 8:378, 379*i*
Sensation, in cornea
esthesiometry in evaluation of, 8:35
reduction of
in herpes simplex epithelial keratitis, 8:144
in neurotrophic keratopathy, 8:102–103, 151
Sense primer, for PCR, 2:230
Sense strand of DNA, 2:195, 201–202
Sensitivity
contrast, in glaucoma, 10:59
flicker, in glaucoma, 10:59
of screening/diagnostic test, 1:292, 354
continuous outcome and, 1:355, 356*i*
likelihood ratio calculation and, 1:358
spatial contrast, in low vision evaluation, 5:97
Sensitivity threshold, in perimetry, 5:91, 92
Sensitization, lymphocyte, 9:22–24, 23*i*. *See also*
Activation
Sensory defects/deprivation
esodeviation and, 6:98*t*, 105–106
exotropia and, 6:115
nystagmus and, 6:164
retinogeniculocortical pathway affected by, 6:49–52,
50*i*, 51*i*
Sensory fusion, 6:43
Sensory nucleus
of cranial nerve V (trigeminal), 2:113, 113*i*, 5:50,
50*i*, 51*i*
of cranial nerve VII (facial), 2:117
Sensory root
of cranial nerve V (trigeminal), 2:113
of cranial nerve V$_1$ (ophthalmic), 2:13, 14*i*
of cranial nerve VII (facial), 2:117
Sensory visual system, 6:41–65
abnormalities of binocular vision and, 6:52–53, 53*i*
testing, 6:93–94

adaptations in strabismus and, **6:**53–65, 54*i*
neurophysiological aspects of, **6:**44–52, 45*i*, 47*i*, 48*i*
physiology of normal binocular vision and, **6:**41–44, 42*i*, 43*t*
Sentinel vessels, **4:**159
Septata, keratoconjunctivitis caused by, **8:**190
Septate filamentous fungi, **8:**129, 129*i*, 130. *See also* Fungi
Septo-optic dysplasia (de Morsier syndrome), **2:**175, 176*i*, **5:**139, **6:**362, 454
Septra. *See* Trimethoprim-sulfamethoxazole
Sequence (congenital anomalies), **6:**205
Sequence-tagged sites, **2:**195
Sequencing, DNA, **2:**231, 232*i*
Ser-Ap-Es. *See* Reserpine
Serevent. *See* Salmeterol
Seroepidemiology, of HIV infection/AIDS, **1:**39
Seronegative spondyloarthropathies, **1:**175–179. *See also specific type*
uveitis in, **9:**129–132
Seroquel. *See* Quetiapine
Serositis, in systemic lupus erythematosus, **1:**181*t*
Serotonin
antipsychotic mechanism of action and, **1:**271
as inflammatory mediator, **9:**77
Serotonin receptor agonists, for migraine, **5:**296
Serotonin reuptake inhibitors, selective, **1:**274–276, 275*t*
Serpasil. *See* Reserpine
Serpiginous choroidopathy (geographic choroiditis/ helicoid peripapillary choroidopathy), **9:**177*t*, 182–184, 184*i*, **12:**174*t*, 176–177, 177*i*
Serratia, **8:**126
endogenous bacterial endophthalmitis caused by, **12:**183
marcescens, **9:**211, 211*i*
postoperative endophthalmitis caused by, **9:**211, 211*i*
Sertaconazole, **1:**76
Serum, **1:**159
Serum drops, for neurotrophic keratopathy, **8:**104
Serum sickness, **9:**59
Serzone. *See* Nefazodone
Setting sun sign, **5:**211
Seventh nerve (facial) palsy. *See* Facial paralysis/ weakness
Severe acute respiratory syndrome (SARS), **1:**33–35
Sex (gender), primary angle closure/angle-closure glaucoma and, **10:**11, 123
Sex chromosomes, **2:**242
aneuploidy of, **2:**249
mosaicism and, **2:**252
Sex-determining region Y (SRY/testis-determining factor/TDF), **2:**266
Sex linked inheritance (sex linked genes), **2:**195, 266–269. *See also* X-linked inheritance; Y-linked inheritance
Sexual abuse, gonococcal conjunctivitis in children and, **6:**225
SFU. *See* Subretinal fibrosis and uveitis syndrome
Shafer's sign ("tobacco dust"/pigment granules), **12:**268, 276, 288
Shaffer system, for gonioscopic grading, **10:**40
Shagreen, crocodile, **8:**370
Shagreen patch, in tuberous sclerosis, **5:**338–339, **6:**410
Shaker-1 (sh1) gene, **2:**221

Shaking injury (shaken baby syndrome), **6:**442–445, 443*i*, 444*i*, **12:**301–302, 302*i*
Shallow anterior chamber. *See* Anterior chamber, flat or shallow
Sharps containers, in infection control, **8:**50
Shave biopsy, **7:**176*i*, 181, **8:**250, 251*i*
Shearing intraocular lens, **11:**142*i*
Sheathing, retinal vascular, in sarcoidosis, **9:**199, 200*i*
Sheathotomy, arteriovenous, for branch retinal vein occlusion, **12:**140–141
Sheehan syndrome (postpartum pituitary necrosis), **5:**345
Sherrington's law of reciprocal innervation, **6:**35
Shield ulcer, **6:**235, **8:**210
Shigella, **8:**126
invasive capability of, **8:**117
Shingles. *See* Herpes zoster
Shock, **1:**317–320. *See also specific type*
assessment of, **1:**318
classification of, **1:**317–318
treatment of, **1:**318–319
Shock value, in functional visual disorder evaluation, **5:**305–306
"Shock wave theory," in central island formation, **13:**101–102
Shoelace suture, **11:**100*i*
Short (p) arm, **2:**192, 205
Short arm 11 deletion syndrome (11p13 syndrome), **2:**254–255
Short ciliary nerves, **2:**15, 110
ciliary muscle supplied by, **2:**69
iris sphincter supplied by, **2:**66
posterior, **2:**38
Short interfering (small interference) RNAs (siRNA), **2:**202
Short interspersed elements, **2:**203
Short tandem repeats, **2:**196, 223, 225*i*
Short tau inversion recovery (STIR) image, **5:**63
signal intensity on, **5:**65*t*
Short-term fluctuation, in perimetry, **5:**96
Short-wavelength automated perimetry (SWAP), **10:**58, 70, 71*i*
Shunting surgery
glaucoma tube, **10:**201–204. *See also* Tube-shunt surgery
lumboperitoneal, for idiopathic intracranial hypertension, **5:**119–120
Sialic acid, in microbial adherence, **8:**116
Sialidoses, **6:**436*t*
cherry-red spot in, **12:**243–244
dysmorphic, **8:**342
Sickle cell disease (sickle cell anemia), **1:**163, **12:**119–124, 120*t*
genetic testing for, **1:**159, 163
ophthalmic manifestations of, **12:**120–124, 121*i*, 122*i*, 123*i*. *See also* Sickle cell retinopathy
angioid streaks, **12:**83, 123
traumatic hyphema and, **6:**447, 448*i*, **8:**402–403
point mutation causing, **2:**256
racial and ethnic concentration of, **2:**260
Sickle cell hemoglobin (SC), **12:**120, 120*t*
Sickle cell preparations ("preps"), **12:**120
Sickle cell retinopathy, **12:**119–124, 120*t*, 122*i*, 123*i*
incidence of, **12:**120*t*
nonproliferative, **12:**121, 121*i*

pathogenetic sequence of, 12:122, 122*i*
photocoagulation for, 12:123–124
proliferative, 12:122, 122*i*, 123*i*
treatment of, 12:123–124
vitreoretinal surgery for, 12:124
Sickle cell thalassemia, 12:120, 120*t*
Sickle cell trait (hemoglobin AS), 12:120, 120*t*
Sideroblastic anemia, 1:162
Siderosis/siderosis bulbi, 4:99, 11:58, 59*i*, 12:299, 299*t*
corneal pigmentation in, 8:377*t*
electroretinogram in evaluation of, 12:36, 299
Siegrist streaks, 12:98
sIGA. *See* Secretory IgA
Sigmoid sinus, 5:22
Sigmoidoscopy, in cancer screening, 1:295*t*, 298
Signal transduction, 2:310–311
in iris–ciliary body, 2:308–310, 310–312, 312*i*, 313*i*
in tear secretion, 2:292–293, 292*i*
Significance, statistical, 1:366–367. *See also P* value
Silastic rods, for frontalis suspension, 7:222
Sildenafil, visual changes caused by, 1:324, 325*t*, 12:251
Silicone acrylate, 3:183–184
Silicone foldable intraocular lenses, 3:213–214
Silicone intubation
for acquired nasolacrimal obstruction, 7:278
for canalicular constriction, 7:275
for canalicular trauma, 7:277
for congenital lacrimal duct obstruction/tearing,
6:246–247, 7:263–264, 266*i*
Silicone oil, for tamponade in retinal detachment,
12:340, 341
Silicone punctal plugs, for dry eye, 8:76, 76*i*, 77
Silicone Study, 12:340, 341
Silicone suspension sling, for paralytic ectropion, 7:199
Silver compounds, corneal pigmentation caused by,
8:376, 377*t*
Silver nitrate, for ophthalmia neonatorum prophylaxis,
6:223
chemical conjunctivitis caused by, 6:223
SIM K (simulated keratometry), 3:303, 304*i*
Simple cells, 5:29
Simple episcleritis, 4:89, 8:235
Simple lentigines (lentigo simplex), 7:171
Simple megalocornea, 6:250
Simple (physiologic/school) myopia, 3:120
Simplex, definition of, 2:196, 240
Simplex retinitis pigmentosa, 12:209
Simulated divergence excess exotropia, 6:112
Simultanagnosia, 5:194, 195*i*, 208
in Alzheimer disease, 1:288
Simultaneous prism and cover test, 6:82
Simvastatin
cataract risk and, 11:54
for hypercholesterolemia, 1:149*t*, 150*t*
Sinemet. *See* Levodopa/carbidopa
SINEs. *See* Short interspersed elements
Single binocular vision
Panum's area of, 6:42*i*, 43, 52
testing field of, 6:89–90, 90*i*
Single-flash cone response (photopic/light-adapted
electroretinogram), 12:28*i*, 29, 205, 206*t*
in hereditary retinal/choroidal degenerations, 12:205,
206*t*
Single-gene disorder (mendelian disorder), 2:190, 257
Single-pedicle (racquet) flaps, 8:438

Single-photon emission computed tomography
(SPECT), 5:69
in ischemic heart disease, 1:119, 294
Single-plane incisions, for cataract surgery, 11:99
Single-stranded conformational polymorphism, 2:230
Single-vision reading glasses, for induced anisophoria,
3:162
Singulair. *See* Montelukast
Sinoatrial (SA) node, 1:133
Sinskey hook, 11:152
Sinskey intraocular lens, 11:142*i*
Sinus arrest (sinus block/SA block), 1:133
Sinus bradycardia, 1:133
Sinus tachycardia, 1:136
Sinus thrombosis, 5:357–358
cavernous, 5:357–358
orbital infections and, 7:42, 44
dural, 5:357–358
lateral (transverse), 5:358
superior sagittal, 5:358
Sinuses
ethmoid, 5:9, 9*i*, 7:20, 21*i*
frontal, 5:9, 9*i*, 7:9*i*, 20, 20*i*, 21*i*
maxillary, 5:9, 7:20–21, 20*i*, 21*i*
paranasal, 2:12, 13*i*, 5:9, 9*i*, 7:7, 20–21, 21*i*
Aspergillus causing infection of, 7:46–47
orbital cellulitis caused by infection of, 6:231,
232*i*, 7:42, 44*t*
orbital tumors originating in, 7:92–93, 93*i*
preseptal cellulitis caused by infection of, 6:230,
7:41–42
tuberculous infection of, orbital involvement and,
7:47
periorbital, 2:12, 13*i*
sphenoid, 5:9, 9*i*, 7:10*i*, 20, 21*i*
Sinusitis
allergic aspergillosis, 7:46–47
orbital cellulitis caused by, 6:231, 232*i*, 7:42, 44*t*
preseptal cellulitis caused by, 6:230, 7:41–42
tuberculous, orbital infection and, 7:47
Sipple-Gorlin syndrome, enlarged corneal nerves in,
8:357, 358*t*
siRNA. *See* Small interference (short interfering) RNAs
Sister chromatids, 2:183, 205
Sixth cranial nerve. *See* Cranial nerve VI
Sixth nerve (abducens) palsy, 5:234–235, 6:98*t*,
107–108, 148, 148*i*
divergence spasm initiating, 5:211
incomitant esodeviation caused by, 6:98*t*, 107–108
Sjögren-Larsson syndrome, ichthyosis in, 12:237
Sjögren syndrome, 1:186, 187*t*, 8:78–80
aqueous tear deficiency and, 8:72*t*, 78–80
cataract surgery in patients with, 11:206–207
classification of, 8:78, 79*t*
laboratory evaluation in diagnosis of, 8:73–74
Sjögren Syndrome Foundation, 8:74
Skeletal disorders. *See also* Connective tissue disorders
corneal changes in, 8:351–353*t*
Skew, of retinal reflex, in axis determination, 3:131,
131*i*
Skew deviation, 5:223–224
alternating, 5:223
in infants, 6:451
in multiple sclerosis, 5:321

Skin
  disorders of
    in Behçet syndrome, 1:193
    cataracts associated with, 11:66
    in dermatomyositis, 1:186, 187, 188*i*
    desquamating, ocular surface involved in, 8:89
    retinal degeneration and, 12:237
    in scleroderma, 1:185
    in systemic lupus erythematosus, 1:179, 181*t*, 182
    eyelid, 2:22, 4:167–168, 167*i*, 7:139, 140*i*, 141*i*, 8:6, 245–246
      microanatomy of, 8:245, 245*i*
    laser resurfacing of, 7:237–238
    tumors of, medial canthal/lacrimal sac involvement and, 7:284
Skin grafts. *See* Flaps; Grafts
Skin tests, tuberculin, 1:23–25, 301–302
Skipped generation (incomplete penetrance), 2:266
Skull base, in craniosynostosis, 6:421, 422*i*, 424
Skull fracture, arteriovenous fistula caused by, 7:70
Slab-off (bicentric grinding), for induced anisophoria, 3:160–161, 161*i*
  reverse, 3:160–161
SLE. *See* Systemic lupus erythematosus
Sleep disorders, hypertension and, 1:95
Sleep test, for myasthenia gravis, 5:326, 327, 6:151
Sliding flap, for wound closure after pterygium excision, 8:429, 430*i*
Slipped muscle, in extraocular muscle surgery, 6:23, 191, 191*i*
  esodeviations and, 6:98*t*, 106–107
Slit illumination, for slit-lamp biomicroscopy, 8:16–17, 17*i*
Slit-lamp biomicroscopy/examination. *See* Biomicroscopy, slit-lamp
Slit-lamp photography, 8:35. *See also* Biomicroscopy, slit-lamp
SLK. *See* Superior limbic keratoconjunctivitis
SLO. *See* Scanning laser ophthalmoscopy
Slo-Phyllin. *See* Theophylline
Slow-acting (disease-modifying) antirheumatic drugs, 1:174
Slow-channel calcium-blocking agents, for angina, 1:120–121
Slow inactivators, isoniazid use in, 2:279
Slow-reacting substance of anaphylaxis, 8:200*t*
Slow-twitch fibers, 2:20, 21, 21*t*, 5:41
Sly syndrome, 6:436*t*
Small-angle approximation, 3:58–60
Small interference (short interfering) RNAs (siRNA), 2:202
Smallest region of overlap, 2:196
Smallpox vaccination, ocular complications of, 8:162
Smart System II PC Plus test, 6:94
SmartLens, 13:180
SMAS. *See* Superficial musculoaponeurotic system
Smith-Indian operation, 11:91
Smokestack, in central serous chorioretinopathy, 12:52
Smoking
  cancer and, 1:252, 296, 297
  cataract development and, 11:64, 73–74
  cessation of, 1:155–156
  heart disease and, 1:111
  hypertension and, 1:85
  optic neuropathy and, 5:152

  thyroid disease and, 1:201, 225, 5:331, 7:53
Smooth muscle tumors, 8:269
Smooth pursuit system, 5:34, 35–36*i*, 6:39
Snapback test, 7:202
Snellen acuity, 3:111–112. *See also* Visual acuity
  in children, 6:78*t*, 79
  contrast sensitivity and, 3:112–113
  in low vision, 3:251
  spatial frequency and, 3:113, 114*i*
Snellen charts, 3:111–112, 112*t*
  in children, 6:78*t*, 79
  monofixation assessment and, 6:58
Snell's law (law of refraction), 3:44–46, 46*i*, 47, 47*i*, 8:39–40
  contact lens power and, 3:174
  Fermat's principle and, 3:51–52
  small-angle approximation and, 3:59–60
Snow blindness, 8:388
Snowballs
  in intermediate uveitis/pars planitis, 9:105, 147, 148*i*, 12:182
  in sarcoidosis, 9:198
Snowbank formation, in intermediate uveitis/pars planitis, 9:106, 147, 12:182
Snowflake cataract, 11:60–61, 61*i*
Snowmen, in intermediate uveitis/pars planitis, 9:147
SNRPN gene, imprinting of, 2:210
SO. *See* Superior oblique muscles; Sympathetic ophthalmia
Social history
  in cataract surgery evaluation, 11:80
  keratorefractive surgery and, 13:40
  in uveitis, 9:122
Socket contraction, 7:125–126, 126*i*. *See also* Anophthalmic socket
SOD. *See* Superoxide dismutase
Sodium
  in aqueous humor, 2:316*t*, 317
  dietary
    congestive heart failure and, 1:127
    hypertension and, 1:85, 87*t*
  in lens, 2:328
  in tear film, 2:290
  transport of, 2:361
    carbonic anhydrase inhibitors affecting, 2:411–412
  in vitreous, 2:337
Sodium balance, in lens, pump-leak theory of maintenance of, 11:20–21, 21*i*
Sodium bicarbonate. *See* Bicarbonate
Sodium chloride, for ocular edema, 2:451
Sodium ferric gluconate, 1:159, 161
Sodium fluorescein. *See* Fluorescein
Sodium hyaluronate, 2:452
  as viscoelastic, 11:144–145, 159, 160, 161*t*
Sodium-potassium-calcium exchanger (Na^+/K^+-Ca exchanger), in rods, 2:342, 344*t*
Sodium-potassium pump (Na^+,K^+-ATPase)
  in Fuchs endothelial dystrophy, 8:325
  in lens active transport, 11:19–20
    pump-leak theory and, 11:20, 21*i*
  in lens ionic balance, 2:329
  in retinal pigment epithelium, 2:358, 361
  in rods, 2:342, 344*t*
Soemmerring's ring, 4:99*i*, 100, 11:186
Soft contact lenses. *See* Flexible (soft) contact lenses

Soft drusen, **4:**138, 138*i,* **12:**56*i,* 57
Soft exudates. *See* Cotton-wool spots
Soft tissue histiocytosis. *See* Histiocytosis
Soft tissue sarcoma, retinoblastoma associated with, **4:**265*t*
Softperm lens, **3:**200
Solar elastosis, of eyelid, **4:**177, 177*i*
Solar (actinic) keratosis, **4:**176–177, 177*i,* **7:**172–173, 172*i*
Solar lentigo, **7:**171
Solar retinopathy/retinitis (foveomacular retinitis), **12:**307–308
Solid-state lasers, **3:**22. *See also* Lasers
Solu-Cortef. *See* Hydrocortisone sodium succinate
Somatic afferent fibers, **2:**117
Somatic motor nerves, cholinergic drug action and, **2:**394, 395*i*
Somatization disorder, **1:**266
Somatoform disorders, **1:**266
Somatoform pain disorder, **1:**266
Somatotroph adenomas, **1:**228
Somite, **2:**127
Somogyi phenomenon, **1:**210
Sonata. *See* Zaleplon
Sonic hedgehog mutations, cyclopia caused by, **2:**165
Sonography. *See* Ultrasonography/ultrasound
SOOF (suborbicularis oculi fat), **7:**135, 141*i,* 145–146
SOOF lift, **7:**241, 242*i*
Sorbitol/sorbitol pathway
    in cataract formation, **2:**331–332, **11:**14–16, 15*i,* 60
        in children, **6:**343
    diabetic retinopathy and, **2:**354
    in lens glucose/carbohydrate metabolism, **2:**331, 331*i,* **11:**14–16, 15*i*
Sordarins, for *Pneumocystis carinii (Pneumocystis jiroveci)* pneumonia, **1:**47
Sorsby macular dystrophy, **12:**223–224, 223*i*
    retinal pigment epithelium in, **2:**363
    TIMP3 defects causing, **2:**227, 350
SOS. *See* Sands of the Sahara
Southern blot analysis, **2:**196, 224*i,* 230
    in mutation screening, **2:**224*i,* 234*i*
SP. *See* Swelling pressure
Space maintenance, by viscoelastics, **11:**159
Spaeth gonioscopic grading system, **10:**40, 41*i*
Sparfloxacin, **1:**62*t,* 73
Spasm of accommodation (ciliary muscle spasm), **5:**314
    accommodative excess caused by, **3:**148
Spasm of convergence, **5:**211
Spasm of fixation, **5:**194
Spasm of near reflex, **3:**148, **5:**313
Spasms
    benign essential blepharospasm, **7:**226
    habit, **5:**290
    hemifacial, **5:**287*t,* 288–289, 288*i,* **7:**227–228
Spasmus nutans, **5:**243, **6:**165–166
Spastic entropion, **7:**201–202, 202*i*
Spastic paretic facial contracture, **5:**289
Spatial (lateral) coherence, **3:**7–8, 8*i*
Spatial frequency, **3:**113–115, 114*i*
    in contrast sensitivity testing, **12:**45–46, 46*i*
    in low vision evaluation, **5:**97
Specialty charts, in functional visual disorder evaluation, **5:**309

Specific (adaptive) immunity, **9:**9–10. *See also* Adaptive immune response
Specificity
    immunologic, **9:**11
    of screening/diagnostic test, **1:**292, 354
        continuous outcome and, **1:**355, 356*i*
        likelihood ratio calculation and, **1:**358
Specimen collection/handling, **4:**31–36, 36*t*
    communication with health care team and, **4:**31–32
    gross dissection and, **4:**33–34, 34*i*
    for ocular cytology, **8:**63–64
    for ocular microbiology, **8:**134–136, 135*t,* 136*i*
    orientation of globe and, **4:**32, 32*i*
    processing/staining tissues and, **4:**35–36, 36*i,* 36*t*
    special techniques and, **4:**37–41
    transillumination and, **4:**32–33, 33*i*
Speckle, laser, **3:**18
SPECT. *See* Single-photon emission computed tomography
Spectacle crown glass, refractive index of, **3:**40*t*
Spectacle lenses (spectacles). *See also* Lenses
    absorptive, **3:**165–167. *See also* Sunglasses
    accommodation affected by, **3:**149–150
    anophthalmic socket camouflage and, **7:**127
    aphakic. *See* Aphakic spectacles
    convergence affected by, **3:**149–150
    cylindrical correcting, **3:**145. *See also* Cylinders
    for dry eye, **8:**76
    frames for, anophthalmic socket camouflage and, **7:**127
    for high accommodative convergence/accommodative esotropia, **6:**102, 103–104
    high-index glass, **3:**168
    impact-resistant, **3:**168
    for intermittent exotropia, **6:**112
    iseikonic, **3:**145
    magnification for near vision with, **3:**255
    monocular distortion and, **3:**327
    for overcorrection of intermittent exotropia, **6:**113
    for partially accommodative esotropia, **6:**104
    plastic, **3:**168
        bifocal, **3:**152
            reverse slab-off and, **3:**161
            prism calibration for, **3:**85, 86*i*
    polycarbonate, **3:**168–169
    power of, bifocal segment decentration and, **3:**163
    prisms incorporated into, **3:**169–170. *See also* Prisms
    for refractive accommodative esotropia, **6:**101–102
    special materials used for, **3:**168–169
    spherical correcting, **3:**143, 144*i*
    vertex distance and, **3:**143–145, 144*i*
Spectinomycin, for gonococcal conjunctivitis, **8:**172
Spectracef. *See* Cefditoren
Spectral irradiance, **2:**460, 460*t*
Spectral radiant exposure, **2:**460, 460*t*
Specular microscopy/photomicroscopy, **3:**294–295, 295*i,* **8:**18, 36–37, 36*i*
    before cataract surgery, **11:**87
    in Fuchs endothelial dystrophy, **8:**325
    in optical focusing technique for pachymetry, **3:**293
    before phakic intraocular lens insertion, **13:**146
    in posterior polymorphous dystrophy, **8:**328
Specular reflection, **3:**42–44, 42*i,* 44*i*
    for slit-lamp biomicroscopy, **8:**17–18, 18*i*
Specular transmission, **3:**44–46, 45*i,* 46*i*

Spheno-cavernous syndrome, 5:236
Sphenoethmoidal recess, 7:20
Sphenoid bone, 5:5, 6*i*, 10, 7:7, 8*i*, 9*i*, 10*i*
    pterygoid process of, 5:5, 9
Sphenoid sinuses, 5:9, 9*i*, 7:10*i*, 20, 21*i*
Sphenopalatine ganglion, 5:9
Spheres
    amplitude of accommodation measured with, 3:151
    power of, fogging in determination of, 3:141
    refining, in subjective refraction, 3:139–140
Spherical aberration, 3:93, 101–102, 103*i*, 231–232,
    233*i*, 8:43, 13:15–16, 17*i*
Spherical equivalent, 3:94
Spherical lenses, correcting, 3:143–145, 144*i*
    vertex distance and, 3:143–145, 144*i*
Spherocylindrical lenses, 3:94–98. *See also* Cylinders
    combination of, 3:99–100
        at oblique axes, 3:100–101, 101*i*
    conoid of Sturm and, 3:93–94, 95*i*
    notations for, 3:95–98, 97*i*
    toric surfaces of, 3:94–95, 97*i*
    transposition and, 3:98–99
Spherocytosis, hereditary, 1:162
Spheroidal degeneration (actinic/Labrador
    keratopathy), 4:68, 69*i*, 8:368–369
Spherophakia, 2:172, 6:304, 304*i*
Spherule, of rod, 2:79, 83*i*
Sphincter muscle, 2:62*i*, 65–66
    damage to, 5:265
    development of, 2:154
    miotics affecting, 2:309
    muscarinic drugs affecting, 2:394, 400, 401*t*
    mydriatics affecting, 2:310, 400, 401*t*
Sphingolipidoses, corneal changes in, 8:340–344
Spielmeyer-Vogt disease, 6:437*t*, 12:233*t*, 241
Spin echo (SE), definition of, 5:80
Spin-lattice/longitudinal relaxation time (T1), 5:81,
    7:30–31
Spin-spin/transverse relaxation time (T2), 5:81, 7:31
Spinal nucleus and tract, of cranial nerve V
    (trigeminal), 2:113–114, 113*i*, 115*i*, 5:50, 50*i*
Spindle cell carcinoma, 8:261
    conjunctival, 4:53
Spindle cell melanoma, 4:160, 160*i*
Spinocerebellar degenerations, retinal degeneration
    and, 12:235–236
    cone–rod dystrophy, 12:215
Spiradenoma, eccrine, 7:167
Spiral computed tomography, in orbital evaluation,
    7:29
Spiral of Tillaux, 2:16, 17*i*, 5:41, 6:16, 18*i*
Spiramycin, 1:60*t*, 71
    for toxoplasmosis, 9:168
Spirochetes, ocular infection caused by, 8:128
Spironolactone, 1:88*t*, 90*t*
Spitz nevus, 4:184
SPK. *See* Thygeson superficial punctate keratitis
Spleen, 9:16
Splice junction site, 2:196
Spliceosome, 2:196, 209
Splicing, 2:196, 209
    alternative, 2:203, 209
Spondylitis, ankylosing, 1:175–176, 9:127*i*, 129–130,
    130*i*
    cataract surgery in patients with, 11:203, 203*i*

HLA in, 9:94–95, 129
juvenile, 1:178
Spondyloarthropathies, 1:175–179. *See also specific type*
    juvenile, 1:178
    seronegative. *See also specific type*
        uveitis in, 9:129–130
    undifferentiated, 1:175
Spongiosis, definition of, 4:169
Spontaneous emission, in lasers, 3:19–21, 21
Spontaneous vitreous hemorrhage, 12:287
Sporadic, definition of, 2:196, 240
Sporadic Alzheimer disease, 1:286
Sporanox. *See* Itraconazole
Spore-forming intestinal protozoa, gastrointestinal
    infection in HIV/AIDS and, 1:48–49
Spreading depression of Leão, 5:191
Springing pupils, 5:270–271
Sputum cytology, in cancer screening, 1:295*t*, 296
Squamous cell carcinoma
    of conjunctiva, 4:53, 53*i*, 8:255*t*, 257*i*, 260–261, 260*i*
    of eyelid, 4:177–179, 178*i*, 7:179–180, 179*i*
        actinic keratosis and, 4:176–177
        in situ (Bowen disease), 7:173
    medial canthal/lacrimal sac involvement and, 7:284
    of orbit, secondary, 7:92*i*, 93
    retinoblastoma associated with, 4:265*t*
Squamous cell papillomas
    conjunctival, 4:51, 52*i*
    of eyelid, 7:163, 164*i*
    lacrimal sac involvement and, 7:284
Squamous dysplasia, of conjunctiva, 8:257, 257*i*
Square-wave jerks, 5:199, 204, 252, 252*i*
Square-wave oscillations, 5:199
SR. *See* Superior rectus muscles
SR (saturation recovery), 5:81
SRI (surface regularity index), 3:303
SRK formulas, for IOL power selection, 3:217,
    219–220, 220*i*, 11:149, 13:202
    clear lens extraction/refractive lens exchange and,
        13:160
SRO. *See* Smallest region of overlap
SRY. *See* Sex-determining region Y
SS. *See* Sigmoid sinus; Sjögren syndrome
SS antibodies (anti-La and anti-Ro antibodies/SSA and
    SSB antigen antibodies)
    in aqueous tear deficiency, 8:73–74
    in Sjögren syndrome, 1:186, 187*t*, 8:73–74, 79*t*
SSCP. *See* Single-stranded conformational
    polymorphism
SSPE. *See* Subacute sclerosing panencephalitis
SSRIs. *See* Selective serotonin reuptake inhibitors
SSS. *See* Superior sagittal sinus
SST. *See* Submacular Surgery Trial
ST-segment changes, in ischemic heart disease, 1:113,
    114, 116
    management of acute coronary syndrome and,
        1:122–125
Stabbing headache, idiopathic, icepick pains and, 5:297
Stable angina pectoris, 1:113
    management of, 1:120–122
    risk stratification for, 1:121*t*
Staining, fluorescein, 12:20–21, 20*i*. *See also*
    Hyperfluorescence
Stains/staining techniques, 4:35–36, 8:20–22, 21*i*
    for microbial keratitis, 8:137*t*

in ocular cytology, 8:65*t*
Stallard-Wright incision, for lateral orbitotomy, 7:114
Stand magnifiers, 3:259
Standard automated perimetry (SAP), in glaucoma, 10:57
Standard (field) lens, in manual lensmeter, 3:305, 306*i*
Standing potential, 12:36, 37*i*
  chemically induced changes in, 12:39
  light response of, 12:36–37, 38*i*
Stapedial nerve, 5:55
Staphylococcus, 1:5–6, 8:123–124, 123*i*
  aureus, 1:5
    blepharitis caused by, 8:163–168, 164*t*, 165*t*, 166*i*, 167*i*
    blepharoconjunctivitis caused by, 8:164–165, 170–171
    endogenous bacterial endophthalmitis caused by, 12:183
    hordeolum caused by, 8:168
    keratitis caused by, 8:179
    as normal ocular flora, 8:115, 115*t*
    orbital cellulitis in children caused by, 6:231
    postoperative endophthalmitis caused by, 9:208*t*, 210–211
    posttraumatic endophthalmitis caused by, 9:208*t*, 212
    preseptal cellulitis caused by, 7:42
      in children, 6:230
  in bleb-associated endophthalmitis, 9:212–213
  blepharitis caused by, 8:163–168, 164*t*, 165*t*, 166*i*, 167*i*
    marginal infiltrates in, 8:165, 166*i*, 168, 229
  blepharoconjunctivitis caused by, 8:164–165
    keratitis and, 8:165–166, 166*i*, 167*i*
  conjunctivitis in children caused by, 6:225
  endocarditis prophylaxis and, 1:7, 8–11*t*
  epidermidis, 1:5–6
    bleb-associated endophthalmitis caused by, 9:213
    as normal ocular flora, 8:115, 115*t*
    postoperative endophthalmitis caused by, 9:208*t*, 210, 210*i*
    posttraumatic endophthalmitis caused by, 9:208*t*, 211
  ocular infection caused by, 8:123–124, 163–168, 164*t*, 165*t*, 166*i*, 167*i*
  in postoperative endophthalmitis, 9:208*t*, 209–211, 210*i*
  in posttraumatic endophthalmitis, 9:208*t*, 212
  resistant strains of, 1:5, 71
Staphylomas
  in children, 4:65, 92, 6:364
  congenital, 4:65, 8:296, 296*i*
  intraocular lens implantation and, 11:215
  peripapillary, 6:364
  scleral, 4:90–91, 90*i*
Starfish cataract, in children, 6:293*i*
Stargardt disease (juvenile macular degeneration/fundus flavimaculatus), 6:337–339, 338*i*, 339*i*, 12:216–218, 216*i*, 217*i*, 217*t*
  cone–rod dystrophy and, 6:338
  retinal pigment epithelium in, 2:363
  rod ABC transporter mutations causing, 2:349
Starlix. *See* Nateglinide
Static imbalance, of vestibulo-ocular reflex, 5:200

Static perimetry, 5:90–91, 10:59
  automated. *See* Automated perimetry
  in vision rehabilitation, 3:252
Statins
  age-related macular degeneration and, 1:143, 150–151, 349
  Alzheimer disease prevention and, 1:288
  cataracts and, 1:151, 11:54
  heart disease prevention and, 1:111, 143, 148
  for hypercholesterolemia, 1:146, 149*t*, 150*t*
  stroke prevention and, 1:101
Stationary night blindness, congenital, 12:198–200, 199*i*, 200*i*
  electroretinogram patterns in, 12:30*i*, 198–200, 199*i*, 200*i*
  with myopia, ocular findings in carriers of, 2:270*t*
Stationary nyctalopia, rod-specific mutations causing, 2:348, 349
Stationary retinal disease, 12:195–202
Statistics, 1:339–372
  clinical practice applications and, 1:362–370
    data presentation and, 1:368–370, 369*i*, 370*i*, 371*i*
    measurement system design and, 1:363–364
    monitoring system implementation and, 1:364–366
    quality improvement and, 1:370, 371*i*
    results analysis and, 1:366–368
  evaluation of research studies and, 1:339–344
    clinical relevance and, 1:344
    intervention issues and, 1:342
    outcome issues and, 1:342–343
    participants and setting and, 1:341
    sample size and, 1:342
    validity and, 1:343, 363
  interpreting results of studies for patients and, 1:360–362
  study designs and, 1:345–360, 345*i*
STATPAC procedure, 10:70, 71*i*
Status epilepticus, 1:320–321
Stavudine (d4T), 1:41
  for postexposure HIV prophylaxis, 1:46–47*t*
Stay (pull-over) sutures, 6:176
Stearate/stearic acid
  in retinal pigment epithelium, 2:358
  in vitreous, 2:337
Steatoblepharon, 7:228
"Steeper add minus" rule, 3:180, 194
Steinert disease, retinal degeneration and, 12:232*t*
Stellate (sutural) cataracts, 11:35–36, 37*i*
Stem cells, 8:8, 9–10, 58, 108, 246. *See also* Limbal stem cells
  blood cell formation and, 1:160
  conjunctival, 8:59, 108, 246
  corneal, 8:8, 108, 246, 424
  in corneal and conjunctival wound healing/repair, 8:58, 384, 424
Stent placement
  for aneurysm, 5:353–354
  for canalicular trauma, 7:277
  in carotid artery, 5:182
  with PTCA
    for angina, 1:121
    in myocardial infarction management, 1:111, 115, 125

Stereo acuity
    development of, 6:203
    testing, 6:93–94
        in monofixation syndrome, 6:58
Stereo Fly test, 6:93
Stereopsis, 6:42i, 43, 44, 93
    depth perception differentiated from, 6:44
    monocular reduced vision and, 5:308, 309t
    in monofixation syndrome, 6:58
    testing, 6:93–94
        in functional visual disorder evaluation, 5:307
Sterile (noninfectious) endophthalmitis, cataract
        surgery and, 11:176
Steroids. See Corticosteroids
Stevens-Johnson syndrome (erythema multiforme
        major), 8:216–219, 217t, 218i, 219i
    in children, 6:237–238, 238i
    mucous membrane grafting for, 8:439
    scleral contact lenses in management of, 3:202
STGD4 gene, in Stargardt disease, 12:216
Stickler syndrome (hereditary progressive arthro-
        ophthalmopathy), 6:341, 12:283–284, 284i
    childhood glaucoma and, 10:155t
    Pierre Robin sequence (anomaly/deformity) and,
        6:341, 433, 12:284
    radial perivascular lattice degeneration in, 4:128
    retinal degeneration and, 12:232t
    vitreous collapse in, 2:339
Stigmatic imaging, 3:38, 38i, 62, 62i, 116–117
    with single refractive surface, 3:53–54, 54i
    wavefront analysis and, 3:237–238, 237i
Stiles-Crawford effect, 8:39
Still disease (systemic onset juvenile idiopathic
        arthritis), 1:178–179, 9:141
Stimulated emission, in lasers, 3:19–21, 21
Stimulated macrophages, 9:50, 51i, 52–53
Stimulatory antibodies, 9:62
Stimulatory hypersensitivity (type V) reaction, 9:54, 54t
Stimulus, as perimetry variable
    luminance and, 10:63
    size and, 10:64
    speed of movement of, 10:65
    wavelength and, 10:65
Stimulus accommodative convergence/accommodation
        ratio, 6:88
STIR (short tau inversion recovery) image, 5:63
    signal intensity on, 5:65t
Stocker's lines, 4:74, 8:366, 366i, 377t
Stokes-Adams syndrome, 1:134
Stomach cancer, 1:252
Stool guaiac slide test, in cancer screening, 1:295t, 298
Stop and chop (phaco chop technique), 11:132–134,
        133i
Stop codon (termination codon), 2:196, 201, 201i
    frameshift mutation and, 2:186
STOP-ROP (Supplemental Therapeutic Oxygen for
        Prethreshold ROP Trial), 12:132
Storage diseases, 6:435–439, 436–437t, 457t. See also
        specific type
    cherry red spot in, 6:350, 436–437t
    enzyme defects/ocular signs in, 2:262t
Storiform pattern, in fibrous histiocytoma, 4:92
Strabismic amblyopia, 6:68–69, 69i
    visual development and, 6:51–52, 51i

Strabismus, 6:9–196. See also Deviations; Diplopia
    A-pattern, 6:119–125. See also A-pattern deviations
    acquired, 6:11
    amblyopia and, 6:67–75
    botulinum toxin for, 6:195–196
    in Brown syndrome, 6:144–146, 145i
    in chronic progressive external ophthalmoplegia,
        6:150–151, 153t
    classification of, 6:10–11
    congenital, 6:11
    in congenital fibrosis syndrome, 6:152–154
    in congenital ocular motor apraxia, 6:156
    convergent, 6:9
    in craniosynostosis, 6:429
    cyclovertical, surgery planning and, 6:178
    diagnosis of, 5:214, 214i, 215i, 6:77–95. See also
        Ocular motility, assessment of
        screening tests in, 1:353–354, 353i, 354i
    dissociated. See Dissociated horizontal deviation;
        Dissociated vertical deviation
    divergent, 6:9
    in Duane syndrome, 6:141–144, 142i, 143i
    esodeviations, 6:97–108, 98t
    exodeviations, 6:109–117
    extorsional, 6:10
    extraocular muscle anatomy and, 6:13–26, 14i, 17t
    extraocular muscle field of action/activation and,
        6:29
    fixus, 6:153
    in Graves eye disease (thyroid ophthalmology),
        6:148–150, 149i, 153t
    high myopia and, 6:155
    history/presenting complaint in, 6:77–78
    in internuclear ophthalmoplegia, 6:155
    intorsional, 6:10
    manifest, 6:9
        cover tests in assessment of, 6:80–82, 81i
    in Möbius syndrome, 6:154–155, 154i
    motor physiology and, 6:27–39
    in myasthenia gravis, 6:151–152, 151i, 153t
    nystagmus and, 6:162, 164, 171. See also Nystagmus
    paralytic, Hering's law and, 6:36
    in pediatric cataract, 6:294
    prescribing guidelines in children and, 3:146
    refractive surgery and, 13:44
    in retinoblastoma, 4:253, 253t, 254i, 6:391
    secondary, botulinum toxin injections causing, 6:196
    sensory adaptations in, 6:53–65, 54i
    sensory physiology and pathology and, 6:41–65
    in sixth nerve (abducens) palsy, 6:98t, 107–108, 148,
        148i
    in superior oblique myokymia, 6:156–157
    terminology related to, 6:9–10
    in third nerve (oculomotor) palsy, 6:146–148, 147i
    treatment of
        chemodenervation (botulinum toxin), 6:195–196
        surgical. See Strabismus surgery
    V-pattern, 6:119–125. See also V-pattern deviations
    vertical deviations, 6:9
        botulinum toxin injections causing, 6:196
    visual development affected by, 6:51–52, 51i
Strabismus surgery, 6:173–192, 193t. See also
        Extraocular muscle surgery
    adjustable suture techniques for, 6:175–176
    anesthesia for, 6:183

complications of, 6:184–192, 193*t*
conjunctival incisions for, 6:183–184
for esodeviations, 6:178–179, 179*t*
for exodeviations, 6:179–180, 180*t*, 181*t*
extraocular muscle anatomy and, 6:23–26, 24*i*, 25*i*, 173
for Graves ophthalmopathy, 7:54
guidelines for, 6:178–183
indications for, 6:173–174
infections after, 6:185–186, 186*i*
oblique muscle-weakening procedures in, 6:180–181
planning, 6:176–178
prior surgery and, 6:177
rectus muscle procedures in, 6:181–183
strengthening procedures in, 6:174–175
techniques for, 6:174–176, 175*t*
transposition procedures in, 6:176
weakening procedures in, 6:174, 175*t*
Straddling, in axis determination, 3:131–132, 132*i*
Straight sinus, 5:23
Strampelli intraocular lens, 11:140*i*, 143
Stratum album profundum, 5:34
Stratum griseum profundum, 5:34
Strawberry hemangioma. *See* Hemangiomas
Streak projection system, for retinoscope, 3:125, 125*i*
Streak reflex. *See* Retinal reflex
Strengthening procedures (extraocular muscle), 6:174–175
Streptococcus, 1:6–7, 8:124
α-hemolytic, endocarditis prophylaxis and, 1:7, 8–11*t*
β-hemolytic. *See* Streptococcus, *pyogenes*
in bleb-associated endophthalmitis, 9:208*t*, 212–213, 12:331
in endogenous bacterial endophthalmitis, 12:183
keratitis caused by, 8:180, 181*i*
as normal ocular flora, 8:115, 115*t*
ocular infection caused by, 8:124
persistence and, 8:117
pneumoniae (pneumococcus), 1:6–7, 308, 8:124
conjunctivitis caused by, 8:119*t*, 170–171
in children, 6:224–225
immunization against, 1:291, 304*t*, 308
as normal ocular flora, 8:115
orbital cellulitis caused by, in children, 6:231
preseptal cellulitis caused by, 4:170
in children, 6:230
in postoperative endophthalmitis, 9:208*t*, 211
in posttraumatic endophthalmitis, 9:212
pyogenes (group A beta-hemolytic), 1:6, 8:124
orbital cellulitis caused by, in children, 6:231
orbital necrotizing fasciitis caused by, 7:44–45
preseptal cellulitis caused by, in children, 6:230
Streptogramins, 1:63*t*, 74
Streptokinase, 1:172, 2:452
for ST-segment elevation acute coronary syndrome, 1:124
for stroke, 1:104
Streptolysin, 8:124
Streptomycin, 1:49, 61*t*, 70, 2:435
ototoxicity of, mitochondrial DNA mutations and, 2:220
Stress (exercise) tests, in ischemic heart disease, 1:119
echocardiography, 1:118
Stress model, corneal, 8:12, 13*i*, 13:23, 24*i*

Striae, in LASIK flaps, 13:122–126, 124*t*, 125*i*
Striate cortex (Brodmann area 17), 5:29, 30*i*, 6:44, 45, 45*i*, 47*i*. *See also* Visual (calcarine/occipital) cortex
development of, 6:46, 48*i*
abnormal visual experience affecting, 6:49–52, 50*i*, 51*i*, 67–68
Striate keratopathy, intraocular surgery causing, 8:419
Striate melanokeratosis, 8:264
Stroke
carotid artery disease and, 1:107–109
completed, 1:102
dementia after, 1:285
in diabetes, 1:218
diagnosis of, 1:103–104
evolving, 1:102
gaze palsy and, 5:208
hemorrhagic, 1:105–106
homonymous hemianopia caused by, 5:168*i*, 169
hypertension management in prevention of, 1:91*t*, 95, 104
incidence of, 1:101
ischemic, 1:101–105
ocular ischemic syndrome and, 12:151
without paralysis, 5:205
risk factors for, 1:103, 5:180–181, 180*t*
transient visual loss and, 5:177, 179–180
treatment of, 1:104–105
emergency transport and, 1:313
recent developments in, 1:101
Stroke (phacoemulsification), definition of, 11:114
Stroke scale, 1:103
Stroma
choroidal, 4:151
development of, 2:149–150
ciliary body, 2:66–67
conjunctival. *See* Substantia propria
corneal, 4:61–62, 61*i*, 8:9*i*, 10–12, 10*i*, 11*i*
anatomy of, 2:46–47, 298*i*, 300–301
biochemistry and metabolism of, 2:300–301
development of, 2:151, 151*i*, 152*i*, 8:6
inflammation of, 8:29, 31*i*, 32*t*
in systemic infections, 8:189–190
neovascularization of, contact lenses causing, 8:108
wound healing/repair of, 4:20, 8:384
iris, 2:62, 4:149
cysts of, 6:265–266
melanoma involving, 4:157, 158*i*
scleral, 2:50, 4:88, 88*i*
Stromal bed thickness, calculation of after LASIK, 13:49
Stromal degenerations
age-related (involutional) changes and, 8:369–370
peripheral, 8:370–371
postinflammatory changes and, 8:372–374
Stromal dystrophies, 8:316–323, 316*t*. *See also specific type*
congenital hereditary, 6:256*t*, 257, 8:297
posterior amorphous, 8:297
Stromal edema, 8:33
after cataract surgery, 11:166
Stromal graft rejection, isolated, 8:468. *See also* Rejection (graft)
Stromal haze, cataract surgery after PRK and, 11:211
Stromal infiltrates, after PRK/LASEK, 13:104, 104*i*

Stromal keratitis
  in Cogan syndrome, **8:**228, 229
  Epstein-Barr virus causing, **8:**156–157, 156*i*
  herpes simplex virus causing, **8:**146–150, 146*i*, 147*i*,
    148*i*, 149*t*
    penetrating keratoplasty for, **8:**151
  in herpes zoster ophthalmicus, **8:**154, 154*i*, 155*i*
  microsporidial, **8:**190
  necrotizing, **8:**29, 147–148, 148*i*, 150
  nonnecrotizing, **8:**146–147, 146*i*, 147*i*
  nonsuppurative, **8:**25*t*, 29, 31*i*, 32*t*
    systemic infections and, **8:**189–190
  scleritis and, **8:**239
  suppurative, **8:**25*t*, 29, 31*i*, 32*t*
  syphilitic, **8:**227
Stromal micropuncture, for recurrent corneal erosions,
  8:99–100, 100*i*
Stromal nevi, **4:**56
STRs. *See* Short tandem repeats
Structure, care system, **1:**362
STSs. *See* Sequence-tagged sites
Student *t* test, **1:**344
Sturge-Weber disease/syndrome (encephalofacial
  angiomatosis), **5:**336*t*, 340, 341*i*, **6:**278, 402*t*,
  414–416, 414*i*, 415*i*, **10:**154
  choroidal hemangioma in, **4:**164, 244, **12:**170
  glaucoma associated with, **5:**340, **10:**32, 154
    in children, **6:**278, 416, **10:**154
  port-wine stain in, **5:**340, 341*i*, **6:**278, 380, 414–415,
    415*i*
Sturm, conoid of, **3:**93–94, 94*i*, 95*i*
  astigmatic dial refraction and, **3:**134–136, 135*i*
Stye (external hordeolum), **4:**170, **7:**160, **8:**168
Subacute bacterial endocarditis. *See* Endocarditis
Subacute granulomatous thyroiditis, **1:**226
Subacute lymphocytic ("painless") thyroiditis, **1:**226
Subacute sclerosing panencephalitis, **8:**162–163
  posterior uveitis caused by, **9:**159–160
Subarachnoid hemorrhage, **1:**105, 106, **5:**353
  ocular hemorrhage with, **5:**351
  in shaking injury, **6:**443, 444
Subarachnoid peripheral lesions, **5:**227–235
Subarachnoid space, optic nerve, **2:**102
Sub-brow fat pads, **7:**146
Subcapsular cataract
  anterior, **4:**97–100, 99*i*
  posterior (cupuliform cataract), **4:**99, 99*i*, **11:**48–49,
    53*i*
    in children, **6:**291, 292*t*
    corticosteroids causing, **11:**50–52
    in myotonic dystrophy, **11:**62–63
Subclavian artery, proximal, **5:**17
Subclavian steal, **5:**349
Subconjunctival hemorrhage, **8:**90, 91*t*, 396
Subcutaneous nodules, in rheumatoid arthritis, **1:**174
Subcutaneous rhytidectomy, **7:**244
Subcutaneous tissue
  of eyelid, **7:**139
  of face, **7:**135
Subendocardial (non–Q wave, nontransmural)
  infarction, **1:**114, 116
Subepithelial corneal degenerations, **8:**368–369
Subepithelial corneal infiltrate, **8:**25*t*
Subepithelial fibrovascular pannus, **4:**68

Subepithelial graft rejection, **8:**467–468, 468*i*. *See also*
  Rejection (graft)
Subepithelial nevi, **4:**56
Subjective refraction, **3:**134–141
  astigmatic dial technique for, **3:**134–136, 135*i*
  with automated refractors, **3:**313
  binocular balance and, **3:**141
  in children, **3:**146
  cross-cylinder technique for, **3:**136–139, 138*i*
  refining sphere and, **3:**139–140
Subjective visual space, **6:**41
Sublimaze. *See* Fentanyl
Subluxed/subluxated lens, **4:**94, **6:**304, 305*t*, 309, **11:**40.
  See also Ectopia lentis
  cataract surgery and, **11:**226–227, 227*i*, 228*i*
Submacular hemorrhage, **12:**326–327, 328*i*
Submacular surgery
  for hemorrhage, **12:**327
  for ocular histoplasmosis syndrome, **12:**81–82
Submacular Surgery Trial (SST), **12:**81–82, 327
Submandibular ganglion, **2:**119
Suborbicularis fat pads (suborbicularis oculi fat/
  SOOF), **7:**135, 141*i*, 145–146
  midface rejuvenation surgery and (SOOF lift), **7:**241,
    242*i*
Subperiorbital surgical space, **7:**109, 110*i*
Subperiosteal midface lift, **7:**241–242
  endoscopic, **7:**242–243, 243*i*
Subretinal fibrosis and uveitis syndrome (SFU), **9:**177*t*,
  184, 184*i*, 185*i*
Subretinal neovascular membranes, in age-related
  macular degeneration, **4:**139
Subretinal space (interphotoreceptor matrix/IPM), **2:**78
  development of, **2:**137*i*
  retinal pigment epithelium in maintenance of,
    2:361–362
Substance abuse disorders, **1:**267–271, 268*t*. *See also*
  specific substance
  ocular trauma and, **1:**271
Substance P, **8:**198*t*, **9:**82*t*
  in iris–ciliary body, **2:**308
  in tear secretion, **2:**290
Substantia nigra
  in Parkinson disease, **1:**278
  pars reticulata of, **5:**54
Substantia propria (conjunctival stroma), **4:**43, **8:**8
  immune and inflammatory cells in, **8:**196*t*, **9:**33
  wound healing/repair and, **8:**383
Sub-Tenon's approach, for periocular corticosteroid
  injection, **9:**116–117, 117*i*
  in pars planitis, **9:**150
  in pediatric uveitis, **6:**319
Succinate, for Leber hereditary optic neuropathy, **5:**136
Succinylcholine, **2:**402*i*, 403
  malignant hyperthermia caused by, **6:**191
  in patients taking cholinesterase inhibitors, **2:**400
  pharmacogenetics and, **2:**279
Suction ring, placement of for LASIK, **13:**113, 113*i*
Sudden cardiac death, **1:**115–116
  ventricular fibrillation and, **1:**140
Sudoriferous cysts, of eyelid (apocrine hidrocystoma),
  7:168, 169*i*
Sufenta. *See* Sufentanil
Sufentanil, perioperative, **1:**332*t*, 338

"Sugar" cataracts, 2:330–332
  aldose reductase in development of, 2:331–332, 354, 11:14–16, 60
Sugiura's sign, 9:203, 204*i*
Suicide, SSRI use and, 1:276
Suicide induction (cell), by cytotoxic T lymphocytes, 9:68, 69*i*
Sulamyd. *See* Sulfacetamide
Sular. *See* Nisoldipine
Sulbactam, 1:69–70. *See also specific antibiotic combination*
Sulcus/sulci
  optic, 2:127, 136, 140*i*
  temporal, 5:31
Sulf-10. *See* Sulfacetamide
Sulfacetamide, 2:431*t*, 433
  in combination preparations, 2:432*t*
Sulfadiazine, 2:433
  for toxoplasmosis, 6:216, 12:187, 187*t*
Sulfasalazine, 1:174, 199
Sulfatase deficiency, multiple, 8:340–341
Sulfisoxazole, 1:55*t*
Sulfite oxidase deficiency, 2:262*t*, 6:308, 11:42
Sulfonamides, 1:54, 55*t*, 2:433. *See also specific agent*
  for toxoplasmosis, 9:168
Sulfonylureas, 1:211–213
Sulfur metabolism, in sulfite oxidase deficiency, 11:42
Sulindac, 1:197*t*, 2:421*t*
Sunburst lesions, black, in sickle cell disease, 12:121
Sunflower cataract
  in chalcosis, 11:59, 12:299
  in Wilson disease, 11:62
Sunglasses, 3:165, 168
  contrast improvement and, 3:165
  contrast sensitivity and, 3:165
  dark adaptation improvement and, 3:165
  glare reduction and, 3:10, 165
  photochromic, 3:166
  polarizing (polarized/Polaroid lenses), 3:10, 13*i*, 165
  ultraviolet-absorbing, 3:166–167
    cataract prevention and, 11:57
  visual functions improved by, 3:165, 166*i*
Sunlight. *See* Ultraviolet light
Sunset-glow fundus, in Vogt-Koyanagi-Harada syndrome, 9:203, 204*i*
"Sunsetting," in infants, 6:451
Superficial mimetic muscles, 7:135, 138–139
Superficial musculoaponeurotic system (SMAS), 7:135, 136*i*
  subcutaneous rhytidectomy with, 7:244–245, 245*i*
Superficial petrosal nerve, greater, 5:55
Superficial punctate keratitis of Thygeson, 8:224–225, 225*i*
Superficial superior colliculus, 5:34
Superficial temporal artery, 5:11, 11–12*i*, 15–16
Superior cerebellar artery, 5:18
Superior cervical ganglion, 5:57
  dilator muscle innervation and, 2:65
Superior colliculus, 5:27, 31, 54
  superficial, 5:34
Superior displacement of globe, in orbital disorders, 7:23
Superior limbic keratoconjunctivitis, 8:96–98, 97*i*
Superior medullary velum, 2:111
Superior muscular artery, 5:15

Superior oblique muscles, 2:8, 15*i*, 17*i*, 18*t*, 19*i*, 5:41, 42, 42*i*, 6:14*i*, 15, 17*t*, 7:12–13, 140*i*
  action of, 6:15, 17*t*, 30*t*, 31, 34*i*
  anatomy of, 6:14*i*, 15, 17*t*
    surgery and, 6:23, 24*i*
  field of action/activation of, 6:29
  overaction of, 6:129–130, 129*i*
    A-pattern deviations associated with, 6:119, 121*i*
    vertical deviations caused by, 6:129–130, 129*i*
  paresis/palsy of, 6:132–135, 133*i*
    Hering's law and, 6:36–37, 37*i*
    after tenotomy for Brown syndrome, 6:146
  surgery of, 6:180–181
    for A- and V-pattern deviations, 6:122–123, 124–125, 181
    for vertical deviation, 6:130
Superior oblique myokymia, 5:254, 6:156–157
Superior oblique tendon, tucking procedure on, 6:174–175
Superior oblique tendon sheath syndrome (Brown syndrome), 5:219–220, 220*i*, 6:135, 144–146, 145*i*
  iatrogenic, tucking procedure causing, 6:175
  inferior oblique muscle paralysis compared with, 6:137*t*
  surgery for, 6:146, 181
Superior oblique tenotomy
  for Brown syndrome, 6:146, 181
  for third nerve (oculomotor) palsy, 6:148
Superior ophthalmic vein, 5:20, 22*i*
Superior orbital fissure, 2:10–12, 11*i*, 12*i*, 5:8*i*, 7:11, 21
  cranial nerve VI in, 5:43, 45–49*i*
  lesions of, 5:236
Superior orbital vein, 6:16
Superior petrosal sinus, 5:23
Superior punctum, 2:22, 34
Superior rectus muscles, 2:15*i*, 17*i*, 18*t*, 19*i*, 5:42, 42*i*, 6:14, 14*i*, 17*t*, 18*i*, 7:12–13, 140*i*
  action of, 6:14, 17*t*, 30, 30*t*, 32*i*
  anatomy of, 6:14, 14*i*, 17*t*, 18*i*
    surgery and, 6:23, 24*i*
  surgery of
    for dissociated vertical deviation, 6:181
    eyelid position changes after, 6:189
    for superior oblique paralysis, 6:134
  V-pattern deviations associated with dysfunction of, 6:119
Superior rectus subnucleus, 5:45–46
Superior sagittal sinus, 5:20
  thrombosis of, 5:358
Superior sulcus deformity, anophthalmic socket and, 7:124, 124*i*
Superior tarsal muscle of Müller, 2:26, 27*i*, 4:168, 5:57, 58*i*, 7:140*i*, 144
  in congenital Horner syndrome, 7:217
  internal (conjunctival) resection of, for ptosis correction, 7:222
  paresis of, 5:262
Superior transverse ligament (Whitnall's ligament), 2:26, 26*i*, 27*i*, 7:140*i*, 142–143, 144*i*, 253
Superior vena cava syndrome, glaucoma associated with, 10:32
Superior vestibular nerve, 5:32, 54
Supernumerary puncta, 6:240
Superoxide. *See also* Free radicals
  as inflammatory mediator, 9:83

Superoxide dismutase, 9:83
  in lens, 2:368, 11:17
  in retina and retinal pigment epithelium, 2:372
Supplemental Therapeutic Oxygen for Prethreshold
    ROP Trial (STOP-ROP), 12:132
Suppression, 6:53–55, 54i
  testing for, 6:55, 58–65
Suppression (immunologic), in development of
    tolerance, 9:88–89
Suppression scotoma, diplopia after strabismus surgery
    and, 6:185
Suppressor T cells. See also T cells
  class I MHC molecules as antigen-presenting
      platform for, 9:19–22, 21i
  in external eye defense, 8:114, 196t
  in immune processing, 9:23i, 24
Supracapsular phacoemulsification (supracapsular
    phaco), 11:128–129, 134
Suprachoroidal/choroidal hemorrhage, 12:332–334,
    333i
  cataract surgery and, 11:164t, 169–170
    delayed, 11:171
    expulsive, 11:170–171
      patients at risk for, 11:215–217
    flat or shallow anterior chamber and, 11:163, 166
Suprachoroidal detachment, melanoma differentiated
    from, 4:230–232
Suprachoroidal effusion, cataract surgery and, 11:163,
    169–170
  flat or shallow anterior chamber and, 11:163
Supraduction. See Elevation of eye
Supranuclear eye movement systems, 5:33–34, 35–38i,
    39, 6:39
  diplopia associated with lesions of, 5:222–223, 223t
Supranuclear palsy, progressive, 5:199
  slowed saccades in, 5:206
Supranuclear pathways
  lesions of, facial weakness/paralysis caused by, 5:281
  in ocular motility, 5:197
Supraorbital artery, 2:32i, 39i, 5:13, 15
Supraorbital ethmoids, 7:20
Supraorbital foramen/notch, 2:5, 7i, 9
Supraorbital nerve, 5:52, 53i
Supratarsal corticosteroid injections, for vernal
    keratoconjunctivitis, 8:211
Suprathreshold, definition of, 10:59
Suprathreshold testing (perimetry), 10:65–66
Supratrochlear artery, 2:32i, 39i, 5:13, 15
Supratrochlear nerve, 5:52, 53i
Supraventricular tachycardias, 1:136–138
Suprax. See Cefixime
Suprofen, 2:306, 422
Surface asymmetry index (SAI), 3:303
Surface dyslexia, in Alzheimer disease, 1:288
Surface markers
  identification of macrophages/monocytes and, 8:68
  lymphocyte, 9:15
Surface normal, 3:42–44, 43i, 45i, 46i
  determination of position of, 3:51, 52i
Surface regularity index (SRI), 3:303
Surface tension, of viscoelastics, 11:158
Surface-wrinkling retinopathy, 5:105, 12:87
Surfactants, in eyedrops, absorption and, 2:385
Surge, in phacoemulsification, 11:115

Surgery. See also specific procedure and Ocular
    (intraocular) surgery
  in diabetic patients, 1:220–221, 332–333
  in elderly patients, 1:237–238
  in patients with pulmonary disease, 1:329
Surgical instruments
  for ECCE, 11:109
  for ICCE, 11:105
  for intrastromal corneal ring segment placement,
      13:79–80, 79t
  for IOL implantation, 11:152–153
  for LASIK, 13:107–110, 108–109i
  for phacoemulsification, 11:113–121
    settings for, 11:135–137, 135t, 136i
Surgical spaces, orbital, 7:12–13
Sursumduction/sursumversion. See Elevation of eye
Susceptibility testing, antimicrobial, 1:66–67
Suspensory ligament of lens. See Zonules
Suspensory ligament of Lockwood, 2:37–38, 38i, 6:21,
    7:145
Sustained-release preparations
  oral, 2:388
  for topical administration, 2:390
Sustiva. See Efavirenz
Sutural cataracts, 11:35–36, 37i
Sutures (lens), 2:75i, 76, 11:9
  development of, 2:146, 11:27i, 28–29, 28i
  opacification of (sutural/stellate cataract), 11:35–36,
      37i
Sutures (surgical)
  adjustable, for strabismus surgery, 6:175–176
  allergic reaction to, 6:186, 187i
  for cataract surgery, astigmatism and, 11:184
  compression, for corneal astigmatism after
      penetrating keratoplasty, 8:466
  for penetrating keratoplasty, 8:456–459, 457i, 458i,
      459i
    in children, 8:470, 471
    postoperative problems and, 8:462–463, 462i, 463i
  pull-over (stay), 6:176
  Quickert, for involutional entropion, 7:204, 205
  removal of
    after corneoscleral laceration repair, 8:416–417
    after pediatric corneal transplantation, 8:470–471,
        470t
Swabbing, for specimen collection, 8:63–64
Sweat glands, of eyelid, 4:168t, 7:167
  tumors arising in, 7:167, 168i, 169i
Swedish interactive thresholding algorithm (SITA)
    testing (perimetry), 10:67
Swelling pressure, 8:11
Swinging flashlight test
  before cataract surgery, 11:81
  for relative afferent pupillary defect, 5:84–85, 86i
SWS. See Sturge-Weber disease/syndrome
Symadine. See Amantadine
Symblepharon, 7:207
  in ocular cicatricial pemphigoid, 8:220, 221i
  in Stevens-Johnson syndrome, 6:237, 8:218, 219i
Symlin. See Pramlintide
Symmetrel. See Amantadine
Sympathetic nerves/pathway, 5:56–57, 58i
  cholinergic drug action and, 2:394, 395i
  in ciliary ganglion, 2:14–15, 14i
  orbit supplied by, 7:15–16

paravertebral, 5:56
in tear secretion, 2:292–293, 292*i*, 293*i*
Sympathetic ophthalmia, 4:152–153, 153*i*, 154*i*,
    9:67–68, 200–203, 200*i*, 201*i*, 202*t*, 12:300–301
    enucleation in prevention of, 7:119–120, 8:410–411
    HLA association in, 9:94*t*
    surgical procedures/injuries leading to, 9:202*t*
Sympatholytics, for hypertension, 1:94
Sympathomimetic activity, intrinsic, beta-blocker, 1:92
Synchysis scintillans, 12:286
Syndactyly
    in Apert syndrome, 6:426, 427*i*
    in Saethre-Chotzen syndrome, 6:426, 428*i*
Syndrome (genetic), definition of, 6:205
Syndrome of prolonged enlargement of blind spot,
    9:182
Synechiae
    anterior
        in glaucoma, 10:5, 7
            gonioscopy in identification of, 10:39
        in sarcoidosis, 9:198
    posterior
        anisocoria and, 5:262
        in children, 6:270
        mydriasis in prevention of, 2:400
        in sarcoidosis, 6:270, 9:198
        in uveitis, 9:104*i*, 105*i*
Synechiolysis, with penetrating keratoplasty, 8:459
Synercid. *See* Quinupristin/dalfopristin
Syneresis, 4:108, 108*i*
    in posterior vitreous detachment, 12:256
    in young eyes, 12:254
Synergist muscles, 6:35
Synergistins, 1:74. *See also* Streptogramins
Synkinesis, 7:211
    facial, 5:280, 280*i*, 284
    in Marcus Gunn jaw-winking ptosis, 6:214, 7:211,
        217, 218*i*
    near reflex and, 2:111
Synkinetic reflex. *See* Near reflex
Synophthalmia, 2:127
Synteny/syntenic traits, 2:196, 220–221, 245
Syphilis, 1:15–18, 8:128, 9:187–191
    chorioretinitis in, 9:188, 189*i*, 12:190–191, 190*i*
        in HIV infection/AIDS, 9:189, 255
        posterior placoid, 9:255
    congenital/intrauterine, 1:15, 302, 6:220–221,
        9:187–188, 188*i*
        corneal manifestations of, 4:67, 6:220, 260, 260*i*,
            8:226–227, 227*i*, 299, 9:187–188, 188*i*
    in HIV infection/AIDS, 1:18, 5:361–362, 9:189,
        255–256
    interstitial keratitis caused by, 6:220, 260, 260*i*,
        8:226–227, 227*i*, 299, 9:187–188, 188*i*
    screening/testing for, 1:16–17, 17*t*, 302
    secondary, 9:188, 189*i*
    uveitis and, 9:107, 187–191
Syphilitic posterior placoid chorioretinitis, 9:255
Syringomas, 7:167, 168*i*
Systemic drug therapy
    corticosteroid, for uveitis, 9:115*t*, 117
    for ocular disorders, 2:388–389
Systemic lupus erythematosus, 1:179–182, 180*i*, 181*t*,
    9:61, 173, 174*i*
    eyelid manifestations of, 4:173*t*

refractive surgery contraindicated in, 13:198
Systemic sclerosis, progressive (scleroderma),
    1:185–186
    eyelid manifestations of, 4:173*t*
Systole (systolic phase), 1:128
Systolic dysfunction, 1:129
    causes of, 1:128
    management of, 1:130–131

T

T. *See* Transducin
T1 (spin-lattice/longitudinal relaxation time), 5:81,
    7:30–31
T1-weighted images, 5:62–63, 63*i*, 64*i*, 65*i*
    parameters of, 5:64*t*
    signal intensity on, 5:65*t*
T2 (spin-spin/transverse relaxation time), 5:81, 7:31
T2-weighted images, 5:62–63, 63*i*, 64*i*, 65*i*, 66*i*
    parameters of, 5:64*t*
    signal intensity on, 5:65*t*
T$_3$. *See* Triiodothyronine
T$_4$. *See* Thyroxine
T4/T8 ratio, in HIV infection/AIDS, 1:37
T-20. *See* Enfuvirtide
T-1249, 1:42
T-cell antigen receptors, 9:87
    HLA disease associations and, 9:95
T-cell signaling inhibitors, for uveitis, 9:119*t*, 120
T cells (T lymphocytes), 1:4, 4:15, 9:15. *See also specific
    type*
    activation of, 9:19–22, 21*i*, 25
    in cell-mediated immunity, 8:199*i*, 201
    class I MHC molecules as antigen-presenting
        platform for, 9:19–22, 21*i*
    class II MHC molecules as antigen-presenting
        platform for, 9:19, 20*i*
    cytologic identification of, 8:67
    cytotoxic, 9:24, 25, 66–70, 69*i*
    delayed hypersensitivity (DH), 9:25, 63–66, 65*i*, 68*t*
    differentiation of, 9:22–24, 23*i*
    downregulatory, 9:88
    effector, 9:25
    in external eye, 8:114, 196*t*
    helper. *See* T helper cells
    in HIV infection/AIDS, 1:37, 40, 8:122, 9:242–243,
        244*t*, 246–248
    in immune processing, 9:22–24, 23*i*
    killer, 8:200
    maturation of, in thymus, 9:16
    suppressor, 9:23*i*, 24
    tumor immunology and, 8:249
    in viral conjunctivitis, 9:35
T helper cells, 9:22–24, 23*i*
    class II MHC molecules as antigen-presenting
        platform for, 9:19–20, 20*i*
    in delayed hypersensitivity (type IV) reactions, 8:201,
        9:63–66, 65*i*, 68*t*
    differentiation of, 9:22–24, 23*i*
    in external eye, 8:114, 196*t*
    in HIV infection/AIDS, 1:37, 9:242–243
    in immune processing, 9:22–24, 23*i*
T helper 0 cells, 9:22

T helper 1 cells, **8:**201, **9:**22–24, 23*i*
  in delayed hypersensitivity (type IV) reactions,
    9:63–66, 65*i*, 68*t*
  in sympathetic ophthalmia, **9:**67–68
T helper 2 cells, **9:**22–24, 23*i*
  in chronic mast cell degranulation, **9:**73
  in delayed hypersensitivity (type IV) reactions,
    9:63–66, 65*i*
  in *Toxocara* granuloma, **9:**67
t-PA. *See* Tissue plasminogen activator
T pallidum hemagglutination assay (TPHA), **1:**17
T score, in osteoporosis, **1:**243
t-tests, **1:**344
T waves, in myocardial infarction, **1:**116
TABO convention, **3:**98*i*
Taches de bougie, in sarcoidosis, **4:**126, **9:**199
Tachyarrhythmias, **1:**136–140
  heart failure and, **1:**131–132
  supraventricular, **1:**136–138
  ventricular, **1:**138–140
Tachycardia
  junctional, **1:**137
  narrow-complex, **1:**136
  sinus, **1:**136
  supraventricular, **1:**136–138
  ventricular, **1:**138–139
  wide-complex, **1:**138
Tachyzoites, in toxoplasmosis transmission, **6:**215
Tacrolimus
  for allergic conjunctivitis, **8:**209
  for uveitis, **9:**119*t*
Tactile aids, for low-vision patient, **3:**261
Tadalafil, ocular effects of, **1:**325*t*
Tadpole pupil, **5:**259–260
Taenia solium (pork tapeworm), **8:**133, **9:**171
  orbital infection caused by, **7:**47
Takayasu arteritis (aortic arch arteritis/aortitis
    syndrome/pulseless disease), **1:**189*t*, 191
Tambocor. *See* Flecainide
Tamiflu. *See* Oseltamivir
Tamoxifen, **1:**260*t*
  ocular effects of, **1:**325*t*
  retinopathy caused by, **12:**249, 250*i*, 250*t*
Tandem repeats, short, **2:**196, 223, 225*i*
Tandem scanning confocal microscopy, **8:**38
Tangent screen, **5:**91
  in strabismus/amblyopia evaluation, **6:**89–90, 90*i*
Tangential incisions, for keratorefractive surgery,
    corneal biomechanics affected by, **8:**13, 14*i*, 13:19,
    23*i*
Tangential power (instantaneous radius of curvature),
    8:43, 43*i*, 44*i*, **13:**7, 7*i*
Tangier disease, **8:**339–340
TAO (thyroid-associated orbitopathy). *See* Thyroid
    ophthalmopathy
TAP (Treatment of Age-Related Macular Degeneration
    with Photodynamic Therapy) Study, **12:**73–75, 321
Tapazole. *See* Methimazole
Tapeworms
  dog (*Echinococcus granulosus*), orbital infection
    caused by, **7:**47
  eye invaded by, **7:**47, **9:**171, 172*i*
  pork (*Taenia solium*), **8:**133, **9:**171
    orbital infection caused by, **7:**47
Tapioca melanoma, **4:**220*t*

Tarantula hairs, ocular inflammation caused by, **8:**395
Tardive dyskinesia, **5:**286
Target screen testing, in functional visual disorder
    evaluation, **5:**311, 313*i*
Targocid. *See* Teicoplanin
Tarka. *See* Verapamil
Tarsal conjunctiva, **8:**8. *See also* Conjunctiva
Tarsal ectropion, **7:**198
Tarsal fracture operation, for cicatricial entropion,
    7:206, 206*i*
Tarsal glands, **2:**22, 24*i*. *See also* Glands of Wolfring;
    Meibomian glands
Tarsal kink, **7:**157
  congenital, **6:**211, 211*i*
Tarsal muscles
  inferior, **7:**145
  superior (Müller's), **4:**168, **7:**140*i*, 144
    in congenital Horner syndrome, **7:**217
    internal (conjunctival) resection of, for ptosis
      correction, **7:**222
Tarsal plates/tarsus, **2:**26–28, 26*i*, 30*i*, 31*i*, **4:**168, **7:**140*i*,
    141*i*, 145, **8:**7*i*, 8
    internal (conjunctival) resection of, for ptosis
      correction, **7:**222
Tarsal strip procedure
  for cicatricial ectropion, **7:**200–201
  for involutional ectropion, **7:**197–198, 197*i*
  for involutional entropion, **7:**205
Tarsoconjunctival grafts
  for cicatricial entropion, **7:**207
  for eyelid repair, **7:**187, 190*i*, 191*i*, 192
Tarsoconjunctival müllerectomy (Fasanella-Servat
    procedure), for ptosis correction, **7:**222
Tarsorrhaphy, **8:**428–429
  for chemical burns, **8:**392
  for craniosynostosis-induced corneal exposure, **6:**428
  for dry eye, **8:**75*t*, 77
  for exposure keratopathy, **8:**95
  for neurotrophic keratopathy, **8:**104
  for paralytic ectropion, **7:**199, 200*i*
  for persistent corneal epithelial defects, **8:**102
  for thyroid-associated orbitopathy, **5:**331
Tarsotomy
  for cicatricial entropion, **7:**206, 206*i*
  for trichiasis, **8:**104
Tarsus. *See* Tarsal plates/tarsus
Tasmar. *See* Tolcapone
TATA box, **2:**196, 206
TATA-box binding protein, **2:**206
Tattoo, corneal, **8:**377*t*, 442–443
Tau proteins, in Alzheimer disease, **1:**286
Taxol. *See* Paclitaxel
Taxon-specific crystallins, **2:**326*t*, 327
Tay-Sachs disease (GM$_2$ gangliosidosis type I), **2:**262*t*,
    6:350, 437*t*, **8:**340
    racial and ethnic concentration of, **2:**259
    retinal degeneration and, **12:**243–244, 244*i*
Tazicef. *See* Ceftazidime
Tazidime. *See* Ceftazidime
Tazobactam, **1:**69–70. *See also specific antibiotic
    combination*
TBG. *See* Thyroxine-binding globulin
TBP. *See* TATA-box binding protein
TBUT. *See* Tear breakup time
3TC. *See* Lamivudine

Tc-99. *See under Technetium-99*
TCA cycle. *See* Tricarboxylic acid (TCA) cycle
Td vaccine, 1:304*t*, 307
TDF. *See* Testis-determining factor
TE (time to echo), definition of, 5:81
Tear breakup, 8:61
Tear breakup time, 8:61
fluorescein in evaluation of, 8:20, 61
in pseudoepiphora evaluation, 7:273
refractive surgery and, 13:44, 45*i*
Tear deficiency states. *See also specific type and* Dry eye syndrome
aqueous, 2:294, 8:56, 57, 71–80, 72*t*. *See also* Aqueous tear deficiency
refractive surgery and, 13:44, 45*i*
evaporative tear dysfunction, 8:72*t*, 80–90
lipid, 8:56
mucin, 2:291, 294, 8:58
rose bengal in evaluation of, 8:22
tests of, 8:61–63, 62*i*, 62*t*
Tear film (tears), 2:287–296, 288*i*, 288*t*, 289*i*, 8:56–58, 56*i*
aqueous phase of, 2:44, 288*i*, 289–291, 289*i*, 8:56
biochemistry and metabolism of, 2:287–296
composition of, 7:253
assays of, 8:63
contact lens optics and, 3:176, 176*i*, 180–181, 181*i*
dysfunction/alterations of, 2:294–296, 295*i*. *See also* Tear deficiency states
illusions caused by, 5:188
evaluation of, 8:61–63, 62*i*, 62*t*
fluorescein for, 8:20
in external eye defense, 8:113
immunoglobulins in, 8:56, 198
inflammatory mediators in, 8:197
lipid layer of, 2:287–289, 288*i*, 289*i*, 8:56, 56*i*
mucin layer of, 2:44, 288*i*, 291, 8:56–57, 56*i*
osmolarity of, 8:63
pH of, 8:57
physiology of, 8:56–58, 56*i*
precorneal, 2:44, 287, 288*i*
preocular, 2:287
refractive index of, 8:40, 57
secretion of, 2:291–294, 292*i*, 293*i*
solutes in, 2:290
structure of, 8:56–57, 56*i*
Tear (fluid) lens, contact lens creation of, 3:176, 180–181, 181*i*, 194
Tear meniscus (marginal tear strip), 2:287
inspection of, 8:61
in pseudoepiphora evaluation, 7:272
Tear pump, 7:256, 257*i*
Tear sac. *See* Lacrimal sac
"Tear star," 8:378
Tearing (epiphora), 7:251, 259–284. *See also specific cause*
acquired, 7:267–284
evaluation of, 7:267–274
management of, 7:274–284
congenital, 6:241–242, 272, 7:259–267
evaluation of, 7:259
management of, 7:259–267
in congenital/infantile glaucoma, 6:272
in congenital nasolacrimal duct obstruction, 6:241–242

conjunctival inflammation causing, 8:24*t*
in craniosynostosis syndromes, 6:430
definition of, 7:272
diagnostic tests for evaluation of, 7:268–274
in punctal atresia, 6:239
reflex, absorption of ocular medication affected by, 2:381–382, 385
Tears (artificial), 2:449–450, 5:286. *See also* Lubricants
for dry eye, 8:74, 75, 75*t*
for hay fever and perennial allergic conjunctivitis, 8:208
for Stevens-Johnson syndrome, 6:237, 8:218
for Thygeson superficial punctate keratitis, 8:225
Tears (retinal). *See* Retinal tears
Technetium-99 pyrophosphate scintigraphy, in ischemic heart disease, 1:119
Technetium-99m Sestamibi scintigraphy, in ischemic heart disease, 1:119
Tectonic penetrating keratoplasty
for herpetic keratitis complications, 8:151
for keratoglobus, 8:335
for peripheral ulcerative keratitis, 8:232
Teczem. *See* Diltiazem
Teenagers. *See* Adolescents
Tegopen. *See* Cloxacillin
Tegretol. *See* Carbamazepine
Teichoic acid, in bacterial cell wall, 8:123
Teicoplanin, 1:61*t*, 72
Telangiectasias
in ataxia-telangiectasia (Louis-Bar syndrome), 6:417, 8:91–92, 270
capillary, 1:106
conjunctival, 5:342, 342*i*, 6:417
hereditary hemorrhagic (Osler-Weber-Rendu disease), 1:166, 8:91
retinal, 6:332–333, 12:156–157, 157*i*. *See also* Coats disease
parafoveal (juxtafoveal), 4:121–122, 12:157–158, 158*i*, 159*i*
in rosacea, 8:84, 85
in scleroderma, 1:185
Telecanthus, 6:209, 424, 7:25
in blepharophimosis syndrome, 6:213, 213*i*
Telecentricity, 3:81
Teleopsia, 5:189
Telescopes
as afocal systems, 3:82–84, 82*i*, 83*i*
astronomical
in operating microscope, 3:296, 297*i*
in slit-lamp biomicroscope, 3:280, 282*i*
Galilean, 3:82–83, 82*i*, 83*i*
contact lens correction of aphakia and, 3:174, 176*i*
in operating microscope, 3:296, 297*i*
reverse, in slit-lamp biomicroscope, 3:280–281
in slit-lamp biomicroscope, 3:280–281, 283*i*
Keplerian, 3:82–84, 83*i*
in operating microscope, 3:296, 297*i*
in slit-lamp biomicroscope, 3:280–281, 282*i*, 283*i*
in vision rehabilitation, 3:82–84
Television, closed circuit, 3:261
Telithromycin, 1:60*t*, 71, 75
Teller acuity cards, in amblyopia evaluation, 6:69, 69*i*, 79
Telmisartan, 1:88*t*, 90*t*
Telomerase, 2:205

Telomeres/telomeric DNA, **2**:197, 203, 205
Telorbitism (hypertelorism), **2**:126, **6**:207, 424, **7**:25
  clefting syndromes and, **7**:38
Telzir. *See* Fosamprenavir
Temafloxacin, **1**:62*t*, 73, **2**:431
Temazepam, **1**:273
Temperature, anterior segment injury and, **8**:387–389
Temperature-sensitive albinism, **6**:347*t*
Temporal (giant cell) arteritis. *See* Arteritis, giant cell
Temporal artery
  eyelids supplied by, **7**:147
  superficial, **5**:11, 11–12*i*, 15–16
Temporal bone, **5**:5
Temporal (longitudinal) coherence, **3**:8, 8*i*
Temporal crescent, **5**:29
  occipital lobe lesions causing, **5**:168
Temporal fossa, **5**:9
Temporal lobe
  lesions of
    epilepsy and, **1**:281
    hallucinations and, **5**:190
    retrochiasmal, **5**:166, 167*i*
  resection of, for seizures, **1**:283
Temporal lobe seizures, **1**:281
Temporal nerve, **5**:56
Temporal sulcus, **5**:31
Temporal veins, eyelids drained by, **7**:147, **8**:7
Temporalis fascia, deep, **7**:138
"Temporary polypseudophakia," **11**:200
Temporin A/temporin B, **1**:75
Temporofacial trunk, of cranial nerve VII, **5**:56
Temporomandibular joint disease, **5**:300
TEN. *See* Toxic epidermal necrolysis
Tenacious proximal fusion, in intermittent exotropia,
  6:111
Tendency-oriented perimeter (TOP) algorithm, **10**:67
Tenectomy, **6**:175*t*
Tenex. *See* Guanfacine
Teniposide, **1**:257, 259*t*
Tennant intraocular lens, **11**:143
Tenofovir (PMPA), **1**:41
Tenon's capsule, **2**:20, 37, 37*i*, **6**:20, 20*i*, 21*i*, 22*i*
  extraocular muscle surgery and, **6**:25
    excessive advancement and, **6**:187
    scarring of (adherence syndrome), **6**:188
Tenoretic. *See* Atenolol
Tenormin. *See* Atenolol
Tenotomy, **6**:175*t*
  superior oblique
    for Brown syndrome, **6**:146, 181
    for third nerve (oculomotor) palsy, **6**:148
Tensilon. *See* Edrophonium
Tensilon test. *See also* Edrophonium
  for myasthenia gravis diagnosis, **2**:403, **5**:326–327,
    6:151, 151*i*, **7**:213
Tension ring, endocapsular, **11**:227, 228*i*
Tension-type headache, **5**:296
  treatment of, **5**:297
Tentorium, inferior hypophyseal artery of, **5**:13
Tenzel semicircular rotation flap/modified Tenzel flap,
  in lower eyelid repair, **7**:192
Tequin. *See* Gatifloxacin
Teratogens, **2**:127, 159, **8**:281–282
  congenital anomalies caused by, **2**:159, 160–162,
    160*i*, 161*i*, 162*i*, 163*i*, **8**:281–282

  definition of, **6**:206, **8**:281
Teratoid medulloepitheliomas, **4**:146
Teratomas, **2**:128, **4**:12, 13*i*
  orbital, **2**:166, **7**:64
    in children, **6**:382, 382*i*
Terazosin, **1**:89*t*
Terbinafine, **1**:64*t*, 76
Terbutaline, **1**:157, 157*t*
Terminal arteries, **2**:103
Terminal web, **2**:48
Termination codon (stop codon), **2**:196, 201, 201*i*
  frameshift mutation and, **2**:186
Terrien marginal degeneration, **8**:370–371, 371*i*
Terson syndrome, **5**:351, 352*i*, **12**:95
Tertiary positions of gaze, **6**:28
Tesla, definition of, **5**:81
Test–retest reliability, **1**:363
Testicular cancer, screening for, **1**:296
Testis-determining factor (TDF/sex-determining region
  Y/SRY), **2**:266
Tetanic cataract, **11**:62
Tetanus, immunization against, **1**:307–308
Tetanus and diphtheria toxoid vaccine (Td vaccine),
  1:304*t*, 307
Tetanus immune globulin, **1**:308
Tetracaine, **2**:446*t*, 448
  maximum safe dose of, **1**:322*t*
Tetracyclines, **1**:61*t*, 72, **2**:433–434. *See also specific*
  agent
  for chemical burns, **8**:392
  for chlamydial conjunctivitis, **8**:177
  intravenous administration of, **2**:389
  for Lyme disease, **5**:364
  for meibomian gland dysfunction, **8**:83
  ocular effects of, **1**:324*t*
  for ophthalmia neonatorum prophylaxis, **6**:223
  for persistent corneal defects, **8**:102
  for rosacea, **8**:86
  for trachoma, **8**:177
Tetrahydrotriamcinolone, anti-inflammatory/pressure-
  elevating potency of, **2**:419*t*
Tetrahydrozoline, **2**:451
Tetravac. *See* DTacP-IPV vaccine
Teveten. *See* Eprosartan
TFIIH, **2**:206
TGF-β. *See* Transforming growth factor-β
TGFB1 gene, **8**:305, 307. *See also BIGH3*
  (keratoepithelin) gene
Th0 cells. *See* T helper 0 cells
Th1 cells. *See* T helper 1 cells
Th2 cells. *See* T helper 2 cells
Thalamic esodeviations, **5**:224
Thalamostriate branch, of posterior cerebral artery,
  median, **5**:18
Thalamus, contralateral, **5**:50, 50*i*
Thalassemia, **1**:161
  beta (β), bone marrow transplantation for, **1**:159,
    161
  sickle cell, **12**:120, 120*t*
Thalidomide, for HIV infection/AIDS, **1**:44
Thallium-201 myocardial scintigraphy, **1**:119
Theo-Dur. *See* Theophylline
Theophylline, **1**:156–157, 157*t*
Theques, **4**:56

Therapeutic lifestyle changes (TLCs). *See* Lifestyle modification
Thermal cautery
 for involutional ectropion, **7**:197
 for involutional entropion, **7**:204
 for punctal occlusion, **7**:274, **8**:77, 77*i*
Thermal injury (burns)
 anterior segment, **8**:387
 retinal, light causing, **12**:307
Thermal laser photocoagulation. *See* Photocoagulation
Thermokeratoplasty, **13**:27–28, 28*i*, 50*t*, 137–142
 conductive keratoplasty, **13**:27–28, 139–142, 140*i*, 141*i*, 141*t*, 142*i*
 history of, **13**:137–138
 laser, **13**:27–28, 138–139
 penetrating keratoplasty after, **13**:204
 risks/benefits of, **13**:50*t*, 138
Thermomechanical injury, **2**:459
Thermotherapy, transpupillary, **12**:320
Thiamine deficiency
 optic neuropathy caused by, **5**:152
 Wernicke-Korsakoff syndrome and, **1**:285
Thiazide diuretics
 for diastolic dysfunction, **1**:131
 for hypertension, **1**:81, 86, 87, 88*t*, 89
 ocular effects of, **1**:325*t*
Thiazolidinediones, **1**:212*t*, 213–214
Thick lenses, power approximation for, **3**:78–79, 78*i*
Thickness of retinal reflex, in axis determination, **3**:130, 131*i*
Thiel-Behnke dystrophy, **8**:310*t*, 315
Thimerosal, allergic/sensitivity reactions and, **2**:381, **8**:107
Thin-beam single raytracing, **8**:49
Thin-lens approximation, **3**:66–67
Thin-lens equation (TLE), **3**:66–67
Thin lenses, power approximation for, **3**:66–67
 negative lenses and, **3**:72–74, 73*i*
Thioflavin t stain, **4**:36*t*
Thioridazine
 lens changes caused by, **11**:53
 retinal degeneration caused by, **12**:248–249, 249*t*
 electroretinogram in evaluation of, **12**:36
Third cranial nerve. *See* Cranial nerve III
Third nerve (oculomotor) palsy, **5**:228–232, 229*i*, **6**:146–148, 147*i*
 aberrant regeneration of third nerve and, **5**:232, 232*i*
 aneurysm and, **5**:351
 anisocoria and, **5**:267, 269
 congenital, ptosis in, **7**:217–218
 divisional, **5**:231
 inferior oblique muscle palsy caused by, **6**:135
 pupil-sparing, **5**:230–231
 pupillary involvement in, **5**:228–230, 229*i*
 in younger patients, **5**:231
Third-order neurons
 dilator muscle innervation and, **2**:65
 lesions of, Horner syndrome caused by, **5**:263, 264
13q14 syndrome (long arm 13 deletion syndrome), **2**:253–254, 253*t*
30 Hz flicker response, **12**:28*i*, 29
 in hereditary retinal/choroidal degenerations, **12**:205
Thorazine. *See* Chlorpromazine
Three cone opsins, **2**:345. *See also* Color vision

Three-dimensional computed tomography, in orbital evaluation, **7**:29
3 o'clock and 9 o'clock staining, **3**:193, 208, 208*i*
3-mirror contact lens, Goldmann, for fundus biomicroscopy, **3**:285–288, 288*i*
3-step test, **6**:90–92, 91*i*
 in inferior oblique muscle paralysis, **6**:136
 Parks-Bielschowsky, for fourth nerve palsy, **5**:232–233
 in superior oblique muscle palsy, **6**:132
Threshold
 genetic, **2**:197
 polygenic traits with, **2**:274
 in perimetry, **10**:66, 67–68, 68*i*
 definition of, **10**:59
 visual, **3**:111
Threshold disease, in retinopathy of prematurity, **6**:329–330, 329*t*, 330*i*, 331*i*, **12**:130, 131*i*
Threshold-related strategy (perimetry), **10**:66, 66*i*
Threshold sensitivity, in perimetry, **5**:91, 92
Thrombin, **2**:453
Thrombocytopenia, **1**:167
 capillary hemangiomas and (Kasabach-Merritt syndrome), **7**:66
Thrombocytopenic purpura
 idiopathic, **1**:167
 thrombotic, **1**:167
 choroidal perfusion abnormalities and, **12**:166
Thrombolytic therapy, **1**:172
 for acute ischemic stroke, **1**:104–105
 emergency transport and, **1**:313
 for ST-segment elevation acute coronary syndrome, **1**:124–125
Thrombophilia (thrombotic disorders), **1**:170–172. *See also* Hypercoagulable states
 antiphospholipid antibody syndrome and, **1**:171, 182–184
 fetal loss/preeclampsia and, **1**:159
 risk factors for, **1**:159
Thrombophlebitis, of orbital vein, **7**:61
Thromboplastin time, partial (PTT), **1**:165
Thrombosis. *See also* Hypercoagulable states; Thrombophilia
 branch retinal artery occlusion and, **12**:146
 central retinal artery occlusion and, **12**:148
 central retinal vein occlusion and, **12**:141, 144
 cerebral and dural sinus, **5**:357–358. *See also* Sinus thrombosis
 after PTCA with stenting, **1**:121
 retinal vasculitis and, **12**:153
 stroke and, **1**:102
Thrombotic thrombocytopenic purpura, **1**:167
 choroidal perfusion abnormalities and, **12**:166
Thromboxanes, **2**:305, 306*i*
 aspirin affecting, **2**:422
Thygeson superficial punctate keratitis, **8**:224–225, 225*i*
Thymoxamine, **2**:309, 408
Thymus
 clonal deletion in, **9**:88
 as lymphoid tissue, **9**:16
Thyroid-associated ophthalmopathy. *See* Thyroid ophthalmopathy
Thyroid-associated orbitopathy. *See* Thyroid ophthalmopathy
Thyroid biopsy, **1**:223

Thyroid carcinoma, retinoblastoma associated with, 4:265*t*
Thyroid dermopathy, in Graves ophthalmopathy, 7:53
Thyroid disease, 1:221–227. *See also* Thyroid ophthalmopathy
  in elderly, 1:249
  eyelid fissure changes in, 2:23*i*
  hyperthyroidism, 1:223–225
  hypothyroidism, 1:225–226
  physiology of, 1:221
  screening/testing for, 1:222–223, 301
    in thyroid ophthalmopathy, 7:35–36
  smoking and, 1:201, 225
  thyroiditis, 1:226–227, 7:53
  tumors, 1:227
Thyroid follicles, 1:221
Thyroid function tests, in thyroid ophthalmopathy/orbitopathy, 5:330, 7:35–36
Thyroid hormones, 1:221
  adenomas producing, 1:228
  measurement of, 1:222
Thyroid medications, in perioperative setting, 1:334
Thyroid microsomal antibody, testing for, 1:223
Thyroid nodules, 1:227
Thyroid ophthalmopathy (Graves disease/ophthalmopathy, dysthyroidism, thyroid orbitopathy), 1:224–225, 4:189–190, 190*i*, 5:145, 146*i*, 329–332, 6:148–150, 149*i*, 153*t*, 7:48–56, 48*i*, 49–50*i*
  antithyroid antibodies and, 1:223
  in children, 6:148–150, 149*i*, 153*t*
  clinical presentation and diagnosis of, 5:330–331, 7:48–51, 51*i*, 53
  compressive optic neuropathy in, 5:330, 330*i*
  in elderly, 1:249
  epidemiology of, 7:52–53
  euthyroid, 1:224–225, 5:330, 7:48
  extraocular myopathy in, 5:329*i*, 330, 6:149, 7:48, 53
  eye movements affected in, 7:26
  eyelid abnormalities and, 5:329, 329*i*, 7:26, 48–51, 48*i*, 53
    fissure changes, 2:23*i*
    retraction, 5:274–275, 276*i*, 279, 7:26, 48–51, 48*i*, 53, 223–225, 224*i*
  glaucoma and, 10:32
  incomitant esotropia and, 6:98*t*
  myasthenia gravis and, 7:53, 54
  pathogenesis of, 7:51–52
  prognosis of, 7:53–55
  proptosis and, 5:329, 6:149, 149*i*, 384, 384*i*, 7:26
    in children, 6:149, 149*i*, 384, 384*i*
    eyelid retraction differentiated from, 7:224, 224*i*
  smoking and, 1:201, 225
  strabismus and, 5:217–218, 6:148–150, 149*i*, 153*t*
  thyroid function tests in, 5:330, 7:35–36
  treatment of, 5:331–332, 7:53–55
Thyroid orbitopathy. *See* Thyroid ophthalmopathy
Thyroid-related immune orbitopathy. *See* Thyroid ophthalmopathy
Thyroid scanning, 1:223
  in identification of thyroid tumors, 1:227
Thyroid-stimulating hormone. *See* Thyrotropin
Thyroid storm, 1:224
Thyroid tumors, 1:227
Thyroid ultrasound, 1:223

Thyroiditis, 1:226–227. *See also specific type*
  in Graves ophthalmopathy, 7:53
Thyrotoxic exophthalmos. *See* Thyroid ophthalmopathy
Thyrotoxicosis. *See* Hyperthyroidism
Thyrotropin (thyroid-stimulating hormone/TSH), 1:221
  pituitary adenoma producing, 1:228
  receptor for, antibodies to in Graves disease, 7:49, 51–52
  serum levels of, 1:222–223
Thyrotropin-releasing hormone, 1:221
Thyroxine-binding globulin (TBG), serum levels of, 1:222, 223
  screening, 1:301
Thyroxine (T$_4$), 1:221
  in block-and-replace therapy, for Graves disease, 7:54
  serum levels of, 1:222
TI (interpulse time), 5:81
Tiagabine, 1:283*t*
TIAs. *See* Transient ischemic attacks
Tiazac. *See* Diltiazem
Tic, facial (habit spasm), 5:290
Tic douloureux (trigeminal neuralgia), 5:299
Ticar. *See* Ticarcillin
Ticarcillin, 1:56*t*, 67, 2:428*t*, 429
  with clavulanic acid, 1:56*t*, 69
Ticks, Lyme disease transmitted by, 1:18–19, 9:191, 12:191
Ticlid. *See* Ticlopidine
Ticlopidine
  for carotid disease, 1:107
  for cerebral ischemia/stroke, 1:104
Tigecycline, 1:75
Tight junctions (zonulae occludentes)
  in ciliary body epithelium, 2:66
  in corneal epithelium, 8:9
  in retinal blood vessels, 2:84
  in retinal pigment epithelium, 2:78, 12:12, 13*i*
Tight lens syndrome, 8:407
Tight orbit, 7:107
TIGR/myocilin (TIGR/MYOC) gene, 10:13*t*, 14
  in congenital glaucoma, 6:271, 10:14
TIGR protein, 10:12. *See also* Myocilin
Tilade. *See* Nedocromil
Tillaux, spiral of, 2:16, 17*i*, 5:41, 6:16, 18*i*
Tilted optic disc syndrome (Fuchs coloboma), 5:139–140, 140*i*, 6:360–361, 361*i*
Time to echo (TE), definition of, 5:81
Time integrated radiance, 2:460, 460*t*
Time to repetition (TR), definition of, 5:81
Timentin. *See* Ticarcillin, with clavulanic acid
Timolide. *See* Timolol
Timolol, 2:410, 410*t*, 10:160*t*, 165
  cholesterol levels affected by, 1:150
  in combination preparations, 2:411*t*, 414
  for glaucoma, 2:410, 410*t*, 10:160*t*, 165
    in children, 6:282, 283
  for hypertension, 1:88*t*, 90*t*
  sustained-release preparation of, 2:390
  systemic absorption of, 2:383*i*
Timoptic. *See* Timolol
TIMP3 gene/TIMP3 protein mutation, 2:227, 350
  in Sorsby dystrophy, 12:223

Tinnitus, in peripheral vestibular nystagmus, 5:246
TINU. *See* Tubulointerstitial nephritis and uveitis syndrome
Tiotropium, 1:158
Tiprinavir, 1:42
TIR. *See* Total internal reflection
Tirofiban, for non-ST-segment elevation acute coronary syndrome, 1:123
Tissue addition/subtraction. *See also specific procedure* corneal biomechanics affected by, 13:23, 24*i*, 25*i*
Tissue adhesives, cyanoacrylate. *See* Cyanoacrylate adhesives
Tissue-bound immune complexes, 9:60–62, 60*i*
Tissue factor pathway inhibitor, 1:164, 165
Tissue plasminogen activator, 1:101, 172, 2:393, 452
    for acute ischemic stroke, 1:101, 104
    intraocular administration of, 2:387, 388
    for ST-segment elevation acute coronary syndrome, 1:124–125
    for submacular hemorrhage, 12:326
    in vitreous, 2:337
Tissue preparation, for pathologic examination, 4:35–36
    fixatives for, 4:35
    processing and, 4:37
    special techniques and, 4:37–41
    staining and, 4:35–36, 36*i*, 36*t*
Titmus stereoacuity test, Polaroid glasses with, in functional visual disorder evaluation, 5:307, 308*i*
TK. *See* Transverse keratotomy
TLCs (therapeutic lifestyle changes). *See* Lifestyle modification
TLE. *See* Thin-lens equation
TMAb. *See* Thyroid microsomal antibody
TMC 125, 1:42
TMJ disease. *See* Temporomandibular joint disease
TMP-SMX. *See* Trimethoprim-sulfamethoxazole
TNF. *See* Tumor necrosis factor
TNM staging system
    for conjunctival carcinoma, 4:285*t*
    for conjunctival melanoma, 4:286*t*
    for eyelid cancer, 4:291*t*
    for lacrimal gland carcinoma, 4:292*t*
    for orbital sarcoma, 4:292*t*
    for retinoblastoma, 4:287–288*t*
    for uveal melanoma, 4:289–290*t*
TNO test, 6:93
"Tobacco dust" (Shafer's sign), 12:268, 276, 288
Tobacco use. *See also* Smoking
    optic neuropathy and, 5:152
Tobralcon. *See* Tobramycin
Tobramycin, 1:61*t*, 70, 2:428*t*, 431*t*, 435
    for bacterial keratitis, 8:182*t*
    in combination preparations, 2:432*t*
    for endophthalmitis, 9:217
    ototoxicity of, mitochondrial DNA mutations and, 2:220
Tobrex. *See* Tobramycin
α-Tocopherol. *See* Vitamin E
Todd's paralysis, 1:282, 5:289
Tofranil. *See* Imipramine
Togaviruses, ocular infection caused by, 8:121
Tolbutamide, 1:212*t*
Tolcapone, for Parkinson disease, 1:279
Tolectin. *See* Tolmetin

Tolerance (drug), 1:267
Tolerance (immunologic), 9:87–89
    to lens crystallins, 9:90
Tolmetin, 1:197*t*, 2:421*t*
    for uveitis in children, 6:320
Tolosa-Hunt syndrome, 5:236, 298
    idiopathic orbital inflammation presenting as, 7:56
Tomato catsup fundus, 4:244, 244*i*
Tomography
    computed. *See* Computed tomography
    myocardial perfusion, 1:119
    optical coherence. *See* Optical coherence tomography
    in orbital evaluation, 7:27–28, 28*i*
Tonic cells, 2:353, 353*i*
Tonic-clonic seizures, 1:282, 320
Tonic convergence, 6:38
Tonic eye deviation, 5:211–212
Tonic fibers, 2:20, 21, 21*t*, 5:41
Tonic pupil (Adie's pupil), 5:266–267, 267*i*, 268*i*
    pharmacologic testing for, 2:395–396
Tono-Pen, 6:274
Tonography, in aqueous outflow measurement, 10:22
Tonometry (tonometer)
    applanation. *See* Applanation tonometer/tonometry; Goldmann applanation tonometry
    in children, 6:274
    in congenital/infantile glaucoma, 6:274–275
    corneal thickness affecting, 8:34
    HIV prevention precautions and, 9:262
    infection control and, 8:50, 10:29
    noncontact (air-puff), 10:28–29
    Perkins, in children, 6:274
    pneumatic, 10:28–29
    Schiøtz (indentation), 10:29
        HIV prevention precautions and, 9:262
    sources of error in, 10:28*t*
Tonopen measurement, of intraocular pressure
    after LASIK, 13:208
    after PRK/LASEK, 13:105, 208
Topamax. *See* Topiramate
Topical anesthesia, 2:445–449, 446*t*. *See also* Anesthesia (anesthetics), local
    for adjustable suture technique, 6:176
    for anterior segment surgery, 2:448
    for cataract surgery, 11:94–96
    for extraocular muscle surgery, 6:176, 183
    for phakic IOL insertion, 13:147
Topical medications, 2:381–386, 382*i*, 383*i*, 385*i*. *See also* Eyedrops
    sustained-release devices for, 2:390
Topiramate, 1:283*t*, 284
    ophthalmic side effects of, 1:263, 284, 324*t*
        glaucoma and, 6:279
Topography, 2:43–44, 43*i*, 4:12
    anterior chamber, 4:77–78, 77*i*, 78*i*
    choroidal, 4:151, 151*i*
    ciliary body, 4:150, 150*i*
    conjunctival, 4:43, 44*i*
    corneal, 3:302–303, 303*i*, 304*i*, 4:61–62, 61*i*, 62*i*, 8:38–49, 9:39, 40*i*, 13:6–12. *See also* Cornea, topography of
    eyelid, 4:167, 167*i*, 168*t*
    iris, 4:149, 150*i*
    lens, 4:93–94, 93*i*, 94*i*

optic nerve, 4:203–204, 203*i*, 204*i*
orbital, 4:187–188, 7:7–10, 8*i*, 9*i*, 10*i*
retinal, 4:117–119, 118*i*, 120*i*
scleral, 4:87–88, 87*i*, 88*i*
uveal tract, 4:149–151, 150*i*, 151*i*
vitreous, 4:105–106
Toprol-XL. *See* Metoprolol
Toradol. *See* Ketorolac
TORCHES, 6:215. *See also specific disorder*
reduced vision and, 6:455–456
Torcular Herophili, 5:22
Toric intraocular lenses, 11:147, 13:161–163
Toric LASIK ablations, 13:117–118
Toric photorefractive keratectomy, 13:98–99. *See also*
Photorefractive keratectomy
Toric soft contact lenses, 3:195–197, 197*i*, 197*t*
Toric surfaces, 3:94–95, 97*i*
Tornalate. *See* Bitolterol
Torsades de pointes, 1:140
Torsemide, 1:88*t*
Torsion, 6:28, 29
Torsional fusional vergence, 6:88
Torsional nystagmus, 5:249–250
Torus, 6:42
Total cataract, 11:38
Total internal reflection (TIR), 3:14, 47–49, 48*i*, 50*i*
gonioscopy and, 3:49–50, 50*i*
Total T₄, 1:222
Tourette syndrome, 5:290
Touton giant cells, 4:13, 15*i*
in juvenile xanthogranuloma, 6:389
Toxemia of pregnancy. *See* Eclampsia; Preeclampsia
Toxic conjunctivitis/keratoconjunctivitis
contact lens solutions causing, 8:107
medications causing, 8:393–395
Toxic dementia, 1:285
Toxic epidermal necrolysis, 8:216–217, 217*t*
Toxic goiter
diffuse, 1:224. *See also* Graves hyperthyroidism
nodular, 1:225
Toxic keratitis, 8:394. *See also* Toxic conjunctivitis/
keratoconjunctivitis
Toxic optic neuropathy, 1:271, 5:152
Toxic solutions, exposure to during cataract surgery,
corneal edema caused by, 11:168
Toxic ulcerative keratopathy, 8:101–102, 375–376
Toxicity, drug therapy, 2:379, 380–381
aging and, 2:381
tissue binding and, 2:385–386
Toxocara (toxocariasis), 6:317–318, 318*i*, 8:133,
9:170–171, 170*i*, 171*i*, 171*t*, 12:191–192, 192*i*
canis, 6:317, 8:133, 9:67, 172
cati, 6:317, 8:133
diffuse unilateral subacute neuroretinitis caused by,
12:190
granuloma caused by, 9:67, 170–171, 170*i*, 171*i*, 171*t*
ocular infection/inflammation caused by, 6:317–318,
318*i*, 8:133
retinoblastoma differentiated from, 4:256–257
uveitis in children caused by, 6:317–318, 318*i*
Toxoplasma (toxoplasmosis), 1:26–27, 6:215–217, 217*i*,
8:51*t*, 132, 9:164–169
in children, 6:215–217, 217*i*
congenital, 1:26, 6:215–217, 217*i*, 9:165, 167, 168,
168*i*

gondii, 1:26–27, 6:215, 8:132, 9:164–165, 165*i*
in HIV infection/AIDS, 1:50, 5:362, 9:165, 165*i*, 166*i*,
254–255, 256*i*
ocular infection/inflammation caused by, 1:26, 8:51*t*,
132
during pregnancy, 1:26, 9:165, 167, 168, 168*i*
punctate outer retinal (PORT), 9:166, 167*i*
retinal, 4:124–125, 125*i*, 12:186–187, 186*i*, 187*t*
treatment of, 1:26
uveitis in, 1:26, 6:216, 217*i*, 317, 9:164–169
Toxoplasma dye test, 9:166–167
Toys, for pediatric examination, 6:3, 4*i*
tPA. *See* Tissue plasminogen activator
TPCD. *See* Typical peripheral cystoid degeneration
TPHA (*T pallidum* hemagglutination assay), 1:17
TR (time to repetition), definition of, 5:81
TRAb. *See* TSH receptor antibodies
Trabecular beams, 4:77–78
Trabecular bone, 1:241
Trabecular meshwork, 2:52*i*, 53*i*, 54–61, 56*i*, 57*i*, 58*i*
congenital anomalies of, 4:78–79, 78*i*, 79*i*
corneoscleral, 2:56–57, 57*i*
development of, 2:153
disorders of, 4:77–85. *See also specific type*
neoplastic, 4:84, 85*i*
endothelial, 2:57, 58*i*, 59*i*, 4:77–78
material in, secondary glaucoma and, 4:80–84, 161
pigmentation of, 10:41–42
in pseudoexfoliation, 4:80
topography of, 4:77–78, 77*i*, 78*i*
uveal, 2:56, 57*i*
in uveitis, 9:105
Trabecular outflow, 10:19*i*, 20–22
Trabeculectomy, for glaucoma, 10:186–188, 187–191*i*
in children, 6:281
Trabeculitis, 9:105
Trabeculocytes, 2:54
Trabeculoplasty, laser, for open-angle glaucoma,
10:180–183, 181*i*
selective, 10:182
Trabeculotomy, for childhood glaucoma, 6:281,
10:207–209, 208*i*, 209*i*
Tracheotomy, for anaphylaxis, 1:319
Trachoma, 8:51*t*, 174–177, 175*i*, 176*i*
in children, 6:229
Trachoma-inclusion conjunctivitis (TRIC) agent, 6:222
Tracking devices
for LASIK, 13:114
for PRK, 13:98
Traction retinal tufts, zonular, 12:259, 260, 262*i*
Tractional retinal detachment. *See* Retinal detachment
Trait, 2:260, 8:307
holandric, 2:188, 266
Trandate. *See* Labetalol
Trandolapril, 1:88*t*, 90*t*
Tranexamic acid, 2:453
for hyphema, 6:448
Trans-iris IOL fixation suture (McCannel suture), for
intraocular lens decentration, 11:191, 192*i*
11-*trans* retinaldehyde, 12:14
Transbronchial biopsy, 1:155
Transcaruncular route, for anterior orbitotomy,
7:113–114
Transconjunctival route
for blepharoplasty, 7:232

for inferior anterior orbitotomy, 7:112*i*, 113, 113*i*
for medial anterior orbitotomy, 7:113
for ptosis repair, 7:222
for superior anterior orbitotomy, 7:113
Transconjunctival vitrectomy system, 12:323, 324*i*
Transcranial Doppler, in cerebral ischemia/stroke, 1:103
Transcribed strand of DNA (antisense DNA), 2:182, 202
Transcription (gene), 2:197, 205–210, 207*i*, 208*i*
reverse, 2:195
Transcription factors, 2:202, 206, 207*i*, 208*i*
Transcripts, illegitimate, 2:188
Transcutaneous routes
for inferior anterior orbitotomy, 7:112–113
for medial anterior orbitotomy, 7:112–113
for ptosis correction, 7:222
for superior anterior orbitotomy, 7:109–110
Transducin, rod, 2:343, 343*i*, 344*t*
mutations in, 2:349
Transepithelial ablation, for PRK, 13:93–94, 93*i*
Transesophageal Doppler echocardiography
in amaurosis fugax, 1:107
in cerebral ischemia/stroke, 1:103
Transfer RNA (tRNA), 2:211–212, 8:306
Transferase deficiency, galactosemia caused by,
11:61–62
Transferrin
in aqueous humor, 2:319, 321
in vitreous, 2:337
Transforming growth factor-β, 2:456, 9:82*t*
in aqueous humor, 2:320
cyclopia and, 2:165
homeobox gene expression affected by, 2:131
in ocular development, 2:130
in pterygium, 8:366
in Sjögren syndrome, 8:78
Transfusion-transmitted virus (TTV), 1:32
Transgenic animals, for genetic studies, 2:231–234, 235*i*
Transient amplifying cells, in corneal epithelium, 2:45
Transient ischemic attacks, 1:102
carotid disease causing, 1:107, 5:177
central retinal artery occlusion and, 12:149
diagnosis/management of, 1:103
stroke following, 5:180–181, 180*t*
transient visual loss and, 5:177
vertebrobasilar, 5:348*i*, 349
causes of, 5:349
nonophthalmic symptoms of, 5:347–348
treatment of, 5:349
Transient nerve fiber layer of Chievitz, 2:140, 144
Transient visual loss, 5:171–186. *See also* Amaurosis,
fugax
age of patient and, 5:171
binocular, 5:185–186
monocular visual loss compared with, 5:171
carotid artery disease and, 1:107
in central retinal artery occlusion, 12:149
cerebrovascular causes of, 5:345–346, 345–349
duration of, 5:171–172
examination of, 5:173, 173*i*
hypercoagulability causing, 5:185
hyperviscosity causing, 5:185
monocular, 5:173–184. *See also* Monocular transient
visual loss
binocular visual loss compared with, 5:171

pattern of, 5:172
in pregnancy, 5:343–344, 344*i*, 345*i*
recovery in, 5:172
signs and symptoms associated with, 5:172
vasospasm causing, 5:184–185
Transillumination, 4:32–33, 33*i*
in choroidal/ciliary body melanoma diagnosis, 4:225,
225*i*
iris, 6:270
in albinism, 6:270, 345
in retinal examination, 12:18
Transit amplification, in stem cell differentiation, 8:108
Transitional zone (peripheral zone), 8:38–39, 39*i*
Transitions, 2:214
Transketolase, in cornea, 2:299
Translated strand of DNA (antisense DNA), 2:182, 202
Translation, 2:197, 205, 210–212, 211*i*
gene product changes/modification after
(posttranslational modification), 2:193
of lens proteins, 2:328
Translocation, chromosome, 2:197
Down syndrome caused by, 2:250
Transmigration, in neutrophil recruitment and
activation, 9:48–50, 49*i*
Transmissibility (gas), of contact lens, 3:185
rigid contact lenses and, 3:185
Transmission, light, 3:14
diffuse, 3:41–42, 43*i*
specular, 3:44–46, 45*i*, 46*i*
Transmission (window) defect, of fluorescence, 12:20*i*,
21. *See also* Hyperfluorescence
in angioid streaks, 12:83
Transnasal laser dacryocystorhinostomy, 7:281–282,
282*i*
Transplant rejection. *See* Rejection (graft)
Transplantation. *See also specific type*
amniotic membrane, 8:423*t*, 425, 439
for chemical burns, 8:392–393, 439
indications for, 8:423*t*
conjunctival, 8:423*t*, 424–425, 429–433
for chemical burns, 8:392
indications for, 8:423*t*
for wound closure after pterygium excision, 8:429,
430*i*, 431–432
corneal, 8:447–451, 453–476. *See also* Donor cornea;
Keratoplasty, penetrating
autograft procedures for, 8:471–472
basic concepts of, 8:447–451
for chemical burns, 8:393
clinical approach to, 8:453–476
donor selection and, 8:449–451, 451*t*
eye banking and, 8:449–451, 451*t*
graft rejection and, 9:39, 40*i*, 41
histocompatibility antigens and, 8:447
immune privilege and, 8:195–196, 447–448
immunobiology of, 8:447–448
lamellar keratoplasty (allograft procedure) and,
8:472–476, 473*i*
pediatric, 8:470–471, 470*t*
rabies virus transmission and, 8:163
histocompatibility antigens and, 8:447, 9:93–94
immune privilege and, 8:447–448
immunobiology of, 8:447–448
limbal, 8:423*t*, 425
for chemical burns, 8:392, 393

indications for, **8**:423*t*
mucous membrane, **8**:423*t*, 425, 439
  indications for, **8**:423*t*, 439
organ, for enzyme deficiency disease, **2**:281
retinal/retinal pigment epithelium, **9**:42
Transplantation antigens, **8**:447, **9**:93–94
Transport mechanisms
  lens, **11**:19–21, 21*i*
  retinal pigment epithelium, **2**:361–362
Transposition, of spherocylindrical lens notation,
  3:98–99
Transposition flaps, for lateral canthal defects, **7**:192
Transposition procedures, extraocular muscle, **6**:176
Transpupillary thermotherapy, **12**:320
  for melanoma, **4**:238
Transpupillary Thermotherapy for Choroidal
  Neovascularization (TTT4CNV) study, **12**:76, 320
Transscleral diathermy, for melanoma, **4**:238
Transscleral diode laser cyclophotocoagulation, in
  lowering intraocular pressure, **10**:205
Transscleral laser cycloablation, for childhood
  glaucoma, **6**:282
Transscleral Nd:YAG, in lowering intraocular pressure,
  10:205
Transseptal route, for anterior orbitotomy, **7**:109
Transthyretin (prealbumin)
  amyloid deposits and, **4**:110–111, **8**:347*t*, 349
  serum levels of, **1**:223
Transverse keratotomy, **13**:21*t*, 66–67, 67*i*
Transverse ligament, superior (Whitnall's), , **2**:26, 26*i*,
  27*i*, **7**:140*i*, 142–143, 144*i*, 253
Transverse magnification, **3**:30–34, 30*i*, 65–66, 66*i*
  in afocal system, **3**:81–82
  calculation of, **3**:65–66, 66*i*
Transverse/spin-spin relaxation time (T2), **5**:81, **7**:31
Transverse sinus, **5**:22
Transversions, **2**:214
Trantas dot, in vernal keratoconjunctivitis, **6**:235
Trauma, **12**:289–303. *See also* Blunt trauma;
  Lacerations; Penetrating injuries; Perforating
  injuries; Wound healing/repair
  angle-recession glaucoma and, **10**:113–114, 113*i*
  anterior segment, **8**:387–420
    animal and plant substances causing, **8**:395–396
    chemical injuries, **8**:389–393
    concussive, **8**:396–403
    nonperforating mechanical, **8**:403–407
    perforating, **8**:407–418. *See also* Perforating
      injuries
    surgical, **8**:418–420
    temperature and radiation causing, **8**:387–389
  anterior uveitis caused by, **9**:107
  blunt. *See* Blunt trauma
  canalicular, **7**:276–277
  cataract surgery after, **11**:225–228, 227*i*, 228*i*
  in children, **6**:441–450, 457*t*, **12**:254–255
    abuse and, **6**:442–445, 443*i*, 444*i*, **12**:301–302, 302*i*
    blunt injury and, **6**:447–450, 448*i*, 449*i*
    cataract caused by, **6**:293*i*, 447
    chemical injuries and, **6**:445
    hyphema and, **6**:447–449, 448*i*
    management of, **6**:441–442
    orbital fractures and, **6**:449–450, 449*i*
    penetrating injury and, **6**:446–447, 446*i*

shaking injury and, **6**:442–445, 443*i*, 444*i*,
  12:301–302, 302*i*
  superficial injury and, **6**:445–446
corneal blood staining and, **4**:73, 76*i*, **8**:399,
  400–401, 400*i*, 401*i*, **10**:110, 110*i*
ectopia lentis caused by, **11**:40, 55, 56*i*
  cataract surgery in patients with, **11**:226–227,
    227*i*, 228*i*
endophthalmitis after, **9**:207, 208*t*, 211–212, **12**:300
evaluation of patient after, **12**:289–290
eyelid, **7**:184–188
  repair of, **7**:184–187, 185*i*
    secondary, **7**:186–187
glaucoma and, **4**:81–84, 82*i*, 83*i*
histologic sequelae of, **4**:24–29
hypercoagulability associated with, **1**:171
innate immune response and, **9**:47
lacrimal sac and nasolacrimal duct, **7**:284
LASIK flap dislocation and, **13**:126–127
lens damage/cataracts caused by, **11**:40, 54–60
  glaucoma and, **11**:67–68
  surgery for, **11**:225–228, 227*i*, 228*i*
optic neuropathy caused by, **2**:102, **5**:153–155, 154*i*,
  7:107
orbital fractures and, **2**:8, **7**:21, 97–106, 99*i*, 101*i*,
  103*i*
penetrating. *See* Penetrating injuries
perforating. *See* Perforating injuries
ptosis caused by, **5**:278, **7**:219
pupillary irregularity caused by, **5**:259
Purtscher retinopathy and, **12**:94, 94*i*, 95*t*
retinal detachment and
  electroretinogram in, **12**:36, 273
  in young patient, **12**:254–255
secondary angle-closure glaucoma and, **10**:143
seventh nerve palsy and, **5**:285
surgical, **8**:418–420
  secondary open-angle glaucoma and, **10**:114–115,
    115*i*
sympathetic ophthalmia and, **9**:200–203, 200*i*, 201*i*,
  202*t*
uveal tract, **4**:25, 26*i*, 166
Traumatic hyphema, **8**:398–403, 399*i*, 400*i*
  in children, **6**:447–449, 448*i*
  medical management of, **8**:401–402
  rebleeding after, **8**:399–401, 400*i*, 401*i*
  sickle cell disease and, **6**:447, 448*i*, **8**:402–403, **12**:123
  surgery for, **8**:402, 403*t*
Traumatic iritis, **8**:397–398
Traumatic miosis, **8**:397
Traumatic mydriasis, **8**:397
Traumatic recession of anterior chamber angle, **4**:25,
  25*i*
  glaucoma and, **4**:82–84, 83*i*
Traumatic retinal breaks, **12**:254–256, 255*i*
Traumatic retinoschisis, in shaking injury, **6**:444, 444*i*
Traumatic visual loss with clear media, **7**:106–108
Travatan. *See* Travoprost
Travel immunizations, **1**:309–310
Travoprost, **2**:414, 414*t*, **10**:162*t*, 171–172
  for childhood glaucoma, **6**:283
Trazodone, **1**:276
Treacher Collins/Treacher Collins–Franceschetti
  syndrome (mandibulofacial dysostosis), **6**:432, 433*i*,
  7:38, 38*i*, **8**:353*t*
  eyelid manifestations of, **4**:173*t*

Treatment of Age-Related Macular Degeneration with
 Photodynamic Therapy Study (TAP), **12**:73–75, 321
Tree sap, ocular injuries caused by, **8**:395–396
Trefoil, **3**:93, 233*i*, **13**:16, 18*i*
Tremor, in Parkinson disease, **1**:279
Trephines, for penetrating keratoplasty, **8**:456
Treponema pallidum, **1**:15–18, **6**:220, **8**:128, 299, **9**:187.
 See also Syphilis
Treponemal antibody tests, for syphilis, **1**:17, 302
TRH. *See* Thyrotropin-releasing hormone
Trial contact lens fitting
 disinfection and, **1**:51, **8**:50, **9**:262
 fluorescein patterns in, **3**:195
Trial frames
 for prism correction, **3**:170
 for refraction in aphakia, **3**:164
Trial lens clips
 for overrefraction, **3**:142, 164–165
 for prism correction, **3**:170
Triamcinolone
 for chalazion, **8**:87–88
 for hemangiomas, **7**:66
 in children, **6**:378
 intracameral, **2**:386
 intravitreal, **2**:386, 387
 for branch retinal vein occlusion, **12**:141
 for central retinal vein occlusion, **12**:144
 for pars planitis, **9**:149, 150
 for pulmonary diseases, **1**:157*t*
 supratarsal injection of, for vernal
  keratoconjunctivitis, **8**:211
 for uveitis, **9**:115*t*
Triamterene, **1**:88*t*, 90*t*
Triazolam, **1**:273
Triazoles, **2**:437–439, 438*t*
 for *Acanthamoeba* keratitis, **8**:189
TRIC (trachoma-inclusion conjunctivitis) agent, **6**:222
Tricarboxylic acid (TCA) cycle, in corneal glucose
 metabolism, **2**:297
Trichiasis, **2**:28, **7**:207–208, **8**:104
 in anophthalmic socket, **7**:127
 in staphylococcal blepharitis, **8**:164
Trichilemmal (pilar) cyst, **7**:166
Trichilemmoma, **7**:168–169
Trichinella spiralis (trichinosis), orbital infection caused
 by, **7**:47
Trichoepithelioma, **7**:168, 169*i*
Trichofolliculoma, **7**:168
Trichromats, **12**:195, 196*t*
 anomalous, **12**:195, 196*t*, 197*i*
Tricyclic antidepressants, **1**:275*t*
 apraclonidine/brimonidine interactions and, **2**:408
Trifluridine, **2**:439, 440*t*
 adverse reactions to topical use of, **8**:101
 for herpes simplex virus infections, **8**:142*t*
 epithelial keratitis, **8**:145
 in infants and children, **6**:210, 226
 stromal keratitis, **8**:148, 149*t*
Trifocal lenses, **3**:152, 154*i*, 156*i*
Trigeminal ganglion (Gasserian/semilunar ganglion),
 2:113*i*, 114, **5**:52
Trigeminal nerve. *See* Cranial nerve V
Trigeminal neuralgia (tic douloureux), **5**:299
Trigeminal nucleus, **5**:50

Triglyceride levels
 lowering, **1**:143, 146–147. *See also* Lipid-lowering
  therapy
 risk assessment and, **1**:144, 144*t*
Trigonometry, review of, **3**:32–33, 33*i*
Trihexyphenidyl, for Parkinson disease, **1**:279
Triiodothyronine (T₃), **1**:221
 serum levels of, **1**:222
Triiodothyronine (T₃) resin uptake test, **1**:222
Trilateral retinoblastoma, **4**:260
Trileptal. *See* Oxacarbazepine
Trilisate. *See* Choline magnesium trisalicylate
Trimethaphan, **2**:402*i*
Trimethoprim, **1**:54
 with sulfonamides, **2**:433. *See also* Trimethoprim-
  sulfamethoxazole
Trimethoprim-polymyxin B, **2**:431*t*
Trimethoprim-sulfamethoxazole, **1**:55*t*, 73–74
 for *Pneumocystis carinii* (*Pneumocystis jiroveci*)
  choroiditis, **9**:257
 for *Pneumocystis carinii* (*Pneumocystis jiroveci*)
  pneumonia, **1**:45, 74, **9**:247
 for toxoplasmosis, **6**:217, **9**:168, 169
 for Wegener granulomatosis, **1**:192
Trinucleotide repeats, **2**:190, 197
 expansion/contraction of, anticipation and, **2**:257
TRIO (thyroid-related immune orbitopathy). *See*
 Thyroid ophthalmopathy
Triple procedure, **11**:208–209
Triplet recognition site (anticodon), **2**:211
Tripod (zygomatic-maxillary complex) fractures,
 7:97–100, 99*i*
Trisomy, **2**:249
Trisomy 13 (Patau syndrome), childhood glaucoma
 and, **10**:155*t*
Trisomy 18 (Edwards syndrome/trisomy E syndrome),
 childhood glaucoma and, **10**:155*t*
Trisomy 21 (Down syndrome/trisomy G syndrome),
 2:250–251, 251*t*
 Brushfield spots in, **4**:219*t*, 220*i*, **6**:266
 childhood glaucoma and, **10**:155*t*
 mosaicism in, **2**:252
 pharmacogenetics and, **2**:279
Trisomy 21 mosaicism, **2**:252
Tritan defects (tritanopia), **12**:44, 195, 196*t*
 in dominant optic atrophy, **5**:136, **6**:364
 testing for, in low vision evaluation, **5**:96
Trivariant color vision, **2**:345–347. *See also* Color vision
Trizivir, **1**:41
tRNA. *See* Transfer RNA
Trochlea, **6**:15, 15*i*, 18*i*
Trochlear nerve. *See* Cranial nerve IV
Trochlear nerve palsy. *See* Fourth nerve (trochlear)
 palsy
Troglitazone, withdrawal of from market, **1**:213–214
Trolands, **3**:16*t*
Trophoblast, **2**:134
-tropia (suffix), definition of, **6**:10
Tropias, **6**:10
 amblyopia caused by, **6**:68
 cover tests in assessment of, **6**:80–82, 81*i*
 diplopia after cataract surgery and, **11**:81
 induced, testing visual acuity and, **6**:79
 intermittent, **6**:10
 esotropia, **6**:97

exotropia, **6:**109–114, 110*i*
Tropicamide, **2:**310, 401*t*
  for cycloplegia/cycloplegic refraction, **3:**142*t*, **6:**94, 94*t*
  for uveitis, **9:**115, 128
Troponins, cardiac-specific (troponins T and I), in myocardial infarction, **1:**117, 118*i*
Trovafloxacin, **1:**62*t*, 73
Trovan. *See* Trovafloxacin
True divergence excess exotropia, **6:**112
Trusopt. *See* Dorzolamide
Truvada, **1:**41
Trypan blue, **2:**452
Tryptase, **8:**200*t*
TS. *See* Transverse sinus; Tuberous sclerosis
TSC1/TSC2 genes, in tuberous sclerosis, **6:**409
Tscherning wavefront analysis/aberrometry, **3:**320, 322*i*, **8:**49
TSCM. *See* Tandem scanning confocal microscopy
TSH (thyroid-stimulating hormone). *See* Thyrotropin
TSH receptor antibodies, in Graves disease, **7:**49
TTP. *See* Thrombotic thrombocytopenic purpura
TTT. *See* Transpupillary thermotherapy
TTT4CNV (Transpupillary Thermotherapy for Choroidal Neovascularization) study, **12:**76, 320
TTV. *See* Transfusion-transmitted virus
Tube-shunt surgery, in lowering intraocular pressure, **10:**201–204
  complications of, **10:**203–204, 204*t*
  contraindications to, **10:**203
  described, **10:**201
  devices in, **10:**201, 201*i*, 201*t*
  indications for, **10:**202
  postoperative management, **10:**203
  preoperative considerations for, **10:**203
  techniques for, **10:**203
Tubercles
  "hard," **4:**13, 14*i*
  in sarcoidosis, **9:**197–199, 197*i*, 198*i*
Tuberculin hypersensitivity, **9:**31, 66
Tuberculin skin test, **1:**23–25, 301–302, **9:**31, 195
  in HIV infection/AIDS, **9:**245
  immune response arc and, **9:**31
Tuberculosis, **1:**23–25, 301–302, **9:**193–195, 194*i*, 196*i*
  choroidal involvement and, **9:**194, 194*i*, **12:**184, 184*i*
  in HIV infection/AIDS, **1:**24, 49–50, 301, 302, **5:**361, **9:**193
  immune response arc in, **9:**30–31
  multidrug-resistant, **1:**24, 49, **9:**195
  orbital involvement and, **7:**47
  screening for, **1:**23–24, 301–302
  treatment of, **9:**195
    in HIV infection/AIDS, **1:**49–50
  uveitis in, **9:**193–195, 194*i*, 196*i*
Tuberin, **5:**338
Tuberous sclerosis (Bourneville disease/syndrome), **5:**336*t*, 338–340, 339*i*, **6:**402*t*, 409–412, 410*i*, 411*i*
  glaucoma associated with, **10:**32
Tubocurarine, **2:**402*i*
Tubulin, **2:**327
Tubulointerstitial nephritis and uveitis syndrome (TINU), **6:**315–316
Tucking procedure, **6:**174–175
Tumor antigens, **8:**249

Tumor cells
  biologic behavior of, **8:**245–252
  cytologic identification of, **8:**70, 70*i*
Tumor immunology, **8:**248–249
Tumor necrosis factor
  α, **8:**197, **9:**81*t*
    drugs affecting, **1:**199
    in Sjögren syndrome, **8:**78
  in apoptosis, **9:**68
  β, **9:**81*t*
    in delayed hypersensitivity, **9:**65*i*, 66
Tumor necrosis factor inhibitors, for scleritis, **8:**240
Tumor-suppressor genes, **1:**252, **2:**197, 215. *See also* *specific type*
  in DNA repair, **2:**213
  recessive, Rb locus as, **2:**253
  Wilms tumor, imprinting of, **2:**210
Tumors. *See also specific type and structure or organ affected and* Cancer; Intraocular tumors; Neoplasia
  cellular and tissue reactions and, **8:**247*t*
  in children, **6:**159*t*, 369–399, 457*t*
    classification of, **6:**370–371*t*
  clinical approach to, **8:**253–278
  definition of, **8:**246
  diagnostic approaches to, **8:**250, 251*i*
  glaucoma and, **10:**138
  management of, **8:**252
  oncogenesis and, **8:**248–249, 248*t*
  secondary. *See* Metastatic eye disease
  viral, **8:**162
Tunica vasculosa lentis, **2:**128, **11:**29–30, 29*i*
  in iris development, **2:**154, 155
  remnant of
    epicapsular star, **11:**32, 32*i*
    Mittendorf dot, **2:**91, 92*i*, 175, 177*i*, **4:**107, **6:**361, **11:**29–30, 31, **12:**280
Tuning, in phacoemulsification, **11:**114
Turban tumors, **7:**168
Turbinates (conchae), nasal, **7:**20
  inferior, **5:**10
  infracture of, for congenital tearing/nasolacrimal duct obstruction, **6:**245–246, **7:**263, 265*i*
Turkey gobbler defect, **7:**236
Turner (XO/XX) syndrome, childhood glaucoma and, **10:**155*t*
Turribrachycephaly, in Apert syndrome, **6:**427*i*
Turricephaly, **6:**421
Twin studies, in glaucoma, **10:**15
TWIST gene, in Saethre-Chotzen syndrome, **6:**426
Twitch fibers, **2:**20, 21, 21*t*, **5:**41
2 × 2 table, **1:**353–354, 353*t*, 354*t*
Two-site combined procedure, **11:**221
2-stage (postoperative) adjustment, after strabismus surgery, **6:**176
TXA. *See* Thromboxanes
Tympanic bone, **5:**54
Tympanic cavity, **2:**118
Typhoid immunization, **1:**309–310
Typical degenerative retinoschisis, **4:**126, **12:**276, 276*i*
Typical peripheral cystoid degeneration, **4:**126, 126*i*, **12:**264, 275, 275*i*
Tyrosinase gene mutations, in albinism, **2:**243, 262*t*, **6:**345. *See also* Tyrosinase-negative/positive albinism

Tyrosinase-negative/positive albinism, 2:176, 243, 6:345, 346*t*, 12:240
Tyrosine kinase, in signal transduction, 2:311
Tyrosinemia, 2:262*t*, 8:310*t*, 344–345
Tyrosinosis, 2:262*t*

U

UBM. *See* Ultrasound biomicroscopy
UGH syndrome. *See* Uveitis-glaucoma-hyphema (UGH) syndrome
Uhthoff symptom, 5:172
UKPDS (United Kingdom Prospective Diabetes Study), 1:215, 12:105, 107
Ulcerative colitis, 1:177, 9:131–132
Ulcerative keratitis. *See also* Keratitis
    peripheral, 8:362
        differential diagnosis of, 8:230*t*
        Mooren ulcer and, 8:231, 232–234, 233*i*, 234*i*
        in systemic immune-mediated diseases, 8:203, 229–232, 230*t*, 232*i*
    in rosacea, 8:86
Ulcerative keratopathy, toxic, 8:101–102, 375–376
Ulcers
    conjunctival, 8:25*t*
    corneal. *See* Corneal ulcers; Keratitis
    eyelid, 8:24*t*
    genital and oral, in Behçet syndrome, 1:193
    Mooren, 8:231, 232–234, 233*i*, 234*i*
    neurotrophic, herpetic keratitis and, 8:103, 103*i*, 151
Ultra Thin lens, aphakic, 3:168
Ultrafast computed tomography, in ischemic heart disease, 1:119
Ultrafiltration, in aqueous humor dynamics/formation, 2:304, 10:18
Ultralente insulin, 1:209–210, 209*t*
Ultrasonic, definition of, 11:114
Ultrasonography/ultrasound (echography), 3:308–312, 309*i*, 5:69
    A-scan, 3:309–312, 310*i*, 311*i*
        in IOL selection, 3:217
    in amaurosis fugax, 1:107
    anterior segment, 8:37
    B-scan, 3:310–312, 311*i*
        anterior segment (ultrasound biomicroscopy), 2:54, 55*i*, 8:37, 38*i*
        before cataract surgery, 11:84
        in differentiating drusen from papilledema, 5:131, 132*i*
    in carotid stenosis, 5:179
    in choroidal/ciliary body melanoma, 4:226–227, 228*i*
    in choroidal hemangioma, 4:243*i*, 245
    duplex
        in carotid evaluation, 5:179
        in cerebral ischemia/stroke, 1:103
    intravascular, in ischemic heart disease, 1:119
    in IOL power determination, 11:150
    in iris melanoma, 4:218
    in lymphoma, 4:278
    in metastatic eye disease, 4:273
    in ocular trauma, 12:290
    in orbital evaluation, 7:33–34
    in pachymetry, 3:293, 294*i*, 8:32, 33*i*

for phacoemulsification, 11:115–118, 116*i*, 117*i*, 118*i*
    terminology related to, 11:114
    in posterior vitreous detachment, 12:258, 279–280
    in retinoblastoma, 4:254–255
    thyroid, 1:223
    in uveitis, 9:113
    in vitreous hemorrhage, 12:287, 291
Ultrasound biomicroscopy, 2:54, 55*i*, 8:37, 38*i*
Ultraviolet-absorbing lenses, 3:166–167. *See also* Sunglasses
Ultraviolet-blue phototoxicity, 2:371, 459, 463
Ultraviolet light (ultraviolet radiation), eye disorders/injury associated with, 2:371, 459, 3:167. *See also* Light toxicity
    age-related macular degeneration, 12:61
    ambient exposure and, 12:309
    anterior segment injury, 8:388
    cataracts, 11:56–57
    corneal haze after PRK and, 13:104
    eyelid tumors, 8:248*t*
    pinguecula, 8:365
    pterygium, 8:366
    retinal damage, 12:307–308
    in retinitis pigmentosa, 12:210, 213
    spheroidal degeneration (Labrador/actinic keratopathy), 4:68, 69*i*, 8:368–369, 369
Umbo, 12:8, 9*t*
Unasyn. *See* Ampicillin, with sulbactam
Uncrossed diplopia, 6:58–60, 59*i*
Underactivity disorders, of cranial nerve VII, 5:281–286, 283*t*
Underelevation in adduction, 6:135
Unequal crossing over, 2:197
Unharmonious anomalous retinal correspondence, 6:60, 65, 65*i*
Unilateral visual loss, bilateral visual loss compared with, 5:83
Unilateral wipe-out syndrome (diffuse unilateral subacute neuroretinitis), 6:318, 9:172–173, 172*i*, 173*i*, 12:189–190, 189*i*
Uniparental disomy, 2:197
Unipen. *See* Nafcillin
Uniphyl. *See* Theophylline
Uniretic. *See* Moexipril
Unit magnification, planes of, 3:75
United Kingdom Prospective Diabetes Study (UKPDS), 1:215, 12:105, 107
Univasc. *See* Moexipril
Universal precautions, 8:50, 9:261
Unoprostone, 2:414, 414*t*, 10:164*t*, 172
Unpolarized light, 3:10
Unstable angina, 1:114
Unsuspected melanomas, 4:228–229
Untranslated region, 2:198, 202
Upbeat nystagmus, 5:249
Upgaze. *See* Elevation; Elevation of eye
Upper eyelids. *See* Eyelids, upper
Urea
    in aqueous humor, 2:318
    clinical use of as hyperosmotic, 2:415, 415*t*
    in tear film, 2:290
Urea-insoluble (membrane structural) lens proteins, 11:11*i*, 12
Urea-soluble (cytoskeletal) lens proteins, 11:11*i*, 12
Ureaphil. *See* Urea

Urinalysis, in immune-mediated disease, 8:202t
Urinary sphincter disturbances, in multiple sclerosis, 5:320
Urokinase, 1:172, 2:452
  for cerebral artery occlusion, 1:104
Urologic cancer, screening for, 1:296
Urticaria (hives), from fluorescein angiography, 12:21
Urushiol (poison ivy toxin), immune response arc in response to, 9:29–30
USH1B gene, 2:220–221
USH2A gene, 12:204
USH3A gene, 12:235
Usher syndrome, 12:204, 212, 233t, 235
  genetic defect in, 12:204, 235
  myosin VIIA mutation in, 2:350
  retinal pigment epithelium in, 2:363
  synteny and, 2:220–221
Usherin, in Usher syndrome, 12:235
UTR. *See* Untranslated region
Uvea (uveal tract), 2:43i, 44, 61–73, 9:101. *See also specific structure*
  bilateral diffuse melanocytic proliferation of, 9:233, 12:165–166, 165i
  congenital anomalies of, 4:151–152
  degenerations of, 4:155–156
  disorders of, 4:149–166. *See also specific type*
    neoplastic, 4:156–166, 165i
    Th1 delayed hypersensitivity and, 9:68t
  immune response in, 9:34t, 36–39
  infection/inflammation of, 4:152–155. *See also* Uveitis
  lymphoid proliferation and, 4:165
    masquerade syndromes secondary to, 9:231–232
  lymphoma of, 4:165, 165i
  melanocytoma of, 4:158
  melanomas of, 4:159–163, 167–171, 222–241, 9:72, 232. *See also* Choroidal/ciliary body melanoma
    staging of, 4:289–290t
    uveitis in children differentiated from, 6:320t
  metastatic disease of, 4:163–164, 163i, 269–271, 270i, 271i, 272i, 273–275
  miscellaneous tumors of, 4:164–165
  in neurofibromatosis, melanocytic tumors and, 6:403–404, 404i
  retinoblastoma involving, 4:144
  topography of, 4:149–151, 150i, 151i
  traumatic injury of, 4:25, 26i, 166
  wound healing/repair and, 4:22
Uveal (posterior) bleeding syndrome (polypoidal choroidal vasculopathy), age-related macular degeneration differentiated from, 12:67–68, 69i
Uveal effusions/uveal effusion syndrome, 12:170–172, 172i
  secondary angle-closure glaucoma and, 10:141
Uveal lymphoid infiltration, 4:165, 279–280
Uveal meshwork, 2:56, 57i, 4:77–78
Uveal prolapse, 4:164–165
Uveitis, 4:152–155, 5:299, 9:101–121. *See also specific type and* Endophthalmitis; Uveitis-glaucoma-hyphema (UGH) syndrome
  acute, 9:108
  anterior. *See* Anterior uveitis; Iridocyclitis; Iritis
    associated factors in, 9:108–109, 109t, 122–126
  autoimmune, molecular mimicry and, 9:89
  in Behçet syndrome, 1:193, 12:181

cataracts and, 9:235–237, 11:64, 65i, 223
  after cataract surgery, 11:164t, 178
  surgery in patients with, 11:155, 223
causes of, 9:109–112, 110–111t, 112t
in children, 6:311–322
  anterior, 6:311, 312–316, 312t, 313t, 314i, 316t
  classification of, 6:311, 312t
  diagnosis/differential diagnosis of, 6:312t, 319, 320t, 321t
  intermediate (pars planitis), 6:311, 312t, 316–317, 317i
  laboratory tests for, 6:319, 321t
  masquerade syndromes and, 6:319, 320t
  posterior, 6:311, 312t, 317–319, 318i
  treatment of, 6:319–322
chronic, 9:108
circulating immune complexes and, 9:57
classification of, 9:106–107
  in children, 6:311, 312t
clinical approach to, 9:101–126
complications of, 9:235–240
cystoid macular edema and, 9:239, 12:154
in cytomegalic inclusion disease, 6:218
diagnosis of, 9:122–126
  in children, 6:319, 320t, 321t
differential diagnosis of, 9:109–112, 110–111t, 112t
  in children, 6:312t
diffuse. *See* Panuveitis
diffuse unilateral subacute neuroretinitis and, 6:318
drug-induced, 9:141
experimental, oxygen-mediated damage in, 9:85
familial juvenile systemic granulomatosis (Blau syndrome) and, 6:318
Fuchs. *See* Fuchs heterochromic iridocyclitis/uveitis
glaucoma and, 9:135, 237–238, 238t
granulomatous, 9:104, 108
herpetic, 9:138–140, 139i
  glaucoma in, 9:139
HLA association in, 1:175, 176, 178, 9:93, 94t, 128–132
hypotony and, 9:239
intermediate. *See* Intermediate uveitis
intraocular lenses and, 9:235, 236, 11:224
  postoperative inflammation and, 9:137–138, 137i
intraocular lymphoma and, 4:114
ischemic, 5:183–184
in juvenile idiopathic (chronic/rheumatoid) arthritis, 6:313–315, 313t, 314i, 9:141–144, 142i, 144t
in Kawasaki syndrome, 6:238
laboratory and medical evaluation of, 9:110–111t, 113
  in children, 6:319, 321t
lens-induced/phacoantigenic/phacoanaphylactic, 4:96, 96i, 97i, 9:64, 135–136, 135i, 136i, 10:105–106, 11:64, 67
lipopolysaccharide-induced, 9:45
nongranulomatous, 9:104, 108, 127–141, 127i, 128i
in onchocerciasis, 9:195–197
peripheral. *See* Pars planitis
phacotoxic, 9:135. *See also* Uveitis, lens-induced
posterior. *See* Posterior uveitis
prevalence of, 9:109–112, 112t
Propionibacterium acnes causing, 9:53
in reactive arthritis, 1:177
retinal detachment and, 9:240

sarcoidosis and, 4:154–155, 154i, 6:315, 8:88, 12:180, 180i
scleritis and, 8:239
signs of, 9:102–106, 103t, 104i, 105i
in spondyloarthropathies, 1:175, 178
subretinal fibrosis and (SFU), 9:177t, 184, 184i, 185i
sympathetic ophthalmia and, 4:152–153, 153i, 154i, 9:67–68, 200–203, 200i, 201i, 202t
symptoms of, 9:101–102, 102t
syphilitic, 9:106, 187–191
systemic disease associations and, 9:108, 109
Th1 delayed hypersensitivity and, 9:68t
in toxocariasis, 6:317–318, 318i, 12:191
in toxoplasmosis, 1:26, 6:216, 217i, 317
traumatic iritis and, 8:397
treatment of, 9:114t
in children, 6:319–322
medical, 9:114–121, 114t
antiviral agents in, 9:140
surgical, 9:114t, 121
in tuberculosis, 9:193–195, 194i, 196i
and tubulointerstitial nephritis, 6:315–316
vitreous opacification and vitritis and, 9:239
Vogt-Koyanagi-Harada syndrome and, 4:153–154, 9:203–205, 204i, 205i, 206i
in children, 6:318
Uveitis-glaucoma-hyphema (UGH) syndrome, 5:174, 9:47, 10:115, 115i
intraocular lens implantation and, 3:215, 9:47, 137–138, 11:143, 192
Uveoscleral drainage/outflow, 2:54, 10:22
Uvula, ventral, 5:33

V

V-neck sign, in dermatomyositis, 1:186
V number (Abbe number), 3:50
V-pattern deviations, 6:86, 119–125, 120i
in Brown syndrome, 6:144–145
in craniosynostosis, 6:119–122, 429, 430i
definition of, 6:119, 122
esotropia, 6:87, 120i, 122
treatment of, 6:124
exotropia, 6:120i, 122
treatment of, 6:124
in superior oblique muscle paralysis, 6:133
surgical treatment of, 6:122–124, 123i, 124, 182
V1 to V6 areas of brain. See Visual (calcarine/occipital) cortex
Vaccine-associated paralytic poliomyelitis, 1:307
Vaccine development, 1:291, 310. See also Immunization
for cancer, 1:262
for HIV, 1:44–45
Vaccinia, ocular infection caused by, 8:162
Vaccinia-immune globulin, 8:162
Vacuum, phacoemulsification aspiration pump, 11:119, 120i
definition of, 11:115
settings for, 11:135–137, 135t
Vacuum rise time, 11:115, 119–121, 120i
aspiration flow rate and, 11:121, 122i
Vagal nerve stimulator, for seizures, 1:283

Valacyclovir, 1:65t, 77, 2:389, 440t, 442
for herpes simplex virus infections, 1:28, 77, 8:142t
epithelial keratitis, 8:145–146
stromal keratitis, 8:148
for herpes zoster, 1:28, 77, 8:155
Valdecoxib, 2:307
removal of from market, 1:173, 196
Valganciclovir, 1:65t, 77, 9:252
for cytomegalovirus retinitis, 1:29, 48
Validity, 1:343, 363
Valium. See Diazepam
Valproate/valproic acid
as mood stabilizer, 1:277
for seizures, 1:283t
Valsalva retinopathy, 12:93–94
Valsartan, 1:88t, 90t
Valtrex. See Valacyclovir
Valve of Hasner, 6:239, 7:255i, 256
nasolacrimal duct obstruction and, 7:257, 261
Valve of Rosenmüller, 6:239, 7:254
Van Herick method, 10:34
Vanceril. See Beclomethasone
Vancocin. See Vancomycin
Vancomycin, 1:60t, 71–72, 2:428t, 435–436
for bacterial keratitis, 8:182t, 183
for endocarditis prophylaxis, 1:11t
for endophthalmitis, 9:217, 218t, 219, 12:300, 329
resistance and, 1:3, 5, 71
Vancomycin-intermediate S aureus (VISA), 1:5
Vancomycin-resistant enterococci (VRE), 1:3, 5, 71
Vancomycin-resistant S aureus (VRSA), 1:3, 5, 71
Vantin. See Cefpodoxime
Variability, in genetic disease, 2:257–258
Variable number of tandem repeats (variable tandem repeats/minisatellite), 2:190, 203, 223
Variance (statistical), 1:368
Variant (Prinzmetal) angina, 1:113
Varicella (chickenpox), 1:28, 8:151–153
conjunctivitis in, 6:226–227, 228i
iritis/iridocyclitis in, 9:138
Varicella vaccine (Varivax), 1:28, 291, 304t, 306
Varicella-zoster virus, 1:28–29. See also Herpes zoster
ocular infection caused by, 8:151–156, 152t
acute retinal necrosis, 9:140, 154–156, 155i, 156i
conjunctivitis, 6:226–227, 228i
herpes simplex virus infection differentiated from, 8:152, 152t
uveitis, 9:138–140, 139i
vaccine against, 1:28, 291, 304t, 306
Varices, orbital, 6:379, 7:70–71, 72i
glaucoma associated with, 10:32
Varivax. See Varicella vaccine
Vascular dementia, 1:285
Vascular endothelial growth factor (VEGF), 2:456–457, 8:198t
antibodies against, in cancer therapy, 1:257
in aqueous humor, 2:321
in diabetic retinopathy, 1:217, 12:104
in pterygium, 8:366
in retinal ischemia, 4:130
retinopathy of prematurity and, 6:326
Vascular filling defect, 12:19
Vascular loops, 2:91
peripapillary, 4:107
prepapillary, 12:280, 282i

Vascular malformations. *See also* Cavernous hemangioma
  intracranial hemorrhage caused by, 1:105, 106
  orbital, 6:379–380, 379*i*
Vascular resistance, reduction of in heart failure management, 1:130
Vascular stroke. *See* Stroke
Vascular system
  anatomy of, 5:10–23
    arterial, 5:11–20
    venous, 5:20–23
  of choroid, 2:71–73, 71*i*, 72*i*, 73*i*
    development of, 2:149
  of conjunctiva, 8:8, 59
    development of, 2:155–156
  disorders of, 1:166. *See also* Vasculitis
  of extraocular muscles, 6:16
    surgery and, 6:23–25
  of eyelids, 2:29, 32*i*, 7:147
  of iris, 2:64
  of orbit, 7:15, 16–18*i*
    anatomy of, 2:38–41, 39*i*, 40*i*, 41*i*
    development of, 2:155–156
  of retina. *See* Retinal blood vessels
  tumors arising in. *See* Vascular tumors
Vascular tufts, papillary conjunctivitis causing, 8:23, 27*i*
Vascular tumors
  of eyelid and conjunctiva, 8:269–272, 270*t*
    benign, 8:270–271, 270*t*
    inflammatory, 8:270*t*, 271, 271*i*
    malignant, 8:270*t*, 272
  of orbit, 4:195–196, 197*i*, 7:64–69, 66*i*, 68*i*
    in children, 6:376–380, 377*i*, 378*i*, 379*i*
    masquerading conditions and, 7:69–70, 71*i*, 72*i*
Vasculitis, 1:188–192, 189*t*. *See also specific type and*
    Arteritis
  in Behçet syndrome, 1:193
  connective tissue disorders associated with, 7:60
  essential cryoglobulinemic, 1:189*t*
  giant cell (temporal) arteritis. *See* Arteritis, giant cell
  large vessel, 1:188–191, 189*t*
  medium-sized vessel, 1:189*t*, 191–192
  optic disc (papillophlebitis), 4:133–134, 5:128, 128*i*
    in central retinal vein occlusion, 12:141
  orbital vessels involved in, 7:59–61
  retinal, 12:152–154, 153*i*
    in Behçet syndrome, 9:133, 134*i*, 12:181
    differential diagnosis of, 9:111*t*
    in herpetic disease, 9:140
    HLA association in, 9:94*t*
    in polyarteritis nodosa, 9:175, 176*i*
    in systemic lupus erythematosus, 9:61, 173–175, 174*i*
    in Wegener granulomatosis, 9:62, 175, 176
  small vessel, 1:189*t*, 192–193
  Takayasu arteritis, 1:189*t*, 191
  transient visual loss caused by, 5:183
  Wegener granulomatosis, 1:189*t*, 192
Vasculopathy, polypoidal choroidal (posterior uveal bleeding syndrome), age-related macular degeneration differentiated from, 12:67–68, 69*i*
Vasculotropin. *See* Vascular endothelial growth factor
Vaseretic. *See* Captopril; Enalapril
Vasoactive amines, 8:198*t*, 9:77

Vasoactive intestinal polypeptide (VIP), 9:82*t*
  in tear secretion, 2:287, 290, 293, 293*i*
Vasocon-A. *See* Naphazoline/antazoline
Vasoconstrictors, for hay fever and perennial allergic conjunctivitis, 8:208
Vasodilators, for hypertension, 1:89*t*, 94
Vasopressors, for shock, 1:318
Vasospasm
  cerebral aneurysm and, 5:352
  retinal (migraine), 5:190, 294
  transient visual loss and, 5:184–185
Vasotec. *See* Enalapril
VCTS. *See* Vision-Contrast Test System
VDRL (Venereal Disease Research Laboratory) test, 1:16–17, 17*t*, 302, 9:189–190, 12:190
VECP. *See* Visually evoked cortical potentials
Vectograph Project-O-Chart slide test, 6:94
Vector, 2:198
  cloning, 2:184
  in gene therapy, 2:237
Vector addition of prisms, 3:88–89, 88*i*
Vegetation/plants, ocular injuries caused by, 8:395–396
VEGF. *See* Vascular endothelial growth factor
Vein of Galen, 5:23
Vein of Labbé, 5:22
Veins. *See also specific vein*
  anatomy of, 5:20–23
Velban. *See* Vinblastine
Velocardiofacial syndrome, posterior embryotoxon in, 6:252
Velocity
  of light, 3:4–6
  in saccades testing, 5:202
  zero, in pursuit testing, 5:203
Velosef. *See* Cephradine
Venereal Disease Research Laboratory (VDRL) test, 1:16–17, 17*t*, 302, 9:189–190, 12:190
Venlafaxine, 1:276
Venography, in orbital evaluation, 7:34
Venous beading, in nonproliferative diabetic retinopathy, 12:103, 104*i*
Venous malformations (varices), orbital, 6:379, 7:70–71, 72*i*
  glaucoma associated with, 10:32
Venous occlusive disease, retinal, 12:136–145. *See also specific type*
  branch retinal vein occlusion, 4:134–135, 135*i*, 12:136–141, 137*i*, 139*i*, 140*i*
  carotid occlusive disease and, 12:145
  central retinal vein occlusion, 4:133–134, 134*i*, 12:141–145, 142*i*
  photocoagulation for, wavelength selection and, 12:315*t*
Venous sinuses, 2:119, 120*i*
Venous stasis retinopathy, 5:184, 12:141, 145
Venous system. *See also specific vein*
  anatomy of, 5:20–23
  of extraocular muscles, 6:16
    surgery and, 6:23–25
Venous thrombosis, 1:170–172
  cerebral, 5:357–358
Ventilatory failure, in shock, 1:317, 318
Ventilatory support
  noninvasive, 1:156
  for shock, 1:318

Venting, in phacoemulsification, 11:115
Ventolin. See Albuterol
Ventral uvula, 5:33
Ventricular complexes, premature (PVCs), 1:135–136
Ventricular fibrillation, 1:140
Ventricular tachyarrhythmias, 1:138–140
    tachycardia, 1:138–139
        heart failure and, 1:131–132
Ventriculography, 1:119–120
Venturi pump, for phacoemulsification aspiration, 11:119, 120i
    vacuum rise time for, 11:120i, 121
VEP/VER. See Visually evoked cortical potentials (visual evoked response)
VePesid. See Etoposide
Verapamil
    for angina, 1:120
    for hypertension, 1:89t, 90t
    for non-ST-segment elevation acute coronary syndrome, 1:122
Verelan. See Verapamil
Vergence change on transfer, 3:66
Vergence system, 6:39
    assessment of, 5:203–204, 6:93–94
    disorders of, 5:210–211
Vergences, 3:62–65, 63i, 64i, 6:38. See also specific type
    calculation of, for mirrors, 3:92–93, 92i
    fusional, 6:43, 88–89
    in infants, 6:451
    reduced, 3:62–65
Verhoeff–van Gieson stain, 4:36t
Vermis, dorsal, 5:41
Vernal conjunctivitis/keratoconjunctivitis, 8:209–211, 209i, 210i
    in children, 6:234–235, 235i
    mast cells in, 9:13
Vernier acuity, 3:111
Verruca (wart)
    papillomavirus causing, 8:162
    vulgaris, of eyelid, 7:164, 165i
Versed. See Midazolam
Versican, in vitreous, 2:333
Versions, 6:36–38, 37i. See also specific type
Vertebral artery, 5:17, 178i
    dissection of, 5:355
Vertebrobasilar system, 5:17–18, 19i
    disorders of
        blurred vision with, 5:186
        neuro-ophthalmic signs in, 5:347–349, 348i
Verteporfin, photodynamic therapy with, 2:391, 454, 12:71–72t, 320–322
    in age-related macular degeneration, 12:71t, 75–76
    in ocular histoplasmosis syndrome, 12:72t, 82
Verteporfin in Photodynamic Therapy Trial (VIP), 12:75–76, 321
Vertex distance, correcting lenses and, 3:143–145, 144i
Vertical deviations, 6:9, 127–140. See also specific type
    botulinum toxin causing, 6:16
    comitant, 6:127
    dissociated, 6:116, 116i, 130–132, 131i
        surgery for, 6:131, 181–182
    incomitant (noncomitant), 6:127
        strabismus surgery planning and, 6:177
    inferior oblique muscle overaction and, 6:127–129, 128i

inferior oblique muscle palsy and, 6:135–136, 136i, 137t
monocular elevation deficiency and, 6:137–138, 138i
orbital floor (blowout) fractures and, 6:138–140, 139i
superior oblique muscle overaction and, 6:129–130, 129i
superior oblique muscle paralysis and, 6:132–135, 133i
Vertical diplopia, in blowout fractures, 7:102–104
    surgery and, 7:104
Vertical eyelid splitting, for anterior orbitotomy, 7:110
Vertical fusional vergence, 6:88
Vertical gaze, 5:37i, 39, 40i
Vertical gaze palsy, 5:208–209, 210i
Vertical heterophoria/phoria
    prismatic effects of bifocal lenses and, 3:157, 158i
    prisms for, 3:169–170
Vertical incomitance, 6:127
    strabismus surgery planning and, 6:177
Vertical interpalpebral fissure height, in ptosis, 7:209, 210i
Vertical prism dissociation test, in functional visual disorder evaluation, 5:307
Vertical rectus muscles, 6:14, 14i, 17t, 18i
    A-pattern deviations associated with dysfunction of, 6:119
    action of, 6:14, 17t, 28, 30
    anatomy of, 6:14, 14i, 17t, 18i
    surgery of
        for A- and V-pattern deviations, 6:124
        eyelid position changes after, 6:189–190, 190i
        for hypotropia and hypertropia, 6:181–182
        for superior oblique paralysis, 6:134
    V-pattern deviations associated with dysfunction of, 6:119
Vertical retraction syndrome, 6:153
Vertical strabismus. See Vertical deviations
Vertical traction test, in blowout fractures, 7:103
    surgery and, 7:104
Vertical vergence movement, 6:38
Vertigo, benign paroxysmal positional, 5:247
Vertometer. See Lensmeters
Vesicle
    of eyelid, 8:24t
    lens, 2:137, 145–146, 147i
    optic, 2:127, 136, 8:6
        lens development and, 2:137, 145–146, 147i
Vestibular artery, anterior/posterior, 5:18
Vestibular nerve, inferior/superior, 5:32, 54
Vestibular nuclei, 5:32
Vestibular nystagmus, 5:245–250
    central, 5:246t, 247–250, 247t
    peripheral, 5:245–247, 246t
Vestibular system
    anatomy of, 5:32, 32i
    dynamic function of, 5:200
    imbalance of, brain stem lesions and, 5:205
Vestibulocerebellum, anatomy of, 5:39–40
Vestibulo-ocular reflex, 5:32–33, 33i, 198
    assessment of, 5:200–201
    disorders of, 5:205
    gain of, 5:201
    imbalance of, tests for, 5:200
Vexol. See Rimexolone

VF. *See* Ventricular fibrillation
VF-14 instrument, cataract surgery outcome evaluated
    with, **11**:160
Vfend. *See* Voriconazole
VHL. *See* von Hippel–Lindau disease
VHL gene, **6**:412
Viagra. *See* Sildenafil
Vibramycin. *See* Doxycycline
Vidarabine, **2**:439, 440*t*
    for herpes simplex virus infections, **1**:28, **8**:142*t*, 145
        in infants and children, **6**:220
Video ophthalmoscopy, **3**:279
Videokeratography, in keratoconus, **8**:331, 331*i*
Videokeratoscopy, **3**:303, 303*i*, **8**:41, 41*i*
    in keratoconus, **8**:330
    tear breakup evaluated with, **8**:61
Videomagnifiers, **3**:262
Videophotography, **8**:35
Videx. *See* Didanosine
Vidian nerve, **5**:57
Vieth-Müller circle, **6**:41–42, 42*i*
VIG. *See* Vaccinia-immune globulin
Vigabatrin, ophthalmic side effects of, **1**:263, 284
Vigamox. *See* Moxifloxacin
VIM (Visudyne in Minimally Classic CNV Trial), **12**:75
Vimentin, **2**:327
Vinblastine, **1**:257, 259*t*
Vinca alkaloids, in cancer chemotherapy, **1**:257, 259*t*
Vincristine, **1**:257, 259*t*
VIO (Visudyne in Occult Choroidal Neovascularization
    Trial), **12**:76, 77*t*
Vioxx. *See* Rofecoxib
VIP. *See* Vasoactive intestinal polypeptide
VIP (Verteporfin in Photodynamic Therapy Trial),
    12:75–76, 321
Vira-A. *See* Vidarabine
Viracept. *See* Nelfinavir
Viral capsid, **8**:119–120
Viral inclusions, **8**:69
    in cytomegalovirus infection, **8**:69, 69*i*
Viral load, testing, in HIV infection/AIDS, **1**:40
Viramune. *See* Nevirapine
Virazole. *See* Ribavirin
Virchow's law, **6**:421, 423*i*
Viread. *See* Tenofovir
Virology, **8**:118–122, 119*t*. *See also* Viruses
Viroptic. *See* Trifluridine
Virtual colonoscopy, in cancer screening, **1**:291, 299
Virtual images, **3**:67–69, 68*i*
    displacement of by prisms, **3**:87, 87*i*
Virtual objects, **3**:67–69, 69*i*
Virulence (microbial), **8**:116–117
    mechanisms of, **1**:3–4
Viruses, **8**:118–120. *See also specific organism or type of
    infection*
    cancer and, **1**:254
    conjunctivitis caused by, **4**:46–47, 48*i*
        in children, **6**:225–229
        immune response to, **9**:35
    eyelid infections caused by, **4**:170–171
    ocular infection/inflammation caused by, **8**:118–122,
        119*t*, 139–163
        adherence and, **8**:116
        invasion and, **8**:117
        isolation techniques for diagnosis of, **8**:136

    specimen collection for diagnosis of, **8**:135*t*
    optic nerve infections caused by, **4**:205
    retinal infections caused by, **4**:123, 124*i*
    Sjögren-like syndromes caused by, **8**:79–80
    treatment of infection caused by. *See* Antiviral agents
    tumors caused by, **8**:162, 248*t*
    uveitis and, **9**:140, 154–160
VISA. *See* Vancomycin-intermediate *S aureus*
Visceral afferent fibers, **2**:117
Visceral efferent fibers, **2**:117
Visceral larva migrans, **6**:317, **8**:133. *See also Toxocara
    (toxocariasis)*
Viscoelasticity, definition of, **11**:158
Viscoelastics, **2**:452, **11**:144–145, 157–160
    for capsular rupture during phacoemulsification,
        11:179
    desired properties of, **11**:159
    elevated intraocular pressure and, **11**:172
    for penetrating keratoplasty, **8**:456
    physical properties of, **11**:157–158, 161*t*
Viscosity
    ocular medication absorption affected by, **2**:384
    of viscoelastic substances, **11**:158
Viscosurgery, **11**:144–145, 157–160
Vision
    awareness of, problems with, **5**:195–196
    binocular. *See* Binocular vision
    classification of, **3**:245*t*, 251–252
    color. *See* Color vision
    decreased. *See* Low vision; Visual loss/impairment
    development of, **6**:46–49, 451
        abnormal visual experience affecting, **6**:49–52, 50*i*,
            51*i*, 67–68
        delayed, **6**:456
    diurnal variation in, after radial keratotomy, **13**:63
    double. *See* Diplopia
    loss of/low. *See* Blindness; Low vision; Visual loss/
        impairment
    near-normal, **3**:245*t*, 251
        magnifiers for reading and, **3**:258
        spectacles for reading and, **3**:255
    neurophysiology of, **6**:44–52, 45*i*, 47*i*, 48*i*
    normal, **3**:245*t*, 251
Vision-Contrast Test System (VCTS), **3**:252
Vision rehabilitation, **3**:243–267
    computers in, **3**:262–263
    counseling and support groups in, **3**:264
    definitions in, **3**:244–246
    goals of, **3**:243
    instruction and training for, **3**:264
    large-print material in, **3**:260
    lighting and glare control in, **3**:264
    magnification in
        for distance vision (telescopes), **3**:259–260
        electronic, **3**:261–263, 263*i*
        for near vision, **3**:254–259
    nonoptical aids used in, **3**:260–263
    nonvisual assistance in, **3**:261
    objective of, **3**:243
    optical aids used in, **3**:254–260
    patient assessment in, **3**:248–254
    pediatric issues and, **3**:266–267
    after perforating injury repair, **8**:417
    prisms in, **3**:260
    professionals providing, **3**:264–265

refraction and, **3:**254
services for, **3:**264–265
telescopes in, **3:**259–260
Visken. *See* Pindolol
Vistide. *See* Cidofovir
Visual acuity, **3:**111–112, 112*t*
after accommodating IOL implantation, **13:**178
after adjustable refractive surgery, **13:**156, 157*t*
in albinism, **6:**345
in astigmatic dial refraction, **3:**136
after bioptics, **13:**156, 157*t*
bottom-up, in functional visual disorder evaluation,
5:308–309
in cataract, **11:**77–78, 77*t*
after cataract surgery, **11:**160–162
in children, **11:**198, 199–200
with ECCE, **11:**112
with ICCE, **11:**108
incorrect lens power and, **11:**193
clinical measurement of. *See* Refraction; Visual
acuity, testing
after conductive keratoplasty, **13:**140, 141–142
for presbyopia, **13:**173
contrast sensitivity/contrast sensitivity function and,
3:112–115, 114*i*
development of, **6:**202–203, 451
diffraction affecting, **3:**11
in epiretinal membrane, **12:**88
fusional vergences and, **6:**89
after hyperopic PRK, **13:**99
after intrastromal corneal ring segment placement,
13:81
after lamellar keratoplasty, **8:**474
after laser thermokeratoplasty, **13:**138
after LASIK, **13:**116
in diabetic patients, **13:**197
for high myopia, **13:**117
for hyperopia, **13:**118
for hyperopic astigmatism, **13:**118
for low myopia, **13:**116
for mixed astigmatism, **13:**118
for moderate myopia, **13:**116–117
for myopia with astigmatism, **13:**117–118
in Leber congenital amaurosis, **6:**334
in low vision
assessment of, **3:**245*t*, 248–254
best-corrected, **5:**84
metric notations and, **3:**112, 112*t*
minimum, **3:**111
with monovision, **13:**172
after multifocal IOL insertion, **13:**164, 173
after myopic spherical PRK, **13:**98
in optic nerve hypoplasia, **6:**362, 453–454
periorbital trauma and, **7:**106–108
after phakic intraocular lens implantation, **13:**149,
152*t*
after photoastigmatic keratectomy, **13:**99
pinhole, **3:**109–110
posterior segment trauma evaluation and, **12:**290
in ptosis, **7:**211–212
after radial keratotomy, **13:**63
retained lens material after phacoemulsification and,
12:339
after retinal reattachment surgery, **12:**273
in Stargardt disease, **6:**338, **12:**217

stereopsis and, **5:**309*t*
strabismus surgery planning and, **6:**178
terminology of, **3:**111–112, 112*t*
testing, **3:**111–112, 111*i*, 112*t*, 113*i*, **6:**78–80, 78*t*,
202–203, 451, **8:**15. *See also* Refraction
in amblyopia, **6:**71, 78–80, 78*t*
before cataract surgery, **11:**84
in children, **6:**78–80, 78*t*, 202–203, 451
in nystagmus, **6:**161–162
after perforating injury, **8:**408
before refractive surgery, **13:**42–43
Snellen chart for, **3:**111–112, 111*i*, 112*t*
in strabismus, **6:**78–80, 78*t*
in vision rehabilitation, **3:**247, 249–254
visual function and, **3:**245
after thermokeratoplasty, **13:**138
after wavefront-guided ablation, **13:**134–135
Visual aids. *See* Low vision aids
Visual allesthesia, **5:**195
Visual aura. *See* Aura
Visual axis, **6:**29–30, 41
Visual confusion, **6:**52, 53*i*
Visual (calcarine/occipital) cortex, **2:**108, **5:**28–29, 30*i*,
31, 31*i*, **6:**44, 45, 45*i*, 47*i*
development of, **6:**46, 48*i*
abnormal visual experience affecting, **6:**49–52, 50*i*,
51*i*, 67–68
disorders of, **5:**191–196, 193*t*
hallucinations and, **5:**170
object recognition problems and, **5:**192, 193*i*, 194
vision or vision deficit awareness in, **5:**195–196
visual-spatial relationships in, **5:**194–195, 195*i*
Visual cycle, vitamin A, **2:**359, 360*i*, 361*t*
Visual deficits. *See also* Low vision; Visual loss/
impairment
central field, **3:**246
classification of, **3:**246–248
cloudy media, **3:**246
peripheral field, **3:**248
problems with awareness of, **5:**195–196
Visual field. *See also* Visual field defects
clinical evaluation of. *See* Visual field testing
with contact lenses, **3:**177
definition of, **10:**57
Visual field defects
bilateral, **5:**113*t*
in branch retinal artery occlusion, **12:**146
characteristics of, **5:**113*t*
in chiasmal lesions, **5:**158, 159*i*, 160*i*, 161*i*
congruous, **5:**29
evaluation of. *See also* Visual field testing
as functional disorder, **5:**309–311, 311*i*, 312*i*, 313*i*
neuroimaging in, **5:**73, 73*i*
in glaucoma, **10:**4, 60, 61–64*i*
primary open-angle (POAG), **10:**84–86, 85*t*,
87–90*t*
incongruous, **5:**29
in optic nerve hypoplasia, **6:**362
in optic neuropathy, **5:**111, 112*i*, 113*t*, 114*i*
in retinitis pigmentosa, **12:**205–206, 207*i*
in retrochiasmal lesions, **5:**164
in Stargardt disease, **12:**217
terms describing, **5:**113*t*
Visual field testing, **5:**89–96
Amsler grid in, **5:**90

before cataract surgery, 11:85
in cone dystrophies, 12:214
confrontation test in, 5:89–90
in glaucoma, 10:57–81
 contrast sensitivity in, 10:59
 decibel in, 10:60
 depression in, 10:60
 electroretinography in, 10:59
 flicker sensitivity in, 10:59
 isopter in, 10:60
 kinetic testing in, 10:59
 static testing in, 10:59
 suprathreshold in, 10:59
 threshold in, 10:59
 visually evoked cortical potentials in, 10:59
Goldmann perimetry in, 5:91–92
 in children, 6:89–90, 90i
in hereditary retinal/choroidal degenerations, 12:205
perimetry in, 5:90–96. See also Perimetry
 tangent screen for, 5:91
in ptosis, 7:212
in retinitis pigmentosa, 12:205–206, 207i
silent, in functional visual disorder evaluation, 5:310
in vision rehabilitation, 3:252–253
Visual function, 3:243, 245–246
 measuring, 3:249–254
  before cataract surgery, 11:84–85
  after cataract surgery, 11:160
Visual handicap. See Low vision; Visual loss/
 impairment
 reducing. See Vision rehabilitation
Visual loss/impairment. See also specific cause and
 Blindness; Low vision
 acquired, in children, 6:456–459, 457t
 in albinism, 6:345
 in Alzheimer disease, 1:288
 amblyopia causing, 6:67–75
 assessment of, 3:248–254, 5:83–102
  adjunctive testing in, 5:96–102
  best-corrected visual acuity in, 5:84
  color vision testing in, 5:96
  electrophysiologic testing in, 5:99–102
  electroretinography in, 5:101–102, 102i
  examination in, 5:84–102
  fluorescein angiography in, 5:98, 99i
  fundus examination in, 5:87–89, 88i, 89i, 89t
  history in, 5:83–84
  objective visual deficit and, 3:245t, 248–254
  photostress recovery test in, 5:97
  potential acuity meter testing in, 5:97–98
  pupillary testing in, 5:84–87, 86i
  spatial contrast sensitivity testing in, 5:97
  visual evoked potential testing in, 5:100–101
  visual field testing in, 5:89–96. See also Visual field
   testing
 bilateral versus unilateral involvement in, 5:83
 after blepharoplasty, 7:232–233
 in blepharoptosis, 7:208
 in blowout fractures, 7:102–105
 carotid dissection and, 5:354
 cataract and, 11:75–76, 77t
 in central retinal artery occlusion, 12:148
 in childhood glaucoma, 6:284, 453
 in craniofacial syndromes, 6:429
 in diabetic retinopathy, 12:99, 102

in elderly, 1:235
in endophthalmitis, 9:207, 211, 219–220
functional, 1:266, 5:303–315
 categories of, 5:303
 diagnosis of, 5:304
 examination techniques in, 5:305–315
 identification of patient with, 5:303–304
 management of, 5:315
in hereditary retinal disease, 6:333
in juvenile idiopathic (chronic/rheumatoid) arthritis,
 6:315
in leukemia, 6:344
nonorganic/nonphysiologic. See Visual loss/
 impairment, functional
in nystagmus, 6:161
in ocular ischemic syndrome, 12:150
after orbital surgery, 7:117
after parasellar tumor therapy, 5:163
in pediatric cataract, 6:294, 453
in retinitis pigmentosa, 12:205–206, 207i, 210, 212
in retinopathy of prematurity, 6:330–332, 331i
symptoms associated with, 5:83–84
time course in, 5:83
transient. See Amaurosis, fugax; Transient visual loss
traumatic, with clear media, 7:106–108
Visual pathways, 2:103i
 afferent, 5:23–31, 269. See also Afferent visual
  pathways
  in functional visual disorder evaluation, 5:305–311
 anatomy of, 5:5–60
  bony anatomy of head and, 5:5–10
  facial motor and sensory fibers and, 5:49–56
  ocular autonomic pathways and, 5:56–60
  vascular anatomy and, 5:10–23
 efferent (ocular motor), 5:32–49. See also Ocular
  motor pathways
  ocular motility and, 5:197
Visual pigments
 absorption spectra of, 12:313, 314i
 regeneration of, retinal pigment epithelium in,
  2:359, 360i, 361t
Visual processing stream, dorsal, in pursuit system,
 5:203
Visual radiations (geniculocalcarine pathways), 2:102
Visual rehabilitation. See Vision rehabilitation
Visual resolution. See Resolution
Visual space, objective and subjective, 6:41
Visual-spatial relationships, disorders of, 5:194–195,
 195i
Visual thresholds, 3:111
Visually evoked cortical potentials (visual evoked
 response), 12:39–41, 40i
 before cataract surgery, 11:86
 in glaucoma, 10:59
 in infants and children, 6:78t, 202, 451
 in low vision evaluation, 5:100–101
Visudyne. See Verteporfin
Visudyne in Combination with Triamcinolone
 acetonide (VisIT), 12:76, 77t
Visudyne in Minimally Classic CNV Trial (VIM), 12:75
Visudyne in Occult Choroidal Neovascularization Trial
 (VIO), 12:77t
Visudyne and Triamcinolone Acetonide (VISTA),
 12:76, 77t
Visuscope, for strabismic amblyopia testing, 6:69

VIT1, in vitreous, 2:333, 337
Vitamin A
  for abetalipoproteinemia, 2:281, 12:241
  for cicatricial pemphigoid, 8:223
  deficiency of, 8:92–94, 92*t*, 93*i*, 12:242
  metabolism of, 8:92*t*
    in retinal pigment epithelium, 2:359
  ocular development/congenital anomalies and, 2:131, 160
  for retinitis pigmentosa, 12:213
  in visual cycle, 2:359, 360*i*, 361*t*
Vitamin B$_6$ (pyridoxine)
  for gyrate atrophy, 12:225–226
  for homocystinuria, 2:281, 6:438
Vitamin B$_{12}$ deficiency, 1:162
  in elderly, 1:247
  optic neuropathy caused by, 5:152
Vitamin B$_{12}$ supplements, for homocystinuria, 6:438
Vitamin C (ascorbic acid)
  for age-related macular degeneration, 12:60–61
  in aqueous humor, 2:316*t*, 317–318
  for chemical burns, 8:94, 392
  deficiency of (scurvy), 1:166, 8:94
  in lens, 2:369, 11:17
  oral supplements and, 2:373, 374*t*, 454
  in retina and retinal pigment epithelium, 2:372
  in tear film, 2:290
Vitamin D, for osteoporosis, 1:244
Vitamin E
  abetalipoproteinemia and, 2:281, 12:241
  age-related macular degeneration and, 12:60–61
  antioxidant effect of
    in lens, 2:369, 369*i*, 11:17
    oral supplements and, 2:373, 374*t*, 454
    in retina and retinal pigment epithelium, 2:372
  cataract surgery in patient taking, 11:202
  retinopathy of prematurity and, 6:326, 12:132
  structure of, 2:373*i*
Vitamin E, Cataract and Age-Related Maculopathy Trial, 2:369
Vitamin K deficiency, coagulation disorders and, 1:168–169
Vitamin deficiency, cataracts caused by, 11:63
Vitamin supplements
  in age-related macular degeneration management, 12:60–61
  antioxidant, 2:373–375, 374*t*, 454
  in genetic disorders, 2:281
  in retinitis pigmentosa management, 12:212–213
Vitelliform/vitelliruptive degeneration/dystrophy. *See* Adult-onset vitelliform lesions; Best disease
Vitelliform exudative macular detachment, 12:220, 220*i*
Vitelliform macular dystrophy gene *(VMD2)*, 6:340, 12:218
Vitiliginous chorioretinitis (birdshot retinochoroidopathy), 9:177*t*, 180–181, 180*i*, 181*i*, 12:174*t*, 177–178, 178*i*
  HLA association in, 9:94*t*, 180
Vitiligo, in Vogt-Koyanagi-Harada syndrome, 9:203, 204*i*
Vitrasert. *See* Ganciclovir
Vitravene. *See* Fomivirsen
Vitrectomy, 12:323–342
  for acute retinal necrosis, 9:155
  anterior
    for capsular rupture during phacoemulsification, 11:179
    for congenital cataract, 11:197
  in *Aspergillus* endophthalmitis, 12:189, 189*i*
  for branch retinal vein occlusion, 12:140–141
  for capsular rupture during phacoemulsification, 11:179
  with capsulectomy, for pediatric cataract
    lensectomy without intraocular lens implantation and, 6:295–296, 298*i*
    lensectomy with intraocular lens implantation and, 6:299–300, 300*i*
  cataract surgery after, 11:224
  for choroidal neovascularization, 12:327, 328*i*
  complications of, 12:342, 342*t*
  for cystoid macular edema, postoperative, 12:154, 332, 333*i*
  in diabetic patients, 12:111–112, 112*t*, 116–117
    macular edema and, 12:116
    for tractional retinal detachments, 12:341
  for dislocated posterior chamber intraocular lenses, 12:340
  for endophthalmitis, 9:217, 219, 226
    acute-onset, 12:329, 330
    bleb-associated, 12:331, 332*i*
    postoperative, 11:177
      chronic (delayed-onset), 12:329–331, 331*i*
  endophthalmitis after, 9:207
  for epiretinal membranes, 12:88, 323–324, 325*i*
  exploratory, sympathetic ophthalmia prevention and, 12:300–301
  for foreign-body removal, 12:298
  for idiopathic macular hole, 12:93, 325–326, 327*i*
  for intraocular lymphoma diagnosis, 4:278
  for macular diseases, 12:323–327
  after needle penetration/perforation of globe, 12:296, 336, 337*i*
  pars plana. *See* Pars plana vitrectomy
  for pars planitis, 9:150, 12:182
  after penetrating injury, 12:295–296
  after perforating injury, 12:296
  for posterior segment complications of anterior segment surgery, 12:328–340
  for primary central nervous system lymphoma, 9:228
  for retained lens fragments after phacoemulsification, 11:183, 12:338–339, 338*t*, 339*i*
  for retinal detachment, 12:272, 274, 336, 340, 341
    in cytomegalovirus retinitis, 9:253
    refractive surgery after, 13:193
    in retinopathy of prematurity, 6:331
  for retinopathy of prematurity, 6:331, 12:136
  in sickle cell retinopathy, 12:124
  for specimen collection, 9:216
  for submacular hemorrhage, 12:326, 328*i*
  for tractional retinal detachment, 12:274
  transconjunctival, 12:323, 324*i*
  for uveal lymphoid infiltration diagnosis, 4:280
  for vitreomacular traction syndrome, 12:89, 324, 326*i*
  for vitreous disruption/incarceration in cataract surgery wound, 11:184
  for vitritis, 9:121

Vitreocorneal adherence, after cataract surgery, 8:420, 11:167
Vitreolysis, enzymatic, 2:339
Vitreomacular (vitreous macular) traction syndrome, 12:7, 89, 90*i*, 280, 281*i*, 324, 326*i*
   epiretinal membrane differentiated from, 12:91*t*
   vitrectomy for, 12:89, 324, 326*i*
Vitreoretinal dystrophies, 12:228–229
   Goldmann-Favre, 6:342, 12:201, 202*i*, 229
Vitreoretinal interface abnormalities, 12:87–93. *See also specific type*
Vitreoretinal surgery, 12:323–342. *See also* Vitrectomy
   in sickle cell retinopathy, 12:124
Vitreoretinal traction, in retinopathy of prematurity, 6:330, 331*i*
Vitreoretinal tufts, 12:259–260, 261*i*, 262*i*
Vitreoretinopathies. *See also specific type*
   familial exudative, 6:324, 341–342, 12:284–285, 285*i*
     glaucoma and, 6:279
   hereditary, 6:340–342
   proliferative, 4:112, 12:270, 270*i*
     classification of, 12:270, 271*t*
     in retinal detachment, 12:268, 270*i*, 271*t*
Vitreous, 2:43*i*, 44, 89–91, 90*i*, 92*i*
   aging affecting, 2:338–339
   amyloidosis involving, 4:110–111, 111*i*, 12:286–287
   anatomy of, 2:43*i*, 44, 89–91, 90*i*, 92*i*, 12:7, 279
   as angiogenesis inhibitor, 2:338–339
   biochemistry and metabolism of, 2:333–339
   cataract surgery complications and, 11:164*t*, 183–184, 12:288
     in glaucoma patient, 11:219
     with ICCE, 11:104–105
     posterior vitreous detachment, 12:257, 279
   in cholesterolosis, 12:286
   collagen in, 2:89, 147, 333–335, 334*t*, 335*i*
   composition of, 2:333–337
   congenital anomalies of, 4:106–107, 106*i*, 12:280–283
   cortex of, 4:105, 12:279
   cysts of, 4:107
   degenerations of, 4:108–114
   development of, 2:146–149, 148*i*
     abnormalities of, 4:106–107, 106*i*, 12:280–283
   disorders of, 4:105–115, 12:279–288. *See also specific type*
     biochemical changes associated with, 2:338–339
     in children, 6:323–357. *See also specific type*
     decreased vision with, 5:104
     neoplastic, 4:114–115, 115*i*
   genetic disease involving, 2:339
   hyaluronan/hyaluronic acid in, 2:147, 335–336, 336*i*
   immune response in, 9:34*t*, 36–39
   inflammatory processes affecting, 2:339, 4:107–108, 108*i*. *See also* Endophthalmitis; Vitritis
   injury to, 2:339
   in leukemia, 4:281, 281*i*, 282*i*
   lipids in, 2:337
   liquefaction of, 2:338
   macula interface with, abnormalities of, 12:87–93. *See also specific type*
   macular hole formation and, 2:339
   myopia caused by changes in, 2:338
   opacification of
     amyloidosis causing, 12:286–287
     in asteroid hyalosis, 12:285, 286*i*

     in toxoplasmosis, 9:166, 166*i*, 239
     in uveitis, 9:239
   optically empty, hereditary hyaloideoretinopathies with, 12:283–284, 284*i*
   pigment granules in ("tobacco dust"/Shafer's sign), 12:268, 276, 288
   primary, 2:146, 148*i*, 4:106
     persistent hyperplasia of. *See* Persistent fetal vasculature
   proteins in, 2:337
   refractive index of, 3:40*t*
   secondary, 2:147, 4:106
   specimen collection from, 9:215–216, 12:329
   tertiary, 2:149, 4:106
   topography of, 2:43*i*, 44, 4:105–106
     in uveitis, 9:103*t*
   wound healing/repair and, 4:24
   zonular fibers in, 2:337
Vitreous base, 2:89, 12:256, 279
   avulsion of (anterior vitreous detachment), 12:254
Vitreous biopsy
   in intraocular lymphoma, 4:278
   for specimen collection, 9:216
   in uveitis, 9:109
Vitreous cellular reaction, in uveitis, 9:102
Vitreous detachment
   anterior, contusion injury causing, 12:254
   hallucinations and, 5:189
   posterior, 2:89, 90*i*, 338, 4:111, 112*i*, 12:256–258, 256*i*, 257*i*, 279–280
     idiopathic macular holes and, 12:89, 92*i*
Vitreous hemorrhage, 2:339, 4:108, 109*i*
   blunt trauma causing, 12:291, 292*i*
   in branch retinal vein occlusion, 12:138
     photocoagulation for, 12:140
   in diabetic retinopathy, 12:111–112, 116–117, 287
   in pars planitis, 12:182
   in posterior vitreous detachment, 12:257–258
   retinal cavernous hemangioma causing, 12:164
   in retinopathy of prematurity, 12:129
   scleral perforation during strabismus surgery and, 6:185
   in shaking injury, 6:443
   spontaneous, 12:287
   vitrectomy for, in diabetic patients, 12:111–112, 116–117
Vitreous macular traction syndrome. *See* Vitreomacular (vitreous macular) traction syndrome
Vitreous membrane, tractional retinal detachment and, 12:274
Vitreous opacities. *See* Vitreous, opacification of
Vitreous seeds, in retinoblastoma, 4:253–254, 254*i*, 6:392, 393*i*
Vitreous tap, for specimen collection, 9:216, 12:329
Vitreous traction, 12:7
   in posterior vitreous detachment, 12:280
   retinal cavernous hemangioma and, 12:164
Vitritis. *See also* Endophthalmitis
   in birdshot retinochoroidopathy, 12:177
   chorioretinitis with/without, differential diagnosis of, 9:111*t*
   in cystoid macular edema, 12:154
   in intraocular lymphoma, 4:278
   in Lyme disease, 9:191, 192, 192*i*, 12:191

in multifocal choroiditis and panuveitis syndrome, 12:178
in pars planitis, 9:148, 152, 12:182
in primary central nervous system lymphoma, 9:228
in uveitis, 9:111*t*
in Vogt-Koyanagi-Harada syndrome, 12:181
Vittaforma corneae, ocular infection caused by, 8:190
VKC. *See* Vernal conjunctivitis/keratoconjunctivitis
VKH. *See* Vogt-Koyanagi-Harada (VKH) syndrome
VLM. *See* Visceral larva migrans
VM-26. *See* Teniposide
VMD2 (vitelliform macular dystrophy) gene, 6:340, 12:218
VMT. *See* Vitreomacular (vitreous macular) traction syndrome
VNTRs. *See* Variable number of tandem repeats
Vogt
　palisades of, 8:8
　white limbal girdle of, 8:369
Vogt-Koyanagi-Harada (VKH) syndrome, 4:153–154, 9:203–205, 204*i*, 205*i*, 206*i*, 12:181
　in children, 6:318
　HLA association in, 9:94*t*, 205
Vogt lines, in keratoconus, 8:330
Vogt triad, in tuberous sclerosis, 6:409
Voltaren. *See* Diclofenac
Volume expansion
　for anaphylaxis, 1:319
　for shock, 1:318
Volume overload, 1:129
Voluntary convergence, 6:38
Voluntary nystagmus, 5:253–254, 312
Vomiting. *See* Nausea and vomiting
von Basedow disease. *See* Hyperthyroidism; Thyroid ophthalmopathy
von Graefe knife, 11:90, 98
von Helmholtz keratometers, 3:300, 301*i*, 302*i*
von Hippel, internal ulcer of. *See* Keratoconus, posterior
von Hippel disease/syndrome (retinal angiomatosis), 4:246–247, 246*i*, 5:336*t*, 340, 342*i*, 6:402*t*, 412–413, 413*i*, 12:160–163, 161*i*, 162*i*
　with hemangioblastomas (von Hippel–Lindau disease/syndrome), 5:336*t*, 340, 342*i*, 6:402*t*, 412–413, 413*i*
　retinoblastoma differentiated from, 6:394
　photocoagulation for, 12:163
　wavelength selection and, 12:316*t*
von Hippel lesions, 12:161
von Hippel–Lindau disease/syndrome, 5:336*t*, 340, 342*i*, 6:402*t*, 412–413, 413*i*. *See also* von Hippel disease/syndrome
　retinoblastoma differentiated from, 6:394
von Kossa stain, 4:36*t*
von Recklinghausen disease. *See* Neurofibromatosis, von Recklinghausen
von Willebrand disease, 1:168
von Willebrand factor, 1:168
VOR. *See* Vestibulo-ocular reflex
Voriconazole, 1:64*t*, 76
Vortex (hurricane) keratopathy, 8:394
Vortex veins, 2:36, 40–41, 40*i*, 41*i*, 5:20, 6:16, 12:15
　extraocular muscle surgery and, 6:25
Vossius ring, 4:25, 11:55
Voxel, definition of, 5:81

VP-16. *See* Etoposide
VRE. *See* Vancomycin-resistant enterococci
VRSA. *See* Vancomycin-resistant *S aureus*
VSR. *See* Venous stasis retinopathy
VT. *See* Ventricular tachyarrhythmias
VTRs. *See* Variable number of tandem repeats
VZV. *See* Varicella-zoster virus

W

Waardenburg syndrome, 6:209, 209*i*
　retinal degeneration and, 12:232*t*
Wagner disease/Wagner hereditary vitreoretinal degeneration, 12:232*t*, 283
WAGR syndrome, 2:255, 6:262, 11:33
Waite-Beetham lines, 8:34, 338
Wald cycle (vitamin A cycle of vision), 2:359, 360*i*, 361*t*
Waldenström macroglobulinemia, corneal deposits in, 8:350
Wall-eyed bilateral internuclear ophthalmoplegia, 5:224, 225*i*
Wallenberg syndrome, 5:207, 263
　lateropulsion in, 5:205
Warfarin/warfarin derivatives, 1:171
　for antiphospholipid antibody syndrome, 1:184
　cataract surgery in patient taking, 11:202
　for heart failure, 1:132
　ocular effects of, 1:325*t*
　in perioperative setting, 1:332
Wart (verruca)
　papillomavirus causing, 8:162
　vulgaris, of eyelid, 7:164, 165*i*
Wasp stings, ocular injury caused by, 8:395
Water, refractive index of, 3:40*t*
Water and electrolyte balance, in lens, maintenance of, 11:19–21, 21*i*
Water-insoluble lens proteins, 11:11, 11*i*
　aging affecting, 11:12–13
Water-jets, for coronary revascularization, 1:122
Water-soluble lens proteins, 11:11, 11*i*. *See also* Crystallins
　conversion of to water-insoluble, 11:12–13
Watershed zone, 2:103, 106*i*
Watt, 3:14–15, 16*t*
　laser power reading in, 3:18, 18*t*
Wave theory, 3:3–7, 4*i*, 5*i*. *See also* Light waves
Wavefront aberrations, 3:238–241. *See also* Wavefront analysis
　coma, 3:93, 233*i*, 239, 13:16, 17*i*
　higher-order, 3:93, 101–102, 103*i*, 238–241, 13:15–17, 17*i*, 18*i*, 19*i*
　　wavefront-guided ablation and, 13:133–134, 135
　hyperopia producing (negative defocus), 13:15
　irregular astigmatism producing, 13:13–17
　lower-order, 13:15, 15*i*, 16*i*
　measurement of, 13:14–15, 14*i*
　　before LASIK, 13:112
　myopia producing (positive defocus), 13:15, 15*i*
　regular astigmatism producing, 13:15, 16*i*
　representation of, 13:14–15, 14*i*
　　three-dimensional, 13:14–15
　spherical, 13:15–16, 17*i*
　trefoil, 13:16, 18*i*

Wavefront aberrometry, **3:**93, 318–320, 319*i*, 321*i*, 322*i*
Wavefront analysis/wavefront visual analysis, **8:**15, 49,
    13:13–17, 49. *See also* Irregular astigmatism;
    Wavefront aberrations
  Fermat's principle and, **13:**13–14
  geometric wavefront and, **3:**238, **13:**14
  before LASIK, **13:**112
  before wavefront-guided ablation, **13:**134
Wavefront-designed optic, for intraocular lenses,
    11:147
Wavefront-guided laser ablation, **13:**30, 49, 90, 133–135
  LASIK, **13:**112, 133–135
  PRK, **13:**21*t*, 90, 133–135
Wavefront-guided photorefractive keratectomy, **13:**21*t*,
    90
Wavefront technology, contact lenses and, **3:**205–206
Wavelength, **3:**3, 4*i*, 39
  laser, **3:**24*i*
  phototoxicity and, **2:**461–462
  refractive index and, **3:**40
  relationship of to frequency, **3:**7
Weakening procedures (extraocular muscle), **6:**174,
    175*t*
  inferior oblique muscle, **6:**180
    for V-pattern deviations, **6:**122, 124
    for vertical deviations, **6:**128–129
  superior oblique muscle, **6:**180–181
    for A-pattern deviations, **6:**122–123, 124–125
    for vertical deviation, **6:**130
Wear-and-tear pigment (lipofuscin granules), **2:**79, 86
Weber syndrome, **5:**227
WEBINO. *See* Wall-eyed bilateral internuclear
    ophthalmoplegia
Wedge resection, for astigmatism after penetrating
    keratoplasty, **8:**465*t*, 466, 467*i*, **13:**67*i*, 187
Wedl (bladder) cells, **4:**99, 99*i*, **11:**49, 186
Wegener granulomatosis, **1:**189*t*, 192, **7:**60–61, 61*i*
  choroidal perfusion abnormalities and, **12:**166, 169*i*
  diagnosis of, **7:**36, 60–61
  eyelid manifestations of, **4:**173*t*
  scleritis/retinal vasculitis and, **9:**62, 175–176, 176*i*
Weight reduction
  diabetes management/prevention and, **1:**201, 207,
    208–209
  hypertension management and, **1:**87*t*
  for idiopathic intracranial hypertension, **5:**119
Weighted value, **2:**462
Weill-Marchesani syndrome, **6:**308
  microspherophakia in, **2:**172, **11:**33
Weiss ring, **12:**256, 256*i*, 279
Welch-Allyn retinoscope, **3:**125
Welding, occupational light injury and, **12:**309
Wellbutrin. *See* Bupropion
Wenckebach type atrioventricular block, **1:**134
Werner syndrome, **8:**353*t*
Wernicke-Korsakoff syndrome, **1:**285
WESDR (Wisconsin Epidemiologic Study of Diabetic
    Retinopathy), **12:**100–101
Wessely immune ring, **8:**202
West Nile virus, **1:**35
Western blot analysis, **2:**198, 230
  in HIV infection/AIDS, **1:**39, **9:**245–246
  in Lyme disease, **1:**20
Wetting angle, of contact lens, **3:**176, 176*i*
WFVA. *See* Wavefront analysis/wavefront visual analysis

Wheezing, **1:**153
Whipple disease, **5:**255
White blood cells, **1:**159, **9:**13–16. *See also specific type*
White coat hypertension, **1:**82
White dot syndromes, **9:**176–185, 177*t*, **12:**173–179,
    174*t*. *See also specific type and*
    Retinochoroidopathies
  multiple evanescent (MEWDS), **5:**107, 108*i*, **9:**177*t*,
    181–182, 182*i*, **12:**174*t*, 175–176, 176*i*
White limbal girdle, **8:**369
White matter lesions, in multiple sclerosis, **5:**143
  treatment of, **5:**143–144
White pupil. *See* Leukocoria
White ring, Coats, **8:**368, 368*i*
"White spot" (hypopigmented macule/ash-leaf spot),
    in tuberous sclerosis, **5:**339, **6:**409–410, 410*i*
Whitnall's ligament (superior transverse ligament),
    2:26, 26*i*, 27*i*, **7:**140*i*, 142–143, 144*i*, 253
Whitnall's tubercle, **2:**9
Whole nucleus emulsification, **11:**129–131, 129*i*, 130*i*
Wide-complex tachycardias, **1:**138
Wide-temple sunglasses, for glare reduction, **3:**165
Width (thickness), of retinal reflex, in axis
    determination, **3:**130, 131*i*
Wies repair
  for involutional entropion, **7:**204, 204*i*
  for lash margin entropion of anophthalmic socket,
    7:127
Wilbrand's knee, **2:**105, **5:**27, 158
Wilcoxon rank sum test, **1:**344
Wild type, **2:**198
Wildervanck syndrome, Duane syndrome and, **6:**141
Willis, circle of, **2:**102, 103*i*, 119–121, 121*i*, **5:**16
Wilms tumor, aniridia and, **4:**151, **6:**262, 277–278
Wilms tumor–suppressor gene, imprinting of, **2:**210
Wilms tumor *(WT1)* gene, aniridia and, **6:**262
Wilson disease (hepatolenticular degeneration), **6:**260,
    8:355–356, 356*i*, **11:**62
  cataracts associated with, **6:**288*t*
  penicillamine for, **2:**281, **8:**356
Window (transmission) defect, of fluorescence, **12:**20*i*,
    21. *See also* Hyperfluorescence
  in angioid streaks, **12:**83
"Wing" cells, **2:**45, 46*i*
Wisconsin Epidemiologic Study of Diabetic
    Retinopathy (WESDR), **12:**100–101
"With" motion, in retinoscopy, **3:**127–128, 128*i*
  finding neutrality and, **3:**129, 130*i*
With-the-rule astigmatism, **3:**117–118
Withdrawal (abstinence) syndrome, **1:**267. *See also*
    specific drug
  hypertension and, **1:**97–98
Wofflin nodules, **6:**266
Wolff-Parkinson-White syndrome, **1:**137
Wolfring, glands of, **2:**24*i*, 29*t*, 34, 290, **4:**168*t*, **7:**140*i*,
    145, 253
  aqueous component/tears secreted by, **8:**56
Working distance
  bifocal segment decentration and, **3:**163
  magnifiers for low vision and, **3:**258–260
  for operating microscope, **3:**296, 297*i*
  spectacle magnification for low vision and,
    3:255–258
"Working distance" lens, in retinoscopy, **3:**128–129
Worst intraocular lens, **11:**140*i*, 143

Worth 4-dot test, **6:**60, 61*i*, 93
  in binocular sensory cooperation evaluation, **6:**93
  in suppression/anomalous retinal correspondence
      evaluation, **6:**60, 61*i*
Wound closure, after cataract surgery
  after ECCE with nucleus expression, **11:**112
  scleral tunnel incisions and, **11:**99–100, 100*i*
  single-plane incisions and, **11:**99
Wound construction, for cataract surgery, **11:**98–103.
  See also Incisions, for cataract surgery
Wound contraction, **4:**19
Wound healing/repair, **4:**19–29, 20*i*, **8:**383–386, 424.
  See also specific tissue
  of conjunctiva, **8:**383, 424
  of cornea, **8:**383–386, 424, **13:**28–29
  general aspects of, **4:**19, 20*i*
  histologic sequelae of trauma and, **4:**24–29
  ocular surface response to, **8:**424–425
  poor, cataract surgery in patients at risk for, **11:**200
  of sclera, **8:**386
Wound leaks
  after cataract surgery, **11:**181
      flat anterior chamber and, **11:**165–166
  after penetrating keratoplasty, **8:**460
WPW syndrome. *See* Wolff-Parkinson-White syndrome
Wreath sign, in multiple evanescent white dot
    syndrome, **9:**182*i*
WT1 (Wilms tumor) gene, aniridia and, **6:**262
Wyburn-Mason syndrome (racemose angioma), **4:**248,
    249*i*, **5:**336*t*, 342–343, 343*i*, **6:**402*t*, 419–420, 420*i*,
    12:163

X

x-axis of Fick, **6:**27, 27*i*
X chromosome, **2:**242
  genes for color vision on, **2:**222, 346
  inactivation of (Lyonization), **2:**190, 210, 242,
      269–273
X-linked disorders, **2:**243
  Aicardi syndrome, **6:**337, 338*i*
  albinism (Nettleship-Falls), **6:**345, 347*t*
      ocular findings in carriers of, **2:**270*t*, 271*i*, 272
  blue-cone monochromatism, **6:**336, **12:**198
      electroretinogram patterns in, **12:**30*i*
      ocular findings in carriers of, **2:**270*t*
  dominant, **2:**268–269
  familial exudative vitreoretinopathy, **6:**341–342,
      12:284
  gene therapy for, **2:**237
  ichthyosis, **8:**89, 309*t*
  Lisch corneal dystrophy, **8:**310*t*, 313–315, 314*i*
  megalocornea, **8:**289, 309*t*
  Norrie disease, **6:**342
  ocular findings in carriers of, **2:**270–271*i*, 270*t*
  pigmentary retinopathies, **12:**233*t*
  retinitis pigmentosa, **12:**211
      ocular findings in carriers of, **2:**270*i*, 270*t*
  retinoschisis (juvenile retinoschisis), **6:**340, 341*i*,
      12:228–229, 228*i*
      electroretinogram patterns in, **12:**30*i*, 228–229
X-linked inheritance (X-linked genes), **2:**198, 220,
    266–269, 268*t*. *See also* X-linked disorders
  dominant, **2:**268, 268*t*

  recessive, **2:**267–268, 268*t*
X-rays. *See* Radiography
Xalatan. *See* Latanoprost
Xanax. *See* Alprazolam
Xanthelasma. *See also* Xanthomas
  in dyslipoproteinemia/hyperlipoproteinemia, **1:**293,
      8:338, 339*t*
  of eyelid, **4:**171, 173*i*, 173*t*, **7:**166
Xanthine derivatives, for pulmonary diseases, **1:**157*t*
Xanthogranuloma, juvenile (nevoxanthoendothelioma),
    6:389, 389*i*, **8:**271, **9:**233
  glaucoma associated with, **10:**32
  of iris, **4:**219*t*, **6:**264, 389, 389*i*
      leukemic involvement differentiated from, **6:**345
  of orbit, **7:**88–89
  uveitis in children differentiated from, **6:**320*t*
Xanthomas
  fibrous (fibrous histiocytoma), **8:**271
      orbital, **4:**199, 199*i*, **7:**81
  scleral, **4:**92
  in hyperlipoproteinemias, **4:**171, 173*t*
Xanthophylls (carotenoids)
  absorption spectrum for, **12:**313, 314*i*
  in lens, **2:**369, 369*i*
  in macula, **12:**7–8
  in retina, **2:**373
  structure of, **2:**373*i*
Xenon fluoride excimer laser, **3:**23. *See also* Lasers
Xeroderma pigmentosum, **7:**174, **8:**90, 310*t*
Xerophthalmia, **8:**92. *See also* Vitamin A, deficiency of
Xerophthalmic fundus, **8:**92
Xerosis
  Corynebacterium xerosis found in, **8:**92, 125
  in vitamin A deficiency, **8:**83, 92, 93*i*
  in vitamin C deficiency, **8:**94
Xibrom. *See* Bromfenac
XLRP. *See* X-linked disorders, retinitis pigmentosa
XLRS. *See* X-linked disorders, retinoschisis
XP. *See* Xeroderma pigmentosum
Xylocaine. *See* Lidocaine

Y

y-axis of Fick, **6:**27, 27*i*, 29–30
Y chromosome, **2:**242
  inheritance/traits determined by (holandric
      inheritance/trait), **2:**188, 266
Y-linked inheritance (Y-linked genes), **2:**188, 198, 266
Y-sutures, lens, **2:**75*i*, 76, **11:**9
  development of, **2:**146, **11:**28–29, 28*i*
  opacification of (sutural/stellate cataract), **11:**35–36,
      37*i*
Y-V-plasties, for blepharophimosis syndrome, **7:**153
YAC. *See* Yeast artificial chromosome
Yeast artificial chromosome (YAC), **2:**198
Yeasts, **5:**365, **8:**128–129, 129–130, 129*t*, 130*i*
  Candida albicans, **1:**25, **9:**163–164
  as normal ocular flora, **8:**115*t*
  ocular infection caused by, **8:**129–130, 130*i*
      endogenous endophthalmitis, **12:**187–188, 188*i*
      keratitis, **8:**185, 186
Yellow fever vaccination, **1:**309
Yellow lasers, **12:**315–316*t*, 317

Yoke muscles, 6:36, 86
  cardinal positions of gaze and, 6:28*i*, 36, 86
  Hering's law of motor correspondence and, 6:36

Z

z-axis of Fick, 6:27–28, 27*i*
z-height, 8:44–45, 13:8, 8*i*
Z-plasties
  for blepharophimosis syndrome, 7:153
  for eyelid repair, 7:187
  for symblepharon, 7:207
Z score, in osteoporosis, 1:243
Zaditor. *See* Ketotifen
Zafirlukast, 1:157*t*
Zagam. *See* Sparfloxacin
Zalcitabine, 1:41
Zaleplon, 1:273
Zanamivir, 1:65*t*, 77, 305
Zarontin. *See* Ethosuximide
Zaroxolyn. *See* Metolazone
Zeaxanthin, 2:86
  antioxidant effect of, 2:373
  cataract risk affected by, 11:63
  in macula, 12:7
  structure of, 2:373*i*
Zebeta. *See* Bisoprolol
Zefazone. *See* Cefmetazole
Zeis, glands of, 2:22, 24*i*, 29*t*, 4:168*t*, 7:166, 8:6, 7*i*
  chalazion caused by obstruction of, 8:87
  sebaceous adenocarcinoma arising in, 7:180
  in tear film-lipids/tear production, 2:289
Zeiss 4-mirror goniolens, for fundus biomicroscopy, 3:288, 288*i*
Zeiss fundus camera, schematic of, 3:277
Zeiss-type lens, 10:39
Zellweger (cerebrohepatorenal) syndrome, 12:233*t*, 234, 236, 242
  childhood glaucoma and, 10:155*t*
Zerit. *See* Stavudine
Zernicke polynomials, for wavefront aberration specification, 3:240–241, 240*i*, 13:15
Zero velocity, in pursuit testing, 5:203
Zestoretic. *See* Lisinopril
Zestril. *See* Lisinopril
Ziac. *See* Bisoprolol
Ziagen. *See* Abacavir
Zidovudine, 1:41, 2:444
  for HIV prophylaxis
    postexposure, 1:45, 46–47*t*
    during pregnancy, 1:45
  with lamivudine, 1:41
Zileuton, 1:157*t*
Zimmerman tumor (phakomatous choristoma), 4:169, 8:277
Zinacef. *See* Cefuroxime
Zinc
  in age-related macular degeneration management, 12:60–61
  antioxidant effect of, oral supplements and, 2:374, 374*t*, 454
  in aqueous humor, 2:317
  foreign body of, 12:299
Zinc finger motif, 2:206, 207*i*

Zinn
  annulus of, 2:10–12, 16, 17*i*, 18*t*, 101, 5:26, 41, 7:14, 14*i*, 15
  zonules of (zonular fibers), 2:75*i*, 76, 323, 4:94, 94*i*, 11:5, 6, 7*i*
    in accommodation, 13:167–171, 168*i*, 169*i*, 170*i*
    development of, 2:146, 11:30
Zinn-Haller, circle of, 2:103, 5:15, 10:48, 49
Ziracin. *See* Evernimicin
Zithromax. *See* Azithromycin
ZMC fractures. *See* Zygomatic-maxillary complex (tripod) fractures
Zocor. *See* Simvastatin
Zofran. *See* Ondansetron
Zolpidem, 1:273
Zonal granuloma, 4:96
Zonegran. *See* Zonisamide
Zones of discontinuity, 2:76
Zonisamide, 1:283*t*
Zonulae adherentes, in retinal pigment epithelium, 2:78
Zonulae occludentes (tight junctions)
  in ciliary body epithelium, 2:66
  in corneal epithelium, 8:9
  in retinal blood vessels, 2:84
  in retinal pigment epithelium, 2:78, 12:12, 13*i*
Zonular apparatus, 2:146
Zonular (lamellar) cataracts, 11:37–38, 39*i*
  in children, 6:289, 290*i*, 292*t*
  hereditary factors in, 6:287*t*
Zonular dehiscence, cataract surgery and, 11:226–227, 227*i*, 228*i*
Zonular fibers
  lens (zonules of Zinn), 2:75*i*, 76, 323, 4:94, 94*i*, 11:5, 6, 7*i*
    in accommodation, 13:167–171, 168*i*, 169*i*, 170*i*
    development of, 2:146, 11:30
  tertiary vitreous, 4:106
  vitreous, 2:337
Zonular lamella, 11:6
Zonular traction retinal tufts, 12:259, 260, 262*i*
Zonules
  occluding, corneal, 2:45
  of Zinn (zonular fibers), 2:75*i*, 76, 323, 4:94, 94*i*, 11:5, 6, 7*i*
    in accommodation, 13:167–171, 168*i*, 169*i*, 170*i*
    development of, 2:146, 11:30
Zoom Galilean telescopes, in operating microscope, 3:296
Zoster. *See* Herpes zoster
Zoster sine herpete, 5:300
Zosyn. *See* Piperacillin, with tazobactam
Zovirax. *See* Acyclovir
Zyflo. *See* Zileuton
Zygomatic bone, 5:5, 6–7*i*, 7*i*, 10, 7:7, 8*i*, 10*i*
  fractures of, 7:97–100, 99*i*
Zygomatic foramen, 2:10
Zygomatic-maxillary complex (tripod) fractures, 7:97–100, 99*i*
Zygomatic nerve, 5:52, 53*i*, 56
  in reflex tear arc, 7:253
Zygomaticofacial canal, 7:11
Zygomaticofacial nerve, 5:52, 53*i*
Zygomaticomaxillary suture, 5:10
Zygomaticotemporal artery, 5:13

Zygomaticotemporal canal, 7:11
Zygomaticotemporal nerve, 5:52, 53*i*
    in reflex tear arc, 7:253
Zygomycetes (zygomycosis), 4:189

Zygote, 2:244
Zymar. *See* Gatifloxacin
Zyprexa. *See* Olanzapine
Zyvox. *See* Linezolid